Obesity and Diabetes: Diagnosis and Management

Obesity and Diabetes: Diagnosis and Management

Editor: Alexander Cullen

FOSTER ACADEMICS
www.fosteracademics.com

www.fosteracademics.com

FOSTER ACADEMICS

Cataloging-in-Publication Data

Obesity and diabetes : diagnosis and management / edited by Alexander Cullen.
p. cm.
Includes bibliographical references and index.
ISBN 978-1-64646-594-1
1. Diabetes. 2. Obesity. 3. Diabetes--Diagnosis. 4. Diabetes--Treatment.
5. Obesity--Diagnosis. 6. Obesity--Treatment. I. Cullen, Alexander.
RC660 .O24 2023
616462--dc23

Foster Academics,
118-35 Queens Blvd., Suite 400,
Forest Hills, NY 11375, USA

ISBN 978-1-64646-594-1 (Hardback)

Contents

Preface

Obesity is a medical condition in which the body gains an excessive amount of fat. It is a complex disease that is associated with other health complications, such as heart disease, diabetes, high blood pressure and certain cancers. Diabetes is a metabolic health condition that affects the mechanism through which the body uses blood sugar. Obesity can affect the mechanism of the body with which it uses insulin to manage blood sugar levels. This leads to an increased risk of insulin resistance and diabetes. The diagnosis of obesity involves skinfold thickness tests, waist-to-hip comparisons, and screening tests such as ultrasounds, CT scans and MRI scans. Blood tests which examine cholesterol and glucose levels, liver function tests, diabetes screening, thyroid tests, and heart tests are performed to diagnose health risks linked with diabetes. Treatment for obesity may include weight loss medications, eating and exercise plans, whereas insulin injections, carbohydrate counting, and frequent blood sugar checks help in the management of diabetes. This book outlines the diagnosis and management of obesity and diabetes in detail. It is a vital tool for all researching and studying these medical conditions.

The researches compiled throughout the book are authentic and of high quality, combining several disciplines and from very diverse regions from around the world. Drawing on the contributions of many researchers from diverse countries, the book's objective is to provide the readers with the latest achievements in the area of research. This book will surely be a source of knowledge to all interested and researching the field.

In the end, I would like to express my deep sense of gratitude to all the authors for meeting the set deadlines in completing and submitting their research chapters. I would also like to thank the publisher for the support offered to us throughout the course of the book. Finally, I extend my sincere thanks to my family for being a constant source of inspiration and encouragement.

Editor

1

Impact of Metabolic Syndrome on Neuroinflammation and the Blood–Brain Barrier

Peter Van Dyken[1] and Baptiste Lacoste[1,2,3]*

[1] Neuroscience Program, Ottawa Hospital Research Institute, Ottawa, ON, Canada, [2] Department of Cellular and Molecular Medicine, Faculty of Medicine, University of Ottawa, Ottawa, ON, Canada, [3] Brain and Mind Research Institute, University of Ottawa, Ottawa, ON, Canada

***Correspondence:**
Baptiste Lacoste
blacoste@uottawa.ca

Metabolic syndrome, which includes diabetes and obesity, is one of the most widespread medical conditions. It induces systemic inflammation, causing far reaching effects on the body that are still being uncovered. Neuropathologies triggered by metabolic syndrome often result from increased permeability of the blood–brain-barrier (BBB). The BBB, a system designed to restrict entry of toxins, immune cells, and pathogens to the brain, is vital for proper neuronal function. Local and systemic inflammation induced by obesity or type 2 diabetes mellitus can cause BBB breakdown, decreased removal of waste, and increased infiltration of immune cells. This leads to disruption of glial and neuronal cells, causing hormonal dysregulation, increased immune sensitivity, or cognitive impairment depending on the affected brain region. Inflammatory effects of metabolic syndrome have been linked to neurodegenerative diseases. In this review, we discuss the effects of obesity and diabetes-induced inflammation on the BBB, the roles played by leptin and insulin resistance, as well as BBB changes occurring at the molecular level. We explore signaling pathways including VEGF, HIFα, PKC, Rho/ROCK, eNOS, and miRNAs. Finally, we discuss the broader implications of neural inflammation, including its connection to Alzheimer's disease, multiple sclerosis, and the gut microbiome.

Keywords: blood–brain barrier, neuroinflammation, obesity, diabetes, brain homeostasis

INTRODUCTION

Metabolic syndrome is one of the most wide-spread diseases in North America, with a prevalence of 34% amongst adults in the United States (Aguilar et al., 2015). It is perhaps the leading avoidable cause of premature death (Hennekens and Andreotti, 2013). Metabolic syndrome is an umbrella term encompassing conditions such as obesity, dyslipidemia, hyperglycemia, and hypertension. These often occur together and result in insensitivity to hormones such as leptin, adiponectin, and insulin (Kaur, 2014). Insulin resistance underlies type 2 diabetes mellitus (T2DM). While the causes of metabolic syndrome are complex, high fat diet (HFD), inactive life styles and genetic predispositions are important risk factors. The components of metabolic syndrome result in wide-ranging effects, many of which impact the central nervous system (CNS) and result in neurodegenerative diseases linked to dysfunction of the BBB. Metabolic syndrome also alters blood pressure and arterial stiffness which, in turn, can damage the BBB. However, given that this review focuses on the effects of inflammation on the BBB, this point will not be discussed.

The BBB is a conserved structure preventing and controlling the passage of most blood components into the central nervous system (CNS) (Andreone et al., 2015; Chow and Gu, 2015; O'Brown et al., 2018). Endothelial cells (ECs) joined together by tight junctions (TJs) form its basic structure (Reese and Karnovsky, 1967), while the basement membrane (BM), pericytes, and astrocytes perform supporting and regulatory functions (Andreone et al., 2015; Daneman and Prat, 2015). The integrity of the BBB is central to neural health, and many autoimmune neurological disorders are associated with its breakdown (Garg and Smith, 2015; Zhao et al., 2015; Chakraborty et al., 2017). BBB opening has been largely linked to inflammation. The maturation and invasion of leukocytes, the release of cytokines, and destruction of targeted cells are effects associated with CNS inflammation that can quickly lead to neuronal damage (Varatharaj and Galea, 2017). Although a sealed BBB normally prevents the passage of immune cells into the CNS, inflammation induces BBB opening by altering its various components (Ransohoff et al., 2015), as we will discuss in this review.

Components of the BBB

In peripheral organs like the liver or kidneys, capillaries contain fenestrae, little gaps in the vessel wall that allow passage of nutrients, proteins, and even cells into surrounding tissues (Claesson-Welsh, 2015; Augustin and Koh, 2017). In most brain areas, however, ECs are connected by TJs that prevent proteins and cells from crossing the vessel wall. Endothelial TJs are formed by the transcellular proteins claudin, occludin, and junctional adhesion molecules (JAMs) (Daneman and Prat, 2015). Claudins are particularly important for barrier function, as loss of claudins greatly increases barrier permeability (Hartsock and Nelson, 2008). Occludins are highly enriched at the BBB, but they do not appear to be essential to barrier function, as occludin-deficient mice retain normal BBB functioning. Nevertheless, occludins are implicated in calcium flux across the BBB (Hartsock and Nelson, 2008). JAMs, particularly JAM4, regulate passage of leukocytes across the BBB and paracellular permeability. In addition to transcellular proteins, zona occludens-1 (ZO-1), ZO-2, and ZO-3 are important for localizing claudins to the TJs and for connecting them to the cytoskeleton (Hartsock and Nelson, 2008; Daneman and Prat, 2015).

Due to a lack of plasmalemma vesicles, brain ECs have very low rates of transcytosis (Ben-Zvi et al., 2014; Andreone et al., 2017; Chow and Gu, 2017). They display low expression of leukocyte adhesion molecules (LAMs) and of ligand-specific transporters. Passage across the BBB is mostly controlled by these transporter proteins. The luminal and abluminal sides possess different proteomic profiles, allowing the BBB to isolate the vascular and perivascular environments (Daneman and Prat, 2015). Many of these transporters, such as the glucose transporter-1 (GLUT1) are passive, allowing their substrates to flow down their concentration gradients (Zhao et al., 2015). Other transporters consume energy, using ATP hydrolysis to fuel the transport of substrates against their concentration gradient. *P*-glycoprotein, for instance, removes toxins from the brain, including β-amyloid (Aβ), a major player in AD (Deo et al., 2014). This tight control on transport across ECs creates strict regulation and polarization of the vascular and perivascular environments (Chow and Gu, 2015; Daneman and Prat, 2015).

Other structures involved in the BBB include astrocytes, pericytes, and the BM. The latter is made of collagens, laminin, nidogen, heparin, and other glycoproteins. It forms a further barrier in the BBB, but can be disrupted by matrix metalloproteinases (Thomsen et al., 2017). Pericytes are embedded within the endothelial BM and form direct connections with ECs. They are involved in the regulation of angiogenesis and vascular stability, and in controlling the BBB (Armulik et al., 2010; ElAli et al., 2014). Astrocytes are the most abundant glial cell type and play important roles in neurovascular regulation. Their processes ensheathe parenchymal blood vessels with their endfeet. They regulate vasomotor responses and cerebral blood flow in response to changes in neural activity in a given region (Attwell et al., 2010; Petzold and Murthy, 2011; Lacoste and Gu, 2015). They also release factors regulating the maturation and maintenance of the BBB (MacVicar and Newman, 2015; Zhao et al., 2015).

Inflammation and BBB Disruption

CNS Immune Privilege and Leukocyte Invasion

Unlike most organs, the healthy CNS contains very few immune cells, parenchymal microglial cells being the sole population. In the healthy CNS, microglia are maintained without reconstitution from the bone marrow and have no contact with plasma proteins, allowing the CNS to maintain an immunosuppressed environment (Ransohoff and Engelhardt, 2012). The CNS tightly controls, and generally prevents, the passage of immune cells into the perivascular space. This 'CNS immune privilege' is largely accomplished by the BBB, which limits leukocyte extravasation (i.e., diapedesis) across the endothelium (Zhao et al., 2015). Undue leukocyte extravasation into neural spaces can result in autoimmune disorders such as multiple sclerosis (MS) (Ransohoff and Engelhardt, 2012).

Leukocyte extravasation requires interactions between adhesion molecules on ECs and leukocytes. LAMs expressed by ECs include P-selectin, E-selectin, intercellular adhesion molecule-1 (ICAM-1) and vascular cell adhesion molecule-1 (VCAM-1) (Su et al., 2012). The selectins bind to P-selectin glycoprotein ligand (PSGL-1), while ICAM-1 and VCAM-1 bind to α4-integrins on leukocytes. After the initial binding event, immune cells roll along the vessel wall releasing chemokines that strengthen their binding interactions. This dramatically reduces cell motility, allowing immune cells to crawl along the vessel in search of a point for extravasation (Engelhardt, 2008; Engelhardt and Ransohoff, 2012). Most transmigration occurs via a paracellular route, which depends on interactions with platelet endothelial cell adhesion molecule (PECAM) and JAM-A (Muller, 2011; Engelhardt and Ransohoff, 2012; Tietz et al., 2018). It can also happen transcellularly, generally when the leukocyte is unable to find an endothelial junction and is strongly activated. The immune cell extends pseudopods and passes right through the endothelium. This phenomenon involves clustering of ICAM-1 and can be inhibited by blocking PECAM. Calveolin-1 plays an important role, especially in the migration of Th1 cells (Lutz et al., 2017). Microtubules are also critical in both types of movement, transporting molecules involved in extravasation to required sites (Muller, 2011).

Leukocyte adhesion molecules are suppressed in the neurovasculature, limiting the opportunity for leukocyte invasion (Chow and Gu, 2015; Daneman and Prat, 2015). The BM forms a second barrier to immune entry. To pass through, leukocytes must be helped by matrix metalloproteinases, such as MMP-9, which clear away membrane filaments. Inflammatory factors open the BBB by upregulating these various factors (Engelhardt and Ransohoff, 2012).

A process called immunosurveillance monitors antigens in the brain and mounts an immune response if foreign bodies are detected. This largely takes place in the cerebrospinal fluid (CSF). Immune cells enter the ventricles through the choroid plexus (CP), a structure in the cerebral ventricles that produces CSF (Ghersi-Egea et al., 2018). There, they are exposed to antigen presenting cells (APC) and drain through meningeal lymphatic vessels into the to the deep cervical lymph node (Louveau et al., 2018). Cells activated in the CSF activate a pro-inflammatory signaling pathway that triggers opening of the BBB and allows leukocyte infiltration, as reviewed elsewhere (Ransohoff and Engelhardt, 2012). Proper functioning of the CP is highly important for neuronal health (Gelb et al., 2018). More recently, a direct route of immune cell infiltration was identified between the bone of the skull and brain meninges by means of microscopic vascular channels (Herisson et al., 2018).

Inflammation and the BBB

Inflammation acts through various pathways to affect gene expression. NF-κB, one of the most important factors, is activated by pro-inflammatory cytokines such as TNF-α and IL-1β. Toll-like receptor-4 (TLR4) binds to microbial molecular patterns and activates myeloid differentiation primary response gene 88 (My88), which also leads to NF-κB activation (Lawrence, 2009). The JAK\STAT pathway is activated by a wide variety of signaling molecules, including interferons (IFNα/β/γ), interleukins (IL-2/3/4/5/6 etc.), and growth factors. These ligands bind to their receptors, leading to activation of STATs which affect gene regulation (O'Shea et al., 2015). Mitogen-activated protein kinase (MAPK) has a role in three separate pathways, including extracellular-signal-regulated kinases (ERKs), Jun amino-terminal kinases (JNK), and p38/stress-activated protein kinases (SAPKs). JNK leads to the activation of c-Jun and c-Fos, which dimerize and form activator protein 1 (AP-1) (Morrison, 2012). Receptors involved in inflammatory responses include cytokine and growth factor receptors, receptor tyrosine kinases, G-coupled protein receptors, and integrins (Morrison, 2012).

Reactive oxygen species are important mediators of inflammation. They are produced as a natural biproduct of aerobic respiration in the mitochondria, through NADPH oxidase activity in phagocytes, and through uncoupled nitric oxide (NO) production (Mittal et al., 2014). Through their oxidative activity, they promote the formation of disulfide bonds between cysteine residues on proteins, affecting protein function (Mittal et al., 2014). In particular, signaling pathways including NF-κB, JNK, and JAK/STAT can be altered by ROS (Nakano et al., 2006; Ray et al., 2012; Hoesel and Schmid, 2013), leading to upregulation of inflammatory cytokines such as transforming growth factor beta (TGF-β), IL-1, IL-6, IL-18, and TNF-α (Elmarakby and Sullivan, 2012). This leads to further inflammation and leukocyte infiltration.

Increased inflammation leads to disruption of the BBB (**Figure 1** and **Table 1**). TJ proteins, including claudin-5, ZO-1, occludins, and caveolin are downregulated (Chehade et al., 2002; Argaw et al., 2009; Pfeiffer et al., 2011; Sajja et al., 2014; Yoo et al., 2016; Varatharaj and Galea, 2017; Xu et al., 2017). Transcytosis is also altered, together with downregulation of *P*-glycoprotein, leptin, and amino acid transporters (Ransohoff et al., 2015), but upregulation of influx transporters for TNF-α, lysosomal enzymes, Aβ, and monoamines (Varatharaj and Galea, 2017). Fibrin is transported across the disrupted BBB and deposits as insoluble fibrin, a key activator of immune responses (Davalos and Akassoglou, 2012). Interestingly, a recent study successfully targeted fibrin with 5B8 antibody, which inhibited fibrin-induced inflammation without affecting clotting (Ryu et al., 2018). In response to inflammation, leukocyte extravasation increases, with upregulation of VCAM-1 and ICAM-1 (Chai and Song, 2014), as well as P and E-selectin (Carvalho-Tavares et al., 2000). Upregulated MMPs degrade the BM, allowing leukocyte passage (Thomsen et al., 2017). Astrocyte endfeet are disrupted, impairing their ability to maintain BBB integrity (Fan et al., 2014). Astrocyte gene expression shifts toward a pro-inflammatory and cytotoxic state, including production of interleukin-1β (IL-1β), interleukin-6 (IL-6), tumor necrosis factor-alpha (TNF-α), and prostaglandins (Zamanian et al., 2012). TNF-α further promotes inflammatory responses, inducing extravasation of macrophages by acting through NF-κB (Skelly et al., 2013). TNF-α and IL-1β both induce expression of chemokines CXCL1 and CCL2, which are involved in immune cell recruitment to brain ECs. Other pathways become affected by pro-inflammatory states. For example, Wnt/β-catenin is regulated by NF-κB activation, as reviewed elsewhere (Ma and Hottiger, 2016). Inhibition of Wnt/β-catenin leads to increased expression of VCAM and Caveolin-1, proteins critical for transmembrane trafficking (Lengfeld et al., 2017). Overall, inflammation increases BBB permeability, promoting leukocyte extravasation, increasing diffusion of solutes across the BBB, and allowing entry of pathogens and toxins into the CNS. This further stimulates inflammatory responses in a vicious cycle.

Conditions that increase systemic inflammation impacts many of the systems in the body, including the brain. As such, inflammation is increasingly being implicated in neuropathology, as we will explain below.

OBESITY AND THE BBB

Obesity is the excess accumulation of body fat caused by an imbalance between energy intake and consumption. It results

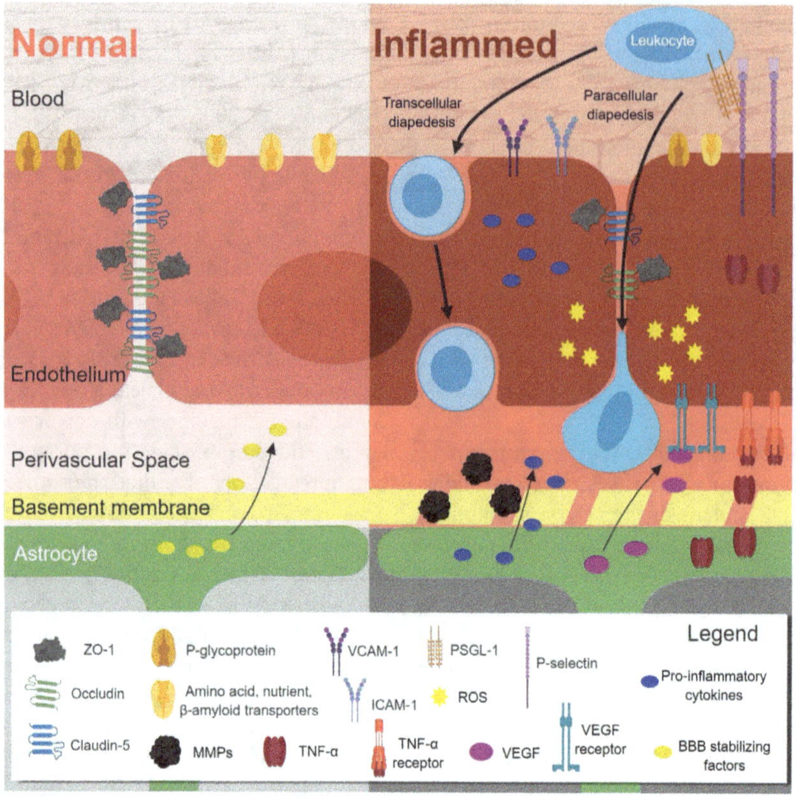

FIGURE 1 | Effects of inflammation on the blood–brain-barrier (BBB). Downregulation of claudin-5, occludin, ZO-1, leptin and amino acid transporters, and P-glycoprotein occurs in conjunction with upregulation of VCAM-1, ICAM-1, P-selectin, MMPs, and pro-inflammatory cytokines. Leukocyte extravasation (diapedesis) increases. Astrocytic gene expression shifts away from BBB stabilizing factors toward VEGF and pro-inflammatory cytokines. The basement membrane is also disrupted. *Figure made with BioRender*.

in high levels of adipose tissue, a hormonally active tissue that secretes adipokines and cytokines. As the number of adipose cells increase, more of these regulating proteins are secreted, causing tissues to develop resistance to their effects. For example, leptin resistance prevents proper satiety so that hunger still occurs despite excess fat. Insulin resistance prevents proper intake and use of blood glucose, causing hyperglycemia. These hormones, and their disruption, affect nearly every organ in the body, making obesity a contributing factor in many diseases, including cardiovascular disease, fatty lipid disease, and neurological disorders like AD (Blüher, 2013).

Obesity and Cerebral Inflammation

The effects of obesity are largely mediated through inflammation (**Figure 2**). High fat diet (HFD) is commonly used to study obesity in mice, and neural inflammation can be seen even before significant weight gain in these murine models. Saturated fatty acids (SFAs), like palmitate, play an important role in activating these early inflammatory pathways. SFAs interact with toll-like receptor 4 (TLR4) and activate myeloid differentiation primary response gene 88 (MyD88) (Milanski et al., 2009), which leads to activation of NF-κB. This pathway is linked to inhibition of anorexic hormones insulin and leptin, partially through increased expression of NF-κB-induced expression of suppressor of cytokine signaling 3 (Kievit et al., 2006; Zhang et al., 2008). NF-κB also upregulates pro-inflammatory cytokines including Il-1β, TNF-α, and IL-6 (Yudkin et al., 1999; De Souza et al., 2005; Zhang et al., 2005; Hommelberg et al., 2009; Lawrence, 2009; Jais and Brüning, 2017), causing a decrease in TJ protein expression and an decrease in BBB integrity (Gustafson et al., 2007). Metabolic, housekeeping, and structural genes are downregulated in mice with diet-induced obesity (Ouyang et al., 2014b). Amplified ROS production results from increased mitochondrial respiration, upregulated expression of NADPH oxidase, and the action of inflammatory cytokines (Zhang et al., 2005; Tucsek et al., 2014; Jais and Brüning, 2017). They further promote cytokine expression and oxidative stress (De Souza et al., 2005; Dorfman and Thaler, 2015). Microglia are activated and upregulate their Fcγ receptors, priming them for response to IgGs (Tucsek et al., 2014). Immune cells are also activated, and macrophages infiltrate the brain parenchyma (Stranahan et al., 2016).

One of the earliest regions to experience HFD-induced inflammation is the hypothalamus (Prada et al., 2005). As a major control center for energy and weight balance, its impairment contributes to the development of obesity (Jais and Brüning, 2017). Hypothalamic inflammation precedes weight gain by a few days in mice on HFD (Thaler et al., 2012). As described above, SFAs promotes leptin and insulin resistance through the

TABLE 1 | The effects caused by inflammation, obesity, and T2DM on the BBB.

Effects of inflammation on BBB	
Downregulation of TJ proteins claudin-5, ZO-1, and occludin	Chehade et al., 2002 ; Argaw et al., 2009; Pfeiffer et al., 2011; Sajja et al., 2014; Yoo et al., 2016; Varatharaj and Galea, 2017; Xu et al., 2017
Downregulation of *P*-glycoprotein and of leptin and amino acid transporters	Ransohoff et al., 2015
Upregulation of influx transporters for TNF-α, lysosomal enzymes, Aβ, monoamines	Varatharaj and Galea, 2017
Transport of fibrin and deposition as insoluble fibers	Davalos and Akassoglou, 2012; Ryu et al., 2018
Upregulation of VCAM-1 and ICAM-1	Chai and Song, 2014
Upregulation of P and E-selectins	Carvalho-Tavares et al., 2000
Upregulation of MMPs	Thomsen et al., 2017
Disruption of astrocytic endfeet	Fan et al., 2014
Shift in astrocytic gene expression toward pro-inflammatory cytokines	Zamanian et al., 2012
Increased extravasation of macrophages	Skelly et al., 2013
Dysregulation of Wnt/β-catenin pathway	Ma and Hottiger, 2016; Lengfeld et al., 2017
Effects of obesity on BBB	
Increased activation of NF-κB through TLR4 mediated SFA signaling	Milanski et al., 2009
Upregulation of pro-inflammatory cytokines	Yudkin et al., 1999; De Souza et al., 2005; Zhang et al., 2005; Hommelberg et al., 2009; Lawrence, 2009; Jais and Brüning, 2017
Downregulation of metabolic and housekeeping genes	Ouyang et al., 2014b
Amplified ROS production	Zhang et al., 2005; Tucsek et al., 2014; Jais and Brüning, 2017
Activation of microglia	Tucsek et al., 2014
Infiltration of macrophages into the parenchyma	Stranahan et al., 2016
Insensitivity to anorexic hormones leptin and insulin	Kievit et al., 2006; Zhang et al., 2008
Disruption of the hypothalamus	Prada et al., 2005; Horvath et al., 2010; Jais and Brüning, 2017
Disruption of the hippocampus and cognitive impairment	Kanoski et al., 2010; Davidson et al., 2012, 2013; Hargrave et al., 2016
Effects of T2DM on BBB	
Increased ROS production	Wang et al., 2012
Upregulation of pro-inflammatory cytokines	Elmarakby and Sullivan, 2012
Downregulation of TJ proteins	Chehade et al., 2002; Argaw et al., 2009; Sajja et al., 2014; Yoo et al., 2016; Xu et al., 2017
Increased permeability of BBB	Hawkins et al., 2007; Fujihara et al., 2016
Upregulation of VCAM-1 and ICAM-1	Janelidze et al., 2017
Thickening of the BM	Junker et al., 1985
Increased MMP activity	Hawkins et al., 2007; Thomsen et al., 2017
Increased levels of AGEs	Kowluru et al., 2004

NF-κB pathway, impairing the hypothalamus' ability to lower hunger and regulate blood sugar (Boden and Shulman, 2002; Jais and Brüning, 2017). Long term HFD reduces the number of synapses on hypothalamic neurons and increases neural apoptosis (Horvath et al., 2010).

High fat diet also leads to cognitive deficits (Pistell et al., 2010). Several studies by Davidson et al. (2012, 2013) have looked at the impact of HFD on the hippocampus, a major center for learning and memory (Kanoski et al., 2010; Hargrave et al., 2016). In one, mice were challenged to determine if they could associate external landmarks with a food reward, an operation dependent on the hippocampus. Mice on HFD were less able to make the association compared with controls fed on a regular diet (Hargrave et al., 2016). Further experiments tested their ability to discriminate between similar stimuli. While mice with diet-induced obesity performed as well as the control in the hippocampus-independent test, they performed poorly on the hippocampus-dependent discrimination test (Davidson et al., 2012, 2013). Interestingly, cognitive impairment occurred before obesity developed, and while it was a good predictor of obesity, the latter was a poor predictor of impairment. Even further, cognitive deficits could be identified before significant BBB leakiness occurred (Davidson et al., 2013). This raises questions about the development and time course of BBB pathology. Cognitive deficits and corresponding BBB disruption can be detected as early as 24 days after HFD (Davidson

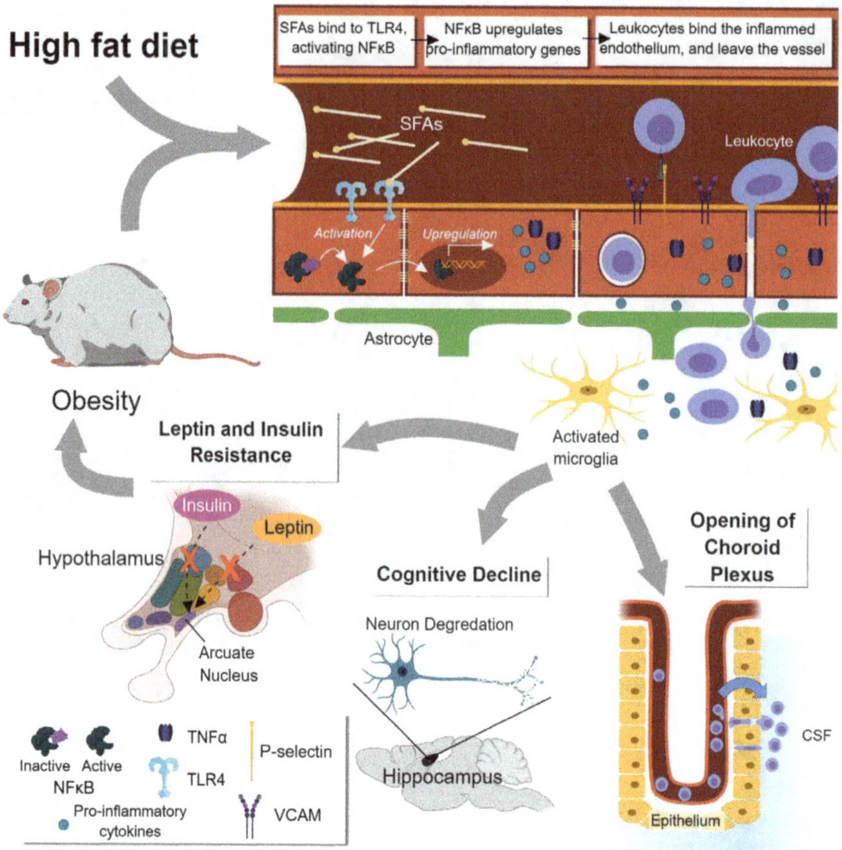

FIGURE 2 | Effects of obesity on the BBB and the brain. Increased saturated fatty acids (SFA) concentration caused by high fat diet (HFD) or obesity enhance NF-κB-mediated inflammation at the BBB via TLR4 receptor. This causes increased leukocyte extravasation, release of pro-inflammatory cytokines, and activation of microglia. The hypothalamus is disrupted, leading to leptin and insulin insensitivity and greater obesity. Disruption of the hippocampus leads to cognitive impairment. Opening of the choroid plexus leads to enhanced leukocyte influx into the cerebrospinal fluid (CSF), more antigen sampling, and greater risk of immune response. *Figure made with BioRender*.

et al., 2013). However, plasma triglyceride and free fatty acid levels do not appear significantly altered that early. There are a number of possible contributing factors. Cognitive deficits were associated with elevated blood glucose levels, and obese rats show decreased GLUT1, a deficiency correlated to impaired cognitive performance (De Vivo et al., 1991). Insulin resistance may also play a role (Hargrave et al., 2016). Indeed, insulin resistance of brain ECs is known as type III diabetes, and it is strongly associated with AD. It is possible that increased Aβ levels may play a role, as this is caused by increased levels of circulating fats and is associated with BBB disruption (Hargrave et al., 2016). None of these factors, however, have been definitively linked with early BBB decline in response to HFD.

Many studies on BBB integrity have looked at regulatory regions like the hypothalamus or memory and learning regions like the hippocampus. A few, however, have looked at the CP, a structure found in the ventricles of the brain that produces the CSF. While it doesn't possess a tight barrier, the CP largely controls the flow of immune cells into the CSF, hence playing a major role in brain immunosurveillance (Schulz and Engelhardt, 2005; Engelhardt, 2006; Ransohoff and Engelhardt, 2012; Ghersi-Egea et al., 2018). In one study, rats exposed to HFD showed a decrease in TJ integrity and corresponding increase in CP leakiness (Kanoski et al., 2010). Another study showed decreased passage of insulin-like growth factor-1 (IGF-1), a neuroprotective factor related to neuropathologies, across the CP barrier (Dietrich et al., 2007). These point to a direct link between neuroimmune disorders and HFDs.

Obesity, Leptin, and Cerebral Inflammation

Many obesity-associated pathologies result from increased production of adipocytes. These, in addition to being the body's predominant fat storage cell, secrete a number of signaling molecules called adipokines. One of these, leptin, is produced by adipose tissue when the body's energy needs are met, acting on the hypothalamus to increase satiety. An increase in adipocyte number leads to higher secretion of leptin, however, despite the high plasma concentration of leptin in obese individuals, they continue to feel hunger. Indeed, the brain develops a leptin resistance, preventing the hormone from exerting its usual effect. Leptin resistance, and factors causing it, has been reviewed elsewhere (Sáinz et al., 2015).

One of the primary possible causes for leptin resistance is ineffective transport across the BBB. Leptin receptors at the BBB are responsible for modulating leptin transport into the parenchyma [although they do not necessarily transport it (Banks and Lebel, 2002)], and they seem to be easily saturated. Obese mice have higher plasma levels of leptin than WT counterparts, but similar levels of leptin in the CSF, suggesting that leptin transport, while not diminished by obesity, does not increase with higher plasma concentrations of leptin (Burguera et al., 2000; Nave et al., 2003). Administering leptin into the plasma of an obese mouse has no effect, but delivering it directly to the brain produces a robust leptin response (Van Heek et al., 1997). Further research, however, has shown that leptin transport can be reduced in obesity. Mice treated with triglycerides in milk displayed a 44% decrease in leptin transport across the BBB compared to mice given fat-free milk (Banks et al., 2004). Increased plasma triglyceride levels are a key feature of obesity (Musunuru, 2010) and would play an important role in leptin resistance.

Leptin has been implicated in many roles beyond signaling satiety, including modulation of immunity. For example, endothelial leptin signaling plays a role in leukocyte extravasation in the spinal cord and other CNS areas. Knocking out leptin receptors prevents this migration, preserves TJ integrity, and attenuates the progression of experimental autoimmune encephalomyelitis (EAE), a mouse model of MS (Lang and Ratke, 2009). Leptin also acts directly on immune cell populations. It promotes the development and activation of Th1 leukocytes, cells associated with the development of EAE (Lord et al., 1998; Matarese et al., 2001b). Conversely, the Th2 immune response, which plays a protective role in EAE, is diminished by leptin (Zamvil and Steinman, 1990; Matarese et al., 2001b). Increased leptin also correlates with a decreased number of Tregs, a regulatory T cell that inhibits inflammation and immune response (Matarese et al., 2005; De Rosa et al., 2007).

These effects of leptin on immune cells are at least partially mediated by the mTOR signaling pathway (Galgani et al., 2010; Procaccini et al., 2012). mTOR-mediated leptin signaling leads to a reduction in Treg production, and Tregs will themselves release leptin to control their own responsiveness (De Rosa et al., 2007; Procaccini et al., 2010). mTOR activation also enhances the development and survival of CD4+CD25- (non-regulatory, helper) T cells by upregulating Bcl-5, a factor involved in T cell differentiation (Galgani et al., 2010). This induced shift toward a pro-inflammatory environment has implicated leptin as an essential player in the development of EAE. Indeed, EAE will not develop in leptin deficient mice (Matarese et al., 2001a; Ouyang et al., 2014a). This also accounts for evidence suggesting increased risk of contracting MS amongst obese adolescents (Hedström et al., 2016). On the other hand, leptin acts on astrocyte leptin receptors to enhance beneficial EAE immune response and decrease disease severity (Mishra et al., 2013). Thus, leptin has a multifaceted role in neuroinflammation, the details of which remain to clarified.

TYPE 2 DIABETES

An important consequence of obesity is type 2 diabetes mellitus (T2DM). Caused by loss of insulin sensitivity in adipocytes, muscles, and other insulin-dependent cells, T2DM results in a loss of effective glucose control (Pandey et al., 2015). If patients do not regulate their sugar levels through diet and/or exercise, they easily become hyperglycemic. This results in increased inflammation, perturbed metabolic pathways, and a number of complications including retinopathy, nephropathy, neuropathy, and degradation of the BBB (Ennis and Keep, 2007; Campos, 2012; Blake and Trounce, 2014; Mapanga and Essop, 2016).

T2DM and Inflammation

As in HFD models of obesity, T2DM mediates many of its effects through inflammation (Brownlee, 2005) (**Figure 3**). The hyperglycemia caused by T2DM leads to increased mitochondrial respiration in ECs, pericytes, and astrocytes. This promotes ROS production and oxidative stress. Enhanced ROS activate NF-κB, activator protein-1 (AP-1), and STAT pathways (Wang et al., 2012). This, in turn, leads to upregulation of inflammatory cytokines (Elmarakby and Sullivan, 2012). ROS also interfere with astrocyte communication by inhibiting the folding of gap junction proteins. Damage to astrocytes can be rescued using antioxidants and chaperone proteins (Gandhi et al., 2010). The damage caused by ROS also eventually leads to pericytes loss, BBB breakdown, and astrocytic endfeet degeneration (Brownlee, 2005). Left untreated, this inflammation can lead to cognitive impairment, just as observed in obesity models (Luchsinger et al., 2007).

The impact of T2DM-induced inflammation in the BBB is readily measurable at the molecular level. T2DM downregulates TJ proteins including claudin-5, ZO-1, occludin, and caveolin (Chehade et al., 2002; Argaw et al., 2009; Sajja et al., 2014; Yoo et al., 2016; Xu et al., 2017). This allows greater influx of blood components into the perivascular space, as shown by studies on albumin and (14)C sucrose penetration (Hawkins et al., 2007; Fujihara et al., 2016). CAMs, including ICAM-1 and VCAM-1, are upregulated (Janelidze et al., 2017). The BM also becomes thicker (Junker et al., 1985), an effect associated with angiopathy leading to increased vascular permeability (Roy et al., 2015). BM thickening is promoted by activation of PKC, AGEs, and growth factors such as TGF-β and connective tissue growth factor. It leads to a compositional change in the extracellular matrix. The upregulation of fibronectin, collagen IV, and laminin compromises cell attachment to the BM and BBB permeability, while downregulation of heparin sulfate proteoglycans removes anionic protein binding sites, destabilizing the BM (Roy et al., 2010; Chronopoulos et al., 2011). MMP activity also increases, and while its protease activity does not offset the increased BM synthesis, it is important for leukocyte extravasation (Hawkins et al., 2007; Thomsen et al., 2017).

The rate at which inflammation causes damage is brain region-dependent. A longitudinal study by Huber et al. (2006) found that increased BBB permeability first occurred in the midbrain, 28 days after T2DM was induced. This was followed by the hippocampus, the cerebral cortex, and the basal ganglia

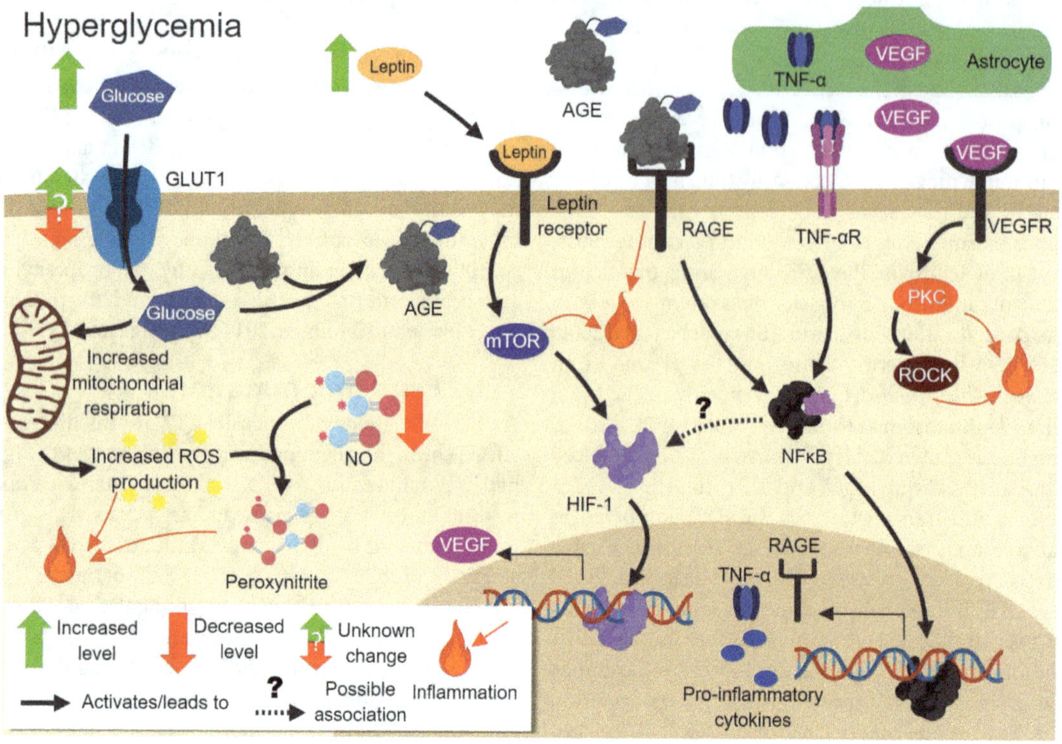

FIGURE 3 | Pathways involved in hyperglycemia-induced neuroinflammation. Increased glucose concentration in cells leads to amplified oxidative respiration and reactive oxygen species (ROS) production. ROS react with NO to produce peroxynitrite. Increased glucose also leads to formation of advanced glycation end products (AGEs), which act on RAGE to increase NF-κB activation. Activated NF-κB increases pro-inflammatory gene expression, including RAGE itself and cytokines. Increased leptin leads to mTOR and HIF-1 pathway activation, increasing vascular endothelial growth factor (VEGF) production. VEGF released from astrocytes activates protein kinase C (PKC) and Rho-associated kinase (ROCK), which further promotes inflammation. *Figure made with BioRender*.

(Huber et al., 2006). Whole brain MRI scans found most brain atrophy in the hippocampus and the temporal, frontal, and limbic gray matter. Damage was also seen in frontal and temporal white matter, but to a lesser extent (Moran et al., 2013). Interestingly, damage to the microvasculature continues even after the hyperglycemia is controlled (Huber et al., 2006). This is partially due to the accumulation of advanced glycation end products (AGEs), which have detrimental effects on the brain (Ceriello, 2012).

Inflammatory Mediators in T2DM

Hyperglycemia and Insulin

Pathways mediating the effects of hyperglycemia are complex and not fully understood. Most seem to be an immediate result of increased glucose levels. Unlike many organs, the brain endothelium uses GLUT1 as glucose transporter, which is not directly regulated by insulin (Shah et al., 2012). In theory, hyperglycemia would lead to increased glucose absorption by the BBB. Whether this actually happens is a matter of debate. Much of the early evidence suggested that hyperglycemia lowered GLUT1 (*Slc2a1*) expression, normalizing brain glucose transport (Pardridge et al., 1990; Cornford et al., 1995). However, other research suggested that there was no difference in glucose transport between normoglycemic and hyperglycemic rats (Pelligrino et al., 1992; Jacob et al., 2002). The answer seems to depend largely on the conditions, models, and brain region. For example, one study found downregulated GLUT1 in the retina, but not in the cerebral cortex (Badr et al., 2000). Another found decreased GLUT1 expression in chronic, but not acute, hyperglycemia (Duelli et al., 2000). This controversy has been reviewed in depth (Shah et al., 2012; Prasad et al., 2014). A study by Jais et al. (2016) found that GLUT1 production and glucose uptake decreased in mice on a HFD. However, the resulting inflammation caused upregulation of VEGF, which led to recovery of GLUT1 levels (Jais et al., 2016). This opens new doors for the study of signaling processes involved in BBB response to hyperglycemia.

Perhaps more important than glucose transport is brain glucose concentration. Here, the preponderance of evidence shows increased glucose uptake through the BBB (Shah et al., 2012). This higher glucose concentration and metabolic rate explains the inflammatory phenotype described above. Note that this has no bearing on the GLUT1 debate. While GLUT1 is the most important glucose transporter, there are many others (GLUT3, GLUT4, GLUT8, and SGLT1) that can modulate neural glucose levels. Few studies have been done on human glucose levels, and their results are mixed, suggesting either no change or an increase in glucose concentration (Kreis and Ross, 1992; Seaquist et al., 2005). Some of these have been done on T1DM patients, but not T2DM (Shah et al., 2012). More work is needed to address this gap.

Surprisingly, studies suggest that altered insulin signaling does not play a critical role in type 2 diabetic pathology. For example, in T1DM, where pancreatic insulin production has been cut off and insulin levels are very low, hyperglycemic patients display the same oxidative stress as their type 2 counterparts (Garg et al., 2014; Yorulmaz et al., 2015). Cell transport and permeability are similarly disrupted in each type. Mice lacking brain endothelial insulin receptors maintain normal BBB function and permeability (Kondo et al., 2004). T2DM patients, on the other hand, display insulin resistance. Thus, despite higher insulin levels, patients with type 2 diabetes show little reactivity to insulin, making them functionally equivalent to patients with type 1 diabetes.

Role of VEGF

The effects of hyperglycemia involve stimulation of *vascular endothelial growth factor* (VEGF), a factor classically associated with both angiogenesis and vascular permeability.

Vascular endothelial growth factor stimulates vasculogenesis, resulting in immature, unstable vessels. Signaling molecules such as Angiopoietin-1 promote vessel maturation and stabilization (Yancopoulos et al., 2000). VEGF also regulates angiogenesis in response to hypoxia via hypoxia-induced factors (Masoud and Li, 2015).

Because VEGF increases BBB permeability, it is associated with inflammation. For example, chronic intracerebral infusion of VEGF in mice was found to upregulate ICAM-1 and major histocompatibility complex I and II, increasing the opportunity for immune response (Proescholdt et al., 1999). Treatment with VEGF also disrupts claudin-5, occludin, and ZO-1, important TJ proteins (Fischer et al., 2002; Argaw et al., 2009). When given after stroke, VEGF triggers rapid (within minutes) stimulation of caveolae-mediated transcytosis, increasing transcellular transport and permeability (Feng et al., 1999; Chen et al., 2002).

Studies of VEGF expression in T2DM have focused on diabetic retinopathy. Increased VEGF production was found in response to hyperglycemia, an effect linked to the increased retinal vascularization (Cai et al., 2014; Capitão and Soares, 2016; Caprnda et al., 2017). The effects of hyperglycemia on VEGF expression in the rest of the brain are less known. One study found that cultured astrocytes exposed to higher glucose had increased VEGF expression (Wang et al., 2012). Astrocytic VEGF is released directly into the parenchyma, allowing it to act on the abluminal VEGF receptors of the endothelium.

The effects of plasma VEGF depend to a certain extent on the state of the BBB. VEGF receptors are located on the abluminal side of blood vessels, so VEGF must be able to cross the barrier in order to exert its effects (Qu Hong et al., 1995). Since the BBB is more permeable in diabetic conditions, the pro-angiogenic and vascular permeability effects of VEGF are most clearly observed in those conditions. A study found that inhibiting early VEGF release from ECs could promote stroke recovery in diabetic mice (Reeson et al., 2015). Interestingly, the most commonly prescribed drug for acute management of stroke, rtPA, generates adverse side effects including increased BBB permeability (Suzuki et al., 2016), in great part via activation of VEGF signaling and increased transcytosis (Benchenane et al., 2005; Turner and Vink, 2012).

One of the upstream players regulating VEGF is HIF-1, a transcriptional factor normally upregulated in hypoxic conditions, which increases oxygen supply, glucose transport, and blood vessel formation (Fischer et al., 2002; Argaw et al., 2009; Balamurugan, 2016). It is also upregulated in response to hyperglycemia and to the resulting advanced glycation endproducts (AGEs) and ROS (Treins et al., 2001). Inhibiting HIF-1 activity reduced the hyperglycemic increase in BBB permeability and decreased expression of VEGF (Yan et al., 2012). Mechanisms by which hyperglycemia can dysregulate HIF-1 are reviewed elsewhere (Catrina, 2014). Further upstream, mTOR regulates HIF-1 activity. Inhibiting mTOR lessens the severity of BBB disruption and decreases the upregulation of both HIF-1 and VEGF (Land and Tee, 2007; Wei et al., 2016). As discussed previously, mTOR shifts the immune system away from Tregs and stabilizes Th1 and Th2 cell, priming the immune system for reaction (Matarese et al., 2001b). mTOR is responsive to nutritional status and blood sugar levels. HFD is linked to higher mTOR activity, which is associated with a more active immune system and higher rates of autoimmunity. mTOR is regulated by leptin which, like in obesity, is upregulated in diabetes due to higher levels of fat and blood glucose (Galgani et al., 2010; Bandaru and Shankar, 2011). NF-κB has also been suggested to mediate TNF-α stimulated upregulation of HIF-1 in muscle cells (Remels et al., 2015). This connection remains to be elucidated in the brain context.

Downstream, VEGF activates PKC, enzyme involved in endothelial permeability (Fleegal et al., 2005; Titchenell et al., 2012; Shao and Bayraktutan, 2013). PKC-β plays an especially important role, and hyperglycemia promotes dysfunction in its pathway, causing an increase in NADPH oxidase and MMP-2, and a decrease in occludin (Shao and Bayraktutan, 2013). PKC-β regulates the Rho-kinase (ROCK)/myosin light chain kinase (MLCK) pathway, which plays an important role in vascular smooth muscle tone. ROCK signaling inhibits expression of endothelial nitric oxide synthase (eNOS), which reduces the availability of NO, an effect associated with endothelial dysfunction. ROCK also inhibits eNOS phosphorylation and its resulting activation by inhibiting Akt activity (protein kinase B), as reviewed elsewhere (Yao et al., 2010). Pathological RhoA/ROCK activation in ECs also promotes an association between caveolin-1 and eNOS and their translocation to membrane caveolae compartments (Zhu et al., 2003, 2013). There, eNOS is inhibited (Ju et al., 1997; Drab et al., 2001; Ming et al., 2002), impairing BBB permeability (Siddiqui et al., 2011). Pathological activation of ROCK also promotes oxidative stress (Rivera et al., 2007; Soliman et al., 2012). Pharmacological blockade of ROCK reduces hyperpermeability via inhibition of oxidative stress in ECs (Allen et al., 2010; Gibson et al., 2014). Interestingly, it has been recently demonstrated that genetic or pharmacological blockage of ROCK prevents BBB breakdown following brain injury, opening new possibilities for treatment (Sadeghian et al., 2018).

Role of eNOS and NO

Nitric oxide (NO) plays autocrine and paracrine roles in the blood stream. It is synthesized by nitric oxide synthases (NOS), enzymes including neuronal NOS (nNOS), inducible NOS (iNOS), and eNOS. The latter constitutively releases a small amount of NO from ECs, which maintains smooth muscle tone (Kumar et al., 2017). It is also implicated in BBB permeability modulation and angiogenesis (Murohara et al., 1998). eNOS is activated by phosphorylation of serine 1177 in humans. This is modulated by VEGF signaling through a number of pathways. VEGF activates phospholipase C, which induces IP_3 synthesis and release of Ca^{2+} into the cytoplasm, followed by activation of calmodulin. This pathway leads to activation of PKC, AMP-dependent kinase (AMPK), and Akt (protein kinase B). VEGF can also activate Akt through PI3K. PKC, Akt, and AMPK can all phosphorylate eNOS.

Depending on the model of inflammation used, eNOS has been found to be up or down-regulated. Inflammatory and stroke models show overexpression of NO leading to detrimental effects (Murohara et al., 1998; Mohammadi et al., 2011). Diabetic models, however, show decreased eNOS expression (Safiah Mokhtar et al., 2013). This partly involves ROCK signaling, but control of eNOS is very complex. For example, insulin activates eNOS through the PI3K/Akt pathway. In hyperglycemia, however, the high amount of glucose increases the activity of the hexosamine pathway, which increases the concentration of UDP-β-*N*-acetylglucosamine (UDP-GlcNAc). This factor glycosylates members of the Pl3K/Akt pathway, limiting eNOS activation and subsequent NO activity (Patti et al., 1999; Federici et al., 2002). AGEs can also limit the production of NO by modifying gene expression, glycosylating eNOS, or quenching NO (Xu et al., 2003; Rojas et al., 2010). This creates a strong case for lowered eNOS activity in diabetes.

Nitric oxide has a half-life of a only few seconds but can diffuse freely through the cytoplasm and cell membranes, making it an effective signaling molecule for the local environment (Pacher et al., 2007). NO directly activates cGMP production, which decreases both P-selectin in endothelium and its ligand, β-2 adhesion molecule, in neutrophils. eNOS null mice show persistent upregulation in inflammatory pathways, with 9-10 times more leukocytes binding to the endothelium following an inflammatory stimulus (Cirino et al., 2003). eNOS is also associated with downregulation of MMPs (Tronc et al., 2000).

Nitric oxide plays an inflammatory role in an oxidative environment. It reacts with superoxide to form peroxynitrite, a highly reactive oxidant responsible for many detrimental effects, including disruption of DNA and protein structure (Pacher et al., 2007). Many studies have implicated peroxynitrite as a key player in BBB degradation (Mayhan, 2000; Tan et al., 2004; Parathath et al., 2006; Phares et al., 2007). The peroxynitrite-dependent IFN-γ pathway is sufficient to increase BBB permeability (Phares et al., 2007), and blocking peroxynitrite or superoxide ameliorates inflammation-induced BBB disruption (Mayhan, 2000; Tan et al., 2004). Peroxynitrite also activates latent MMPs (Rajagopalan et al., 1996) and inhibits the MMP inhibitor, TIMP (Frears et al., 1996), causing degradation of the BM.

The role of NO is still somewhat unclear. One study found inactivation of eNOS attenuated the downregulation of claudin-5 and occludin and decreased the BBB permeability caused by VEGF signaling from reactive astrocytes (Argaw et al., 2012). However, this report did not specify whether peroxynitrite was involved. The same can be said for studies that connected eNOS activation with increased BBB permeability in connection with VEGF activation or induced stroke (Fukumura et al., 2001; Mohammadi et al., 2011). Clarification of the precise mechanism responsible for these effects is necessary to evaluate their significance. In addition, peroxynitrite has a multifaceted role, with one study suggesting it protected neurons against nitric-oxide mediated apoptosis (García-Nogales et al., 2003). Thus, more work is needed to elucidate the role of NO in inflammation-induced BBB breakdown.

Role of AGEs

AGEs, primary mediators of diabetes-associated pathologies, result from hyperglycemia. Glucose combines with a protein to form a Schiff base that undergoes further modification to become an AGE. AGEs alter protein structure and function, affecting enzyme activity, reducing protein half-life and weakening ligand binding (Vlassara and Palace, 2002). Certain AGEs can cross-link proteins, creating matrixes that inhibit normal protein function. Their production leads to ROS formation that cause damage to the cell by oxidative stress. DNA and lipids are vulnerable to AGE formation. For review see (Ahmed, 2005; Ceriello, 2012).

AGEs act on a variety of receptors, the most common of which is the receptor for AGE (RAGE). RAGE activates an immune response by modulating a number of cytokines, including pro-inflammatory cytokines IL-8, TGF-β1, TNF-α, interferon γ (IFN-γ), IL-2, and IL4, and basement membrane modifying proteins COL-1, COL-III, and MMP-2 (Shimizu et al., 2013; Serban et al., 2016). Many of RAGE's effects are mediated through NF-κB (Ahmed, 2005). NF-κB activation leads to increased expression of IL-6, IL-1α, and TNF-α. It promotes coagulation and vasoconstriction through the upregulation of tissue factor, thrombomodulin, and endothelin-1. It also increases VCAM-1 and ICAM-1 expression, allowing for enhanced penetration of leukocytes (Lawrence, 2009; Hoesel and Schmid, 2013). Perhaps most importantly, NF-κB promotes further expression of RAGE, creating a positive feedback loop. This has implicated RAGE in metabolic memory, a phenomenon in which oxidative damage and inflammatory gene expression continue even after hyperglycemia has been normalized (Ceriello, 2012). In one study, as little as 2 months of hyperglycemia before glucose control was re-established was enough to cause permanent changes to NF-κB activity (Kowluru et al., 2004). Hyperglycemia greatly alters gene expression, and many oxidation controlling genes are downregulated. These modifications may persist after glucose levels are normalized, further contributing to metabolic memory (Ceriello, 2012). As a result, the inflammatory state induced by hyperglycemia can persist long after blood glucose levels are controlled, increasing the severity of hyperglycemia.

Role of miRNAs

Micro RNAs (miRNAs) have also been shown to play a role in BBB disruption. miRNAs are short, 15–20 nucleotide-long RNAs that bind to messenger RNAs, preventing their translation or marking them for degradation (Hammond, 2015). They are increasingly recognized to play an important role in many pathologies, including inflammatory diseases. Pro-inflammatory cytokines TNFα and IFNγ have been shown to downregulate several miRNAs. One of them, miR-125a-5p, regulates barrier tightness and prevents leukocyte extravasation (Reijerkerk et al., 2013). Another, miR-143, is associated with T2DB. It downregulates oxysterol-binding protein-related protein 8, impairing the ability of insulin to induce Akt activation. This creates a miRNA-linked mechanism for insulin insensitivity (Li et al., 2018). miR-143 also downregulates PUMA, a pro-apoptotic molecule. PUMA is associated with BBB damage and permeability, and it decreases TJ protein expression (Bai et al., 2016). These studies open a new mechanistic approach to inflammation, necessitating further investigation.

IMPACT OF METABOLIC SYNDROME ON NEURAL HEALTH

Connections to Aging

The inflammatory effects of metabolic syndrome described above are, in many respects, comparable to effects of aging. While aging is a very complex process not well understood to date, its features appear to be the products of inflammation caused by cell senescence and deterioration, with the accumulation of AGEs and other harmful waste products (Lucke-Wold et al., 2014). Metabolic syndrome often accompanies the aging process, with 46.7% prevalence amongst those over 60 compared to 18.3% amongst those aged 20–39 (Aguilar et al., 2015). It leads to less healthy aging and poorer quality of life. Hypertension and cardiovascular disease have long been known to increase risk of ischemic stroke, and obesity and diabetes are also known risk factors (Lucke-Wold et al., 2014). Metabolic syndrome is also associated with reduced cognitive performance and exacerbates the risk and outcomes of neurodegenerative disease, such as AD and MS (Hassing et al., 2009).

Both obesity and diabetes, through the mechanisms described above, lead to increased neuroinflammation, essentially accelerating the aging process. For example, AGEs produced because of diabetes contributes to production of ROS which causes protein and DNA damage, cell death, and the activation of immune pathways (Ahmed, 2005). High concentrations of leptin induced by obesity lead to immune cell activation (Lord et al., 1998; Matarese et al., 2001b). The damage caused to endothelial cells by increased inflammation and ROS are more susceptible to binding platelets and forming clots (McEwen, 2014).

Astrocytes succumb to the pressures of oxidative stress and telomeric replication exhaustion, becoming unable to meet their role of maintaining ion and neurotransmitter homeostasis, and the BBB (Bhat et al., 2012). The BBB begins to decay, with occludin and ZO-1 significantly reduced (Mooradian et al., 2003), and endothelial cell structure becoming less robust (Lee et al., 2012). Meanwhile, inflammatory pathways are increasingly active. In their review on aging and metabolic syndrome, Lucke-Wold et al. (2014) described a positive feedback loop in which activated microglia produce ROS, leading to cell death and increased local glutamate levels. This, in turn, leads to increased secretion of pro-inflammatory cytokines and further microglial activation. This process would be interrupted in a younger brain by astrocytes buffering excess glutamate (Lucke-Wold et al., 2014).

Connections to Alzheimer's Disease

Neuroinflammation is implicated in many neurological disorders, and inflammation caused by metabolic syndrome increases the likelihood and severity of these pathologies. The link between obesity, diabetes and AD is now well established and has been studied extensively (Nguyen et al., 2014; Pugazhenthi et al., 2017). Both obesity and diabetes can lead to insulin resistance in the CNS, a disorder known as type 3 diabetes (de la Monte and Wands, 2008). The resulting lack of insulin and insulin-like growth factors signaling is identical to that seen in AD. Both lead to neuronal death and glial activation. They also result in mitochondrial dysfunction, oxidative stress, and increased ROS levels. The inflammasome, a protein complex leading to pro-inflammatory cytokine secretion, caspase-1, and proteolytic cleavage, gets upregulated and increases inflammation (Pugazhenthi et al., 2017). As described above, this leads to degradation of the BBB and the influx of leukocytes. Aβ formation is upregulated in AD, and the damaged BBB is less able to remove it, causing accumulation in the parenchyma (Bell and Zlokovic, 2009; Zlokovic, 2011; Sagare et al., 2012). In addition, leptin has been implicated in AD pathogenesis. It decreases Aβ production by blocking β-secretase and increasing Aβ uptake, and it deactivates glycogen synthase kinase beta, the protein primarily responsible for tau hyperphosphorylation (Folch et al., 2015). Although leptin levels increase in obesity, insensitivity prevents it from fulfilling its function. Lastly, adiponectin, an anti-inflammatory molecule with protective effects against AD, is decreased in obesity (Letra et al., 2014).

Connections to Multiple Sclerosis

An association exists between MS and T1DM, however, this is more related to their common origin as autoimmune diseases, and less to an inflammatory environment created by T1DM (Tettey et al., 2015). Links between MS and T2DM are more tenuous. In their review, Tettey et al. (2014) reported evidence for vascular comorbidities in MS, including T2DM. An epidemiological study was unable to find any difference in MS prevalence between diabetic, hypertensive, or hyperlipidemic populations and the general population from 1984 to 2006 (Marrie et al., 2012). More recently, Hou et al. (2017) showed a small, albeit significant, association between T2DM and MS incidence. Another study focusing on MS patients between found that diabetes, obstructive lung disease and hypertension affected clinical outcomes such as walking speed, self-reported disability, and depression (Conway et al., 2017). However, none of these studies provide strong evidence that T2DM increases risk of contracting MS.

As with T2DM, investigations on links between obesity and MS have produced mixed results. The prevalence of obesity amongst MS patients has been found either increased (Slawta et al., 2003), decreased (Markianos et al., 2013; Pinhas-Hamiel et al., 2015), or unchanged (Khurana et al., 2009). A systemic review by Wens et al. (2013) found evidence for increased risk of cardiovascular disease in MS, but the precise connection remains unclear. However, several studies have associated obesity during adolescence with a higher risk of contracting MS (Hedström et al., 2012, 2016). A mendelian randomization study by Mokry et al. (2016) found significant association between genetically induced obesity and MS, with low risk of pleiotropic effects (i.e., the genes in question influence the two conditions through separate pathways).

Possible mechanistic links between obesity and MS has been reviewed elsewhere (Guerrero-García et al., 2016; Palavra et al., 2016). These focus on a few factors, including a possible confounding role played by serum levels of vitamin D, dyslipidemia, and adipokines such as leptin. An increased inflammatory state may be a very important link between obesity, T2DM, and MS. HFDs have been shown to open the CP, which would allow for greater immune sampling and, presumably, greater immune sensitivity (Kanoski et al., 2010). In addition, systemic inflammation would open the BBB, allowing for easier immune penetration (Varatharaj and Galea, 2017). These effects would decrease the threshold required for autoimmune activation, allowing the stimulation of myelin reactive cells.

METABOLIC SYNDROME AND THE GUT MICROBIOME-BBB AXIS

The gut microbiome has been implicated as an important player in neural health, as well as with obesity and T2DM. Imbalance of the microbiome, known as dysbiosis, has long been known to play a role in the development of metabolic syndrome and obesity (Barlow et al., 2015). For example, germ free (GF) mice gain significantly less weight than specific-pathogen-free (SPF) counterparts, despite higher food intake. Reintroducing bacteria to the GF mice results in further weight gain (Bäckhed et al., 2004). Substantial work has explored the specific contributions of various bacterial phyla to obesity and diabetes, as reviewed elsewhere (Barlow et al., 2015).

More recently, dysbiosis has been shown to be comorbid with neuropathologies including autism spectrum disorder, Parkinson's disease, MS, and chronic pain (Martin et al., 2018). The microbiota communicate with the brain by interacting with endocrine and enterochromaffin cells, which secrete hormones and neuromodulatory molecules. They also directly signal the brain through peptides, inflammatory molecules, and bacterial metabolites (Martin et al., 2018). Aberration of these signaling pathways leads to neural dysfunction, and gut microbiota profiles have been linked to specific brain profiles, including the size of structures like the hypothalamus, caudate nucleus, and hippocampus (Fernandez-Real et al., 2015; Labus et al., 2017). GF mice showed cognitive deficits, as did *Citrobacter rodentium* infected mice exposed to acute stress (Gareau et al., 2011; Fernandez-Real et al., 2015). In humans, female subjects put on a probiotic milk product for 4 weeks had altered neural activity in affective, viscerosensory, and somatosensory cortices (Tillisch et al., 2013). The microbiota also influences the BBB. GF mice display increased BBB permeability compared to SPF mice, with downregulation of claudin-5 and occludin. Exposure of GF mice to the SPF microbiota decreased BBB permeability and upregulated TJ proteins (Braniste et al., 2014). These findings highlight the importance of the gut microbiota for neural health, but many questions remain unresolved. The microbiota-to-BBB connection has been discovered very recently, and more work is required to elucidate the pathways involved. In addition, most of the work in this area has been done on rodents, and translation to humans remain unclear (Martin et al., 2018).

THE POSITIVE EFFECTS OF INFLAMMATION

Despite all the harmful consequences of inflammation, it still serves vitally important functions in the brain that are worth mentioning. Interestingly, many of these functions center around MS, a disease notorious for autoimmune attack driven by inflammation. For example, myelin reactive T cells are normally implicated in neural decline, but when they were injected into rats following partial crush injury of the optic nerve, the rats retained 300% more retinal ganglion cells (Moalem et al., 1999). This beneficial response is specific to anti-myelin T cells. Immune deficient mice given CNS trauma showed improved recovery following treatment with myelin reactive cells, whereas treatment with ovalbumin reactive cells did not have any effect (Yoles et al., 2001). These effects seem to come largely from Th1 and Th2 cells. One study immunizing mice with Th1 and Th2 myelin reactive cells opened the BBB using an antiseptic approach, instead of pertussis toxin, to induce EAE. Instead of a pathological response, Th1 and Th2 both accelerated re-vascularization and healing (Hofstetter et al., 2003), suggesting Th1 and Th2 in a non-inflammatory environment are beneficial for EAE recovery. Another study observed the progression of MS in the mouse brain. Areas with initial oligodendrocyte and myelin loss had high phagocyte count but low B or T cell count. Areas with complete demyelination had high T cell count, an observation apparently connected to oligodendrocyte regeneration (Henderson et al., 2009). Several mechanisms underlying this effect have been explored, and a likely candidate is the release of neurotrophins from activated immune cells that beneficially affect brain recovery. These include compounds like neural growth factor, which modulates B cell proliferation, immunoglobulin production, and cell survival, and brain derived neurotrophic factor, involved in neuronal survival (Hohlfeld et al., 2006; Schwartz and Raposo, 2014).

Such studies contradict the idea that autoreactive T cells are accidental biproducts of failed T cell sorting in the thymus. Indeed, Schwartz and Raposo (2014) defined "protective autoimmunity" as an essential component of CNS health. In their model, an active population of

CNS-reactive T cells are essential for proper neuronal development and protection against neurodegenerative diseases such as AD. These cells must be carefully controlled by Tregs, which limit the immune response. While low Treg activity will result in chronic inflammation, high activity of Tregs would lead to neurodegenerative diseases. Such model implies that effective treatment for diseases like MS cannot unselectively suppress the immune system. Instead, it must suppress aspects of the immune system that are destructive, while promoting those that are regenerative.

CONCLUSION

Metabolic syndrome and the resulting insulin and leptin resistance and hyperglycemia have pro-inflammatory effects with profound consequences on the BBB. Breakdown of the BBB leads to immune infiltration into the parenchyma and neuronal death. This carries many implications, depending on the brain region affected. Impact on the hypothalamus leads to hormonal disbalance (Boden and Shulman, 2002; Horvath et al., 2010; Jais and Brüning, 2017), damage to the hippocampus leads to cognitive decline (Davidson et al., 2012), and injury to the CP leads to increased immune sensitivity (Kanoski et al., 2010). Many signaling pathways have been implicated in these processes, including VEGF, PKC, RhoA/ROCK, HIF, mTOR, eNOS, AGEs, and miRNA, all of which intersect each other (Fischer et al., 2002; Cirino et al., 2003; Land and Tee, 2007; Yao et al., 2010; Reijerkerk et al., 2013; Shao and Bayraktutan, 2013; Balamurugan, 2016; Serban et al., 2016). Anti-inflammatory drugs target these pathways, but because of the complexity of the picture, it is difficult to predict what side effects they may produce. Given that a certain amount of inflammation is necessary (Moalem et al., 1999), it is vital to carefully select drug targets that will modulate the patient's immune response in a protective way. Resolving metabolic memory may be one of the more relevant therapeutic approaches, as it causes continued inflammation even after blood glucose levels are resolved (Ceriello, 2012). Furthermore, the effects of glucose on GLUT1 expression levels in the human brain have not been fully resolved. Since hyperglycemia is one of the most important factors causing the conditions described above, understanding why its flux across the barrier increases is essential to understanding and preventing its effects. miRNAs remain a largely unexplored factor in systemic inflammation. Given the increasingly important role miRNAs play in cellular physiology, further study is warranted. Finally, the microbiota has been implicated as a key player in BBB integrity, but remains poorly understood. More work is needed to elucidate this connection.

AUTHOR CONTRIBUTIONS

PVD prepared the draft following BL's instructions. BL chose the theme, edited and corrected the manuscript.

REFERENCES

Aguilar, M., Bhuket, T., Torres, S., Liu, B., and Wong, R. J. (2015). Prevalence of the metabolic syndrome in the united states, 2003-2012. *JAMA* 313, 1973–1974. doi: 10.1001/jama.2015.4260

Ahmed, N. (2005). Advanced glycation endproducts—role in pathology of diabetic complications. *Diabetes Res. Clin. Pract.* 67, 3–21. doi: 10.1016/J.DIABRES. 2004.09.004

Allen, C., Srivastava, K., and Bayraktutan, U. (2010). Small GTPase RhoA and its effector Rho kinase mediate oxygen glucose deprivation-evoked in vitro cerebral barrier dysfunction. *Stroke* 41, 2056–2063. doi: 10.1161/STROKEAHA. 109.574939

Andreone, B. J., Chow, B. W., Tata, A., Lacoste, B., Ben-Zvi, A., Bullock, K., et al. (2017). Blood-brain barrier permeability is regulated by lipid transport-dependent suppression of caveolae-mediated transcytosis. *Neuron* 94, 581–594.e5. doi: 10.1016/j.neuron.2017.03.043

Andreone, B. J., Lacoste, B., and Gu, C. (2015). Neuronal and vascular interactions. *Annu. Rev. Neurosci.* 38, 25–46. doi: 10.1146/annurev-neuro-071714-033835

Argaw, A. T., Asp, L., Zhang, J., Navrazhina, K., Pham, T., Mariani, J. N., et al. (2012). Astrocyte-derived VEGF-A drives blood brain barrier disruption in CNS inflammatory disease. *J. Clin. Invest.* 122, 2454–2468. doi: 10.1172/ JCI60842

Argaw, A. T., Gurfein, B. T., Zhang, Y., Zameer, A., and John, G. R. (2009). VEGF-mediated disruption of endothelial CLN-5 promotes blood-brain barrier breakdown. *Proc. Natl. Acad. Sci. U.S.A.* 106, 1977–1982. doi: 10.1073/pnas. 0808698106

Armulik, A., Genové, G., Mäe, M., Nisancioglu, M. H., Wallgard, E., Niaudet, C., et al. (2010). Pericytes regulate the blood-brain barrier. *Nature* 468, 557–561. doi: 10.1038/nature09522

Attwell, D., Buchan, A. M., Charpak, S., Lauritzen, M., MacVicar, B. A., and Newman, E. A. (2010). Glial and neuronal control of brain blood flow. *Nature* 468, 232–243. doi: 10.1038/nature09613

Augustin, H. G., and Koh, G. Y. (2017). Organotypic vasculature: from descriptive heterogeneity to functional pathophysiology. *Science* 357:eaal2379. doi: 10. 1126/science.aal2379

Bäckhed, F., Ding, H., Wang, T., Hooper, L. V., Koh, G. Y., Nagy, A., et al. (2004). The gut microbiota as an environmental factor that regulates fat storage. *Proc. Natl. Acad. Sci. U.S.A.* 101, 15718–15723. doi: 10.1073/pnas.0407076101

Badr, G. A., Tang, J., Ismail-Beigi, F., and Kern, T. S. (2000). Diabetes downregulates GLUT1 expression in the retina and its microvessels but not in the cerebral cortex or its microvessels. *Diabetes* 49, 1016–1021. doi: 10.2337/ diabetes.49.6.1016

Bai, Y., Zhang, Y., Hua, J., Yang, X., Zhang, X., Duan, M., et al. (2016). Silencing microRNA-143 protects the integrity of the blood-brain barrier: implications for methamphetamine abuse. *Sci. Rep.* 6:35642. doi: 10.1038/srep35642

Balamurugan, K. (2016). HIF-1 at the crossroads of hypoxia, inflammation, and cancer. *Int. J. Cancer* 138, 1058–1066. doi: 10.1002/ijc.29519

Bandaru, P., and Shankar, A. (2011). Association between plasma leptin levels and diabetes mellitus. *Metab. Syndr. Relat. Disord.* 9, 19–23. doi: 10.1089/met.2010. 0037

Banks, W. A., Coon, A. B., Robinson, S. M., Moinuddin, A., Shultz, J. M., Nakaoke, R., et al. (2004). Triglycerides induce leptin resistance at the blood-brain barrier. *Diabetes* 53, 1253–1260. doi: 10.2337/diabetes.53.5.1253

Banks, W. A., and Lebel, C. R. (2002). Strategies for the delivery of leptin to the CNS. *J. Drug Target.* 10, 297–308. doi: 10.1080/10611860290031895

Barlow, G. M., Yu, A., and Mathur, R. (2015). Role of the gut microbiome in obesity and diabetes mellitus. *Nutr. Clin. Pract.* 30, 787–797. doi: 10.1177/ 0884533615609896

Bell, R. D., and Zlokovic, B. V. (2009). Neurovascular mechanisms and blood–brain barrier disorder in Alzheimer's disease. *Acta Neuropathol.* 118, 103–113. doi: 10.1007/s00401-009-0522-3

Benchenane, K., Berezowski, V., Fernández-Monreal, M., Brillault, J., Valable, S., Dehouck, M.-P., et al. (2005). Oxygen glucose deprivation switches the transport of tPA across the blood–brain barrier from an LRP-dependent to an increased LRP-independent process. *Stroke* 36, 1059–1064. doi: 10.1161/01.STR.0000163050.39122.4f

Ben-Zvi, A., Lacoste, B., Kur, E., Andreone, B. J., Mayshar, Y., Yan, H., et al. (2014). Mfsd2a is critical for the formation and function of the blood-brain barrier. *Nature* 509, 507–511. doi: 10.1038/nature13324

Bhat, R., Crowe, E. P., Bitto, A., Moh, M., Katsetos, C. D., Garcia, F. U., et al. (2012). Astrocyte senescence as a component of Alzheimer's disease. *PLoS One* 7:e45069. doi: 10.1371/journal.pone.0045069

Blake, R., and Trounce, I. A. (2014). Mitochondrial dysfunction and complications associated with diabetes. *Biochim. Biophys. Acta* 1840, 1404–1412. doi: 10.1016/j.bbagen.2013.11.007

Blüher, M. (2013). Adipose tissue dysfunction contributes to obesity related metabolic diseases. *Best Pract. Res. Clin. Endocrinol. Metab.* 27, 163–177. doi: 10.1016/J.BEEM.2013.02.005

Boden, G., and Shulman, G. I. (2002). Free fatty acids in obesity and type 2 diabetes: defining their role in the development of insulin resistance and beta-cell dysfunction. *Eur. J. Clin. Invest.* 32(Suppl. 3), 14–23. doi: 10.1046/j.1365-2362.32.s3.3.x

Braniste, V., Al-Asmakh, M., Kowal, C., Anuar, F., Abbaspour, A., Tóth, M., et al. (2014). The gut microbiota influences blood-brain barrier permeability in mice. *Sci. Transl. Med.* 6:263ra158. doi: 10.1126/scitranslmed.3009759

Brownlee, M. (2005). The pathobiology of diabetic complications: a unifying mechanism. *Diabetes* 54, 1615–1625. doi: 10.2337/diabetes.54.6.1615

Burguera, B., Couce, M. E., Curran, G. L., Jensen, M. D., Lloyd, R. V., Cleary, M. P., et al. (2000). Obesity is associated with a decreased leptin transport across the blood-brain barrier in rats. *Diabetes* 49, 1219–1223. doi: 10.2337/diabetes.49.7.1219

Cai, Y., Li, X., Wang, Y.-S., Shi, Y.-Y., Ye, Z., Yang, G.-D., et al. (2014). Hyperglycemia promotes vasculogenesis in choroidal neovascularization in diabetic mice by stimulating VEGF and SDF-1 expression in retinal pigment epithelial cells. *Exp. Eye Res.* 123, 87–96. doi: 10.1016/J.EXER.2014.04.012

Campos, C. (2012). Chronic hyperglycemia and glucose toxicity: pathology and clinical sequelae. *Postgrad. Med.* 124, 90–97. doi: 10.3810/pgm.2012.11.2615

Capitão, M., and Soares, R. (2016). Angiogenesis and inflammation crosstalk in diabetic retinopathy. *J. Cell. Biochem.* 117, 2443–2453. doi: 10.1002/jcb.25575

Caprnda, M., Kubatka, P., Saxena, S., Valaskova, J., Stefanickova, J., Kobyliak, N., et al. (2017). The impact of hyperglycemia on VEGF secretion in retinal endothelial cells. *Folia Med.* 59, 183–189. doi: 10.1515/folmed-2017-0029

Carvalho-Tavares, J., Hickey, M. J., Hutchison, J., Michaud, J., Sutcliffe, I. T., and Kubes, P. (2000). A role for platelets and endothelial selectins in tumor necrosis factor-α-induced leukocyte recruitment in the brain microvasculature. *Circ. Res.* 87, 1141–1148. doi: 10.1161/01.RES.87.12.1141

Catrina, S.-B. (2014). Impaired hypoxia-inducible factor (HIF) regulation by hyperglycemia. *J. Mol. Med.* 92, 1025–1034. doi: 10.1007/s00109-014-1166-x

Ceriello, A. (2012). The emerging challenge in diabetes: the "metabolic memory." *Vascul. Pharmacol.* 57, 133–138. doi: 10.1016/J.VPH.2012.05.005

Chai, J., and Song, Q. (2014). Quantitative and multiplexed study of endothelial cell inflammation. *Cell Biochem. Biophys.* 70, 1783–1790. doi: 10.1007/s12013-014-0129-8

Chakraborty, A., de Wit, N. M., van der Flier, W. M., and de Vries, H. E. (2017). The blood brain barrier in Alzheimer's disease. *Vascul. Pharmacol.* 89, 12–18. doi: 10.1016/j.vph.2016.11.008

Chehade, J. M., Haas, M. J., and Mooradian, A. D. (2002). Diabetes-related changes in rat cerebral occludin and zonula occludens-1 (ZO-1) expression. *Neurochem. Res.* 27, 249–252. doi: 10.1023/A:1014892706696

Chen, J., Braet, F., Brodsky, S., Weinstein, T., Romanov, V., Noiri, E., et al. (2002). VEGF-induced mobilization of caveolae and increase in permeability of endothelial cells. *Am. J. Physiol. Cell Physiol.* 282, C1053–C1063. doi: 10.1152/ajpcell.00292.2001

Chow, B. W., and Gu, C. (2015). The molecular constituents of the blood–brain barrier. *Trends Neurosci.* 38, 598–608. doi: 10.1016/J.TINS.2015.08.003

Chow, B. W., and Gu, C. (2017). Gradual suppression of transcytosis governs functional blood-retinal barrier formation. *Neuron* 93, 1325–1333.e3. doi: 10.1016/j.neuron.2017.02.043

Chronopoulos, A., Trudeau, K., Roy, S., Huang, H., Vinores, S. A., and Roy, S. (2011). High glucose-induced altered basement membrane composition and structure increases trans-endothelial permeability: implications for diabetic retinopathy. *Curr. Eye Res.* 36, 747–753. doi: 10.3109/02713683.2011.585735

Cirino, G., Fiorucci, S., and Sessa, W. C. (2003). Endothelial nitric oxide synthase: the Cinderella of inflammation? *Trends Pharmacol. Sci.* 24, 91–95. doi: 10.1016/S0165-6147(02)00049-4

Claesson-Welsh, L. (2015). Vascular permeability–the essentials. *Ups. J. Med. Sci.* 120, 135–143. doi: 10.3109/03009734.2015.1064501

Conway, D. S., Thompson, N. R., and Cohen, J. A. (2017). Influence of hypertension, diabetes, hyperlipidemia, and obstructive lung disease on multiple sclerosis disease course. *Mult. Scler. J.* 23, 277–285. doi: 10.1177/1352458516650512

Cornford, E. M., Hyman, S., Cornford, M. E., and Clare-Salzler, M. (1995). Down-regulation of blood-brain glucose transport in the hyperglycemic nonobese diabetic mouse. *Neurochem. Res.* 20, 869–873. doi: 10.1007/BF00969700

Daneman, R., and Prat, A. (2015). The blood-brain barrier. *Cold Spring Harb. Perspect. Biol.* 7:a020412. doi: 10.1101/cshperspect.a020412

Davalos, D., and Akassoglou, K. (2012). Fibrinogen as a key regulator of inflammation in disease. *Semin. Immunopathol.* 34, 43–62. doi: 10.1007/s00281-011-0290-8

Davidson, T. L., Hargrave, S. L., Swithers, S. E., Sample, C. H., Fu, X., Kinzig, K. P., et al. (2013). Inter-relationships among diet, obesity and hippocampal-dependent cognitive function. *Neuroscience* 253, 110–122. doi: 10.1016/j.neuroscience.2013.08.044

Davidson, T. L., Monnot, A., Neal, A. U., Martin, A. A., Horton, J. J., and Zheng, W. (2012). The effects of a high-energy diet on hippocampal-dependent discrimination performance and blood-brain barrier integrity differ for diet-induced obese and diet-resistant rats. *Physiol. Behav.* 107, 26–33. doi: 10.1016/j.physbeh.2012.05.015

de la Monte, S. M., and Wands, J. R. (2008). Alzheimer's disease is type 3 diabetes-evidence reviewed. *J. Diabetes Sci. Technol.* 2, 1101–1113. doi: 10.1177/193229680800200619

De Rosa, V., Procaccini, C., Calì, G., Pirozzi, G., Fontana, S., Zappacosta, S., et al. (2007). A key role of leptin in the control of regulatory T cell proliferation. *Immunity* 26, 241–255. doi: 10.1016/J.IMMUNI.2007.01.011

De Souza, C. T., Araujo, E. P., Bordin, S., Ashimine, R., Zollner, R. L., Boschero, A. C., et al. (2005). Consumption of a fat-rich diet activates a proinflammatory response and induces insulin resistance in the hypothalamus. *Endocrinology* 146, 4192–4199. doi: 10.1210/en.2004-1520

De Vivo, D. C., Trifiletti, R. R., Jacobson, R. I., Ronen, G. M., Behmand, R. A., and Harik, S. I. (1991). Defective glucose transport across the blood-brain barrier as a cause of persistent hypoglycorrhachia, seizures, and developmental delay. *N. Engl. J. Med.* 325, 703–709. doi: 10.1056/NEJM199109053251006

Deo, A. K., Borson, S., Link, J. M., Domino, K., Eary, J. F., Ke, B., et al. (2014). Activity of P-glycoprotein, a β-amyloid transporter at the blood-brain barrier, is compromised in patients with mild Alzheimer disease. *J. Nucl. Med.* 55, 1106–1111. doi: 10.2967/jnumed.113.130161

Dietrich, M. O., Muller, A., Bolos, M., Carro, E., Perry, M. L., Portela, L. V., et al. (2007). Western style diet impairs entrance of blood-borne insulin-like growth factor-1 into the brain. *Neuromolecular Med.* 9, 324–330. doi: 10.1007/s12017-007-8011-0

Dorfman, M. D., and Thaler, J. P. (2015). Hypothalamic inflammation and gliosis in obesity. *Curr. Opin. Endocrinol. Diabetes Obes.* 22, 325–330. doi: 10.1097/MED.0000000000000182

Drab, M., Verkade, P., Elger, M., Kasper, M., Lohn, M., Lauterbach, B., et al. (2001). Loss of caveolae, vascular dysfunction, and pulmonary defects in caveolin-1 gene-disrupted mice. *Science* 293, 2449–2452. doi: 10.1126/science.1062688

Duelli, R., Maurer, M. H., Staudt, R., Heiland, S., Duembgen, L., and Kuschinsky, W. (2000). Increased cerebral glucose utilization and decreased glucose transporter Glut1 during chronic hyperglycemia in rat brain. *Brain Res.* 858, 338–347. doi: 10.1016/S0006-8993(00)01942-9

ElAli, A., Thériault, P., and Rivest, S. (2014). The role of pericytes in neurovascular unit remodeling in brain disorders. *Int. J. Mol. Sci.* 15, 6453–6474. doi: 10.3390/ijms15046453

Elmarakby, A. A., and Sullivan, J. C. (2012). Relationship between oxidative stress and inflammatory cytokines in diabetic nephropathy. *Cardiovasc. Ther.* 30, 49–59. doi: 10.1111/j.1755-5922.2010.00218.x

Engelhardt, B. (2006). Molecular mechanisms involved in T cell migration across the blood–brain barrier. *J. Neural Transm.* 113, 477–485. doi: 10.1007/s00702-005-0409-y

Engelhardt, B. (2008). Immune cell entry into the central nervous system: involvement of adhesion molecules and chemokines. *J. Neurol. Sci.* 274, 23–26. doi: 10.1016/J.JNS.2008.05.019

Engelhardt, B., and Ransohoff, R. M. (2012). Capture, crawl, cross: the T cell code to breach the blood–brain barriers. *Trends Immunol.* 33, 579–589. doi: 10.1016/J.IT.2012.07.004

Ennis, S. R., and Keep, R. F. (2007). Effect of sustained-mild and transient-severe hyperglycemia on ischemia-induced blood–brain barrier opening. *J. Cereb. Blood Flow Metab.* 27, 1573–1582. doi: 10.1038/sj.jcbfm.9600454

Fan, L., Wang, T., Chang, L., Song, Y., Wu, Y., and Ma, D. (2014). Systemic inflammation induces a profound long term brain cell injury in rats. *Acta Neurobiol. Exp.* 74, 298–306.

Federici, M., Menghini, R., Mauriello, A., Hribal, M. L., Ferrelli, F., Lauro, D., et al. (2002). Insulin-dependent activation of endothelial nitric oxide synthase is impaired by O-linked glycosylation modification of signaling proteins in human coronary endothelial cells. *Circulation* 106, 466–472. doi: 10.1161/01.CIR.0000023043.02648.51

Feng, Y.-Q., Seibler, J., Alami, R., Eisen, A., Westerman, K. A., Leboulch, P., et al. (1999). Site-specific chromosomal integration in mammalian cells: highly efficient CRE recombinase-mediated cassette exchange. *J. Mol. Biol.* 292, 779–785. doi: 10.1006/jmbi.1999.3113

Fernandez-Real, J.-M., Serino, M., Blasco, G., Puig, J., Daunis-i-Estadella, J., Ricart, W., et al. (2015). Gut microbiota interacts with brain microstructure and function. *J. Clin. Endocrinol. Metab.* 100, 4505–4513. doi: 10.1210/jc.2015-3076

Fischer, S., Wobben, M., Marti, H. H., Renz, D., and Schaper, W. (2002). Hypoxia-induced hyperpermeability in brain microvessel endothelial cells involves VEGF-mediated changes in the expression of zonula occludens-1. *Microvasc. Res.* 63, 70–80. doi: 10.1006/mvre.2001.2367

Fleegal, M. A., Hom, S., Borg, L. K., and Davis, T. P. (2005). Activation of PKC modulates blood-brain barrier endothelial cell permeability changes induced by hypoxia and posthypoxic reoxygenation. *Am. J. Physiol. Circ. Physiol.* 289, H2012–H2019. doi: 10.1152/ajpheart.00495.2005

Folch, J., Patraca, I., Martínez, N., Pedrós, I., Petrov, D., Ettcheto, M., et al. (2015). The role of leptin in the sporadic form of Alzheimer's disease. Interactions with the adipokines amylin, ghrelin and the pituitary hormone prolactin. *Life Sci.* 140, 19–28. doi: 10.1016/j.lfs.2015.05.002

Frears, E. R., Zhang, Z., Blake, D. R., O'Connell, J. P., and Winyard, P. G. (1996). Inactivation of tissue inhibitor of metalloproteinase-1 by peroxynitrite. *FEBS Lett.* 381, 21–24. doi: 10.1016/0014-5793(96)00065-48

Fujihara, R., Chiba, Y., Nakagawa, T., Nishi, N., Murakami, R., Matsumoto, K., et al. (2016). Albumin microvascular leakage in brains with diabetes mellitus. *Microsc. Res. Tech.* 79, 833–837. doi: 10.1002/jemt.22708

Fukumura, D., Gohongi, T., Kadambi, A., Izumi, Y., Ang, J., Yun, C. O., et al. (2001). Predominant role of endothelial nitric oxide synthase in vascular endothelial growth factor-induced angiogenesis and vascular permeability. *Proc. Natl. Acad. Sci. U.S.A.* 98, 2604–2609. doi: 10.1073/pnas.041359198

Galgani, M., Procaccini, C., De Rosa, V., Carbone, F., Chieffi, P., La Cava, A., et al. (2010). Leptin modulates the survival of autoreactive $CD4^+$ T cells through the nutrient/energy-sensing mammalian target of rapamycin signalling pathway. *J. Immunol.* 185, 7474–7479. doi: 10.4049/jimmunol.1001674

Gandhi, G. K., Ball, K. K., Cruz, N. F., and Dienel, G. A. (2010). Hyperglycaemia and diabetes impair gap junctional communication among astrocytes. *ASN Neuro* 2:AN20090048. doi: 10.1042/AN20090048

García-Nogales, P., Almeida, A., and Bolaños, J. P. (2003). Peroxynitrite protects neurons against nitric oxide-mediated apoptosis. A key role for glucose-6-phosphate dehydrogenase activity in neuroprotection. *J. Biol. Chem.* 278, 864–874. doi: 10.1074/jbc.M206835200

Gareau, M. G., Wine, E., Rodrigues, D. M., Cho, J. H., Whary, M. T., Philpott, D. J., et al. (2011). Bacterial infection causes stress-induced memory dysfunction in mice. *Gut* 60, 307–317. doi: 10.1136/gut.2009.202515

Garg, M., Thamotharan, M., Becker, D. J., and Devaskar, S. U. (2014). Adolescents with clinical type 1 diabetes display reduced red blood cell glucose transporter isoform 1 (GLUT1). *Pediatr. Diabetes* 15, 511–518. doi: 10.1111/pedi.12127

Garg, N., and Smith, T. W. (2015). An update on immunopathogenesis, diagnosis, and treatment of multiple sclerosis. *Brain Behav.* 5:e00362. doi: 10.1002/brb3.362

Gelb, S., Stock, A. D., Anzi, S., Putterman, C., and Ben-Zvi, A. (2018). Mechanisms of neuropsychiatric lupus: the relative roles of the blood-cerebrospinal fluid barrier versus blood-brain barrier. *J. Autoimmun.* 91, 34–44. doi: 10.1016/j.jaut.2018.03.001

Ghersi-Egea, J.-F., Strazielle, N., Catala, M., Silva-Vargas, V., Doetsch, F., and Engelhardt, B. (2018). Molecular anatomy and functions of the choroidal blood-cerebrospinal fluid barrier in health and disease. *Acta Neuropathol.* 135, 337–361. doi: 10.1007/s00401-018-1807-1

Gibson, C. L., Srivastava, K., Sprigg, N., Bath, P. M. W., and Bayraktutan, U. (2014). Inhibition of Rho-kinase protects cerebral barrier from ischaemia-evoked injury through modulations of endothelial cell oxidative stress and tight junctions. *J. Neurochem.* 129, 816–826. doi: 10.1111/jnc.12681

Guerrero-García, J. J., Carrera-Quintanar, L., López-Roa, R. I., Márquez-Aguirre, A. L., Rojas-Mayorquín, A. E., and Ortuño-Sahagún, D. (2016). Multiple sclerosis and obesity: possible roles of adipokines. *Mediators Inflamm.* 2016:4036232. doi: 10.1155/2016/4036232

Gustafson, D. R., Karlsson, C., Skoog, I., Rosengren, L., Lissner, L., and Blennow, K. (2007). Mid-life adiposity factors relate to blood-brain barrier integrity in late life. *J. Intern. Med.* 262, 643–650. doi: 10.1111/j.1365-2796.2007.01869.x

Hammond, S. M. (2015). An overview of microRNAs. *Adv. Drug Deliv. Rev.* 87, 3–14. doi: 10.1016/j.addr.2015.05.001

Hargrave, S. L., Davidson, T. L., Zheng, W., and Kinzig, K. P. (2016). Western diets induce blood-brain barrier leakage and alter spatial strategies in rats. *Behav. Neurosci.* 130, 123–135. doi: 10.1037/bne0000110

Hartsock, A., and Nelson, W. J. (2008). Adherens and tight junctions: structure, function and connections to the actin cytoskeleton. *Biochim. Biophys. Acta Biomembr.* 1778, 660–669. doi: 10.1016/J.BBAMEM.2007.07.012

Hassing, L. B., Dahl, A. K., Thorvaldsson, V., Berg, S., Gatz, M., Pedersen, N. L., et al. (2009). Overweight in midlife and risk of dementia: a 40-year follow-up study. *Int. J. Obes.* 33, 893–898. doi: 10.1038/ijo.2009.104

Hawkins, B. T., Lundeen, T. F., Norwood, K. M., Brooks, H. L., and Egleton, R. D. (2007). Increased blood-brain barrier permeability and altered tight junctions in experimental diabetes in the rat: contribution of hyperglycaemia and matrix metalloproteinases. *Diabetologia* 50, 202–211. doi: 10.1007/s00125-006-0485-z

Hedström, A., Olsson, T., and Alfredsson, L. (2016). Body mass index during adolescence, rather than childhood, is critical in determining MS risk. *Mult. Scler. J.* 22, 878–883. doi: 10.1177/1352458515603798

Hedström, A. K., Olsson, T., and Alfredsson, L. (2012). High body mass index before age 20 is associated with increased risk for multiple sclerosis in both men and women. *Mult. Scler. J.* 18, 1334–1336. doi: 10.1177/1352458512436596

Henderson, A. P. D., Barnett, M. H., Parratt, J. D. E., and Prineas, J. W. (2009). Multiple sclerosis: distribution of inflammatory cells in newly forming lesions. *Ann. Neurol.* 66, 739–753. doi: 10.1002/ana.21800

Hennekens, C. H., and Andreotti, F. (2013). Leading avoidable cause of premature deaths worldwide: case for obesity. *Am. J. Med.* 126, 97–98. doi: 10.1016/j.amjmed.2012.06.018

Herisson, F., Frodermann, V., Courties, G., Rohde, D., Sun, Y., Vandoorne, K., et al. (2018). Direct vascular channels connect skull bone marrow and the brain surface enabling myeloid cell migration. *Nat. Neurosci.* 21, 1209–1217. doi: 10.1038/s41593-018-0213-2

Hoesel, B., and Schmid, J. A. (2013). The complexity of NF-κB signalling in inflammation and cancer. *Mol. Cancer* 12:86. doi: 10.1186/1476-4598-12-86

Hofstetter, H. H., Sewell, D. L., Liu, F., Sandor, M., Forsthuber, T., Lehmann, P. V., et al. (2003). Autoreactive T cells promote post-traumatic healing in the central nervous system. *J. Neuroimmunol.* 134, 25–34. doi: 10.1016/S0165-5728(02)00358-2

Hohlfeld, R., Kerschensteiner, M., Stadelmann, C., Lassmann, H., and Wekerle, H. (2006). The neuroprotective effect of inflammation: implications for the therapy of multiple sclerosis. *Neurol. Sci.* 27, s1–s7. doi: 10.1007/s10072-006-0537-7

Hommelberg, P. P., Plat, J., Langen, R. C., Schols, A. M., and Mensink, R. P. (2009). Fatty acid-induced NF-κB activation and insulin resistance in skeletal muscle are chain length dependent. *Am. J. Physiol. Metab.* 296, E114–E120. doi: 10.1152/ajpendo.00436.2007

Horvath, T. L., Sarman, B., Garcia-Caceres, C., Enriori, P. J., Sotonyi, P., Shanabrough, M., et al. (2010). Synaptic input organization of the melanocortin system predicts diet-induced hypothalamic reactive gliosis and obesity. *Proc. Natl. Acad. Sci. U.S.A.* 107, 14875–14880. doi: 10.1073/pnas.1004282107

Hou, W.-H., Li, C.-Y., Chang, H.-H., Sun, Y., and Tsai, C.-C. (2017). A population-based cohort study suggests an increased risk of multiple sclerosis incidence in patients with type 2 diabetes mellitus. *J. Epidemiol.* 27, 235–241. doi: 10.1016/j.je.2016.06.006

Huber, J. D., VanGilder, R. L., and Houser, K. A. (2006). Streptozotocin-induced diabetes progressively increases blood-brain barrier permeability in specific brain regions in rats. *Am. J. Physiol. Circ. Physiol.* 291, H2660–H2668. doi: 10.1152/ajpheart.00489.2006

Jacob, R. J., Fan, X., Evans, M. L., Dziura, J., and Sherwin, R. S. (2002). Brain glucose levels are elevated in chronically hyperglycemic diabetic rats: no evidence for protective adaptation by the blood brain barrier. *Metabolism* 51, 1522–1524. doi: 10.1053/meta.2002.36347

Jais, A., and Brüning, J. C. (2017). Hypothalamic inflammation in obesity and metabolic disease. *J. Clin. Invest.* 127, 24–32. doi: 10.1172/JCI88878

Jais, A., Solas, M., Backes, H., Chaurasia, B., Kleinridders, A., Theurich, S., et al. (2016). Myeloid-cell-derived VEGF maintains brain glucose uptake and limits cognitive impairment in obesity. *Cell* 165, 882–895. doi: 10.1016/j.cell.2016.03.033

Janelidze, S., Hertze, J., Nägga, K., Nilsson, K., Nilsson, C., Wennström, M., et al. (2017). Increased blood-brain barrier permeability is associated with dementia and diabetes but not amyloid pathology or APOE genotype. *Neurobiol. Aging* 51, 104–112. doi: 10.1016/j.neurobiolaging.2016.11.017

Ju, H., Zou, R., Venema, V. J., and Venema, R. C. (1997). Direct interaction of endothelial nitric-oxide synthase and caveolin-1 inhibits synthase activity. *J. Biol. Chem.* 272, 18522–18525. doi: 10.1074/jbc.272.30.18522

Junker, U., Jaggi, C., Bestetti, G., and Rossi, G. L. (1985). Basement membrane of hypothalamus and cortex capillaries from normotensive and spontaneously hypertensive rats with streptozotocin-induced diabetes. *Acta Neuropathol.* 65, 202–208. doi: 10.1007/BF00686999

Kanoski, S. E., Zhang, Y., Zheng, W., and Davidson, T. L. (2010). The effects of a high-energy diet on hippocampal function and blood-brain barrier integrity in the rat. *J. Alzheimers Dis.* 21, 207–219. doi: 10.3233/JAD-2010-091414

Kaur, J. (2014). A comprehensive review on metabolic syndrome. *Cardiol. Res. Pract.* 2014:943162. doi: 10.1155/2014/943162

Khurana, S. R., Bamer, A. M., Turner, A. P., Wadhwani, R. V., Bowen, J. D., Leipertz, S. L., et al. (2009). The prevalence of overweight and obesity in veterans with multiple sclerosis. *Am. J. Phys. Med. Rehabil.* 88, 83–91. doi: 10.1097/PHM.0b013e318194f8b5

Kievit, P., Howard, J. K., Badman, M. K., Balthasar, N., Coppari, R., Mori, H., et al. (2006). Enhanced leptin sensitivity and improved glucose homeostasis in mice lacking suppressor of cytokine signalling-3 in POMC-expressing cells. *Cell Metab.* 4, 123–132. doi: 10.1016/j.cmet.2006.06.010

Kondo, T., Hafezi-Moghadam, A., Thomas, K., Wagner, D. D., and Kahn, C. R. (2004). Mice lacking insulin or insulin-like growth factor 1 receptors in vascular endothelial cells maintain normal blood–brain barrier. *Biochem. Biophys. Res. Commun.* 317, 315–320. doi: 10.1016/J.BBRC.2004.03.043

Kowluru, R. A., Chakrabarti, S., and Chen, S. (2004). Re-institution of good metabolic control in diabetic rats and activation of caspase-3 and nuclear transcriptional factor (NF-kB) in the retina. *Acta Diabetol.* 41, 194–199. doi: 10.1007/s00592-004-0165-8

Kreis, R., and Ross, B. D. (1992). Cerebral metabolic disturbances in patients with subacute and chronic diabetes mellitus: detection with proton MR spectroscopy. *Radiology* 184, 123–130. doi: 10.1148/radiology.184.1.1319074

Kumar, S., Singh, R. K., and Bhardwaj, T. R. (2017). Therapeutic role of nitric oxide as emerging molecule. *Biomed. Pharmacother.* 85, 182–201. doi: 10.1016/J.BIOPHA.2016.11.125

Labus, J. S., Hollister, E. B., Jacobs, J., Kirbach, K., Oezguen, N., Gupta, A., et al. (2017). Differences in gut microbial composition correlate with regional brain volumes in irritable bowel syndrome. *Microbiome* 5:49. doi: 10.1186/s40168-017-0260-z

Lacoste, B., and Gu, C. (2015). Control of cerebrovascular patterning by neural activity during postnatal development. *Mech. Dev.* 138(Pt 1), 43–49. doi: 10.1016/j.mod.2015.06.003

Land, S. C., and Tee, A. R. (2007). Hypoxia-inducible factor 1α is regulated by the mammalian target of rapamycin (mTOR) via an mTOR signalling motif. *J. Biol. Chem.* 282, 20534–20543. doi: 10.1074/jbc.M611782200

Lang, K., and Ratke, J. (2009). Leptin and Adiponectin: new players in the field of tumor cell and leukocyte migration. *Cell Commun. Signal.* 7:27. doi: 10.1186/1478-811X-7-27

Lawrence, T. (2009). The nuclear factor NF-kappaB pathway in inflammation. *Cold Spring Harb. Perspect. Biol.* 1:a001651. doi: 10.1101/cshperspect.a001651

Lee, S. W., Clemenson, G. D., and Gage, F. H. (2012). New neurons in an aged brain. *Behav. Brain Res.* 227, 497–507. doi: 10.1016/J.BBR.2011.10.009

Lengfeld, J. E., Lutz, S. E., Smith, J. R., Diaconu, C., Scott, C., Kofman, S. B., et al. (2017). Endothelial Wnt/β-catenin signalling reduces immune cell infiltration in multiple sclerosis. *Proc. Natl. Acad. Sci. U.S.A.* 114, E1168–E1177. doi: 10.1073/pnas.1609905114

Letra, L., Santana, I., and Seiça, R. (2014). Obesity as a risk factor for Alzheimer's disease: the role of adipocytokines. *Metab. Brain Dis.* 29, 563–568. doi: 10.1007/s11011-014-9501-z

Li, B., Fan, J., and Chen, N. (2018). A novel regulator of type II diabetes: MicroRNA-143. *Trends Endocrinol. Metab.* 29, 380–388. doi: 10.1016/J.TEM.2018.03.019

Lord, G. M., Matarese, G., Howard, J. K., Baker, R. J., Bloom, S. R., and Lechler, R. I. (1998). Leptin modulates the T-cell immune response and reverses starvation-induced immunosuppression. *Nature* 394, 897–901. doi: 10.1038/29795

Louveau, A., Herz, J., Alme, M. N., Salvador, A. F., Dong, M. Q., Viar, K. E., et al. (2018). CNS lymphatic drainage and neuroinflammation are regulated by meningeal lymphatic vasculature. *Nat. Neurosci.* 21, 1380–1391. doi: 10.1038/s41593-018-0227-9

Luchsinger, J. A., Reitz, C., Patel, B., Tang, M.-X., Manly, J. J., and Mayeux, R. (2007). Relation of diabetes to mild cognitive impairment. *Arch. Neurol.* 64, 570–575. doi: 10.1001/archneur.64.4.570

Lucke-Wold, B. P., Logsdon, A. F., Turner, R. C., Rosen, C. L., and Huber, J. D. (2014). Aging, the metabolic syndrome, and ischemic stroke: redefining the approach for studying the blood-brain barrier in a complex neurological disease. *Adv. Pharmacol.* 71, 411–449. doi: 10.1016/bs.apha.2014.07.001

Lutz, S. E., Smith, J. R., Kim, D. H., Olson, C. V. L., Ellefsen, K., Bates, J. M., et al. (2017). Caveolin1 is required for Th1 cell infiltration, but not tight junction remodeling, at the blood-brain barrier in autoimmune neuroinflammation. *Cell Rep.* 21, 2104–2117. doi: 10.1016/j.celrep.2017.10.094

Ma, B., and Hottiger, M. O. (2016). Crosstalk between Wnt/β-catenin and NF-κB signalling pathway during inflammation. *Front. Immunol.* 7:378. doi: 10.3389/fimmu.2016.00378

MacVicar, B. A., and Newman, E. A. (2015). Astrocyte regulation of blood flow in the brain. *Cold Spring Harb. Perspect. Biol.* 7:a020388. doi: 10.1101/cshperspect.a020388

Mapanga, R. F., and Essop, M. F. (2016). Damaging effects of hyperglycemia on cardiovascular function: spotlight on glucose metabolic pathways. *Am. J. Physiol. Circ. Physiol.* 310, H153–H173. doi: 10.1152/ajpheart.00206.2015

Markianos, M., Evangelopoulos, M.-E., Koutsis, G., Davaki, P., and Sfagos, C. (2013). Body mass index in multiple sclerosis: associations with CSF neurotransmitter metabolite levels. *ISRN Neurol.* 2013, 1–6. doi: 10.1155/2013/981070

Marrie, R. A., Yu, B. N., Leung, S., Elliott, L., Caetano, P., Warren, S., et al. (2012). Rising prevalence of vascular comorbidities in multiple sclerosis: validation of administrative definitions for diabetes, hypertension, and hyperlipidemia. *Mult. Scler. J.* 18, 1310–1319. doi: 10.1177/1352458512437814

Martin, C. R., Osadchiy, V., Kalani, A., and Mayer, E. A. (2018). The brain-gut-microbiome axis. *Cell. Mol. Gastroenterol. Hepatol.* 6, 133–148. doi: 10.1016/J.JCMGH.2018.04.003

Masoud, G. N., and Li, W. (2015). HIF-1α pathway: role, regulation and intervention for cancer therapy. *Acta Pharm. Sin. B* 5, 378–389. doi: 10.1016/j.apsb.2015.05.007

Matarese, G., Carrieri, P. B., La Cava, A., Perna, F., Sanna, V., De Rosa, V., et al. (2005). Leptin increase in multiple sclerosis associates with reduced number of CD4+CD25+ regulatory T cells. *Proc. Natl. Acad. Sci. U.S.A.* 102, 5150–5155. doi: 10.1073/pnas.0408995102

Matarese, G., Di Giacomo, A., Sanna, V., Lord, G. M., Howard, J. K., Di Tuoro, A., et al. (2001a). Requirement for leptin in the induction and progression of autoimmune encephalomyelitis. *J. Immunol.* 166, 5909–5916. doi: 10.4049/jimmunol.166.10.5909

Matarese, G., Sanna, V., Giacomo, A. D., Lord, G. M., Howard, J. K., Bloom, S. R., et al. (2001b). Leptin potentiates experimental autoimmune encephalomyelitis in SJL female mice and confers susceptibility to males. *Eur. J. Immunol.* 31, 1324–1332.

Mayhan, W. G. (2000). Nitric oxide donor-induced increase in permeability of the blood–brain barrier. *Brain Res.* 866, 101–108. doi: 10.1016/S0006-8993(00)02254-X

McEwen, B. (2014). The influence of diet and nutrients on platelet function. *Semin. Thromb. Hemost.* 40, 214–226. doi: 10.1055/s-0034-1365839

Milanski, M., Degasperi, G., Coope, A., Morari, J., Denis, R., Cintra, D. E., et al. (2009). Saturated fatty acids produce an inflammatory response predominantly through the activation of TLR4 signalling in hypothalamus: implications for the pathogenesis of obesity. *J. Neurosci.* 29, 359–370. doi: 10.1523/JNEUROSCI.2760-08.2009

Ming, X.-F., Viswambharan, H., Barandier, C., Ruffieux, J., Kaibuchi, K., Rusconi, S., et al. (2002). Rho GTPase/Rho kinase negatively regulates endothelial nitric oxide synthase phosphorylation through the inhibition of protein kinase B/Akt in human endothelial cells. *Mol. Cell. Biol.* 22, 8467–8477. doi: 10.1128/MCB.22.24.8467-8477.2002

Mishra, P. K., Hsuchou, H., Ouyang, S., Kastin, A. J., Wu, X., and Pan, W. (2013). Loss of astrocytic leptin signalling worsens experimental autoimmune encephalomyelitis. *Brain Behav. Immun.* 34, 98–107. doi: 10.1016/J.BBI.2013.07.176

Mittal, M., Siddiqui, M. R., Tran, K., Reddy, S. P., and Malik, A. B. (2014). Reactive oxygen species in inflammation and tissue injury. *Antioxid. Redox Signal.* 20, 1126–1167. doi: 10.1089/ars.2012.5149

Moalem, G., Leibowitz-Amit, R., Yoles, E., Mor, F., Cohen, I. R., and Schwartz, M. (1999). Autoimmune T cells protect neurons from secondary degeneration after central nervous system axotomy. *Nat. Med.* 5, 49–55. doi: 10.1038/4734

Mohammadi, M. T., Shid Moosavi, S. M., and Dehghani, G. A. (2011). Contribution of nitric oxide synthase (NOS) activity in blood-brain barrier disruption and edema after acute ischemia/reperfusion in aortic coarctation-induced hypertensive rats. *Iran. Biomed. J.* 15, 22–30.

Mokry, L. E., Ross, S., Timpson, N. J., Sawcer, S., Davey Smith, G., and Richards, J. B. (2016). Obesity and multiple sclerosis: a mendelian randomization study. *PLoS Med.* 13:e1002053. doi: 10.1371/journal.pmed.1002053

Mooradian, A. D., Haas, M. J., and Chehade, J. M. (2003). Age-related changes in rat cerebral occludin and zonula occludens-1 (ZO-1). *Mech. Ageing Dev.* 124, 143–146. doi: 10.1016/S0047-6374(02)00041-6

Moran, C., Phan, T. G., Chen, J., Blizzard, L., Beare, R., Venn, A., et al. (2013). Brain atrophy in type 2 diabetes. *Diabetes Care* 36, 4036–4042. doi: 10.2337/dc13-0143

Morrison, D. K. (2012). MAP kinase pathways. *Cold Spring Harb. Perspect. Biol.* 4:a011254. doi: 10.1101/cshperspect.a011254

Muller, W. A. (2011). Mechanisms of leukocyte transendothelial migration. *Annu. Rev. Pathol.* 6, 323–344. doi: 10.1146/annurev-pathol-011110-130224

Murohara, T., Asahara, T., Silver, M., Bauters, C., Masuda, H., Kalka, C., et al. (1998). Nitric oxide synthase modulates angiogenesis in response to tissue ischemia. *J. Clin. Invest.* 101, 2567–2578. doi: 10.1172/JCI1560

Musunuru, K. (2010). Atherogenic dyslipidemia: cardiovascular risk and dietary intervention. *Lipids* 45, 907–914. doi: 10.1007/s11745-010-3408-1

Nakano, H., Nakajima, A., Sakon-Komazawa, S., Piao, J.-H., Xue, X., and Okumura, K. (2006). Reactive oxygen species mediate crosstalk between NF-κB and JNK. *Cell Death Differ.* 13, 730–737. doi: 10.1038/sj.cdd.4401830

Nave, H., Kuhlmann, S., Brabant, G., and Pabst, R. (2003). Changes in cerebral endothelial barrier antigen, without alteration of permeability for intravenously injected leptin in diet-induced obesity in rats. *Exp. Toxicol. Pathol.* 55, 45–49. doi: 10.1078/0940-2993-00300

Nguyen, J. C. D., Killcross, A. S., and Jenkins, T. A. (2014). Obesity and cognitive decline: role of inflammation and vascular changes. *Front. Neurosci.* 8:375. doi: 10.3389/fnins.2014.00375

O'Brown, N. M., Pfau, S. J., and Gu, C. (2018). Bridging barriers: a comparative look at the blood–brain barrier across organisms. *Genes Dev.* 32, 466–478. doi: 10.1101/gad.309823.117

O'Shea, J. J., Schwartz, D. M., Villarino, A. V., Gadina, M., McInnes, I. B., and Laurence, A. (2015). The JAK-STAT pathway: impact on human disease and therapeutic intervention. *Annu. Rev. Med.* 66, 311–328. doi: 10.1146/annurev-med-051113-024537

Ouyang, S., Hsuchou, H., Kastin, A. J., Mishra, P. K., Wang, Y., and Pan, W. (2014a). Leukocyte infiltration into spinal cord of EAE mice is attenuated by removal of endothelial leptin signalling. *Brain Behav. Immun.* 40, 61–73. doi: 10.1016/j.bbi.2014.02.003

Ouyang, S., Hsuchou, H., Kastin, A. J., Wang, Y., Yu, C., and Pan, W. (2014b). Diet-induced obesity suppresses expression of many proteins at the blood-brain barrier. *J. Cereb. Blood Flow Metab.* 34, 43–51. doi: 10.1038/jcbfm.2013.166

Pacher, P., Beckman, J. S., and Liaudet, L. (2007). Nitric oxide and peroxynitrite in health and disease. *Physiol. Rev.* 87, 315–424. doi: 10.1152/physrev.00029.2006

Palavra, F., Almeida, L., Ambrósio, A. F., and Reis, F. (2016). Obesity and brain inflammation: a focus on multiple sclerosis. *Obes. Rev.* 17, 211–224. doi: 10.1111/obr.12363

Pandey, A., Chawla, S., and Guchhait, P. (2015). Type-2 diabetes: current understanding and future perspectives. *IUBMB Life* 67, 506–513. doi: 10.1002/iub.1396

Parathath, S. R., Parathath, S., and Tsirka, S. E. (2006). Nitric oxide mediates neurodegeneration and breakdown of the blood-brain barrier in tPA-dependent excitotoxic injury in mice. *J. Cell Sci.* 119, 339–349. doi: 10.1242/jcs.02734

Pardridge, W. M., Triguero, D., and Farrell, C. R. (1990). Downregulation of blood-brain barrier glucose transporter in experimental diabetes. *Diabetes* 39, 1040–1044. doi: 10.2337/diab.39.9.1040

Patti, M.-E., Virkamäki, A., Landaker, E. J., Kahn, C. R., and Yki-Järvinen, H. (1999). Activation of the hexosamine pathway by glucosamine in vivo induces insulin resistance of early postreceptor insulin signaling events in skeletal muscle. *Diabetes* 48, 1562–1571. doi: 10.2337/diabetes.48.8.1562

Pelligrino, D. A., LaManna, J. C., Duckrow, R. B., Bryan, R. M., and Harik, S. I. (1992). Hyperglycemia and blood-brain barrier glucose transport. *J. Cereb. Blood Flow Metab.* 12, 887–899. doi: 10.1038/jcbfm.1992.126

Petzold, G. C., and Murthy, V. N. (2011). Role of astrocytes in neurovascular coupling. *Neuron* 71, 782–797. doi: 10.1016/j.neuron.2011.08.009

Pfeiffer, F., Schäfer, J., Lyck, R., Makrides, V., Brunner, S., Schaeren-Wiemers, N., et al. (2011). Claudin-1 induced sealing of blood-brain barrier tight junctions ameliorates chronic experimental autoimmune encephalomyelitis. *Acta Neuropathol.* 122, 601–614. doi. 10.1007/s00401-011-0883-2

Phares, T. W., Fabis, M. J., Brimer, C. M., Kean, R. B., and Hooper, D. C. (2007). A peroxynitrite-dependent pathway is responsible for blood-brain barrier permeability changes during a central nervous system inflammatory response: TNF-alpha is neither necessary nor sufficient. *J. Immunol.* 178, 7334–7343. doi: 10.4049/JIMMUNOL.178.11.7334

Pinhas-Hamiel, O., Livne, M., Harari, G., and Achiron, A. (2015). Prevalence of overweight, obesity and metabolic syndrome components in multiple sclerosis patients with significant disability. *Eur. J. Neurol.* 22, 1275–1279. doi: 10.1111/ene.12738

Pistell, P. J., Morrison, C. D., Gupta, S., Knight, A. G., Keller, J. N., Ingram, D. K., et al. (2010). Cognitive impairment following high fat diet consumption is associated with brain inflammation. *J. Neuroimmunol.* 219, 25–32. doi: 10.1016/J.JNEUROIM.2009.11.010

Prada, P. O., Zecchin, H. G., Gasparetti, A. L., Torsoni, M. A., Ueno, M., Hirata, A. E., et al. (2005). Western diet modulates insulin signalling, c-Jun N-terminal kinase activity, and insulin receptor substrate-1 ser307 phosphorylation in a tissue-specific fashion. *Endocrinology* 146, 1576–1587. doi: 10.1210/en.2004-0767

Prasad, S., Sajja, R. K., Naik, P., and Cucullo, L. (2014). Diabetes mellitus and blood-brain barrier dysfunction: an overview. *J. Pharmacovigil.* 2:125. doi: 10.4172/2329-6887.1000125

Procaccini, C., De Rosa, V., Galgani, M., Abanni, L., Calì, G., Porcellini, A., et al. (2010). An oscillatory switch in mTOR kinase activity sets regulatory T cell responsiveness. *Immunity* 33, 929–941. doi: 10.1016/J.IMMUNI.2010.11.024

Procaccini, C., De Rosa, V., Galgani, M., Carbone, F., Cassano, S., Greco, D., et al. (2012). Leptin-induced mTOR activation defines a specific molecular and transcriptional signature controlling $CD4^+$ effector T cell responses. *J. Immunol.* 189, 2941–2953. doi: 10.4049/jimmunol.1200935

Proescholdt, M. A., Heiss, J. D., Walbridge, S., Mühlhauser, J., Capogrossi, M. C., Oldfield, E. H., et al. (1999). Vascular endothelial growth factor (VEGF)

modulates vascular permeability and inflammation in rat brain. *J. Neuropathol. Exp. Neurol.* 58, 613–627. doi: 10.1097/00005072-199906000-00006

Pugazhenthi, S., Qin, L., and Reddy, P. H. (2017). Common neurodegenerative pathways in obesity, diabetes, and Alzheimer's disease. *Biochim. Biophys. Acta* 1863, 1037–1045. doi: 10.1016/j.bbadis.2016.04.017

Qu-Hong, Nagy, J. A., Senger, D. R., Dvorak, H. F., and Dvorak, A. M. (1995). Ultrastructural localization of vascular permeability factor/vascular endothelial growth factor (VPF/VEGF) to the abluminal plasma membrane and vesiculovacuolar organelles of tumor microvascular endothelium. *J. Histochem. Cytochem.* 43, 381–389. Available at: http://www.ncbi.nlm.nih.gov/pubmed/7534783

Rajagopalan, S., Meng, X. P., Ramasamy, S., Harrison, D. G., and Galis, Z. S. (1996). Reactive oxygen species produced by macrophage-derived foam cells regulate the activity of vascular matrix metalloproteinases in vitro. Implications for atherosclerotic plaque stability. *J. Clin. Invest.* 98, 2572–2579. doi: 10.1172/JCI119076

Ransohoff, R. M., and Engelhardt, B. (2012). The anatomical and cellular basis of immune surveillance in the central nervous system. *Nat. Rev. Immunol.* 12, 623–635. doi: 10.1038/nri3265

Ransohoff, R. M., Schafer, D., Vincent, A., Blachère, N. E., and Bar-Or, A. (2015). Neuroinflammation: ways in which the immune system affects the brain. *Neurotherapeutics* 12, 896–909. doi: 10.1007/s13311-015-0385-3

Ray, P. D., Huang, B.-W., and Tsuji, Y. (2012). Reactive oxygen species (ROS) homeostasis and redox regulation in cellular signalling. *Cell. Signal.* 24, 981–990. doi: 10.1016/j.cellsig.2012.01.008

Reese, T. S., and Karnovsky, M. J. (1967). Fine structural localization of a blood-brain barrier to exogenous peroxidase. *J. Cell Biol.* 34, 207–217. doi: 10.1083/jcb.34.1.207

Reeson, P., Tennant, K. A., Gerrow, K., Wang, J., Weiser Novak, S., Thompson, K., et al. (2015). Delayed inhibition of VEGF signaling after stroke attenuates blood–brain barrier breakdown and improves functional recovery in a comorbidity-dependent manner. *J. Neurosci.* 35, 5128–5143. doi: 10.1523/JNEUROSCI.2810-14.2015

Reijerkerk, A., Lopez-Ramirez, M. A., van Het Hof, B., Drexhage, J. A. R., Kamphuis, W. W., Kooij, G., et al. (2013). MicroRNAs regulate human brain endothelial cell-barrier function in inflammation: implications for multiple sclerosis. *J. Neurosci.* 33, 6857–6863. doi: 10.1523/JNEUROSCI.3965-12.2013

Remels, A. H. V., Gosker, H. R., Verhees, K. J. P., Langen, R. C. J., and Schols, A. M. W. J. (2015). TNF-α-Induced NF-κB activation stimulates skeletal muscle glycolytic metabolism through activation of HIF-1α. *Endocrinology* 156, 1770–1781. doi: 10.1210/en.2014-1591

Rivera, P., Ocaranza, M. P., Lavandero, S., and Jalil, J. E. (2007). Rho kinase activation and gene expression related to vascular remodeling in normotensive rats with high angiotensin I converting enzyme levels. *Hypertens* 50, 792–798. doi: 10.1161/HYPERTENSIONAHA.107.095117

Rojas, A., Gonzalez, D., Figueroa, H., Morales, M., and Romero, J. (2010). Modulation of nitric oxide pathway by multiligands/RAGE axis: a crossing point on the road to microvascular complication in diabetes. *Curr. Enzym. Inhib.* 6, 34–45. doi: 10.2174/157340810790712050

Roy, S., Bae, E., Amin, S., and Kim, D. (2015). Extracellular matrix, gap junctions, and retinal vascular homeostasis in diabetic retinopathy. *Exp. Eye Res.* 133, 58–68. doi: 10.1016/j.exer.2014.08.011

Roy, S., Ha, J., Trudeau, K., and Beglova, E. (2010). Vascular basement membrane thickening in diabetic retinopathy. *Curr. Eye Res.* 35, 1045–1056. doi: 10.3109/02713683.2010.514659

Ryu, J. K., Rafalski, V. A., Meyer-Franke, A., Adams, R. A., Poda, S. B., Rios Coronado, P. E., et al. (2018). Fibrin-targeting immunotherapy protects against neuroinflammation and neurodegeneration. *Nat. Immunol.* 19, 1212–1223. doi: 10.1038/s41590-018-0232-x

Sadeghian, H., Lacoste, B., Qin, T., Toussay, X., Rosa, R., Oka, F., et al. (2018). Spreading depolarizations trigger caveolin-1-dependent endothelial transcytosis. *Ann. Neurol.* 84, 409–423. doi: 10.1002/ana.25298

Safiah Mokhtar, S., Vanhoutte, M. P., Leung, W. S. S., Imran Yusof, M., Wan Sulaiman, W. A., Zaharil Mat Saad, A., et al. (2013). Reduced expression of prostacyclin synthase and nitric oxide synthase in subcutaneous arteries of type 2 diabetic patients. *Tohoku J. Exp. Med.* 231, 217–222. doi: 10.1620/tjem.231.217

Sagare, A. P., Bell, R. D., and Zlokovic, B. V. (2012). Neurovascular dysfunction and faulty amyloid -peptide clearance in Alzheimer disease. *Cold Spring Harb. Perspect. Med.* 2:a011452. doi: 10.1101/cshperspect.a011452

Sáinz, N., Barrenetxe, J., Moreno-Aliaga, M. J., and Martínez, J. A. (2015). Leptin resistance and diet-induced obesity: central and peripheral actions of leptin. *Metabolism* 64, 35–46. doi: 10.1016/J.METABOL.2014.10.015

Sajja, R. K., Prasad, S., and Cucullo, L. (2014). Impact of altered glycaemia on blood-brain barrier endothelium: an in vitro study using the hCMEC/D3 cell line. *Fluids Barriers CNS* 11:8. doi: 10.1186/2045-8118-11-8

Schulz, M., and Engelhardt, B. (2005). The circumventricular organs participate in the immunopathogenesis of experimental autoimmune encephalomyelitis. *Cerebrospinal Fluid Res.* 2:8. doi: 10.1186/1743-8454-2-8

Schwartz, M., and Raposo, C. (2014). Protective autoimmunity: a unifying model for the immune network involved in CNS repair. *Neuroscientist* 20, 343–358. doi: 10.1177/1073858413516799

Seaquist, E. R., Tkac, I., Damberg, G., Thomas, W., and Gruetter, R. (2005). Brain glucose concentrations in poorly controlled diabetes mellitus as measured by high-field magnetic resonance spectroscopy. *Metabolism* 54, 1008–1013. doi: 10.1016/j.metabol.2005.02.018

Serban, A. I., Stanca, L., Geicu, O. I., Munteanu, M. C., and Dinischiotu, A. (2016). RAGE and TGF-β1 cross-talk regulate extracellular matrix turnover and cytokine synthesis in AGEs exposed fibroblast cells. *PLoS One* 11:e0152376. doi: 10.1371/journal.pone.0152376

Shah, K., DeSilva, S., Abbruscato, T., Shah, K., DeSilva, S., and Abbruscato, T. (2012). The role of glucose transporters in brain disease: diabetes and Alzheimer's disease. *Int. J. Mol. Sci.* 13, 12629–12655. doi: 10.3390/ijms131012629

Shao, B., and Bayraktutan, U. (2013). Hyperglycaemia promotes cerebral barrier dysfunction through activation of protein kinase C-β. *Diabetes Obes. Metab.* 15, 993–999. doi: 10.1111/dom.12120

Shimizu, F., Sano, Y., Tominaga, O., Maeda, T., Abe, M., and Kanda, T. (2013). Advanced glycation end-products disrupt the blood-brain barrier by stimulating the release of transforming growth factor-β by pericytes and vascular endothelial growth factor and matrix metalloproteinase-2 by endothelial cells in vitro. *Neurobiol. Aging* 34, 1902–1912. doi: 10.1016/j.neurobiolaging.2013.01.012

Siddiqui, M. R., Komarova, Y. A., Vogel, S. M., Gao, X., Bonini, M. G., Rajasingh, J., et al. (2011). Caveolin-1-eNOS signalling promotes p190RhoGAP-A nitration and endothelial permeability. *J. Cell Biol.* 193, 841–850. doi: 10.1083/jcb.201012129

Skelly, D. T., Hennessy, E., Dansereau, M.-A., and Cunningham, C. (2013). A systematic analysis of the peripheral and CNS effects of systemic LPS, IL-1B, TNF-α and IL-6 challenges in C57BL/6 mice. *PLoS One* 8:e69123. doi: 10.1371/journal.pone.0069123

Slawta, J. N., Wilcox, A. R., McCubbin, J. A., Nalle, D. J., Fox, S. D., and Anderson, G. (2003). Health behaviors, body composition, and coronary heart disease risk in women with multiple sclerosis. *Arch. Phys. Med. Rehabil.* 84, 1823–1830. doi: 10.1016/S0003-9993(03)00466-0

Soliman, H., Gador, A., Lu, Y.-H., Lin, G., Bankar, G., and MacLeod, K. M. (2012). Diabetes-induced increased oxidative stress in cardiomyocytes is sustained by a positive feedback loop involving Rho kinase and PKCβ2. *Am. J. Physiol. Circ. Physiol.* 303, H989–H1000. doi: 10.1152/ajpheart.00416.2012

Stranahan, A. M., Hao, S., Dey, A., Yu, X., and Baban, B. (2016). Blood-brain barrier breakdown promotes macrophage infiltration and cognitive impairment in leptin receptor-deficient mice. *J. Cereb. Blood Flow Metab.* 36, 2108–2121. doi: 10.1177/0271678X16642233

Su, Y., Lei, X., Wu, L., and Liu, L. (2012). The role of endothelial cell adhesion molecules P-selectin, E-selectin and intercellular adhesion molecule-1 in leucocyte recruitment induced by exogenous methylglyoxal. *Immunology* 137, 65–79. doi: 10.1111/j.1365-2567.2012.03608.x

Suzuki, Y., Nagai, N., and Umemura, K. (2016). A review of the mechanisms of blood-brain barrier permeability by tissue-type plasminogen activator treatment for cerebral ischemia. *Front. Cell. Neurosci.* 10:2. doi: 10.3389/fncel.2016.00002

Tan, K. H., Harrington, S., Purcell, W. M., and Hurst, R. D. (2004). Peroxynitrite mediates nitric oxide-induced blood-brain barrier damage. *Neurochem. Res.* 29, 579–587. doi: 10.1023/B:NERE.0000014828.32200.bd

Tettey, P., Simpson, S., Taylor, B. V., and van der Mei, I. A. F. (2014). Vascular comorbidities in the onset and progression of multiple sclerosis. *J. Neurol. Sci.* 347, 23–33. doi: 10.1016/j.jns.2014.10.020

Tettey, P., Simpson, S., Taylor, B. V., and van der Mei, I. A. F. (2015). The co-occurrence of multiple sclerosis and type 1 diabetes: shared aetiologic features and clinical implication for MS aetiology. *J. Neurol. Sci.* 348, 126–131. doi: 10.1016/j.jns.2014.11.019

Thaler, J. P., Yi, C.-X., Schur, E. A., Guyenet, S. J., Hwang, B. H., Dietrich, M. O., et al. (2012). Obesity is associated with hypothalamic injury in rodents and humans. *J. Clin. Invest.* 122, 153–162. doi: 10.1172/JCI59660

Thomsen, M. S., Routhe, L. J., and Moos, T. (2017). The vascular basement membrane in the healthy and pathological brain. *J. Cereb. Blood Flow Metab.* 37, 3300–3317. doi: 10.1177/0271678X17722436

Tietz, S., Périnat, T., Greene, G., Enzmann, G., Deutsch, U., Adams, R., et al. (2018). Lack of junctional adhesion molecule (JAM)-B ameliorates experimental autoimmune encephalomyelitis. *Brain Behav. Immun.* 73, 3–20. doi: 10.1016/j.bbi.2018.06.014

Tillisch, K., Labus, J., Kilpatrick, L., Jiang, Z., Stains, J., Ebrat, B., et al. (2013). Consumption of fermented milk product with probiotic modulates brain activity. *Gastroenterology* 144, 1394–1401.e4. doi: 10.1053/J.GASTRO.2013.02.043

Titchenell, P. M., Lin, C.-M., Keil, J. M., Sundstrom, J. M., Smith, C. D., and Antonetti, D. A. (2012). Novel atypical PKC inhibitors prevent vascular endothelial growth factor-induced blood-retinal barrier dysfunction. *Biochem. J.* 446, 455–467. doi: 10.1042/BJ20111961

Treins, C., Giorgetti-Peraldi, S., Murdaca, J., and Van Obberghen, E. (2001). Regulation of vascular endothelial growth factor expression by advanced glycation end products. *J. Biol. Chem.* 276, 43836–43841. doi: 10.1074/jbc.M106534200

Tronc, F., Mallat, Z., Lehoux, S., Wassef, M., Esposito, B., and Tedgui, A. (2000). Role of matrix metalloproteinases in blood flow-induced arterial enlargement: interaction with NO. *Arterioscler. Thromb. Vasc. Biol.* 20, E120–E126. doi: 10.1161/01.ATV.20.12.e120

Tucsek, Z., Toth, P., Sosnowska, D., Gautam, T., Mitschelen, M., Koller, A., et al. (2014). Obesity in aging exacerbates blood-brain barrier disruption, neuroinflammation, and oxidative stress in the mouse hippocampus: effects on expression of genes involved in beta-amyloid generation and Alzheimer's disease. *J. Gerontol. Ser. A Biol. Sci. Med. Sci.* 69, 1212–1226. doi: 10.1093/gerona/glt177

Turner, R. J., and Vink, R. (2012). Combined tissue plasminogen activator and an NK1 tachykinin receptor antagonist: an effective treatment for reperfusion injury following acute ischemic stroke in rats. *Neuroscience* 220, 1–10. doi: 10.1016/j.neuroscience.2012.06.047

Van Heek, M., Compton, D. S., France, C. F., Tedesco, R. P., Fawzi, A. B., Graziano, M. P., et al. (1997). Diet-induced obese mice develop peripheral, but not central, resistance to leptin. *J. Clin. Invest.* 99, 385–390. doi: 10.1172/JCI119171

Varatharaj, A., and Galea, I. (2017). The blood-brain barrier in systemic inflammation. *Brain Behav. Immun.* 60, 1–12. doi: 10.1016/J.BBI.2016.03.010

Vlassara, H., and Palace, M. R. (2002). Diabetes and advanced glycation endproducts. *J. Intern. Med.* 251, 87–101. doi: 10.1046/j.1365-2796.2002.00932.x

Wang, J., Li, G., Wang, Z., Zhang, X., Yao, L., Wang, F., et al. (2012). High glucose-induced expression of inflammatory cytokines and reactive oxygen species in cultured astrocytes. *Neuroscience* 202, 58–68. doi: 10.1016/J.NEUROSCIENCE.2011.11.062

Wei, J., Jiang, H., Gao, H., and Wang, G. (2016). Blocking mammalian target of rapamycin (mTOR) attenuates HIF-1α pathways engaged-vascular endothelial growth factor (VEGF) in diabetic retinopathy. *Cell. Physiol. Biochem.* 40, 1570–1577. doi: 10.1159/000453207

Wens, I., Dalgas, U., Stenager, E., and Eijnde, B. O. (2013). Risk factors related to cardiovascular diseases and the metabolic syndrome in multiple sclerosis – a systematic review. *Mult. Scler. J.* 19, 1556–1564. doi: 10.1177/1352458513504252

Xu, B., Chibber, R., Ruggiero, D., Kohner, E., Ritter, J., and Ferro, A. (2003). Impairment of vascular endothelial nitric oxide synthase activity by advanced glycation end products. *FASEB J.* 17, 1289–1291. doi: 10.1096/fj.02-0490fje

Xu, Z., Zeng, W., Sun, J., Chen, W., Zhang, R., Yang, Z., et al. (2017). The quantification of blood-brain barrier disruption using dynamic contrast-enhanced magnetic resonance imaging in aging rhesus monkeys with spontaneous type 2 diabetes mellitus. *Neuroimage* 158, 480–487. doi: 10.1016/j.neuroimage.2016.07.017

Yan, J., Zhang, Z., and Shi, H. (2012). HIF-1 is involved in high glucose-induced paracellular permeability of brain endothelial cells. *Cell. Mol. Life Sci.* 69, 115–128. doi: 10.1007/s00018-011-0731-5

Yancopoulos, G. D., Davis, S., Gale, N. W., Rudge, J. S., Wiegand, S. J., and Holash, J. (2000). Vascular-specific growth factors and blood vessel formation. *Nature* 407, 242–248. doi: 10.1038/35025215

Yao, L., Romero, M. J., Toque, H. A., Yang, G., Caldwell, R. B., and Caldwell, R. W. (2010). The role of RhoA/Rho kinase pathway in endothelial dysfunction. *J. Cardiovasc. Dis. Res.* 1, 165–170. doi: 10.4103/0975-3583.74258

Yoles, E., Hauben, E., Palgi, O., Agranov, E., Gothilf, A., Cohen, A., et al. (2001). Protective autoimmunity is a physiological response to CNS trauma. *J. Neurosci.* 21, 3740–3748. doi: 10.1523/JNEUROSCI.21-11-03740.2001

Yoo, D. Y., Yim, H. S., Jung, H. Y., Nam, S. M., Kim, J. W., Choi, J. H., et al. (2016). Chronic type 2 diabetes reduces the integrity of the blood-brain barrier by reducing tight junction proteins in the hippocampus. *J. Vet. Med. Sci.* 78, 957–962. doi: 10.1292/jvms.15-0589

Yorulmaz, H., Kaptan, E., Seker, F. B., and Oztas, B. (2015). Type 1 diabetes exacerbates blood-brain barrier alterations during experimental epileptic seizures in an animal model. *Cell Biochem. Funct.* 33, 285–292. doi: 10.1002/cbf.3113

Yudkin, J. S., Stehouwer, C. D. A., Emeis, J. J., and Coppack, S. W. (1999). C-reactive protein in health subjects: association with obesity, insulin resistance, and endothelial dysfunction. *Arterioscler. Thromb. Vasc. Biol.* 19, 972–978. doi: 10.1161/01.ATV.19.4.972

Zamanian, J. L., Xu, L., Foo, L. C., Nouri, N., Zhou, L., Giffard, R. G., et al. (2012). Genomic analysis of reactive astrogliosis. *J. Neurosci.* 32, 6391–6410. doi: 10.1523/JNEUROSCI.6221-11.2012

Zamvil, S. S., and Steinman, L. (1990). The T lymphocyte in experimental allergic encephalomyelitis. *Annu. Rev. Immunol.* 8, 579–621. doi: 10.1146/annurev.iy.08.040190.003051

Zhang, X., Dong, F., Ren, J., Driscoll, M. J., and Culver, B. (2005). High dietary fat induces NADPH oxidase-associated oxidative stress and inflammation in rat cerebral cortex. *Exp. Neurol.* 191, 318–325. doi: 10.1016/J.EXPNEUROL.2004.10.011

Zhang, X., Zhang, G., Zhang, H., Karin, M., Bai, H., and Cai, D. (2008). Hypothalamic IKKβ/NF-κB and ER stress link overnutrition to energy imbalance and obesity. *Cell* 135, 61–73. doi: 10.1016/j.cell.2008.07.043

Zhao, Z., Nelson, A. R., Betsholtz, C., and Zlokovic, B. V. (2015). Establishment and dysfunction of the blood-brain barrier. *Cell* 163, 1064–1078. doi: 10.1016/J.CELL.2015.10.067

Zhu, X.-Y., Li, P., Yang, Y.-B., and Liu, M.-L. (2013). Xuezhikang, extract of red yeast rice, improved abnormal hemorheology, suppressed caveolin-1 and increased eNOS expression in atherosclerotic rats. *PLoS One* 8:e62731. doi: 10.1371/journal.pone.0062731

Zhu, Y., Liao, H.-L., Niu, X.-L., Yuan, Y., Lin, T., Verna, L., et al. (2003). Low density lipoprotein induces eNOS translocation to membrane caveolae: the role of RhoA activation and stress fiber formation. *Biochim. Biophys. Acta* 1635, 117–126. doi: 10.1016/j.bbalip.2003.10.011

Zlokovic, B. V. (2011). Neurovascular pathways to neurodegeneration in Alzheimer's disease and other disorders. *Nat. Rev. Neurosci.* 12, 723–738. doi: 10.1038/nrn3114

2

Pituitary Gland Functional Connectivity and BMI

Paige Rucker[1] and Toshikazu Ikuta[2]*

[1] School of Medicine, The University of Mississippi Medical Center, Jackson, MS, United States, [2] Department of Communication Sciences and Disorders, The University of Mississippi, Oxford, MS, United States

***Correspondence:**
Toshikazu Ikuta
tikuta@olemiss.edu

The pituitary gland (PG) influences body weight through hormonal releases; however, the relation between body weight and PG's co-activities with other brain regions remains unclear. Here, we aimed to identify (1) the functional connectivity of the PG and (2) PG functional connectivity associated with body mass index by examining resting state functional magnetic resonance imaging data. Using enhanced Nathan Kline Institute-Rockland Sample, PG functional connectivity of 494 individuals was analyzed to assess in voxel-wise fashion. A negative association was found between BMI and PG functional connectivity with the orbitofrontal cortex, hippocampus, putamen, and temporal lobe. Our results show PG dysconnectivity to these regions is associated with higher BMI and implicate that the connectivity between these dopaminergic regions and PG may be associated with body weight maintenance through feeding behavior and growth.

Keywords: pituitary gland, functional connectivity, resting state fMRI, gustatory cortex, caudate head

INTRODUCTION

The hypothalamic-pituitary-adrenal (HPA) axis including the pituitary gland (PG) has been shown to be associated with obesity (Pasquali et al., 2006). In obesity, responses to growth hormone releasing factor are impaired (Williams et al., 1984). Chronic stress has been implicated to promote obesity through the HPA axis (Bose et al., 2009). Genetic variation in leptin receptors also shows association with obesity (Clement et al., 1998). The PG synthesizes and secretes hormones that regulate body weight, including somatotropins and oxytocin; however, the brain regions responsible for associating the PG activity and obesity are not clearly known.

Functional connectivity analysis using resting state fMRI (Fox and Raichle, 2007; Biswal et al., 2010) has provided newer insights into brain coactivity and obesity. The default mode network (DMN) and temporal lobe network have been found to be associated with obesity (Kullmann et al., 2012). In obesity, the precuneus shows an increased functional connectivity in the DMN while that of the anterior cingulate cortex is decreased. The insular cortex shows reduced connectivity in the temporal lobe network. Dysconnectivity between the hypothalamus and left insula has been found in obesity (Wijngaarden et al., 2015). After 48 h of fasting, connectivity of the hypothalamus to the dorsal anterior cingulate cortex increases in lean populations and decreases in the obese populations, suggesting a differential influence of obesity to functional connectivity of the hypothalamus (Wijngaarden et al., 2015). The putamen has been found to have elevated functional connectivity in obesity, while cognitive processing speed was negatively associated with the connectivity of the putamen to the salience network, suggesting an altered processing of salience detection (García-García et al., 2013). Obesity-preventive eating tendency has been found to be associated with caudate-precuneus functional connectivity (Nakamura and Ikuta, 2017). Caudate-precuneus connectivity inversely predicts the personal characteristics of avoiding obesity-inducing behaviors, suggesting the functional connectivity signature of avoiding causes of obesity independent of current body weight status. Surgical and behavioral weight loss has been found to differentially influence functional connectivity (Lepping et al., 2015). Despite its strong relationships to obesity, the influence of functional connectivity of the PG to body weight has not been yet studied.

Resting state functional connectivity of the PG is minimally studied, although functional connectivity is associated with adrenocorticotropic hormone (ACTH) levels. Cortisol concentrations have been found to predict interhemispheric connectivity, and ACTH concentrations were shown to be associated with the subcallosal anterior cingulate cortex (Kiem et al., 2013). Nonetheless, the resting state PG connectivity remains unclear. In this study, we (1) examined the resting state functional connectivity of the PG and (2) aimed to isolate resting state functional connectivity of the PG associated with BMI.

MATERIALS AND METHODS

Data Acquisition

The MRI images, the clinical data, and the demographic data of the enhanced Nathan Kline Institute-Rockland Sample (Nooner et al., 2012) were obtained from Collaborative Informatics and Neuroimaging Suite (Biswal et al., 2010). This data subset consisted of 494 individuals without known neurological preconditions (such as stroke, tumor, and traumatic brain damage) and MRI counter indications (43.46 $\pm$ 20.81 years old), 310 females and 184 males, six Native Americans, 25 Asians, 102 Black or African Americans, two Native Hawaiians, 346 Caucasians, and 13 other races, with the mean BMI of 27.32 $\pm$ 6.35 (between 15.29 and 56.28), for whom resting state and structural data were both available. Participants in the sample were recruited from Rockland County, NY, whose demographics represent the United States (Nooner et al., 2012). The subjects with known pituitary conditions (such as pituitary tumor) were not included in the analysis data.

Resting state echo planar image (EPI) volumes had 64 slices of 2 mm 112 $\times$ 112 matrix with 2 mm thickness (voxel size = 2 mm $\times$ 2 mm $\times$ 2 mm), FOV = 224 mm, with repetition time (TR) of 1400 ms and echo time (TE) of 30 ms. A total of 404 volumes ($\sim$10 min) were used in the analysis. High-resolution structural T1 volume was acquired as 176 sagittal slices of with 1 mm thickness (voxel size = 1 mm $\times$ 1 mm $\times$1 mm, TR = 1900 ms and TE = 2.52 ms, FOV = 256).

Data Processing

Data processing followed previous publication (Kiparizoska and Ikuta, 2017). Data preprocessing and statistical analyses were conducted using FMRIB Software Library (FSL,) as well as Analysis of Functional NeuroImages (AFNI). The anatomical volume for each subject was skull stripped, segmented (gray matter, white matter, and CSF), and registered to the MNI 2 mm standard brain. First four EPI volumes were removed. Transient signal spikes were removed by de-spiking interpolation. To correct head motion, the volumes were linearly registered to the then first volume, through which six motion parameters and displacement distance between two consecutive volumes were estimated. The first volume is registered to the standard MNI152 2 mm brain. Through this registration, 12 affine parameters were created between rs-fMRI volume and MNI152 2 mm space, so that the processed EPI volume can later be registered to the MNI space. Each of the resting state volumes was regressed by white matter and cerebrospinal fluid signal fluctuations as well as the six motion parameters. After smoothing with a 6 mm FWHM Gaussian kernel, the volumes were resampled, spatially transformed and aligned to the MNI 2 mm standard brain space. To perform scrubbing where the volumes with excess motion are removed, as a displacement distance between two EPI volumes, the root mean square deviation was calculated from motion correction parameters, at an r = 40 mm spherical surface using FSL's rmsdiff tool (Power et al., 2012, 2015). Volumes whose displacement distance exceeded the threshold (0.3 mm) were removed (*scrubbed*) from further statistical analyses (Siegel et al., 2014).

The PG ROI was manually defined in the MNI 2 mm space centered approximately at [MNI: 0, 2, −32] (**Figure 2**: Red), following previous MRI literature (Klomp et al., 2012). Data were excluded if the PG was located outside of the acquisition. Voxel-wise connectivity analysis was conducted in each individual brain. The time course was spatially averaged within the PG ROI that was registered to the EPI space so that correlations could be tested between the ROI and each individual voxel across the brain. The Z-scores representing the correlations between the ROI and a voxel were used for group level analysis after registration to the MNI 2 mm brain space.

In order to elucidate the regions which showed functional connectivity and dysconnectivity, one-sample t test was conducted assessing correlation (positive connectivity) and anti-correlation (negative connectivity) to the PG. Using *randomize* script in FSL, contrast images were estimated with cluster threshold of $Z > 3.72$. The association between BMI and whole brain functional connectivity to the PG was tested in a voxel-wise fashion using *randomize* script in FSL, taking age as a covariate. Contrast images were estimated with voxel-wise threshold of $p < 0.05$ (family wise error corrected), and minimum cluster size of 10 voxels.

RESULTS

In one-sample t test, in addition to the hypothalamus, the ventral and medial prefrontal cortex, inferior temporal gyrus, postcentral gyrus, insular cortex, parahippocampal gyrus, putamen, caudate head, and midbrain (periaqueductal gray), bilaterally showed positive connectivity with the PG (yellow/red in **Figure 1**). The dorsolateral prefrontal, parietal, occipital, and anterior cingulate cortices, hippocampus, caudate body, thalamus, pons medulla, and cerebellum showed bilateral negative connectivity (blue in **Figure 1**).

No regions showed positive association between the PG functional connectivity and BMI. The left orbitofrontal cortex,

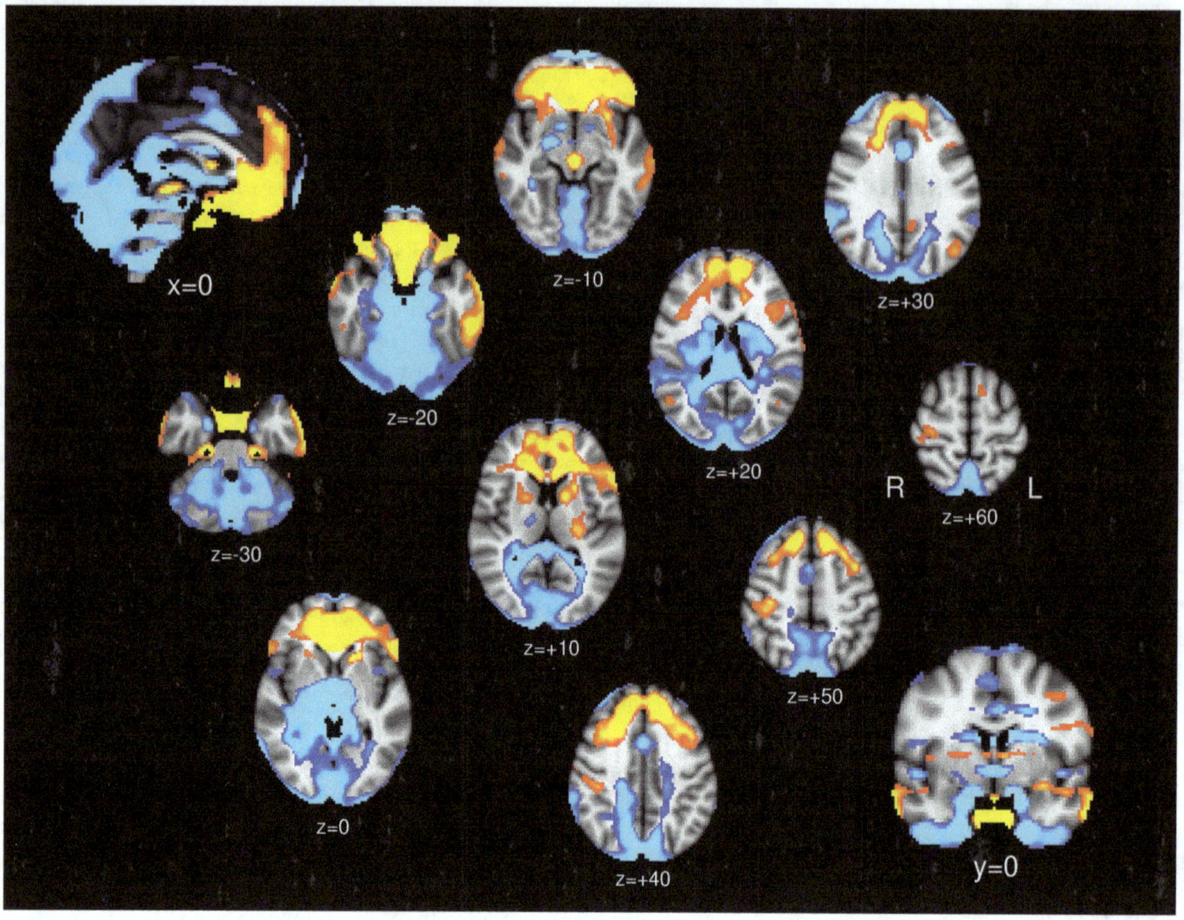

FIGURE 1 | One-sample *t* test; Brain regions show significant positive connectivity (yellow/red) and negative connectivity (blue) to the PG.

TABLE 1 | Regions whose PG connectivity showed negative association with BMI.

	Voxels	Peak *p* (corrected)	Cluster *p* (corrected)	MNI coordinates			Cluster Region
				x	y	z	
1	45	0.0002	0.015	−26	12	−20	Left Orbitofrontal Cortex
2	41	0.0012	0.019	−24	−12	−20	Left Hippocampus
3	33	0.0064	0.046	40	−26	−4	Right Superior Temporal Gyrus
4	23	0.0024	0.019	16	10	−4	Right Putamen
5	22	0.006	0.022	26	−2	−4	Right Putamen/Pallidum
6	21	0.013	0.030	−44	16	−30	Left Temporal Pole
7	14	0.009	0.024	16	−36	0	Right Hippocampus
8	10	0.023	0.035	−14	8	−10	Left Putamen

bilateral hippocampus, bilateral putamen, and right superior temporal gyrus showed functional connectivity with the PG inversely associated with BMI (**Table 1** and **Figure 2**).

DISCUSSION

This study aimed to identify (1) the functional connectivity of the PG and (2) brain regions whose functional connectivity to the PG shows associations with Body Mass Index. In one-sample *T*-test, the hypothalamus showed positive associations with the PG. This conforms to their close relationship classically know as a part of the HPA axis, which is known to be associated with obesity (Chalew et al., 1995). In this current study, however, the hypothalamus-PG functional connectivity did not show significant association with BMI.

Given their close relationship, we conducted an ROI-ROI connectivity analysis between the hypothalamus and PG. To

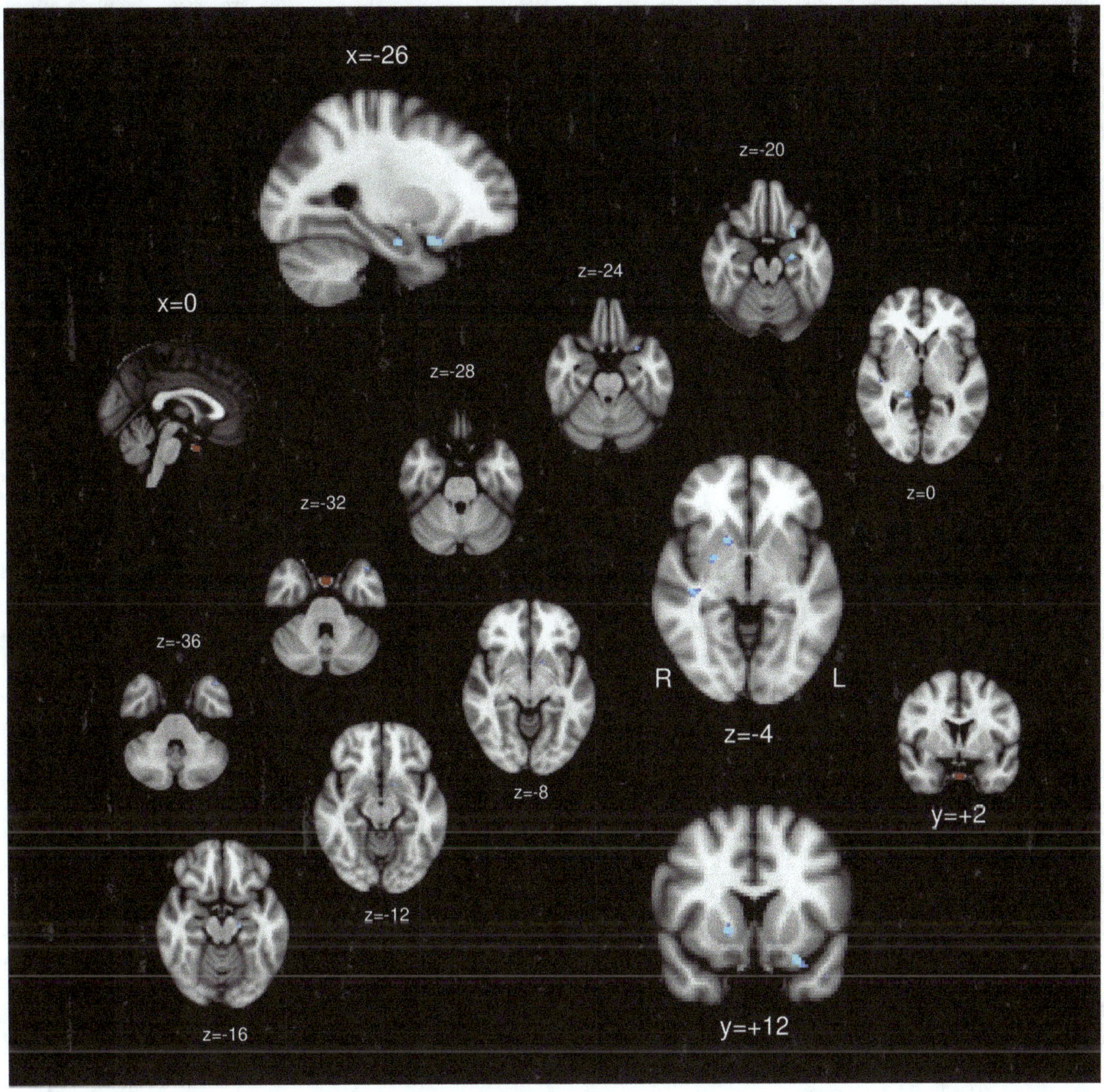

FIGURE 2 | The pituitary ROI (red) and regions whose pituitary connectivity showed negative association with BMI (blue).

assess the association between the BMI and hypothalamus-PG connectivity, a multiple linear regression was calculated to predict the hypothalamus-PG connectivity based on BMI, age, and sex. The regression was not significant, suggesting that the connectivity between hypothalamus-PG connectivity is constant across BMI, while PG and hypothalamus connectivity to the other parts of the brain identified in our voxel-wise analysis are associated with BMI. That is, the PG and hypothalamus are, similarly, influenced by the rest of the brain, resulting in the hypothalamus-PG connectivity remaining constant across BMI. Since the hypothalamus and PG are strongly positively connected, it is expected that the functional connectivity of the hypothalamus would show similar pattern with the PG in its association with BMI.

The orbitofrontal cortex (OFC) showed positive functional connectivity with the PG and inverse association with the BMI in its connectivity to the PG. It is implicated that lesser connectivity between the PG and OFC is associated with BMI. The OFC has been shown to be associated with obesity, as well as being responsible for taste and flavor processing (Small et al., 2007) and food choice (Cohen et al., 2011). Reduced OFC gray matter volume has been found in both adolescent (Ross et al., 2015) and midlife obesity (Driscoll et al., 2011). The OFC volume has been found to predict the risk for obesity (Smucny et al., 2012). More specifically, the OFC has been implicated in its role in preventing overeating. The OFC has been shown to be responsible for disinhibition of eating (Maayan et al., 2012), implicating its importance in preventing obesity. OFC volume has also been found to be associated with reward response in obesity (Shott et al., 2015). Reduced connectivity between the PG and OFC in a more obese population may suggest downregulated control of the OFC over PG.

The putamen showed inverse association between PG connectivity and BMI. That is, lesser PG-putamen connectivity is implicated in higher BMI. The association between pituitary-putamen dysconnectivity and BMI may be also accounted for by its role in the reward processing since the putamen and PG are both rich in dopamine D2 receptors. Striatal D2 receptors were shown to be reduced in individuals with obesity (Wang et al., 2004) and deficits of D2 receptor availability predicts future weight gain (Michaelides et al., 2012). Antipsychotics, whose pharmacological mechanism is represented by D2 antagonism, is widely known to induce weight gain (Correll et al., 2011). A D2 agonist bromocriptine has been found to counteract obesity (Kok et al., 2006). On the genetic level, polymorphisms in the D2 receptor gene (*DRD2*) have been implicated in its association to obesity (Nisoli et al., 2007; Ariza et al., 2012), as well as the weight gain response to antipsychotics (Lencz et al., 2010). The D2R profiles in the PG also show association with obesity. Disrupting D2 receptors in the pituitary lactotropes results in weight gain (Perez Millan et al., 2014). Dopaminergic modulations in the PG and striatum are both implicated in their association with BMI.

The PG receives dopaminergic projections from the hypothalamic arcuate nucleus as the terminal of the tuberoinfundibular pathway. Although this may partially account for their lack of BMI-differentiated association, it does not account for the associations with the striatal regions which are independently dopaminergic as the terminal of mesolimbic dopaminergic pathway originating in the substantia niagra. While the striatum and PG are independently dopaminergic in their primary source of their dopaminergic afferents, prolactin has been shown to upregulate both tuberoinfundibular and striatal dopamine neurons. While dopamine is inhibitory against secretion of prolactin (Ben-Jonathan, 1985; Liang et al., 2014), prolactin has been found to promote dopamine discharge in the tuberoinfundibular pathway (Lyons et al., 2012), forming a loop to regulate serum prolactin. In the striatum, rat prolactin increases dopamine turnover in the striatum (Fuxe et al., 1977). Prolonged intake of excessive sucrose has been found to upregulate striatal prolactin, thus showing implication to induce compulsive eating behavior (Ahmed et al., 2014). The prolactin-mediated dopaminergic response may be the underlying factor in the association between pituitary-caudate/NAcc functional dysconnectivity and BMI, whereby dopaminergic neurons in the PG and striatum are downregulated by prolactin.

It has to be noted that prolactin would not be the only mechanism that could both interact with the PG and striatum in the complex HPA axis. A voxel-based morphometric study showed a reduced volume of the putamen in obesity and a negative correlation between fasting plasma leptin concentrations and obesity (Pannacciulli et al., 2006), suggesting leptin mediated role of the putamen in regulating food intake. Dysconnectivity between the putamen and PG in obesity could be associated through the mechanism for leptin regulation.

The hippocampus also showed inverse association in its connectivity with the PG, while the hippocampi showed anti-correlation with the PG in the one-sample T-test. It is implicated that the anti-correlation is positively associated with BMI. Whilst the hippocampi also receive dopaminergic afferent from the ventral tegmental area, the association between hippocampus and food intake manipulation as well as physical exercise has been well documented. Physical exercise, which is shown to prevent excessive weight gain, acutely increases hippocampal volume, while hippocampal reduction is found after a series of cafeteria-diet in mice (Sack et al., 2017). Calorie restriction has been shown to improve cognition by upregulating brain-derived neurotrophic factor (BDNF) and downregulating oxidative stress in the hippocampus (Kishi et al., 2015). The hippocampus has been shown to be activated when images of high-calorie food are presented and this activation has been found to be a function of fasting plasma levels of insulin (Wallner-Liebmann et al., 2012), suggesting that the hippocampi respond to energy stimuli under the influence of hunger status. Our PG-hippocampus dysconnectivity finding may implicate that the PG is regulated by the hippocampus based on the hunger status and food availability.

Several limitations of the current study need to be addressed. First, as this study is based on functional connectivity, where functional connectivity is estimated by co-activations of two regions, causal relationships are not illuminated, although it could be inferred through known endocrinological properties of the PG. Second, despite the known subdivisions within the PG, such as the anterior and posterior pituitary, we avoided to make distinctions due to the imaging resolution of 2 mm^3 voxels and smoothing employed in processing. These two regions that showed functional dysconnectivity associated with BMI may arise from two distinct sub-regions of the PG.

It needs to be also addressed that the current study does not make distinction whether the PG connectivity influences BMI or BMI influences PG connectivity. While brain connectivity has been shown to influence body weight specifically in the context of the reward system, body weight status induced by surgical procedures has also been shown to influence functional brain connectivity (Lepping et al., 2015). It remains unclear whether our connectivity findings are the cause or results of the body weight.

In this study, we found functional dysconnectivity between the PG and dopaminergic regions including the putamen, hippocampus, and OFC. The results implicate dopaminergic modulation between the PG and these regions that influences body weight.

ETHICS STATEMENT

This study was approved by the University of Mississippi Institutional Review Board. This study had no direct involvement of human or animal subjects. All human subjects gave written informed consent.

AUTHOR CONTRIBUTIONS

PR and TI designed the study and drafted the manuscript. TI analyzed the data.

REFERENCES

Ahmed, S., Kashem, M. A., Sarker, R., Ahmed, E. U., Hargreaves, G. A., and McGregor, I. S. (2014). Neuroadaptations in the striatal proteome of the rat following prolonged excessive sucrose intake. *Neurochem. Res.* 39, 815–824. doi: 10.1007/s11064-014-1274-1276

Ariza, M., Garolera, M., Jurado, M. A., Garcia-Garcia, I., Hernan, I., Sánchez-Garre, C., et al. (2012). Dopamine genes (DRD2/ANKK1-TaqA1 and DRD4-7R) and executive function: their interaction with obesity. *PLoS One* 7:e41482. doi: 10.1371/journal.pone.0041482

Ben-Jonathan, N. (1985). Dopamine: a prolactin-inhibiting hormone. *Endocr. Rev.* 6, 564–589. doi: 10.1210/edrv-6-4-564

Biswal, B. B., Mennes, M., Zuo, X.-N., Gohel, S., Kelly, C., Smith, S. M., et al. (2010). Toward discovery science of human brain function. *Proc. Natl. Acad. Sci.* 107, 4734–4739. doi: 10.1073/pnas.0911855107

Bose, M., Oliván, B., and Laferrère, B. (2009). Stress and obesity: the role of the hypothalamic–pituitary–adrenal axis in metabolic disease. *Curr. Opin. Endocrinol. Diabetes Obes.* 16, 340–346. doi: 10.1097/MED.0b013e32832fa137

Chalew, S., Nagel, H., and Shore, S. (1995). The hypothalamic-pituitary-adrenal axis in obesity. *Obes. Res.* 3, 371–382. doi: 10.1002/j.1550-8528.1995.tb00163.x

Clement, K., Vaisse, C., Lahlou, N., Cabrol, S., Pelloux, V., Cassuto, D., et al. (1998). A mutation in the human leptin receptor gene causes obesity and pituitary dysfunction. *Nature* 392, 398–401. doi: 10.1038/32911

Cohen, J. I., Yates, K. F., Duong, M., and Convit, A. (2011). Obesity, orbitofrontal structure and function are associated with food choice: a cross-sectional study. *BMJ Open* 1:e000175. doi: 10.1136/bmjopen-2011-2175

Correll, C. U., Lencz, T., and Malhotra, A. K. (2011). Antipsychotic drugs and obesity. *Trends Mol. Med.* 17, 97–107. doi: 10.1016/j.molmed.2010.10.010

Driscoll, I., Beydoun, M. A., An, Y., Davatzikos, C., Ferrucci, L., Zonderman, A. B., et al. (2011). Midlife obesity and trajectories of brain volume changes in older adults. *Hum. Brain Mapp.* 33, 2204–2210. doi: 10.1002/hbm.21353

Fox, M. D., and Raichle, M. E. (2007). Spontaneous fluctuations in brain activity observed with functional magnetic resonance imaging. *Nat. Rev. Neurosci.* 8, 700–711.

Fuxe, K., Eneroth, P., Gustafsson, J.-A., Löfström, A., and Skett, P. (1977). Dopamine in the nucleus accumbens: preferential increase of DA turnover by rat prolactin. *Brain Res.* 122, 177–182. doi: 10.1016/0006-8993(77)90677-90671

García-García, I., Jurado, M. Á, Garolera, M., Segura, B., Sala-Llonch, R., Marqués-Iturria, I., et al. (2013). Alterations of the salience network in obesity: a resting-state fMRI study. *Hum. Brain Mapp* 34, 2786–2797. doi: 10.1002/hbm.22104

Kiem, S. A., Andrade, K. C., Spoormaker, V. I., Holsboer, F., Czisch, M., and Sämann, P. G. (2013). Resting state functional MRI connectivity predicts hypothalamus-pituitary-axis status in healthy males. *Psychoneuroendocrinology* 38, 1338–1348. doi: 10.1016/j.psyneuen.2012.11.021

Kiparizoska, S., and Ikuta, T. (2017). Disrupted olfactory integration in schizophrenia: functional connectivity study. *Int. J. Neuropsychopharmacol.* 20, 740–746. doi: 10.1093/ijnp/pyx045

Kishi, T., Hirooka, Y., Nagayama, T., Isegawa, K., Katsuki, M., Takesue, K., et al. (2015). Calorie restriction improves cognitive decline via up-regulation of brain-derived neurotrophic factor. *Int. Heart J.* 56, 110–115. doi: 10.1536/ihj.14-168

Klomp, A., Koolschijn, P. C., Hulshoff Pol, H. E., Kahn, R. S., and Van Haren, N. E. (2012). Hypothalamus and pituitary volume in schizophrenia: a structural MRI study. *Int. J. Neuropsychopharmacol.* 15, 281–288. doi: 10.1017/S1461145711000794

Kok, P., Roelfsema, F., Frölich, M., van Pelt, J., Stokkel, M. P. M., Meinders, A. E., et al. (2006). Activation of dopamine D2 receptors simultaneously ameliorates various metabolic features of obese women. *Am. J. Physiol. Endocrinol. Metab.* 291:E1038. doi: 10.1152/ajpendo.00567.2005

Kullmann, S., Heni, M., Veit, R., Ketterer, C., Schick, F., Häring, H.-U., et al. (2012). The obese brain: association of body mass index and insulin sensitivity with resting state network functional connectivity. *Hum. Brain Mapp.* 33, 1052–1061. doi: 10.1002/hbm.21268

Lencz, T., Robinson, D. G., Napolitano, B., Sevy, S., Kane, J. M., Goldman, D., et al. (2010). DRD2 promoter region variation predicts antipsychotic-induced weight gain in first episode schizophrenia. *Pharmacog. Genom.* 20:569. doi: 10.1097/FPC.0b013e32833ca24b

Lepping, R. J., Bruce, A. S., Francisco, A., Yeh, H.-W., Martin, L. E., Powell, J. N., et al. (2015). Resting-state brain connectivity after surgical and behavioral weight loss. *Obesity* 23, 1422–1428. doi: 10.1002/oby.21119

Liang, S.-L., Hsu, S.-C., and Pan, J.-T. (2014). Involvement of dopamine D2 receptor in the diurnal changes of tuberoinfundibular dopaminergic neuron activity and prolactin secretion in female rats. *J. Biomed. Sci.* 21, 37–37. doi: 10.1186/1423-0127-21-37

Lyons, D. J., Hellysaz, A., and Broberger, C. (2012). Prolactin regulates tuberoinfundibular dopamine neuron discharge pattern: novel feedback control mechanisms in the lactotrophic axis. *J. Neurosci.* 32:8074. doi: 10.1523/JNEUROSCI.0129-12.2012

Maayan, L., Hoogendoorn, C., Sweat, V., and Convit, A. (2012). Disinhibited eating in obese adolescents is associated with orbitofrontal volume reductions and executive dysfunction. *Obesity* 19, 1382–1387. doi: 10.1038/oby.2011.15

Michaelides, M., Thanos, P. K., Kim, R., Cho, J., Ananth, M., Wang, G.-J., et al. (2012). PET imaging predicts future body weight and cocaine preference. *NeuroImage* 59, 1508–1513. doi: 10.1016/j.neuroimage.2011.08.028

Nakamura, Y., and Ikuta, T. (2017). Caudate-precuneus functional connectivity is associated with obesity preventive eating tendency. *Brain Connect.* 7, 211–217. doi: 10.1089/brain.2016.0424

Nisoli, E., Nisoli, E., Brunani, A., Borgomainerio, E., and Tonello, C. (2007). D2 dopamine receptor (DRD2) gene Taq1A polymorphism and the eatingrelated psychological traits in eating disorders (anorexia nervosa and bulimia) and obesity. *Eat. Weight Disord.* 12, 91–96. doi: 10.1007/BF03327583

Nooner, K. B., Colcombe, S. J., Tobe, R. H., Mennes, M., Benedict, M. M., Moreno, A. L., et al. (2012). The NKI-rockland sample: a model for accelerating the pace of discovery science in psychiatry. *Front. Neurosci.* 6:152. doi: 10.3389/fnins.2012.00152

Pannacciulli, N., Del Parigi, A., Chen, K., Le, D. S., Reiman, E. M., and Tataranni, P. A. (2006). Brain abnormalities in human obesity: a voxel-based morphometric study. *NeuroImage* 31, 1419–1425. doi: 10.1016/j.neuroimage.2006.01.047

Pasquali, R., Vicennati, V., Cacciari, M., and Pagotto, U. (2006). The hypothalamic-pituitary-adrenal axis activity in obesity and the metabolic syndrome. *Ann. N. Y. Acad. Sci.* 1083, 111–128. doi: 10.1196/annals.1367.009

Perez Millan, M. I., Luque, G. M., Ramirez, M. C., Noain, D., Ornstein, A. M., Rubinstein, M., et al. (2014). Selective disruption of dopamine D2 receptors in pituitary lactotropes increases body weight and adiposity in female mice. *Endocrinology* 155, 829–839. doi: 10.1210/en.2013-1707

Power, J. D., Barnes, K. A., Snyder, A. Z., Schlaggar, B. L., and Petersen, S. E. (2012). Spurious but systematic correlations in functional connectivity MRI networks arise from subject motion. *NeuroImage* 59, 2142–2154. doi: 10.1016/j.neuroimage.2011.10.018

Power, J. D., Schlaggar, B. L., and Petersen, S. E. (2015). Recent progress and outstanding issues in motion correction in resting state fMRI. *NeuroImage* 105, 536–551. doi: 10.1016/j.neuroimage.2014.10.044

Ross, N., Yau, P. L., and Convit, A. (2015). Obesity, fitness, and brain integrity in adolescence. *Appetite* 93, 44–50. doi: 10.1016/j.appet.2015.03.033

Sack, M., Lenz, J. N., Jakovcevski, M., Biedermann, S. V., Falfán-Melgoza, C., Deussing, J., et al. (2017). Early effects of a high-caloric diet and physical exercise on brain volumetry and behavior: a combined MRI and histology study in mice. *Brain Imag. Behav.* 11, 1385–1396. doi: 10.1007/s11682-016-9638-y

Shott, M. E., Cornier, M.-A., Mittal, V. A., and Pryor, T. L. (2015). Orbitofrontal cortex volume and brain reward response in obesity. *Int. J. Obes.* 39, 214–221. doi: 10.1038/ijo.2014.121

Siegel, J. S., Power, J. D., Dubis, J. W., Vogel, A. C., Church, J. A., Schlaggar, B. L., et al. (2014). Statistical improvements in functional magnetic resonance imaging analyses produced by censoring high-motion data points. *Hum. Brain Mapp.* 35, 1981–1996. doi: 10.1002/hbm.22307

Small, D. M., Bender, G., Veldhuizen, M. G., Rudenga, K., Nachtigal, D., and Felsted, J. (2007). The role of the human orbitofrontal cortex in taste and flavor processing. *Ann. N. Y. Acad. Sci.* 1121, 136–151. doi: 10.1196/annals.1401.002

Smucny, J., Cornier, M.-A., Eichman, L. C., Thomas, E. A., Bechtell, J. L., and Tregellas, J. R. (2012). Brain structure predicts risk for obesity. *Appetite* 59, 859–865. doi: 10.1016/j.appet.2012.08.027

Wallner-Liebmann, S., Deisseroth, K., Reishofer, G., Sorantin, E., Blaschitz, B., Kruschitz, R., et al. (2012). Insulin and hippocampus activation in response to images of high-calorie food in normal weight and obese adolescents. *Obesity* 18, 1552–1557. doi: 10.1038/oby.2010.26

Wang, G.-J., Volkow, N. D., Thanos, P. K., and Fowler, J. S. (2004). Similarity between obesity and drug addiction as assessed by neurofunctional imaging. *J. Addict. Dis.* 23, 39–53. doi: 10.1300/J069v23n03_04

Wijngaarden, M. A., Veer, I. M., Rombouts, S. A. R. B., van Buchem, M. A., Willems van Dijk, K., Pijl, H., et al. (2015). Obesity is marked by distinct functional connectivity in brain networks involved in food reward and salience. *Behav. Brain Res.* 287, 127–134. doi: 10.1016/j.bbr.2015.03.016

Williams, T., Berelowitz, M., Joffe, S. N., Thorner, M. O., Rivier, J., Vale, W., et al. (1984). Impaired growth hormone responses to growth hormone-releasing factor in obesity. *N. Engl. J. Med.* 311, 1403–1407. doi: 10.1056/NEJM198411293112203

3

Brain Innate Immune Response in Diet-Induced Obesity as a Paradigm for Metabolic Influence on Inflammatory Signaling

Felipe Macedo, Lucas Souza dos Santos, Isaias Glezer and Fernanda Marques da Cunha**

Departamento de Bioquímica, Escola Paulista de Medicina, Universidade Federal de São Paulo, São Paulo, Brazil

***Correspondence:**
Isaias Glezer
iglezer@unifesp.br
Fernanda Marques da Cunha
fmcunha@unifesp.br

Obesity is a predisposing factor for numerous morbidities, including those affecting the central nervous system. Hypothalamic inflammation is a hallmark of obesity and is believed to participate in the onset and progression of the obese phenotype, by promoting changes in neuronal functions involved in the control of metabolism. The activation of brain immune cells in the hypothalamus, which are represented by microglia and brain macrophages, is associated with obesity and has been the focus of intense research. Despite the significant body of knowledge gathered on this topic, obesity-induced metabolic changes in brain cells involved in innate immune responses are still poorly characterized due, at least in part, to limitations in the existing experimental methods. Since the metabolic state influences immune responses of microglia and other myeloid cells, the understanding and characterization of the effects of cellular metabolism on the functions of these cells, and their impact on brain integrity, are crucial for the development of efficient therapeutic interventions for individuals exposed to a long-term high fat diet (HFD). Here we review and speculate on the cellular basis that may underlie the observed changes in the reactivity and metabolism of the innate immune cells of the brain in diet-induced obesity (DIO), and discuss important points that deserve further investigation.

Keywords: hypothalamus, inflammation, metabolism, microglia, obesity, saturated fatty acids

INTRODUCTION

According to the World Health Organization, obesity has almost tripled since 1975 and is now considered a worldwide epidemic, affecting more than 650 million people[1]. This rapid increase in the number of obese individuals raises profound concerns in the health community, since obesity is a predisposing factor for a wealth of morbidities, many of which are life-threatening (Guh et al., 2009). In fact, obese people have been shown to be more prone to developing central pathologies, including: stroke, depression, and Alzheimer's disease (Bruce-Keller et al., 2009).

[1] http://www.who.int/en/news-room/fact-sheets/detail/obesity-and-overweight

One of the hallmarks of obesity is the presence of metaflammation, an atypical systemic and sterile inflammation. This inflammatory state involves the participation of the innate and adaptive immune systems, resulting in the production of cytokines, chemokines and inflammatory lipids (Iyer et al., 2010; Cooke et al., 2016; Ralston et al., 2017). Metaflammation has been detected in a variety of different tissues, including different areas of the brain (Beilharz et al., 2016; Guillemot-Legris et al., 2016).

Inflammation in brain areas, other than the hypothalamus, might certainly contribute to the onset and progression of some of the central pathologies associated with obesity, however, hypothalamic inflammation was previously shown to play a central role in disease processes, affecting the control of energy intake and energy expenditure (Velloso and Schwartz, 2011). Moreover, these inflammation-induced alterations in the mediobasal hypothalamus (MBH) directly impact the integrity of homeostatic processes, such as hepatic glucose storage and delivery into the blood (Mravec et al., 2018). Interestingly, some brain-related obesity effects are modulated by sex (reviewed in Morselli et al., 2016 and Ávalos et al., 2018). Since *in vivo* experiments tend to employ male animals, this must be taken into consideration when interpreting data obtained from animal studies.

Here we review a variety of factors that contribute to modifications of brain innate immune cell metabolism and reactivity in diet-induced obesity (DIO). In this particular context, it was found that very little is known about the metabolism of microglia and brain macrophages. Thus, since a high fat diet (HFD) impacts pro-inflammatory gene expression, activity and morphology of hypothalamic immune cells, future studies should focus on and investigate which metabolic pathways in these cells are modulated by DIO, and determine how these changes contribute to the progression of obesity.

DIET-INDUCED OBESITY (DIO) LEADS TO HYPOTHALAMIC INFLAMMATION

In 2005, the first report showing evidence demonstrating an association between DIO and hypothalamic inflammation was published (De Souza et al., 2005). Since then, numerous groups have confirmed and extended this finding in both rodents and humans (Thaler et al., 2012; Schur et al., 2015; Valdearcos et al., 2015). It is also well established that a HFD rapidly induces hypothalamic inflammation, with an associated increase in inflammatory gene expression and gliosis, that subsides and returns if the HFD is not interrupted (Thaler et al., 2012; Berkseth et al., 2014). Interestingly, early hypothalamic inflammation can be observed weeks before adipose tissue (AT) expansion and inflammation (Thaler et al., 2012; Gao et al., 2014), suggesting that hypothalamic inflammatory signaling contributes to the genesis of the overt obese phenotype, and is not simply a consequence of peripheral inflammation. The central role hypothalamic inflammation plays in obesity was further supported by two studies reporting that the detrimental HDF-related effects could be alleviated through genetic ablation or pharmacological inhibition of hypothalamic inhibitor of NF-κB[2] kinase subunit β (IKKβ) (Zhang et al., 2008; Posey et al., 2009). Although pro-inflammatory signaling in the hypothalamus is a key event in the onset of DIO, the widespread inflammation and metabolic changes promoted by a HFD may further impact the hypothalamus.

A Different Inflammatory Profile in Obesity

Obesity is characterized by a distinct level of systemic innate immune response, often referred to as "chronic low grade inflammation." Metabolic dysfunction is accompanied by increased levels of non-esterified fatty acids and systemic inflammatory mediators, such as plasma pro-inflammatory cytokines (Iyer et al., 2010). While a discussion on the accurate use of the term inflammation, for a systemic and chronic response, is beyond the scope of this review, the notion of a generalized response from tissues and blood immune cells, as well vascular endothelial cells, is quite commonsense these days. Interestingly, the presence of inflammatory molecules in the blood and CNS induces sickness behavior, as characterized by decreased food intake (reviewed in Thaler et al., 2010). The paradox on how DIO-mediated inflammation results in a different outcome has been discussed (Thaler et al., 2010). According to the authors, it is plausible that the net impact, resulting from the complex cellular interplay between hypothalamic cells, along with factors such as stimulus quality, duration and intensity, could account for these differences. However, it is clear that HFD-induced hypothalamic inflammation diverges from other pro-inflammatory stimuli that promote sickness behavior. Understanding how this diet triggers inflammation and identifying why innate immune cells in the hypothalamus respond differently is essential to combating obesity.

The Unknown Pathway That Triggers Inflammation in the MBH

It is important to note that the typical neurovascular unit that forms the blood-brain barrier (BBB) (Obermeier et al., 2013) is not the only example of vascular organization in the hypothalamus. Structures devoid of blood-barriers, such as fenestrated median eminence (ME) capillaries, or conversely some of the more tightly sealed endothelia in the arcuate nucleus (ARC), are actually surrounded by cellular processes projected from the third ventricle tanycytes (Langlet, 2014). This atypical cellular disposition contributes to the peculiar properties of the MBH in terms of collecting metabolic information carried by the blood stream (**Figure 1**). As an example, circulating pro-inflammatory mediators and biomolecules characterized as pathogen- and damage/danger- associated molecular patterns (PAMPs and DAMPs, respectively) were shown to be readily detected by brain immune cells associated with structures that lack the BBB (Rivest et al., 2000; Mallard, 2012). PAMPs and DAMPS represent an important concept in immunology, since

[2]Nuclear factor kappa-B, a master activator of pro-inflammatory gene expression.

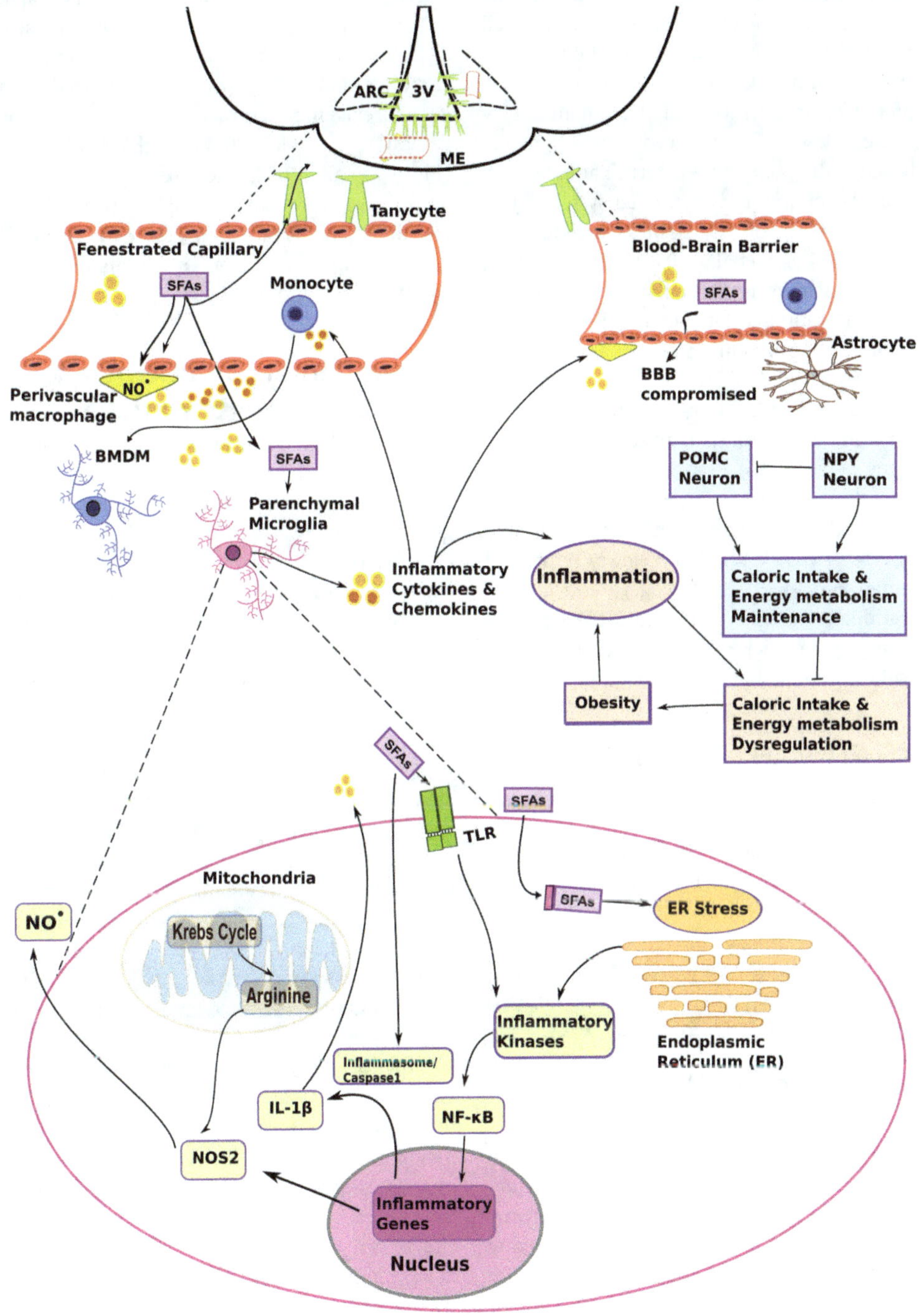

FIGURE 1 | The complex interplay among different myeloid cells and metabolic substrates promotes hypothalamic inflammation in diet-induced obesity (DIO). A high fat diet (HFD) increases the levels of non-esterified saturated fatty acids in the blood and systemic inflammatory mediators, such as plasma pro-inflammatory cytokines. These molecules primarily target fenestrated capillaries in the median eminence (ME), and also influence the mediobasal hypothalamus (MBH) region, including the arcuate nucleus (ARC). Saturated fatty acids (SFAs) and inflammatory molecules activate brain endothelia and its associated immune cells, such as the perivascular macrophages. Changes in vascular permeability due to hypothalamic inflammation and signaling molecules such as nitric oxide (NO˙), act in concert to promote lipid load accumulation in the MBH. Brain myeloid cells are heterogeneous and present particular phenotypes that result from the microenvironment and ontogeny. Resident parenchymal microglia are activated in DIO. Although several mechanisms still remain to be determined, it has been suggested that chronic low-level microglial activation perturbs metabolic control, and that this contributes to the development of the obese phenotype. At the same time, SFAs may influence the metabolic program and inflammatory signaling in microglia. The figure depicts hypothetical metabolic and inflammatory signaling changes in microglia based on data collected from metabolic macrophages (MMe) (see main text for details). Other abbreviations: 3V, third ventricle; BBB, blood brain barrier; BMDM, bone marrow-derived microglia; IL-1β, interleukin 1β. NF-κB, nuclear factor κB; NOS2, nitric oxide synthase 2 (inducible form; iNOS); TLR, *Toll*-like receptor.

these molecules are recognized by germline-encoded non-clonal receptors, and are the primary triggers of innate immune cell responses. However, it remains to be firmly established how an HFD could initiate hypothalamic inflammation.

Studies aiming at the characterization of the inflammatory molecules responsible for HFD-induced hypothalamic inflammation identified fatty acids as determinant factors. Indeed, a key characteristic of obesity is increased systemic free fatty acids, which accumulate in diverse tissues, including the hypothalamus (Boden, 2008; Posey et al., 2009; Valdearcos et al., 2014). In fact, the hypothalamus is particularly prone to the accumulation of long chain saturated fatty acids (SFAs), such as palmitoyl-CoA, thus promoting hypothalamic inflammation in animals fed a HFD. Moreover, while there has been no evidence showing that increased caloric or unsaturated fatty acid intake influences hypothalamic inflammation (Huang et al., 2004; Posey et al., 2009; Valdearcos et al., 2014), the amount of evidence implementing SFAs in this response is growing. With regards to the effects associated with other lipids, including unsaturated fatty acids, the reader is referred to dedicated reviews (White and Marette, 2014; Hammad and Jones, 2017; Rogero and Calder, 2018). A plausible rationale for how SFAs and HFD promote pro-inflammatory signaling in microglia cells—key players in DIO progression—will be presented in the next sections.

MICROGLIA AS PRIMARY TARGETS IN DIO

Of the various cell types that populate the MHB, microglia have been the most studied in terms of DIO-induced hypothalamic inflammation, perhaps due to the fact that they are considered the resident brain macrophages. Indeed, microglial reactivity and inflammatory molecule production were found to be increased in the hypothalamus of animals fed an HFD and obese humans (Thaler et al., 2012; Gao et al., 2014; Valdearcos et al., 2014).

Microglia Cells Respond to HFD and Play an Important Role in DIO

The fact that manipulation of microglia interferes with DIO indirectly shows that an HFD provokes profound effects on these brain myeloid cells, resulting in drastic metabolic consequences. Experimental approaches employing alternative strategies have demonstrated that microglia play a fundamental role in DIO. For example, interventions that impair microglia response (i.e., depleting these cells, restraining their responsivity or inhibiting microglia proliferation) alleviate the DIO phenotype and blunt the HFD-induced inflammation *in vivo*. A similar beneficial effect of microglial inhibition was observed in cultured brain slices stimulated with palmitate (Valdearcos et al., 2014, 2017; André et al., 2017). In contrast, forcing microglial activation by cell-specific deletion of tumor necrosis factor α-induced protein 3 (TNFAIP3), an anti-inflammatory molecule and negative regulator of NF-κB, rapidly induced obesity in mice, even when animals were fed control diets (Valdearcos et al., 2017). While this latter study does not explain how an HFD activates microglia, it certainly implicates hypothalamic microglia as a key player in DIO. Interestingly, persistent secretion of TNF-α by microglia in the MHB of mice fed a high fat/high carbohydrate (HFHC) diet was reported to cause dysfunction in anorexigenic neurons that produce proopiomelanocortin (POMC) (Yi et al., 2017), a characteristic feature of obesity (Pinto et al., 2004; Horvath et al., 2010). Assuming that lipids participate in microglial pro-inflammatory signaling, we direct the reader to **Table 1**, which summarizes the findings supporting a pro-inflammatory effect of SFAs on the hypothalamus and microglia.

Experimental Limitations and Thoughtful Interpretations

While the above-mentioned set of data suggests a prominent role for microglia in the detrimental effects of DIO, it is appropriate to introduce some notes of caution. At first glance, brain myeloid cells are thought to be either pathogen eradicators, or instigators of neuronal dysfuntion and cell death in various neurodegenerative diseases. However, microglia are important for the proper shaping of the brain, and function as a neuroprotective component of the innate immune response, a concept strongly supported by experimental data (Wyss-Coray and Mucke, 2002; Glezer et al., 2007; ElAli and Rivest, 2016). Thus, while experimental results indicate that preventing hypothalamic myeloid cell responses improves the outcome of HFD-treated animals, the consequences of DIO on the unprotected brain for a long period of time are not known. Secondly, due to limitations in experimental tools, "microglia" was frequently used as a generic term for all brain myeloid cells (myeloid as lineage term, not to be confused with bone marrow origin) in the past. Now it is known that in addition to the prototypical parenchymal microglia, other myeloid cells are present in the brain, including the non-parenchymal meningeal, perivascular and choroid-plexus macrophages, and disease-associated monocytes (Prinz et al., 2017). In this sense, it is likely that inflammatory signaling in the hypothalamus is coordinated by a complex interplay between microglia/macrophages, endothelial cells and macroglia (astrocytes, oligodendrocytes and their progenitors). Thus, efforts to target specific pathways and/or microglia/brain macrophage subpopulations are valuable and necessary, but the interpretation of the results should be performed carefully and objectively.

Lastly, it is important to keep in mind that brain myeloid cells do not necessarily influence metabolism through stereotyped responses to noxious stimuli. Indeed, myeloid cell specific *Cx3cr1*-driven ablation of receptors for the "satiety" hormone leptin was shown to result in increased food intake and body weight, dystrophic and less phagocytic microglia, and altered neuronal circuitry in the MBH (Gao et al., 2018). However, this genetic strategy cannot provide a conclusion about the specific role for leptin signaling in microglia/brain macrophages, since this approach may affect myeloid cells from multiple tissues, a commonly encountered experimental

TABLE 1 | Microglia activation induced by high fat diet or fatty acid treatment.

Experimental model	Treatment	Duration of treatment	Results	References
Hypothalamus	Normal diet (ND) HFD	13 and 16 weeks	↑ TNFα ↑ IL-1β ↑ IL-6	De Souza et al., 2005
		16 weeks	↑ TNFα mRNA ↑ IL-1β mRNA	
Hypothalamus	ND HFD	16 weeks	↑ TNFα ↑ IL-1β ↑ IL-6	Milanski et al., 2009
	Intracerebroventricular infusion of oleic acid	3 days	↑ IL-6 and IL-6 mRNA ↑ IL-10 and IL-10 mRNA	
	Intracerebroventricular infusion of stearic acid	3 days	↑ TNFα ↑ IL-1β ↑ IL-10	
	Intracerebroventricular infusion of linolenic acid	3 days	↑ IL-6 ↑ IL-10	
	Intracerebroventricular infusion of arachidic acid	3 days	↑ TNFα ↑ IL-1β ↑ IL-6 ↑ IL-10	
	Intracerebroventricular infusion of behenic acid	3 days	↑ TNFα ↑ IL-1β ↑ IL-6	
Hypothalamus	Intracerebroventricular infusion of palmitate	20 min	↑ pIKKβ ↓ IκBα	Posey et al., 2009
	LFD HFD	7 weeks	↑ pIKKβ	
Primary glial cells	Control serum DIO serum	48 h	↑ CD11b positive cells	Hsuchou et al., 2012
BV-2 microglial cells	Vehicle 0.125 mM Palmitate	24 h	↓ TNFα mRNA ↑ Chi3L3 mRNA ↑ Arg1 mRNA	Kappe et al., 2012
Hypothalamus	ND HFD	4 weeks	↑ TNFα mRNA ↑ IL-6 mRNA	Thaler et al., 2012
BV-2 microglial cells	Vehicle 0.125 mM Palmitate	24 h	↑ Arg1 mRNA	Tracy et al., 2013
Primary microglial cells	Control serum HFD serum	120 min	↑ Iba-1 ↑ TNFα ↑ IL-1β	Gao et al., 2014
Hypothalamus	ND HFD	4 and 16 weeks 4 weeks	↑ Iba-1 positive cells ↑ TNFα mRNA ↑ IL-6 mRNA ↑ IL-1β mRNA	Valdearcos et al., 2014

(Continued)

TABLE 1 | Continued

Experimental model	Treatment	Duration of treatment	Results	References
	Enteric gavage of lauric acid	3 days	↑ TNFα mRNA ↑ IL-6 mRNA	
	Enteric gavage of palmitic acid	3 days	↑ TNFα mRNA ↑ IL-6 mRNA ↑ IL-1β mRNA	
Primary microglial cells	Vehicle 0.1 mM lauric acid	24 h	↑ TNFα ↑ IL-6 ↑ MCP-1	
	Vehicle 0.1 mM myristic acid	24 h	↑ TNFα ↑ IL-6 ↑ MCP-1	
	Vehicle 0.1 mM palmitic acid	24 h	↑ TNFα ↑ IL-6	
	Vehicle 0.1 mM stearic acid	24 h	↑ TNFα ↑ IL-6 ↑ MCP-1	
BV-2 microglial cells	Vehicle 0.1 mM Palmitate	12 h	↑ iNOS mRNA	Duffy et al., 2017
Hypothalamus	ND HFD	4 weeks	↑ Iba-1 ↓ P2Y12	Valdearcos et al., 2017
BV-2 microglial cells	Vehicle 0.3 mM Palmitate	48 h	↑ IL-1β ↑ CD11b mRNA ↑ IL-6 ↑ MCP-1	Yang et al., 2017
Hypothalamus	Low fat diet (LFD) HFD	8 weeks	↑ TNFα mRNA ↑ IL-1β mRNA	

limitation associated with attempting to target, regulate and/or delete a specific gene in microglia (Han et al., 2017). The results, nonetheless, suggest that these cell types are responsive to a vast array of signals. Interestingly, recent data demonstrated that *Cx3cr1*-driven microglia and monocyte ablation in rats disrupts the gustatory circuitry at the paraventricular nucleus of the hypothalamus, leading to anorexia and weight loss (De Luca et al., 2019). Strikingly, it was reported that mice fed an HFD and treated with an intracerebroventricular injection of AraC, to block cell proliferation induced by HFD, presented reduced food intake, weight gain and adiposity, when compared with mice fed the same diet, but without being administered AraC (André et al., 2017). Thus, it is tempting to speculate that the reported benefits of microglia and monocyte ablation/inhibition in the DIO setting is secondary to decreased food intake, and not solely due to a reduction in inflammation.

Although many of the studies cited here indicate that there is a relationship among the HFD-induced increase in SFAs, brain myeloid cells pro-inflammatory response and hypothalamic energy metabolism control, the precise mechanisms linking these events are not definitively established. While improved experimental models and detailed molecular approaches are still necessary in order to unify these pieces of evidence into a compelling and complete model, it is clear that an HFD severely impacts the function of microglia.

LIPIDS ACTIVATE MICROGLIA/MACROPHAGES

Since long chain saturated fatty acids seem to be important for HFD-associated hypothalamic inflammation, *in vitro* studies have been employed, using palmitate as a stimulus, for elucidating the molecular pathways involved in the microglial response to HFD. However, mixed results were reported, ranging from anti-inflammatory responses (Tracy et al., 2013; Kim et al., 2018) to pro-inflammatory ones (Wang et al., 2012). This discrepancy may stem, at least in part, from different lipid loads, since they may be modulated not only by the concentration of lipid used in the assays, but also by the ratio of lipid to the carrier protein albumin (Alsabeeh et al., 2018). Not surprisingly, the mechanisms through which parenchymal microglia respond to an HFD or SFAs are not clear yet, and much is still unknown. It is noteworthy that most of the research in the field has focused on typical macrophage readouts such as cytokine secretion, cellular recruitment, gene expression and cell morphology when exploring the effects of HFD or SFAs on microglia. Furthermore, data related to the mechanisms involved in the parenchymal microglia response to HFD or SFAs are extremely scarce. Therefore, we will summarize the findings related to macrophages, for which more information is available and discuss the extent to which these findings also apply to microglia.

Macrophages and Microglia Do Not Necessarily Respond to HFD in the Same Way

With regards to macrophages, the response to SFAs seems to involve canonical and non-canonical mechanisms. The innate immune signaling is largely dependent on pattern recognition receptors, such as the *toll*-like receptors (TLRs). This family of membrane proteins activates pro-inflammatory transcription upon the recognition of structurally distinct PAMPs, such as lipopolysaccharide (LPS) from gram-negative bacteria (Takeuchi and Akira, 2010). Additionally, this response is complemented by intracellular protein complexes called inflammasomes, which sense PAMPs/DAMPs or relay upstream signaling, and promote the secretion of cytokines such as interleukin (IL)-1β (Sharma and Kanneganti, 2016). While SFAs are far from being considered PAMPs or DAMPs, similar response mechanisms have been described. For example, palmitate, but not unsaturated oleate, has been shown to activate the NLRP3-ASC inflammasome (Wen et al., 2011). Additionally, other studies also point to engagement of TLR4, the same receptor for LPS, by SFAs (Lee et al., 2001; Shi et al., 2006; Huang et al., 2012), suggesting that SFAs present the natural capacity to trigger innate immune cells. However, the evolutionary basis for the controversial idea that the immune system would respond against important caloric nutrients remains to be clarified.

How do the findings reported in macrophages apply to microglia? While it is expected that signals triggered by PAMPs and DAMPs follow quite similar pathways in different myeloid cells, it is important to mention that resident brain cells present unique and remarkable features. Molecular tracing and fate mapping studies revealed that microglia originate from yolk sac erythro-myeloid progenitors (primitive macrophages). Additionally, unlike macrophages from other tissues (that are largely derived from fetal monocytes), microglia and brain macrophages preserve their primitive lineage by means of self-renewal of resident progenitors, which infiltrated the brain during embryo development (Ginhoux et al., 2010; ElAli and Rivest, 2016; Prinz et al., 2017; Hoeffel and Ginhoux, 2018). This is relevant because microglia and brain macrophages maintain distinct repertoires of signaling and function, and long-term brain exposure to macrophage activating molecules will follow different cellular dynamics when compared to other tissues that actively replenish macrophages with bone marrow-derived cells. Furthermore, it is important to point out that environmental factors clearly determine the transcriptional programs that define the identity of microglia. For example, specific transcripts from murine microglia are lost when these cells are removed from the brain and transferred to cell culture (Gosselin et al., 2017). In addition, microglia completely regain their identity when transferred from *in vitro* culture to the brain *in vivo*, an event specific for yolk-sac primitive ontogeny, that cannot be replicated by engrafted macrophages from other tissues (Bennett et al., 2018). The authors of this study identified that the microglia-like cells, and not microglia, have a few unique markers that are found in pathological states of the human brain. The impact of these findings is very clear in terms of how crucial it is to determine which specific brain myeloid cells respond to HFD and SFAs, and the extent to which *in vitro* generated data can be translated to the hypothalamic niche of animals subjected to DIO.

Very recently, perivascular macrophages of the ARC, whose ontogeny has yet to be defined, were shown to proliferate *in situ* and express high levels of inducible nitric oxide synthase (iNOS/NOS2) when mice were fed an HFD (Lee et al., 2018). The same study also showed that hypothalamic NOS2 inhibition diminished several deleterious effects associated with DIO, including BBB permeability and lipid efflux (Lee et al., 2018). The idea that inflammatory cells regulate lipid uptake into the brain is quite attractive, but it is not clear how lipid overload, that occurs with an HFD, upregulates the expression of iNOS and other genes typically involved in pathogen defense. This is of particular relevance, since "chronic low grade inflammation" is commonly observed in obesity.

Due to the emergent nature of the subject, detailed studies describing the ontogeny and neuroanatomical details of the microglia/macrophages that are involved in the *in vivo* response to HFD, as well as studies combining specific gene promoters to drive pro-inflammatory signaling interference without disrupting brain barriers, are awaited. A comprehensive understanding of the molecular and cellular mechanisms involved in the response of microglia/brain macrophage to DIO and SFAs will likely reveal novel therapeutic targets for the prevention and/or treatment of obesity.

DISTINCT METABOLIC PROGRAMS SUPPORT INFLAMMATORY PHENOTYPES IN MACROPHAGES AND (POSSIBLY) MICROGLIA

It is now clear that immune cells have a profound impact on metabolic homeostasis and, that metabolic pathways can also significantly influence immune cell function. Indeed, the transition of immune cells from one phenotype to another is supported by and dependent on specific metabolic programs (reviewed in Van den Bossche et al., 2017). For example, macrophages stimulated with LPS(+ IFNγ) adopt a metabolic program that includes increased flux through glycolysis and the pentose phosphate pathway together with a reduction in oxidative phosphorylation (Rodríguez-Prados et al., 2010), due to a disruption of the citric acid cycle (Jha et al., 2015). This disruption repurposes the intermediary metabolites of the citric acid cycle for specific biosynthetic reactions, which sustain the inflammatory activities of LPS-stimulated macrophages (Tannahill et al., 2013; Littlewood-Evans et al., 2016; Mills et al., 2016; Williams and O'Neill, 2018). Interestingly, inhibition of specific mitochondrial membrane carriers impairs this repurposing and attenuates pro-inflammatory macrophage polarization by LPS, without affecting cell viability (Jha et al., 2015). Thus, indicating that metabolic pathways can influence the phenotype of immune cells and that modulating these pathways may represent a potent therapeutic strategy.

In obesity, macrophages acquire a specific phenotype that is strikingly different from the pro-inflammatory M1 phenotype, elicited by stimulation with LPS(+ IFNγ), and the anti-inflammatory M2 phenotype, induced by IL-4 (Lumeng et al., 2007; Zeyda et al., 2007; Kratz et al., 2014; Coats et al., 2017). In fact, macrophages stimulated with metabolic cues such as high SFAs, insulin and glucose, which are preponderant in obesity, are designated as metabolic macrophages (MMe). The MMe phenotype is associated with the production of cytokines, but presents a different set of surface molecules, when compared with macrophages stimulated with LPS. Additionally, these differences were also detected when macrophages isolated from the AT of obese patients were compared with macrophages isolated from the lungs of patients with cystic fibrosis, a disease in which the patients experience recurrent bacterial infections of the airway (Kratz et al., 2014). To date, little is known about the metabolic landscape of MMe macrophages, but different lipid metabolism programs seem to be important for MMe macrophage polarization and/or activity. In fact, SFAs seem to be important drivers of MMe activation, since macrophages stimulated with SFAs produce IL-1β and express surface markers characteristic of MMe isolated from obese mice (Kratz et al., 2014). The expression of many of the MMe surface markers are under the control of the lipid-engaged receptor PPARγ, reinforcing the idea that lipid metabolism is intimately linked to MMe activation and/or function. Indeed, it was shown that upon internalization, SFAs insert into phospholipid bilayer, changing the degree of membrane saturation. This altered lipid composition induces endoplasmic reticulum stress, a characteristic feature of MMe, which ultimately leads to the production of IL-1β (Robblee et al., 2016). Interestingly, the pharmacological inhibition of PPARγ or genetic inhibition of mitochondrial fatty acid oxidation in macrophages stimulated with SFAs exacerbate inflammation, and PPARγ deletion in macrophages aggravates insulin resistance in mice fed a HFD (Odegaard et al., 2007; Kratz et al., 2014; Namgaladze et al., 2014). Recently, gene expression data indicated that genes involved in glycolysis, oxidative phosphorylation and those related to lactate production were increased in AT macrophages isolated from obese mice, when compared to those isolated from lean animals. This metabolic program seems to be specific for AT macrophages as the expression of genes involved in energy metabolism was unaltered by an HDF in peritoneal macrophages (Boutens et al., 2018), highlighting the importance of the niche for macrophage response. Despite the data gathered so far, much more work is needed before we obtain a clear comprehensive understanding of the different metabolic programs that promote MMe polarization and activity (Namgaladze and Brüne, 2016), and how different niches (i.e., different AT depots) and the origin of the cell influence these responses.

With respect to microglia metabolism and its impact on cell phenotype and function, very little is known. Studies using LPS(+ INFγ) to stimulate microglia in culture reported increased pro-inflammatory cytokine and lactate production, which was accompanied by increased flux through glycolysis and the pentose phosphate pathway and decreased mitochondrial oxygen consumption (Voloboueva et al., 2013; Gimeno-Bayón et al., 2014). Thus, suggesting that there are parallels between macrophages and microglia in terms of their metabolic response to LPS(+INFγ), at least *in vitro*. However, these similarities seem to be limited, since there is still no clear evidence that microglia are responsive to IL-4, revealing the inadequacy of using the bimodal M1/M2 designation to describe the microglial response (Ransohoff, 2016). With regards to microglial metabolism in obesity, it was recently reported that impairing lipid uptake, through the silencing of lipoprotein lipase (LPL), specifically in microglia, exacerbates weight gain and glucose intolerance in mice fed an HFHC diet (Gao et al., 2017). The same study also reported that the absence of LPL in the microglia of mutant mice impaired the cellular responses (i.e., increase in number, changes in morphology and phagocytic capacity) observed in control mice fed an HFHC diet. In fact, this impairment was accompanied by an increased number of dysmorphic mitochondria in the microglia, possibly due to extensive alterations of the lipidome of those cells (Gao et al., 2017). While the work by Gao et al. indicated that lipid metabolism may play a central role in microglia phenotype and/or function in obesity, data related to microglia immunometabolism, especially in the context of obesity, are virtually non-existent. Thus, future studies investigating the modulation of microglia metabolism and, in a broader view, of myeloid cells are urgently needed, since these areas appear to be a promising avenue for treating obesity. It is important to note that although *in vitro* assays are important for providing mechanistic insights, *in vivo* work is crucial for accurately determining the metabolic response of microglia to different stimuli, as the niche exerts a profound influence on the cellular response. It is likely that changes in myeloid cell metabolism promote different outcomes in the MHB. In the context of obesity, more studies are needed to fully understand the impact of myeloid metabolism on cell function and reactivity; however, the origin of the cell and the niche must be taken into account when attempting to elucidate these response mechanisms.

CONCLUDING REMARKS AND FUTURE DIRECTIONS

Although much has been done, very little is known about how microglia cell metabolism affects the function of these brain cells. Additionally, it is unclear whether microglial metabolism is rewired, due to obesity-associated metabolic cues *in vivo*, or how this could occur. Due to the fact that microglia play a central role in obesity, and since obesity has devastating effects on human health, we believe that the metabolic program promoting obesity-induced microglial activation must be understood in detail. It will also be interesting to evaluate whether other brain myeloid cells present different metabolic programs, and to investigate the role each type of cell plays in hypothalamic inflammation. For example, if SFAs and myeloid cell metabolism induce an atypical inflammatory state, would it be possible to metabolically reprogram the microglia and restore normal hypothalamic function during DIO? Moreover, could the anti-inflammatory or deactivated microglia strategies employed in rodents be utilized in humans? Answering these questions, as well as others will pave the way for the development of therapeutic interventions aimed at preventing the onset and progression of obesity, as well as its associated co-morbidities.

AUTHOR CONTRIBUTIONS

All authors listed have made a substantial, direct and intellectual contribution to the work, and approved it for publication.

ACKNOWLEDGMENTS

The authors thank Dr. Bruno Chausse for valuable discussions and suggestions.

REFERENCES

Alsabeeh, N., Chausse, B., Kakimoto, P. A., Kowaltowski, A. J., and Shirihai, O. (2018). Cell culture models of fatty acid overload: problems and solutions. *Biochim. Biophys. Acta Mol. Cell Biol. Lipids* 1863, 143–151. doi: 10.1016/j.bbalip.2017.11.006

André, C., Guzman-Quevedo, O., Rey, C., Rémus-Borel, J., Clark, S., Castellanos-Jankiewicz, A., et al. (2017). Inhibiting microglia expansion prevents diet-induced hypothalamic and peripheral inflammation. *Diabetes* 66, 908L–919L. doi: 10.2337/db16-0586

Ávalos, Y., Kerr, B., Maliqueo, M., and Dorfman, M. (2018). Cell and molecular mechanisms behind diet-induced hypothalamic inflammation and obesity. *J. Neuroendocrinol.* 30:e12598. doi: 10.1111/jne.12598

Beilharz, J. E., Maniam, J., and Morris, M. J. (2016). Short-term exposure to a diet high in fat and sugar, or liquid sugar, selectively impairs hippocampal-dependent memory, with differential impacts on inflammation. *Behav. Brain Res.* 306, 1–7. doi: 10.1016/j.bbr.2016.03.018

Bennett, F. C., Bennett, M. L., Yaqoob, F., Mulinyawe, S. B., Grant, G. A., Hayden Gephart, M., et al. (2018). A Combination of ontogeny and CNS environment establishes microglial identity. *Neuron* 98, 1170.e8–1183.e8. doi: 10.1016/j.neuron.2018.05.014

Berkseth, K. E., Guyenet, S. J., Melhorn, S. J., Lee, D., Thaler, J. P., Schur, E. A., et al. (2014). Hypothalamic gliosis associated with high-fat diet feeding is reversible in mice: a combined immunohistochemical and magnetic resonance imaging study. *Endocrinology* 155, 2858–2867. doi: 10.1210/en.2014-1121

Boden, G. (2008). Obesity and free fatty acids. *Endocrinol. Metab. Clin. North Am.* 37, 635–646. doi: 10.1016/j.ecl.2008.06.007

Boutens, L., Hooiveld, G. J., Dhingra, S., Cramer, R. A., Netea, M. G., and Stienstra, R. (2018). Unique metabolic activation of adipose tissue macrophages in obesity promotes inflammatory responses. *Diabetologia* 61, 942–953. doi: 10.1007/s00125-017-4526-6

Bruce-Keller, A. J., Keller, J. N., and Morrison, C. D. (2009). Obesity and vulnerability of the CNS. *Biochim. Biophys. Acta Mol. Basis Dis.* 1792, 395–400. doi: 10.1016/j.bbadis.2008.10.004

Coats, B. R., Schoenfelt, K. Q., Barbosa-Lorenzi, V. C., Peris, E., Cui, C., Hoffman, A., et al. (2017). Metabolically activated adipose tissue macrophages perform detrimental and beneficial functions during diet-induced obesity. *Cell Rep.* 20, 3149–3161. doi: 10.1016/j.celrep.2017.08.096

Cooke, A. A., Connaughton, R. M., Lyons, C. L., McMorrow, A. M., and Roche, H. M. (2016). Fatty acids and chronic low grade inflammation associated with obesity and the metabolic syndrome. *Eur. J. Pharmacol.* 785, 207–214. doi: 10.1016/j.ejphar.2016.04.021

De Luca, S. N., Sominsky, L., Soch, A., Wang, H., Ziko, I., Rank, M. M., et al. (2019). Conditional microglial depletion in rats leads to reversible anorexia and weight loss by disrupting gustatory circuitry. *Brain. Behav. Immun.* 77, 77–91. doi: 10.1016/j.bbi.2018.12.008

De Souza, C. T., Araujo, E. P., Bordin, S., Ashimine, R., Zollner, R. L., Boschero, A. C., et al. (2005). Consumption of a fat-rich diet activates a proinflammatory response and induces insulin resistance in the hypothalamus. *Endocrinology* 146, 4192–4199. doi: 10.1210/en.2004-1520

Duffy, C. M., Xu, H., Nixon, J. P., Bernlohr, D. A., and Butterick, T. A. (2017). Identification of a fatty acid binding protein4-UCP2 axis regulating microglial mediated neuroinflammation. *Mol. Cell. Neurosci.* 80, 52–57. doi: 10.1016/j.mcn.2017.02.004

ElAli, A., and Rivest, S. (2016). Microglia ontology and signaling. *Front. Cell Dev. Biol.* 4:72. doi: 10.3389/fcell.2016.00072

Gao, Y., Ottaway, N., Schriever, S. C., Legutko, B., García-Cáceres, C., de la Fuente, E., et al. (2014). Hormones and diet, but not body weight, control hypothalamic microglial activity. *Glia* 62, 17–25. doi: 10.1002/glia.22580

Gao, Y., Vidal-Itriago, A., Kalsbeek, M. J., Layritz, C., García-Cáceres, C., Tom, R. Z., et al. (2017). Lipoprotein lipase maintains microglial innate immunity in obesity. *Cell Rep.* 20, 3034–3042. doi: 10.1016/j.celrep.2017.09.008

Gao, Y., Vidal-Itriago, A., Milanova, I., Korpel, N. L., Kalsbeek, M. J., Tom, R. Z., et al. (2018). Deficiency of leptin receptor in myeloid cells disrupts hypothalamic metabolic circuits and causes body weight increase. *Mol. Metab.* 7, 155–160. doi: 10.1016/j.molmet.2017.11.003

Gimeno-Bayón, J., López-López, A., Rodríguez, M. J., and Mahy, N. (2014). Glucose pathways adaptation supports acquisition of activated microglia phenotype. *J. Neurosci. Res.* 92, 723–731. doi: 10.1002/jnr.23356

Ginhoux, F., Greter, M., Leboeuf, M., Nandi, S., See, P., Gokhan, S., et al. (2010). Fate mapping analysis reveals that adult microglia derive from primitive macrophages. *Science* 330, 841–845. doi: 10.1126/science.1194637

Glezer, I., Simard, A. R., and Rivest, S. (2007). Neuroprotective role of the innate immune system by microglia. *Neuroscience* 147, 867–883. doi: 10.1016/j.neuroscience.2007.02.055

Gosselin, D., Skola, D., Coufal, N. G., Holtman, I. R., Schlachetzki, J. C. M., Sajti, E., et al. (2017). An environment-dependent transcriptional network specifies human microglia identity. *Science* 356:eaal3222. doi: 10.1126/science.aal3222

Guh, D. P., Zhang, W., Bansback, N., Amarsi, Z., Birmingham, C. L., and Anis, A. H. (2009). The incidence of co-morbidities related to obesity and overweight: A systematic review and meta-analysis. *BMC Publ. Health* 9:88. doi: 10.1186/1471-2458-9-88

Guillemot-Legris, O., Masquelier, J., Everard, A., Cani, P. D., Alhouayek, M., and Muccioli, G. G. (2016). High-fat diet feeding differentially affects the development of inflammation in the central nervous system. *J. Neuroinflamm.* 13:206. doi: 10.1186/s12974-016-0666-8

Hammad, S. S., and Jones, P. J. (2017). Dietary fatty acid composition modulates obesity and interacts with obesity-related genes. *Lipids* 52, 803–822. doi: 10.1007/s11745-017-4291-9

Han, J., Harris, R. A., and Zhang, X. M. (2017). An updated assessment of microglia depletion: current concepts and future directions. *Mol. Brain* 10:25. doi: 10.1186/s13041-017-0307-x

Hoeffel, G., and Ginhoux, F. (2018). Fetal monocytes and the origins of tissue-resident macrophages. *Cell. Immunol.* 330, 5–15. doi: 10.1016/j.cellimm.2018.01.001

Horvath, T. L., Sarman, B., García-Cáceres, C., Enriori, P. J., Sotonyi, P., Shanabrough, M., et al. (2010). Synaptic input organization of the melanocortin system predicts diet-induced hypothalamic reactive gliosis and obesity. *Proc. Natl. Acad. Sci.* 107, 14875–14880. doi: 10.1073/pnas.1004282107

Hsuchou, H., Kastin, A. J., and Pan, W. (2012). Blood-borne metabolic factors in obesity exacerbate injury-induced gliosis. *J. Mol. Neurosci.* 47, 267–277. doi: 10.1007/s12031-012-9734-4

Huang, S., Rutkowsky, J. M., Snodgrass, R. G., Ono-Moore, K. D., Schneider, D. A., Newman, J. W., et al. (2012). Saturated fatty acids activate TLR-mediated proinflammatory signaling pathways. *J. Lipid Res.* 53, 2002–2013. doi: 10.1194/jlr.D029546

Huang, X. F., Xin, X., McLennan, P., and Storlien, L. (2004). Role of fat amount and type in ameliorating diet-induced obesity: Insights at the level of hypothalamic arcuate nucleus leptin receptor, neuropeptide Y and pro-opiomelanocortin mRNA expression. *Diabetes Obes. Metab.* 6, 35–44. doi: 10.1111/j.1463-1326.2004.00312.x

Iyer, A., Fairlie, D. P., Prins, J. B., Hammock, B. D., and Brown, L. (2010). Inflammatory lipid mediators in adipocyte function and obesity. *Nat. Rev. Endocrinol.* 6, 71–82. doi: 10.1038/nrendo.2009.264

Jha, A. K., Huang, S. C.-C., Sergushichev, A., Lampropoulou, V., Ivanova, Y., Loginicheva, E., et al. (2015). Network integration of parallel metabolic and transcriptional data reveals metabolic modules that regulate macrophage polarization. *Immunity* 42, 419–430. doi: 10.1016/j.immuni.2015.02.005

Kappe, C., Tracy, L. M., Patrone, C., Iverfeldt, K., and Sjöholm, Å. (2012). GLP-1 secretion by microglial cells and decreased CNS expression in obesity. *J. Neuroinflamm.* 9:276. doi: 10.1186/1742-2094-9-276

Kim, S. M., McIlwraith, E. K., Chalmers, J. A., and Belsham, D. D. (2018). Palmitate induces an anti-inflammatory response in immortalized microglial BV-2 and IMG cell lines that decreases TNFα levels in mHypoE-46 hypothalamic neurons in co-culture. *Neuroendocrinology* 107, 387–399. doi: 10.1159/000494759

Kratz, M., Coats, B. R., Hisert, K. B., Hagman, D., Mutskov, V., Peris, E., et al. (2014). Metabolic dysfunction drives a mechanistically distinct proinflammatory phenotype in adipose tissue macrophages. *Cell Metab.* 20, 614–625. doi: 10.1016/j.cmet.2014.08.010

Langlet, F. (2014). Tanycytes: a gateway to the metabolic hypothalamus. *J. Neuroendocrinol.* 26, 753–760. doi: 10.1111/jne.12191

Lee, C. H., Kim, H. J., Lee, Y. S., Kang, G. M., Lim, H. S., Lee, S. H., et al. (2018). Hypothalamic macrophage inducible nitric oxide synthase mediates obesity-associated hypothalamic inflammation. *Cell Rep.* 25, 934.e5–946.e5. doi: 10.1016/j.celrep.2018.09.070

Lee, J. Y., Sohn, K. H., Rhee, S. H., and Hwang, D. (2001). Saturated fatty acids, but not unsaturated fatty acids, induce the expression of cyclooxygenase-2 mediated through toll-like receptor 4. *J. Biol. Chem.* 276, 16683–16689. doi: 10.1074/jbc.M011695200

Littlewood-Evans, A., Sarret, S., Apfel, V., Loesle, P., Dawson, J., Zhang, J., et al. (2016). GPR91 senses extracellular succinate released from inflammatory macrophages and exacerbates rheumatoid arthritis. *J. Exp. Med.* 213, 1655L–1662L. doi: 10.1084/jem.20160061

Lumeng, C. N., Bodzin, J. L., and Saltiel, A. R. (2007). Obesity induces a phenotypic switch in adipose tissue macrophage polarization. *J. Clin. Invest.* 117, 175–184. doi: 10.1172/JCI29881

Mallard, C. (2012). Innate immune regulation by toll-like receptors in the brain. *ISRN Neurol.* 2012:701950. doi: 10.5402/2012/701950

Milanski, M., Degasperi, G., Coope, A., Morari, J., Denis, R., Cintra, D. E., et al. (2009). Saturated fatty acids produce an inflammatory response predominantly through the activation of TLR4 signaling in hypothalamus: implications for the pathogenesis of obesity. *J. Neurosci.* 29, 359–370. doi: 10.1523/JNEUROSCI.2760-08.2009

Mills, E. L., Kelly, B., Logan, A., Costa, A. S. H., Varma, M., Bryant, C. E., et al. (2016). Succinate dehydrogenase supports metabolic repurposing of mitochondria to drive inflammatory macrophages. *Cell* 167, 457.e13–470.e13. doi: 10.1016/j.cell.2016.08.064

Morselli, E., Frank, A. P., Palmer, B. F., Rodriguez-Navas, C., Criollo, A., and Clegg, D. J. (2016). A sexually dimorphic hypothalamic response to chronic high-fat diet consumption. *Int. J. Obes.* 40, 206–209. doi: 10.1038/ijo.2015.114

Mravec, B., Horvathova, L., and Cernackova, A. (2018). Hypothalamic inflammation at a crossroad of somatic diseases. *Cell. Mol. Neurobiol.* 39, 11–29. doi: 10.1007/s10571-018-0631-4

Namgaladze, D., and Brüne, B. (2016). Macrophage fatty acid oxidation and its roles in macrophage polarization and fatty acid-induced inflammation. *Biochim. Biophys. Acta Mol. Cell Biol. Lipids* 1861, 1796–1807. doi: 10.1016/j.bbalip.2016.09.002

Namgaladze, D., Lips, S., Leiker, T. J., Murphy, R. C., Ekroos, K., Ferreiros, N., et al. (2014). Inhibition of macrophage fatty acid β-oxidation exacerbates palmitate-induced inflammatory and endoplasmic reticulum stress responses. *Diabetologia* 57, 1067–1077. doi: 10.1007/s00125-014-3173-4

Obermeier, B., Daneman, R., and Ransohoff, R. M. (2013). Development, maintenance and disruption of the blood-brain barrier. *Nat. Med.* 19, 1584–1596. doi: 10.1038/nm.3407

Odegaard, J. I., Ricardo-Gonzalez, R. R., Goforth, M. H., Morel, C. R., Subramanian, V., Mukundan, L., et al. (2007). Macrophage-specific PPARγ controls alternative activation and improves insulin resistance. *Nature* 447:1116. doi: 10.1038/nature05894

Pinto, S., Roseberry, A. G., Liu, H., Diano, S., Shanabrough, M., Cai, X., et al. (2004). Rapid rewiring of arcuate nucleus feeding circuits by leptin. *Science* 304, 110–115. doi: 10.1126/science.1089459

Posey, K. A., Clegg, D. J., Printz, R. L., Byun, J., Morton, G. J., Vivekanandan-Giri, A., et al. (2009). Hypothalamic proinflammatory lipid accumulation, inflammation, and insulin resistance in rats fed a high-fat diet. *Am. J. Physiol. Metab.* 296, E1003–E1012. doi: 10.1152/ajpendo.90377.2008

Prinz, M., Erny, D., and Hagemeyer, N. (2017). Ontogeny and homeostasis of CNS myeloid cells. *Nat. Immunol.* 18, 385–392. doi: 10.1038/ni.3703

Ralston, J. C., Lyons, C. L., Kennedy, E. B., Kirwan, A. M., and Roche, H. M. (2017). Fatty acids and NLRP3 inflammasome–mediated inflammation in metabolic tissues. *Annu. Rev. Nutr.* 37, 77–102. doi: 10.1146/annurev-nutr-071816-064836

Ransohoff, R. M. (2016). A polarizing question: do M1 and M2 microglia exist? *Nat. Neurosci.* 19:987. doi: 10.1038/nn.4338

Rivest, S., Lacroix, S., Vallières, L., Nadeau, S., Zhang, J., and Laflamme, N. (2000). How the blood talks to the brain parenchyma and the paraventricular nucleus of the hypothalamus during systemic inflammatory and infectious stimuli. *Proc. Soc. Exp. Biol. Med.* 223, 22–28. doi: 10.1046/j.1525-1373.2000.22304.x

Robblee, M. M., Kim, C. C., Abate, J. P., Valdearcos, M., Sandlund, K. L. M., Shenoy, M. K., et al. (2016). Saturated fatty acids engage an IRE1α-dependent pathway to activate the NLRP3 inflammasome in myeloid cells. *Cell Rep.* 14, 2611–2623. doi: 10.1016/j.celrep.2016.02.053

Rodríguez-Prados, J.-C., Través, P. G., Cuenca, J., Rico, D., Aragonés, J., Martín-Sanz, P., et al. (2010). Substrate fate in activated macrophages: a comparison between innate, classic, and alternative activation. *J. Immunol.* 185, 605L–614L. doi: 10.4049/jimmunol.0901698

Rogero, M. M., and Calder, P. C. (2018). Obesity, inflammation, toll-like receptor 4 and fatty acids. *Nutrients* 10:E432. doi: 10.3390/nu10040432

Schur, E. A., Melhorn, S. J., Oh, S.-K., Lacy, J. M., Berkseth, K. E., Guyenet, S. J., et al. (2015). Radiologic evidence that hypothalamic gliosis is associated with obesity and insulin resistance in humans. *Obesity* 23, 2142–2148. doi: 10.1002/oby.21248

Sharma, D., and Kanneganti, T. D. (2016). The cell biology of inflammasomes: mechanisms of inflammasome activation and regulation. *J. Cell Biol.* 213, 617–629. doi: 10.1083/jcb.201602089

Shi, H., Kokoeva, M. V., Inouye, K., Tzameli, I., Yin, H., and Flier, J. S. (2006). TLR4 links innate immunity and fatty acid-induced insulin resistance. *J. Clin. Invest.* 116, 3015–3025. doi: 10.1172/JCI28898

Takeuchi, O., and Akira, S. (2010). Pattern recognition receptors and inflammation. *Cell* 140, 805–820. doi: 10.1016/j.cell.2010.01.022

Tannahill, G. M., Curtis, A. M., Adamik, J., Palsson-McDermott, E. M., McGettrick, A. F., Goel, G., et al. (2013). Succinate is an inflammatory signal that induces IL-1β through HIF-1α. *Nature* 496, 238–242. doi: 10.1038/nature11986

Thaler, J. P., Choi, S. J., Schwartz, M. W., and Wisse, B. E. (2010). Hypothalamic inflammation and energy homeostasis: resolving the paradox. *Front. Neuroendocrinol.* 31, 79–84. doi: 10.1016/j.yfrne.2009.10.002

Thaler, J. P., Yi, C. X., Schur, E. A., Guyenet, S. J., Hwang, B. H., Dietrich, M. O., et al. (2012). Obesity is associated with hypothalamic injury in rodents and humans. *J. Clin. Invest.* 122, 153–162. doi: 10.1172/JCI59660

Tracy, L. M., Bergqvist, F., Ivanova, E. V., Jacobsen, K. T., and Iverfeldt, K. (2013). Exposure to the saturated free fatty acid palmitate alters BV-2 microglia inflammatory response. *J. Mol. Neurosci.* 51, 805–812. doi: 10.1007/s12031-013-0068-7

Valdearcos, M., Douglass, J. D., Robblee, M. M., Dorfman, M. D., Stifler, D. R., Bennett, M. L., et al. (2017). Microglial inflammatory signaling orchestrates the hypothalamic immune response to dietary excess and mediates obesity susceptibility. *Cell Metab.* 26, 185.e3–197.e3. doi: 10.1016/j.cmet.2017.05.015

Valdearcos, M., Robblee, M. M., Benjamin, D. I., Nomura, D. K., Xu, A. W., and Koliwad, S. K. (2014). Microglia dictate the impact of saturated fat consumption on hypothalamic inflammation and neuronal function. *Cell Rep.* 9, 2124–2138. doi: 10.1016/j.celrep.2014.11.018

Valdearcos, M., Xu, A. W., and Koliwad, S. K. (2015). Hypothalamic inflammation in the control of metabolic function. *Annu. Rev. Physiol.* 77, 131–160. doi: 10.1146/annurev-physiol-021014-071656

Van den Bossche, J., O'Neill, L. A., and Menon, D. (2017). Macrophage immunometabolism: where are we (going)? *Trends Immunol.* 38, 395–406. doi: 10.1016/j.it.2017.03.001

Velloso, L. A., and Schwartz, M. W. (2011). Altered hypothalamic function in diet-induced obesity. *Int. J. Obes.* 35, 1455–1465. doi: 10.1038/ijo.2011.56

Voloboueva, L. A., Emery, J. F., Sun, X., and Giffard, R. G. (2013). Inflammatory response of microglial BV-2 cells includes a glycolytic shift and is modulated by mitochondrial glucose-regulated protein 75/mortalin. *FEBS Lett.* 587, 756–762. doi: 10.1016/j.febslet.2013.01.067

Wang, Z., Liu, D., Wang, F., Liu, S., Zhao, S., Ling, E.-A., et al. (2012). Saturated fatty acids activate microglia via Toll-like receptor 4/NF-κB signalling. *Br. J. Nutr.* 107, 229–241. doi: 10.1017/S0007114511002868

Wen, H., Gris, D., Lei, Y., Jha, S., Zhang, L., Huang, M. T. H., et al. (2011). Fatty acid-induced NLRP3-ASC inflammasome activation interferes with insulin signaling. *Nat. Immunol.* 12, 408–415. doi: 10.1038/ni.2022

White, P. J., and Marette, A. (2014). Potential role of omega-3-derived resolution mediators in metabolic inflammation. *Immunol. Cell Biol.* 92, 324–330. doi: 10.1038/icb.2013.112

Williams, N. C., and O'Neill, L. A. J. (2018). A role for the krebs cycle intermediate citrate in metabolic reprogramming in innate immunity and inflammation. *Front. Immunol.* 9:141. doi: 10.3389/fimmu.2018.00141

Wyss-Coray, T., and Mucke, L. (2002). Inflammation in neurodegenerative disease — a double-edged sword. *Neuron* 35, 419–432. doi: 10.1016/S0896-6273(02)00794-8

Yang, J., Kim, C.-S., Tu, H. T., Kim, M.-S., Goto, T., Kawada, T., et al. (2017). Quercetin protects obesity-induced hypothalamic inflammation by reducing microglia-mediated inflammatory responses via HO-1 induction. *Nutrients* 9:E650. doi: 10.3390/nu9070650

Yi, C. X., Walter, M., Gao, Y., Pitra, S., Legutko, B., Kälin, S., et al. (2017). TNFα drives mitochondrial stress in POMC neurons in obesity. *Nat. Commun.* 8:15143. doi: 10.1038/ncomms15143

Zeyda, M., Farmer, D., Todoric, J., Aszmann, O., Speiser, M., Györi, G., et al. (2007). Human adipose tissue macrophages are of an anti-inflammatory phenotype but capable of excessive pro-inflammatory mediator production. *Int. J. Obes.* 31:1420. doi: 10.1038/sj.ijo.0803632

Zhang, X., Zhang, G., Zhang, H., Karin, M., Bai, H., and Cai, D. (2008). Hypothalamic IKK beta/NF-kappa beta and ER stress link overnutrition to energy imbalance and obesity. *Cell* 135, 61–73. doi: 10.1016/j.cell.2008.07.043 doi: 10.1016/j.cell.2008.07.043

4

The Role of Leptin and Adiponectin in Obesity-Associated Cognitive Decline and Alzheimer's Disease

Leticia Forny-Germano[1], Fernanda G. De Felice[1,2] and Marcelo Nunes do Nascimento Vieira[1]*

[1] Institute of Medical Biochemistry Leopoldo de Meis, Federal University of Rio de Janeiro, Rio de Janeiro, Brazil, [2] Centre for Neuroscience Studies, Department of Psychiatry, Queen's University, Kingston, ON, Canada

***Correspondence:**
Marcelo Nunes do Nascimento Vieira
mnunes@bioqmed.ufrj.br

Cross-talk between adipose tissue and central nervous system (CNS) underlies the increased risk of obese people to develop brain diseases such as cognitive and mood disorders. Detailed mechanisms for how peripheral changes caused by adipose tissue accumulation in obesity impact the CNS to cause brain dysfunction are poorly understood. Adipokines are a large group of substances secreted by the white adipose tissue to regulate a wide range of homeostatic processes including, but not limited to, energy metabolism and immunity. Obesity is characterized by a generalized change in the levels of circulating adipokines due to abnormal accumulation and dysfunction of adipose tissue. Altered adipokine levels underlie complications of obesity as well as the increased risk for the development of obesity-related comorbidities such as type 2 diabetes, cardiovascular and neurodegenerative diseases. Here, we review the literature for the role of adipokines as key mediators of the communication between periphery and CNS in health and disease. We will focus on the actions of leptin and adiponectin, two of the most abundant and well studied adipokines, in the brain, with particular emphasis on how altered signaling of these adipokines in obesity may lead to cognitive dysfunction and augmented risk for Alzheimer's disease. A better understanding of adipokine biology in brain disorders may prove of major relevance to diagnostic, prevention and therapy.

Keywords: adipokine, leptin, adiponectin, obesity, Alzheimer's disease, cognitive decline

INTRODUCTION

Lifestyle, nutrition and lack or inefficient exercise to control body weight is making the global population more susceptible to obesity. Food with high sugar and carbohydrate contents are in general cheaper and more readily available for the current busy lives. These factors contribute to a widespread epidemic of overweight and obesity, metabolic disorders characterized by the accumulation of peripheral and/or visceral adipose tissue (Hendrickx et al., 2005; Hill et al., 2012). Obesity is a well established risk factor for a number of other chronic disorders, including type 2 diabetes, cardiovascular diseases, arthritis and some types of cancer (Elias et al., 2005; Haslam and James, 2005; Lengyel et al., 2018). More recently, attention has been drawn to the impact of obesity on central nervous system (CNS) functioning, as growing evidence indicate that the obese population are more susceptible to some neurological conditions. Overweight and, in particular, central obesity during midlife have been associated to a higher risk of developing cognitive disorders, including Alzheimer's disease (AD), later in life (Kivipelto et al., 2005; Rosengren et al., 2005; Whitmer et al., 2005, 2008). In addition, overweight and obese individuals are at higher risk for developing mood disorders, such as major depression disorder (MDD) and bipolar disorder (BD) (Luppino et al., 2010; reviewed in Mather et al., 2009; Vogelzangs et al., 2010; Vannucchi et al., 2014; Mansur et al., 2015). These evidences indicate that changes in the organism that accompany overweight and obesity can ultimately lead to CNS dysfunction. However, the pathophysiological mechanisms and molecular players underlying this connection are poorly known.

The obese body accumulates adipose tissues broadly classified in white (WAT) and brown adipose tissue (BAT) (Caron et al., 2018). Initially considered a fat storage organ, it is now established that the WAT is an endocrine organ secreting a group of substances that act in a pleiotropic manner exerting autocrine, paracrine or endocrine effects on processes in the periphery and CNS (Ahima, 2012). This class of WAT-derived substances are named adipocytokines or adipokines. Adipokines comprehend a wide range of molecules including hormones, cytokines and growth factors (Lehr et al., 2012), and exert a variety of distinct functions in the organism ranging from control of metabolism homeostasis to immune system regulation and behavior (Kiliaan et al., 2014; Fasshauer and Blüher, 2015). Abnormal production and secretion of adipokines resulting from aberrant accumulation of WAT in obesity leads to dysregulation of important homeostatic systems, resulting in the complications of obesity and in an increased risk for comorbidities such as insulin resistance and type 2 diabetes, hypertension, atherosclerosis and other cardiovascular diseases, and neurological disorders such as depression and AD (Kiliaan et al., 2014).

In the following sections, we review the literature for studies on the role of adipokines as the possible mediators of signals from the periphery to the CNS in obesity-associated brain dysfunctions. Specifically, we will focus on two of the most abundant and well studied adipokines – leptin and adiponectin – and their interaction with cognitive processes of the CNS in health and disease.

ADIPOKINES IN OBESITY AND RELATED DISEASES

Disproportional accumulation of white adipose tissue in overweight and obesity is accompanied by a generalized change in the circulating levels of several adipokines. Adipose dysfunction and adipokine dysregulation are thought to be responsible for or, at least, be an important contributor to the increased risk of obese people to develop a number of related diseases. For instance, increased levels of proinflammatory adipokines such as interleukin (IL)-1β, IL-6, TNFα and leptin, and decreased levels of anti-inflammatory adipokines, such as adiponectin, in obesity produce a chronic state of low-grade inflammation which promotes the development of insulin resistance and type-2 diabetes, hypertension, atherosclerosis and other cardiovascular diseases, and some types of cancer (Friedemann et al., 2012; Odegaard and Chawla, 2013; Hotamisligil, 2017). Moreover, since adiponectin also acts as an insulin-sensitizing hormone in muscle and liver, lower levels of adiponectin further contribute to peripheral insulin resistance in obesity (Liu et al., 2016; Saltiel and Olefsky, 2017). Lastly, increased circulating levels of leptin in obesity lead to hypothalamic leptin resistance, turning down anorexigenic and energy expenditure signals and further contributing to aggravate obesity (Waterson and Horvath, 2015).

The CNS is not exempt from negative effects of obesity, as adipose dysfunction associated with obesity have been linked to altered brain metabolism, neuroinflammation, neuronal dysfunction, brain atrophy, impaired mood and cognitive decline (Luppino et al., 2010; Ahima et al., 2017; Arshad et al., 2018). Studies associating obesity to morphometric changes in brain structure are somehow controversial. While the vast majority demonstrates obesity to be associated with lower gray matter and whole brain volumes (Pannacciulli et al., 2006; Gunstad et al., 2007; Raji et al., 2010; Yokum et al., 2011; Marqués-Iturria et al., 2013; Veit et al., 2014), fewer publications showed no association (van Boxtel et al., 2007; Sharkey et al., 2015). This controversy has been recently addressed in a meta-analysis study which found obesity to be consistently associated with lower gray matter volumes in brain areas associated with executive functions, including medial prefrontal cortex, left temporal lobe and bilateral cerebellum. These findings were further validated in the same study in an independent dataset (García-García et al., 2018).

Obesity has also been linked to cognitive disorders. Obese individuals are under greater risk to develop age-related cognitive decline, vascular dementia, mild cognitive impairment (MCI) and AD (Frisardi et al., 2010). Furthermore, animal models of obesity also develop cognitive decline (Winocur et al., 2005; Kleinert et al., 2018; McLean et al., 2018). Mechanisms proposed to underlie obesity associated risk for cognitive disorders include development of brain inflammation (Nguyen et al., 2014; Heneka et al., 2015) and central insulin resistance (de la Monte et al., 2009; Kim and Feldman, 2015). Peripheral inflammation in obesity results from secretion of proinflammatory cytokines by adipocytes and adipose tissue-resident activated macrophages (Lee and Lee, 2014). Proinflammatory cytokines such as TNFα, interleukin (IL)-1β and IL-6, have been shown to cross the blood–brain barrier (BBB) (Banks, 2005) and may act in concert with proinflammatory factors produced locally by microglial cells to foster brain inflammation in AD (De Felice and Ferreira, 2014). Importantly, such cytokines has been shown to modulate synaptic plasticity and cognition both in health and disease states (Nelson et al., 2012; Gruol, 2015; Rizzo et al., 2018). Moreover, as occurs in peripheral tissues in obesity and type 2 diabetes, proinflammatory cytokines, in particular TNFα, mediate the development of neuronal insulin resistance (Bomfim et al., 2012; Lourenco et al., 2013). Since both insulin and cytokine signaling in the brain regulate synaptic plasticity, learning and memory, neuroinflammation and neuronal insulin resistance may be key mediators of obesity-associated cognitive decline (reviewed in De Felice and Ferreira, 2014).

The increased risk for obese individuals to develop CNS pathology reflects the capacity of adipose tissue to communicate with the brain and impact brain function. It is not clear yet how this cross-talk occurs, but growing evidence indicate that adipokines are involved. Adipokines may impact brain physiology through different mechanisms. Some adipokines such as leptin and TNFα can cross the BBB and act directly in the brain while other adipokines would act on endothelial brain cells, regulating BBB permeability and the access of other circulating mediators into the brain. Importantly, in pathological states such as inflammation, the BBB integrity is compromised allowing the penetration of adipokines and other substances to which the brain is normally inaccessible. Finally, local expression of adipokines such as leptin and adiponectin have been reported in the mammalian brain (Denver et al., 2011; Thundyil et al., 2012). Advances on adipokine research have been providing information to understand how obesity affect brain function to cause brain atrophy, cognitive dysfunction, mood disorders and increase the risk for neurological diseases.

In the following sections, we will examine key aspects of leptin and adiponectin - the two most abundant and well studied adipokines - regarding their roles in brain physiology and their involvement in obesity-related cognitive dysfunction, dementia and AD (**Figure 1**).

LEPTIN

Leptin in the Brain

The discovery of leptin in 1994 is considered the cornerstone for adipokine research (Zhang et al., 1994). Leptin is classically related to the central control of food intake and energy homeostasis (Friedman, 2016). However, other neurophysiological functions have been attributed to leptin, including brain development (Ahima et al., 1998; Bouret, 2010) neurogenesis (Garza et al., 2008), neuronal protection (Doherty et al., 2013), mood and stress regulation (Lu et al., 2006; Paz-Filho et al., 2010), reproduction and reproductive behaviors (Caprio et al., 2001; Lu et al., 2006; Chehab, 2014).

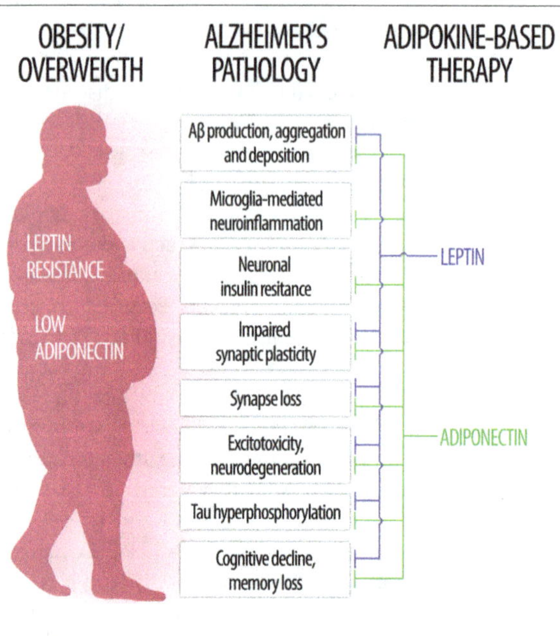

FIGURE 1 | The role of leptin and adiponectin in Alzheimer's disease physiopathology. (Left) In obesity, low levels of circulating adiponectin as well as central leptin resistance may contribute to brain pathology and increased risk for Alzheimer's disease. (Right) Conversely, therapeutic approaches based on leptin (blue) and adiponectin (green) signaling may counteract a wide range of pathological processes associated to AD (center).

Leptin is mainly produced by adipose tissue, more specifically by visceral white adipocytes in rodent and by subcutaneous adipose tissue in human (Trayhurn et al., 1995; Hube et al., 1996). However, local expression of leptin mRNA and protein in CNS has been reported (Morash et al., 1999; Scott et al., 2009; Patterson et al., 2011). Circulating levels of leptin are dynamic and susceptible to different regulatory factors such as metabolism, body fat mass, circadian cycle and sexual dimorphisms (Trayhurn et al., 1995; Licinio et al., 1997; Saad et al., 1997; Park and Ahima, 2015). Leptin crosses the BBB by binding to specific receptors or interacting with BBB. The partially saturate influx of leptin through BBB indicates that membrane proteins facilitate leptin uptake where the entrance is limited by transport dynamics (Banks et al., 1996). There is evidence that leptin transport into the brain can be mediated by megalin at the choroid plexus epithelium (Dietrich et al., 2008; Bartolome et al., 2017) and by short LepR isoforms in tanycytes (Hileman et al., 2002; Balland et al., 2014; Di Spiezio et al., 2018). Therefore, levels of leptin in the brain are subject to regulation by local leptin production, circulating leptin levels and leptin transport across BBB through different mechanisms.

Leptin receptors (LepR or ObR) were first detected in 1995 at the mouse choroid plexus (Tartaglia et al., 1995). Posterior studies revealed that alternative splicing during LepR-coding *db* gene expression result in six different LepR isoforms (LepRa-f) (Lee et al., 1996; Wang et al., 1996). Long leptin receptor (LepRb) is the isoform which best bind to leptin and activate intracellular pathways (Allison and Myers, 2014). LepRs are tyrosine-kinase receptors that undergo autophosphorylation upon leptin binding to activate different signaling cascades, including JAK/STAT, ERK/MAPK and IRS/PI3K pathways. STAT (signal transducer and activator of transcription) is a family of transcription factor which, upon phosphorylation, migrate to the nucleus and regulate transcription of target genes such as the suppressor of cytokine signaling 3 (SOCS3) and protein tyrosine phosphatase 1B (PTP1B). STAT3 is the major signaling pathway recruited by leptin and, due to its responsive property, STAT3 phosphorylation became an alternative way to identify leptin-responsive cells and infer leptin sensitivity (Ramos-Lobo and Donato, 2017; Pan and Myers, 2018).

LepRb is the main isoform of leptin receptor expressed in the brain. Robust expression comprehends the arcuate nucleus (ARC), the paraventricular nucleus and the dorsomedial, lateral and ventromedial regions of the hypothalamus (Schwartz et al., 1996; Wauman and Tavernier, 2011; Mercer et al., 2018). Extrahypothalamic sites also express leptin receptors including hippocampus, cortex, midbrain and hindbrain (Elmquist et al., 2005; Patterson et al., 2011). A transgenic mouse expressing LepRb-cre in combination with cre-inducible enhanced green fluorescent protein (EGFP) and farnesylated EGFP (EGFPf) was used to reveal a detailed distribution of LepRb expressing neurons as well as their projection sites throughout the brain (Patterson et al., 2011). Regions found to contain LepRb expressing neurons were consistent with those previously determined by examination of LepRb mRNA expression via *in situ* hybridization (Elmquist et al., 1998), but this study further identified projections sites of LepRb neurons in the brain. LepRb neurons and projection were observed throughout the prefrontal cortex, while more discrete, circumscribed regions containing both LepRb neurons and projections were found in insular, temporal, auditory, somatosensory and visual cortices (Patterson et al., 2011). The hippocampus displayed few LepRb neurons along with projections from LepRb neurons mostly concentrated in CA1–3 regions and, to a lower extent, in the dentate (Elmquist et al., 2005; Mercer et al., 2018).

The wide variety of leptin effects in the CNS likely reflects the peculiar distribution of leptin receptors through different brain structures as well as the particular signaling cascades activated by these receptors in distinct regions (Bjørbaek and Kahn, 2004).

In the following sections, we review key aspects of brain leptin signaling that are relevant for its role in cognitive decline and AD (**Table 1**).

Leptin in Synaptic Function and Memory

Synaptic plasticity is a crucial event for learning and memory process. Long-term potentiation (LTP) and long-term depression (LTD) of synaptic transmission are pivotal mechanisms in hippocampal memory formation and consolidation (Bliss and Collingridge, 1993). At the molecular level, LTP and LTD are regulated by insertion or removal of NMDA- and AMPA-type glutamate receptors from post-synaptic terminals, thereby modulating synaptic transmission strength (Malenka and Bear, 2004).

There is substantial evidence indicating that leptin regulates hippocampal synaptic plasticity and memory. LepRs in hippocampal neurons are closely associated with somato-dendritic and synaptic regions, indicating the potential for leptin to modulate synaptic function (Harvey, 2015). Recent studies demonstrate that leptin activation of JAK2/STAT3 signaling pathway induces transcription of genes related to LTD (McGregor et al., 2017). Moreover, learning and memory formation are modulated by JAK2/STAT5 signaling (Furigo et al., 2018), a pathway also subject to regulation by leptin receptor signaling in the hippocampus (Gong et al., 2007). Two different LepR-deficient rodent strains (Zucker rats and db/db mice) show impaired LTP in the CA1 region of the hippocampus, which is accompanied by poor performance in the water maze spatial memory test (Li et al., 2002). Conversely, leptin treatment has been shown to improve learning and memory performances in different models (Shanley et al., 2001; Oomura et al., 2006; reviewed in Irving and Harvey, 2013).

Leptin was shown to regulated synaptic plasticity by targeting NMDA- and AMPA-receptors trafficking, particularly in the CA1 region of the hippocampus. Schaffer collaterals (SCs) and temporoammonic (TA) projections to CA1 pyramidal neurons exhibit an age-dependent response to leptin. Interestingly, these functionally distinct circuits appear to respond differently to leptin exposure. In SC-CA1 synapses, leptin was shown to induce depression of synaptic transmission in young rodents

TABLE 1 | Summary of the main findings associating leptin signaling to physiopathological processes relevant to AD.

Finding	Model(s)	Reference
Leptin signaling modulates synaptic function and plasticity	Hippocampal slices from adult rats	Shanley et al., 2001; Xu et al., 2008; Moult et al., 2009, 2010; Luo et al., 2015; McGregor and Harvey, 2017; McGregor et al., 2018
LepR-deficiency causes impairment of LTP and spatial memory	Zucker rats and db/db mice	Li et al., 2002
Leptin treatment improves learning and memory	Hippocampal slices from adult rats; rats ICV-infused with Aβ; AD mouse models (SAMP-8 mice; CRND8 transgenic mice (TgCRND8) and APP/PS1	Shanley et al., 2001; Farr et al., 2006; Oomura et al., 2006; Greco et al., 2010; Pérez-González et al., 2014; Tong et al., 2015
Deficient leptin transport across BBB	Aged mice, APP/PS1 mice	Carro et al., 2005; Dietrich et al., 2008
PTP1B upregulation	APP/PS1 mice; Human AD patients	Pei et al., 1994; Mody et al., 2011; King et al., 2018
SOCS3 upregulation	APP/PS1 mice; human AD patients	Walker et al., 2015; Iwahara et al., 2017; King et al., 2018
Impaired leptin signaling	Human AD patients; Tg 2576 mice; APP/PS1 mice	Bonda et al., 2014; Maioli et al., 2015
Decreased leptin levels in CSF and plasma	Human AD patients	Holden et al., 2009; Lieb et al., 2009; Bigalke et al., 2011; Chakrabarti, 2014; Johnston et al., 2014; Khemka et al., 2014b; Baranowska-Bik et al., 2015
Increased leptin levels in CSF and brain	Human AD patients	Bonda et al., 2014; Yin et al., 2018
Unchanged leptin levels in CSF and brain	Human AD patients	Maioli et al., 2015; Oania and McEvoy, 2015
Aβ disrupts leptin signaling	Human AD patients; rabbit hippocampal slices	Marwarha et al., 2010; Bonda et al., 2014
Leptin reduce Aβ levels	SH-SY5Y cells; Neuro2a cells; primary neuronal cultures from rat embryos; APP/PS1 mice; adult rats	Fewlass et al., 2004; Pérez-González et al., 2014; Tong et al., 2015
Leptin reduce tau hyperphosphorylation	SH-SY5Y cells; NT2 cells; primary rat cortical neurons	Greco et al., 2008

hippocampus (Xu et al., 2008; Moult et al., 2009) whereas, in adult animals, leptin promote synaptic strengthening and LTP (Moult et al., 2010; Moult and Harvey, 2011). Different effects were observed in TA-CA1 synapses, where leptin induces LTP in young (Luo et al., 2015), promote LTD in the adult but had no effect on synaptic transmission in aged rat hippocampus (McGregor et al., 2018). Importantly, the age- and regional-variability of leptin effects on hippocampal synaptic plasticity appears to be driven by the composition of NMDARs subtypes, and to be achieved by regulating the traffic of different subsets of AMPARs toward and away from synapses. Leptin regulation of synaptic plasticity involves several downstream targets, including JAK2-STAT3, PTEN, PI3K, ERK, and CaMKII (for more comprehensive reviews, see Moult and Harvey, 2009; McGregor and Harvey, 2017).

Leptin Resistance

Several studies demonstrated that leptin responsiveness decreases with obesity, aging and neurodegenerative diseases, a phenomenon called leptin resistance. Leptin resistance affects a range of processes such as food intake, insulin sensitivity, inflammation and cognition. In obesity, leptin resistance leads to increased production of leptin by adipocytes and hyperleptinemia, in an attempt of the organism to compensate for low leptin responsiveness. Decreased leptin signaling in the CNS may be related to defective leptin transport across BBB, LepR downregulation and/or deficient leptin signaling downstream LepRs (Myers et al., 2008, 2012; de Git and Adan, 2015; Bluher, 2016; Banks et al., 2018).

Triglycerides can impair BBB leptin transport causing central leptin deficiency (Banks et al., 2004). Furthermore, it was recently demonstrated that triglycerides can cross the BBB to directly induce hypothalamic leptin and insulin receptor resistance, leading to decreased satiety and cognitive impairment in mice (Banks et al., 2018). Interestingly, triglycerides increased leptin binding in different brain regions, suggesting an allosteric or post-receptor rather than a competitive mechanism of inhibition of LepR signaling by triglycerides (Banks et al., 2018). In light of longitudinal studies linking increased mid-life triglyceride levels to the risk for AD (Vemuri et al., 2017; Nägga et al., 2018), the above results suggest that triglycerides may contribute to AD pathogenesis and progression by suppressing leptin signaling in the brain. Deficient leptin transport across BBB by megalin leading to reduced leptin entry into the brain has also been described in aged mice and in mouse models of AD (Carro et al., 2005; Dietrich et al., 2008).

At the intracellular level, leptin signaling is negatively regulated by the suppressor of SOCS3 and by the PTP1B. SOCS3 binds to LepR and JAK2 to inhibit their activities, whereas PTP1B dephosphorylates tyrosine residues deactivating LepR and JAK2. PTP1B have been linked to central leptin resistance in humans (Myers et al., 2010) as well as in a variety of animal models of obesity (Cheng et al., 2002; Zabolotny et al., 2002; White et al., 2009) and aging (Morrison et al., 2007). SOCS3 and PTP1B were also found upregulated in the brains of AD mouse models (Mody et al., 2011; Iwahara et al., 2017; King et al., 2018) and AD patients (Pei et al., 1994; Walker et al., 2015). Therefore, targeting PTP1B and SOCS3 may prove valuable to overcome central leptin resistance in obesity, aging, and AD (Engin, 2017; Vieira et al., 2017).

Central leptin resistance can also be mediated by downregulation of LepRs expression. In this regard, LepR levels were found to be decreased in the hippocampus of AD patients, whereas leptin levels were upregulated both in CSF and locally in the hippocampus, possibly due to a compensatory mechanism for receptor dysfunction (Bonda et al., 2014; Maioli et al., 2015). Age-dependent changes in LepR expression levels were also reported in Tg2576 and APP/PS1 mouse models of AD (Maioli et al., 2015; King et al., 2018). Although the results from these studies are hard to interpret, they are consistent with an impact of AD phenotypes in LepR expression in brain areas relevant to cognition and memory.

Taken together, the results described above indicate that impaired brain leptin signaling may play a role in AD pathophysiology, and that restoring leptin signaling may constitute a valid approach to restore synaptic function and cognition in AD.

Leptin Signaling, Obesity, and Alzheimer's Disease

Several studies indicate that over-weight and obesity during mid-age increases risk to develop AD (Whitmer et al., 2008; Hassing et al., 2009; Xu et al., 2011; Gustafson et al., 2012; Emmerzaal et al., 2014; Alhurani et al., 2016). In contrast, high weight in late-life was shown to be protective against AD and cognitive decline (Hughes and Ganguli, 2009; Gustafson et al., 2012; Emmerzaal et al., 2014; Bell et al., 2017). Surprisingly, weight loss in late age is related to higher risk for dementia and AD (Barrett-Connor et al., 1996; Buchman et al., 2005; Stewart et al., 2005; Johnson et al., 2006; Hughes and Ganguli, 2009; Gao et al., 2011; Joo et al., 2018). This apparently paradoxical influence of body weight on dementia and AD risk is far from being understood. Interestingly, a similarly complex relation is observed between overweight/obesity and other neurodegenerative diseases. For instance, in amyotrophic lateral sclerosis (ALS) patients, mild obesity is associated with increased survival rates, whereas morbid obesity increases mortality rates (Paganoni et al., 2011; Gallo et al., 2013). The influence of body weight on the clinical outcomes of dementia, AD and other neurodegenerative diseases suggest that adipose tissue dysfunction and adipokines dysregulation may play a broad role across the spectrum of neurodegenerative diseases. Moreover, the explanation for this puzzling and somehow paradoxical influence of adiposity on brain diseases may lie in how weight changes impact production and action of adipokines such as leptin and adiponectin.

Evidence regarding how leptin levels are affected in AD are controversial. Several studies show decreased leptin levels in CSF and plasma in AD patients (Holden et al., 2009; Lieb et al., 2009; Bigalke et al., 2011; Chakrabarti, 2014; Johnston et al., 2014; Khemka et al., 2014b; Baranowska-Bik et al., 2015) whereas increased leptin levels (Bonda et al., 2014; Yin et al., 2018) and unaffected levels (Maioli et al., 2015; Oania and McEvoy, 2015) in CSF and cerebral tissue were also reported. Conflicting findings can be associate to variations in dementia score, post-mortem neuropathological analyses to confirm dementia, sample size, stratification in sex, age, and others (Kiliaan et al., 2014; Mcguire and Ishii, 2016).

Leptin signaling was found to interact with several mechanisms associated with AD physiopathology. Aβ disrupt leptin signaling leading to down-regulation of hippocampal leptin and LepR expression (Marwarha et al., 2010; Bonda et al., 2014). Conversely, leptin was reported to be neuroprotective in AD models by suppressing Aβ accumulation and toxicity and attenuating tau pathology. Leptin administration reduce Aβ levels in the Tg2576 mouse model of AD (Fewlass et al., 2004). The anti-amyloidogenic effect of leptin involve inhibition of APP processing by down regulating β-amyloid precursor protein (APP) cleaving enzyme (BACE1) and increase in APOE-dependent Aβ uptake, and seems to be mediated by activation of AMP-activated protein kinase (AMPK) (Fewlass et al., 2004; Marwarha et al., 2010; Pérez-González et al., 2014; Tong et al., 2015).

Tau phosphorylation can be suppressed by leptin modulation of GSK3β activity (Greco et al., 2008). Importantly, leptin treatment also improve memory performance in different mouse models of AD (Farr et al., 2006; Greco et al., 2010; Pérez-González et al., 2014). In a rat model of intracerebroventricular Aβ injection, chronic leptin administration rescued Aβ-induced impairment of spatial memory and late-phase LTP (Tong et al., 2015). Leptin was further shown to enhance hippocampal neurogenesis in AD mice (Pérez-González et al., 2011). Collectively, the above studies provide initial validation for the potential therapeutic applications of leptin signaling enhancement in AD brains.

ADIPONECTIN

Adiponectin is a 30 KDa adipokine encoded by the AdipoQ gene, mainly produced and secreted by adipocytes and highly abundant in human plasma. Adiponectin is known to increase insulin sensitivity of target organs such as liver and muscle, ultimately regulating peripheral glucose and fatty acid metabolism (Hotta et al., 2001; Yamauchi et al., 2001, 2002). Besides being a metabolic regulator, adiponectin is also known for its anti-inflammatory and anti-oxidant activity (Takemura et al., 2007; Liu Y. et al., 2015). These characteristics make adiponectin a protective factor in conditions such as obesity, type 2 diabetes and cardiovascular diseases (Yamauchi et al., 2003a; Spranger et al., 2006; Antoniades et al., 2009). Levels of circulating adiponectin are decreased in obesity and metabolic syndrome, likely contributing to the development of insulin resistance (Arita et al., 1999; Hotta et al., 2001; Yang et al., 2001). Low levels of adiponectin have also been linked to several types of cancer (Miyoshi et al., 2003; Bao et al., 2013; Ma et al., 2016) and cardiovascular diseases (Komatsu et al., 2004).

Adiponectin naturally self-associate to form different types of aggregates. In plasma, adiponectin exists as trimers, hexamers or high molecular weight (HMW) multimers. Adiponectin trimers are mainly stabilized by non-covalent interactions, whereas larger aggregates require crosslinking between subunits by disulfide bonds (Waki et al., 2003). In addition, adiponectin also circulates as biologically active globular fragment generated through proteolysis of full-length adiponectin (Fruebis et al., 2001). Importantly, these post-translational modifications affect biological activity, as distinct adiponectin complexes present tissue-specificity and may activate different signaling pathways (for reviews, see Wang et al., 2008; Liu and Liu, 2014).

Adiponectin acts through binding to three different receptors: adiponectin receptor 1 (AdipoR1), adiponectin receptor 2 (AdipoR2) and T-cadherin. AdipoR1 and AdipoR2 are the most abundant sites for adiponectin binding and mediate most of adiponectin actions through the organism (Yamauchi et al., 2003b, 2007). Activation of AdipoRs by adiponectin leads to the recruitment of the adaptor protein APPL1 (adaptor protein, phosphotyrosine interacting with PH domain and leucine zipper 1) (Mao et al., 2006) which, in turn, mediates downstream adiponectin signaling through a number of different pathways including AMPK, PI3K-Akt, MAPK-Erk1/2, PPARα, p38-MAPK, PTEN and JNK (Cheng et al., 2007; Chandrasekar et al., 2008; Coope et al., 2008; Lee et al., 2008). APPL1 also plays a crucial role in the insulin sensitization effect of adiponectin by interacting with and facilitating the binding of IRS1/2 to the insulin receptor (Ryu et al., 2014).

Adiponectin in the Brain

Data from epidemiological studies demonstrate that diabetes, obesity, and metabolic syndrome increase the risk of developing cognitive problems and dementia (Stewart and Liolitsa, 1999; Baker et al., 2011; Kerwin et al., 2011; McCrimmon et al., 2012; Lehtisalo et al., 2016; Espeland et al., 2017; Pal et al., 2018; Palta et al., 2018). More recently, evidence indicate that insulin signaling dysfunction and chronic neuroinflammation are key factors in cognitive decline, MCI and AD (Steen et al., 2005; Arnold et al., 2018, reviewed in De Felice, 2013; Ferreira et al., 2014; Heneka et al., 2015). In face of these observations, adiponectin has gained attention in the context of such CNS disorders due to its potentially protective actions as an anti-inflammatory and insulin sensitizing hormone.

Adiponectin is present in human and mouse CSF, albeit in much lower concentrations than in blood (Kubota et al., 2007; Kusminski et al., 2007; Neumeier et al., 2007). However, the source(s) for adiponectin in CNS are not completely clear. Initial studies suggested that adiponectin expression was limited to adipocytes and, to a lower extent, other peripheral tissues such as liver, muscle, placenta, and epithelium. More recently, however, some studies reported adiponectin expression at both mRNA and protein levels in the chicken and mammalian brain (Maddineni et al., 2005; Hoyda et al., 2007; Kaminski et al., 2014; Shen et al., 2014). Whether peripheral adiponectin crosses the BBB to reach the brain is a matter of debate. While some studies conclude that adiponectin does not cross the BBB (Pan et al., 2006; Spranger et al., 2006), other studies found evidence suggesting that peripheral adiponectin does reach the brain through the BBB (Qi et al., 2004; Yau et al., 2014). This is an important open question with physiological and potential translational relevance, since adiponectin-based therapies to treat brain conditions would possibly consist of peripheral administration and require adiponectin to reach the CNS. Therefore, further studies are required to clarify whether or not peripheral adiponectin can reach the brain tissue through BBB.

Adiponectin receptors are also expressed in different structures of the brain. The hypothalamus is the best documented site for AdipoRs expression in the mammalian brain, but there is also evidence for expression in endothelial brain cells, cerebral cortex, brain stem and hippocampus (Yamauchi et al., 2003b, 2007) reviewed in (Thundyil et al., 2012). Interestingly, a study in post mortem human brains also revealed intense immunostaining for AdipoR1 in the nucleus basalis magnocellularis (NBM) (Psilopanagioti et al., 2009), a small structure rich in cholinergic neurons projecting diffusely to the whole neocortex and other brain areas, and that is severely affected in AD (Liu A.K. et al., 2015).

Adiponectin functions in the brain are highly diversified. It has been shown to act locally in the brain to control key processes of brain physiology including neuronal excitability and synaptic plasticity, neuroprotection, neurogenesis and regulation of glial cells activation (Yau et al., 2014; Chabry et al., 2015; Song et al., 2015; Nicolas et al., 2017; Shah et al., 2017; Pousti et al., 2018). More recently, adiponectin was found to modulate glucose metabolism in hippocampal neurons, increasing glucose uptake, glycolysis and ATP production rates (Cisternas et al., 2018). Adiponectin also acts on brain to regulate peripheral and systemic processes such as thermogenesis, energy expenditure (Qi et al., 2004) and reproduction (Angelidis et al., 2012). Finally, central adiponectin has been shown to regulate behaviors like food intake (Suyama et al., 2016), locomotor activity (Miyatake et al., 2015) as well as cognition, anxiety and mood (Jeong et al., 2012; Zhang et al., 2017; Cao et al., 2018; Cezaretto et al., 2018; Nicolas et al., 2018; Platzer et al., 2018; Sun et al., 2018). This variety of central effects of adiponectin likely reflects the wide distribution of different adiponectin receptors throughout the brain. For the purpose of this review, the following sections will focus on roles of adiponectin that are most likely relevant to cognitive dysfunction and AD, namely synaptic regulation, insulin sensitivity, neuroinflammation, neuroprotection and neurogenesis (**Table 2**).

Adiponectin in Synaptic Function and Memory

Synapse loss is the best pathological correlate for clinical manifestations of cognitive dysfunction in AD (DeKosky and Scheff, 1990; Terry et al., 1991). Compelling evidence indicate that Aβ oligomers, toxins that accumulate in AD brains, target synapses impairing synaptic function and plasticity and causing synapse loss (reviewed in Lambert et al., 1998; Ferreira and Klein, 2011; Forny-Germano et al., 2014) Aβ oligomers inhibit LTP and promote LTD of hippocampal synapses *in vitro* and *in vivo* (Wang et al., 2002; Shankar et al., 2008; Li et al., 2009; Jürgensen et al., 2011).

Interestingly, recent data indicate that adiponectin signaling directly regulates synaptic function and plasticity, preserving and enhancing cognitive functions in a number of different models. Intracerebroventricular administration of adiponectin in anesthetized rats potentiates high frequency stimulation (HFS)-induced LTP and suppresses low-frequency stimulation (LFS)-induced LTD. Furthermore, adiponectin administration alone induced a chemical LTP, independent of presynaptic stimulus (Pousti et al., 2018). Osmotin, a plant-derived homolog of adiponectin capable of activate AdipoRs, improves LTP impairment and ameliorates memory deficits in a mouse model of AD (Shah et al., 2017). This effect appears to be mediated by AdipoR1 and the Nogo66 receptor 1 (NgR1) and involve promotion of neurite outgrowth and increasing of dendritic spine and synapse density in the hippocampus (Zhang et al., 2016; Yoon et al., 2018). Adiponectin-deficient mice displays increased excitability of hippocampal dentate gyrus (DG) granule neurons, associated with impaired extinction of contextual fear memory. Adiponectin and its mimetic drug AdipoRon restored fear memory extinction via AdipoR2 activation and inhibition of DG neuron excitability (Zhang et al., 2017). Aged adiponectin-deficient mice have reduced levels of synaptic proteins suggesting synapse loss, and also performs poorly in spatial memory and contextual fear conditioning tests (Ng et al., 2016). Importantly, both adiponectin and osmotin treatments ameliorate learning and memory deficits in AD animal models (Ali et al., 2015; Shah et al., 2017). Caloric restriction increases circulating adiponectin levels and improve cognition in mice probably via regulation of the AMPK signaling pathway in mouse hippocampus (Ma et al., 2018). Finally, a recent clinical study found that individuals with higher adiponectin levels tend to perform better in a delayed word recall test, supporting the notion that adiponectin is a protective factor against cognitive decline and represents a promising therapeutic strategy in cognitive disorders (Cezaretto et al., 2018).

Collectively, these recent studies consistently established a previously ignored ability of adiponectin to regulate hippocampal synaptic function and plasticity and to improve cognitive function, learning and memory. This further support a protective role for adiponectin in AD, suggesting that diminished brain adiponectin signaling in obesity may favor AD onset and progression and that adiponectin signaling may be an interesting target in AD therapy.

Adiponectin in Central Insulin Signaling

Neuronal insulin signaling is important for synaptic plasticity and memory, mainly by regulating glutamate receptors trafficking (Beattie et al., 2000; Man et al., 2000; Skeberdis et al., 2001; Zhao et al., 2004). Impaired insulin signaling is well documented both in human AD patients and in a variety of AD animal models (Steen et al., 2005; Bomfim et al., 2012; Talbot et al., 2012) and is considered an important mechanism for neuronal dysfunction and cognitive impairment in AD (Ferreira et al., 2014; Vieira et al., 2018) Synaptotoxicity of Aβ oligomers is accompanied by insulin receptor dysfunction *in vitro* and

TABLE 2 | Summary of the main findings associating adiponectin signaling to physiopathological processes relevant to AD.

Finding	Model(s)	Reference
Adiponectin and AdipoRs signaling modulates synaptic function and plasticity	APP/PS1 mice; NSE-APPsw mice; adiponectin-deficient mice; rats	Zhang et al., 2016, 2017; Shah et al., 2017; Pousti et al., 2018; Yoon et al., 2018
Adiponectin deficiency causes AD-like synapse loss and memory impairment	Adiponectin-deficient mice	Ng et al., 2016
Adiponectin signaling improves memory	Adiponectin-deficient mice; APP/PS1 mice; NSE-APPsw mice; Aβ i.c.v.-infused mice	Ali et al., 2015; Shah et al., 2017; Zhang et al., 2017
High adiponectin levels is associated with better cognitive performance	Middle-aged non-diabetic humans	Cezaretto et al., 2018
Adiponectin signaling deficiency leads to impaired brain insulin signaling	Adiponectin knockout mice; AdipoR1 deficient mice	Ng et al., 2016; Kim et al., 2017
Adiponectin improve neuronal insulin sensitivity	Insulin resistant SH-SY5Y human neuroblastoma cells	Ng et al., 2016
Adiponectin deficiency promote neuroinflammation	Adiponectin knockout mice	Ng et al., 2016
Adiponectin signaling attenuates microglia-mediated neuroinflammation	Environment-enriched mice; adiponectin deficient mice; mouse model of intracerebral hemorrhage; brain sorted microglia; primary microglial cells; BV2 microglial cells exposed to Aβ	Chabry et al., 2015; Nicolas et al., 2015, 2017; Song et al., 2017; Zhao et al., 2018
Adiponectin and AdipoRs agonists are neuroprotective	Primary rat hippocampal neurons; SH-SY5Y cells; rodent models of hemorrhagic and ischemic stroke	Jung et al., 2006; Chen et al., 2009; Jeon et al., 2009; Qiu et al., 2011; Chan et al., 2012; Song et al., 2013, 2015; Guo et al., 2015; Wang et al., 2016; Yang et al., 2017; Ma et al., 2018
Adiponectin and AdipoRs agonists promotes neurogenesis	Exercised mice; adiponectin deficient mice; corticosterone-induced anxiety/depressive-like mice	Yau et al., 2014; Chan et al., 2017; Nicolas et al., 2018
Adiponectin and AdipoRs agonists has antidepressive proporties	Exercised mice; corticosterone-induced anxiety/depressive-like mice	Yau et al., 2014; Zhang et al., 2016; Chan et al., 2017; Nicolas et al., 2018
Adiponectin signaling deficiency produce AD like phenotypes	Adiponectin knockout mice; AdipoR1 deficient mice	Ng et al., 2016; Kim et al., 2017
Adiponectin signaling impairment in AD models	APP/PS1 mice	Várhelyi et al., 2017
Adiponectin reduce Aβ production and aggregation	APP/PS1 mice; SH-SY5Y cells overexpressing APP	Shah et al., 2017
Adiponectin attenuates tau hyperphosphorylation	Streptozotocin injected rats	Xu et al., 2018
Altered levels of adiponectin in AD (conflicting results have been reported, see the Section "Adiponectin in Alzheimer's Disease" for details)	Human subjects	Kamogawa et al., 2010; Une et al., 2010; van Himbergen et al., 2012; Teixeira et al., 2013; Khemka et al., 2014a; García-Casares et al., 2016; Ma et al., 2016

in vivo and can be prevented by treatment with insulin sensitizing drugs and by insulin itself (De Felice et al., 2009; Bomfim et al., 2012; Batista et al., 2018). These discoveries encouraged several groups to evaluate the efficacy of different classes of anti-diabetic drugs in AD models, and positive preclinical results paved the way for human clinical trials (for comprehensive reviews, see De Felice, 2013; Yarchoan and Arnold, 2014; de la Monte, 2017). In this context, interest has recently been directed to the insulin-sensitizing actions of adiponectin to correct aberrant insulin signaling in AD. Impaired brain insulin signaling was observed, along with several other AD-like pathological features, in adiponectin knockout mice and in AdipoR1 deficient mice (Ng et al., 2016; Kim et al., 2017). Conversely, adiponectin increases insulin sensitivity in SH-SY5Y neuronal cell line modeling insulin resistance, through AdipoR1 receptor activation of AMPK (Ng et al., 2016). These data indicate that adiponectin has the potential to restore neuronal insulin signaling, with possible therapeutic implications for AD and other neurodegenerative diseases. However, further translational studies using proper animal models of AD are required to validate adiponectin signaling as a therapeutic approach to overcome brain insulin resistance in AD.

Adiponectin in Neuroinflammation

Adiponectin is well known for its anti-inflammatory activity in peripheral tissues, which include suppression of macrophage activation and secretion of pro-inflammatory cytokines (Yokota et al., 2000; Elfeky et al., 2016, 2018). For that, adiponectin is considered a protective factor against pathological processes such as peripheral insulin resistance and cardiovascular diseases, whereas low levels of adiponectin in obesity contributes to chronic inflammation and obesity-associated risk for related diseases (For recent reviews, see Ohashi et al., 2015; Liu et al., 2016).

Alzheimer's disease is also characterized by a chronic state of low-grade inflammation in the brain. This response is mediated by microglial cells activation and secretion of pro-inflammatory cytokines TNFα, IL-6, and IL-1β (Bamberger et al., 2003; Lourenco et al., 2013; Heneka et al., 2015; reviewed in De Felice and Lourenco, 2015; Sarlus and Heneka, 2017). Proinflammatory cytokines trigger a series of detrimental events in the AD brain, including neuronal insulin resistance, endoplasmic reticulum stress, synaptotoxicity and neurodegeneration (Bomfim et al., 2012; Lourenco et al., 2013; Rizzo et al., 2018).

Adiponectin-knockout mice develop a series of pathological features in the brain resembling AD, including insulin resistance, reduced levels of synaptic proteins and the presence of neuroinflammatory markers such as microgliosis, astrogliosis and elevated levels of the pro-inflammatory cytokines TNFα and IL-1β (Ng et al., 2016). Environmental enrichment, housing conditions that promote physical activity, cognitive engagement and social interactions, has been shown to improve cognitive functions and be protective in AD mouse models. These effects are at least in part due to modulation of microglial response to the insult of Aβ oligomers (Xu et al., 2016; Vieira and Beckman, 2017). Interestingly, it was recently shown that beneficial effects of environmental enrichment to the brain are mediated by adiponectin, and involves the promotion of an anti-inflammatory activation state of microglia with decreased production of pro-inflammatory cytokines (Chabry et al., 2015; Nicolas et al., 2015). The same group also showed that globular adiponectin directly inhibits microglia pro-inflammatory profile *in vivo* and *in vitro* (Nicolas et al., 2017) in a mechanism involving AdipoR1 and NF-κB. Adiponectin also modulates microglial activation profile under Aβ toxicity *in vitro*, via PPARγ activation (Song et al., 2017). Further evidence for the anti-inflammatory actions of adiponectin in the CNS come from a study showing that CTRP9, an AdipoR1 agonist, attenuates neuroinflammation in a mouse model of intracerebral hemorrhage through a AdipoR1/AMPK/NFκB signaling mechanism (Zhao et al., 2018). Moreover, AdipoRon treatment suppresses macrophage recruitment in a model of spinal cord injury (Zhou et al., 2018). Finally, it has been proposed that adiponectin can also modulate neuroinflammation by reducing expression of pro-inflammatory cytokines by brain endothelial cells (Spranger et al., 2006). These evidences support a role for adiponectin in mitigating brain inflammation, and suggest that adiponectin deficiency in obesity may trigger neuroinflammatory events leading to AD and other related CNS disorders.

Adiponectin in Neuroprotection and Neurogenesis

Neurodegeneration in AD is mediated by overactivation of glutamate receptors and excessive neuronal calcium influx, a process called excitotoxicity (Dong et al., 2009; Wang and Reddy, 2017; Arshad et al., 2018). Excitotoxicity can be triggered by toxic amyloid-β aggregates *in vitro* and *in vivo*, and represents an important pathological mechanism in synaptic failure and neuronal death in AD (reviewed in Paula-Lima et al., 2013). Excitotoxicity is commonly associated with mitochondrial dysfunction and oxidative stress (Johnston et al., 2014; Bhat et al., 2015), and also occurs in other pathological conditions such as stroke and brain and spinal cord injuries (Li and Stys, 2000; Ahuja et al., 2017).

In the past few years, a growing number of studies demonstrated the neuroprotective properties of adiponectin and other AdipoRs agonists against a variety of neuronal toxic insults *in vitro* and *in vivo*. *In vitro*, adiponectin was shown to protect SH-SY5Y human neuroblastoma cells against oxidative stress and cytotoxicity induced by Aβ and MPP+, an inhibitor of mitochondrial complex I (Jung et al., 2006; Chan et al., 2012). Adiponectin neuroprotection was also observed in a model of kainic acid (KA)-induced excitotoxicity in primary cultures of rat hippocampal neurons (Jeon et al., 2009; Qiu et al., 2011). A series of studies also reported neuroprotective roles of adiponectin and AdipoRs in different models of hemorrhagic and ischemic stroke. Cellular mechanisms reported to underlie adiponectin and AdipoRs neuroprotection include suppression of oxidative stress, apoptosis and inflammation, and involve a remarkable variety of intracellular targets, including antioxidant enzymes, AMPK, JNK/PI3K/Akt, PKA, GSK3β, NFkappaB, Bax/Bcl-2 and caspase 3 (Chen et al., 2009; Song et al., 2013, 2015; Guo et al., 2015; Wang et al., 2016; Yang et al., 2017; Ma et al., 2018). These neuroprotective actions of adiponectin may be therapeutically applicable in neurodegenerative diseases.

The antidepressant effects of physical exercise are well known and widely used in the clinic as a non-pharmacological treatment for depression. Recently, adiponectin was shown to play a crucial role in antidepressant effects of exercise, by mediating exercise-induced hippocampal neurogenesis (Yau et al., 2014; Chan et al., 2017). The neurogenic and neurotrophic effects of adiponectin signaling were further demonstrated by intracerebroventricular injection of adiponectin in adiponectin-deficient mice (Zhang et al., 2016). Remarkably, chronic intraperitoneal administration of the AdipoRs agonist AdipoRon in an anxiety/depression mouse model reversed depression-like state by modulating several CNS processes, including neurogenesis (Nicolas et al., 2018). This study is of particular translational relevance since AdipoRon, a small-molecule adiponectin-mimetic drug, showed central activity while administered peripherally. It has been suggested that, for its neurogenic and antidepressant actions, adiponectin can be explored as a pharmacological surrogate for physical exercise to treat depression and, possibly, other brain disorders (Li et al., 2015).

Adiponectin in Alzheimer's Disease

Recent studies indicate that adiponectin signaling deficiency is sufficient to induce an AD-like phenotype in mice. Aged adiponectin-knockout mice recapitulate several aspects of AD pathology, including increased Aβ levels and deposition, tau hyperphosporylation, neuroinflammation, synapse loss, neuronal apoptosis and impaired insulin signaling. Importantly, aged adiponectin knockout mice also performed poorly in spatial memory and fear conditioning behavioral tests (Ng et al., 2016). These observations were further corroborated by another recent study showing that gene-therapy induced suppression of AdipoR1 also produces an AD-like phenotype, which includes impaired spatial memory and learning, increased levels of Aβ aggregates and hyperphosphorylated tau, insulin signaling dysfunction, neuroinflammation and neurodegeneration markers (Kim et al., 2017). Collectively, these studies make strong case for a role for adiponectin deficiency in AD pathogenesis. The NBM is a cholinergic nucleus in the basal forebrain which is severely affected in AD and other neurodegenerative diseases. It is well documented that neuronal loss of NBM cholinergic neurons contributes to cholinergic dysfunction and, most importantly, it correlates with clinical measures of dementia (Arendt et al., 1983; Whitehouse et al., 1986; Iraizoz et al., 1999; reviewed in Liu A.K. et al., 2015). Interestingly, NBM was found to be a prominent site of expression of AdipoR1 (Psilopanagioti et al., 2009). Therefore, it is possible that adiponectin deficiency contributes to the onset and progression of AD by promoting NBM dysfunction and degeneration. This hypothesis, however, remain to be tested.

Conversely, impairment in adiponectin function is also observed in amyloid-based AD models, whereas activating adiponectin signaling reduces AD-like pathology. In APP/PS1 mice, changes in AdipoRs expression levels were less responsive to a stress-inducing paradigm as compared to wild-type mice (Várhelyi et al., 2017). In the same model, the adiponectin-homolog osmotin ameliorated AD-like neuropathological features such as Aβ production and aggregation, synaptic dysfunction and impaired LTP, memory and cognitive deficits. AdipoR1 silencing abolished osmotin beneficial effects and further aggravated brain pathology in AD-mice (Shah et al., 2017). Osmotin was further shown to reduce Aβ deposition in cultured SH-SY5Y human neuroblastoma cells overexpressing APP. Osmotin effects were mediated by activation of AMPK, an enzyme downregulated by Aβ oligomers in hippocampal neurons (Seixas da Silva et al., 2017). In a rat model of streptozotocin-induced brain pathology, intracerebroventricular injection of adiponectin rescued cognitive deficits and attenuated GSK3β-mediated tau hyperphosphorylation in AD-relevant sites (Xu et al., 2018). These results suggest boosting adiponectin signaling, particularly through AdipoR1, as a potential therapeutic approach in AD (Ng and Chan, 2017). In this regard, chronic treatment with donepezil, an acetylcholinesterase inhibitor widely use to treat AD, was recently shown to increase serum levels of adiponectin (Pákáski et al., 2013). Moreover, thiazolidinediones (TZDs) such as rosiglitazone and pioglitazone, PPARγ agonists used for decades to treat type 2 diabetes due to its insulin sensitization activity (Saltiel and Olefsky, 1996; Malinowski and Bolesta, 2000; Hong et al., 2018) were recently repurposed to treat AD. The insulin-sensitizing effect of TZDs is in part mediated by induction of peripheral adiponectin and AdipoRs expression (Yu et al., 2002; Tsuchida et al., 2005; Nie and Li, 2017). Therefore, it is possible that adiponectin mediate part of the observed beneficial effects of donepezil and TZDs.

AdipoRon, an orally bioavailable small-molecule agonist of adiponectin receptors (Okada-Iwabu et al., 2013), was shown to modulate hippocampal synaptic transmission and to facilitate fear memory extinction in rodents (Zhang et al., 2017). AdipoRon was further shown to regulate activity of dopaminergic neurons in the ventral-tegmental area (Sun et al., 2018) and to act as an antidepressant and metabolic regulator in a mouse model of depression (Nicolas et al., 2018). Importantly, central AdipoRon effects were obtained by peripheral administration, and it was shown that it crosses the BBB to activate AdipoRs in the brain. However, to our knowledge, there are no available data on AdipoRon effects in AD models. It should be interesting to investigate the efficacy of this adiponectin-mimetic drug with translational potential in AD models.

Studies relating adiponectin levels to AD in humans are controversial. Increased baseline adiponectin levels in plasma have been associated with a higher risk of women, but not men, to develop AD and other types of dementia (van Himbergen et al., 2012). Furthermore, elevated adiponectin levels were reported in the plasma and CSF of subjects with MCI and sporadic AD (Une et al., 2010; Khemka et al., 2014a), whereas plasma levels of adiponectin positively correlated with the degree of dementia. The correlation between high blood adiponectin and AD has been replicated and supported by meta-analysis study (Ma et al., 2016). However, while the studies described above suggest increased adiponectin levels to be associated with AD and dementia, opposite results have also been reported. One study found lower levels of circulating adiponectin in MCI and AD subjects. Moreover, adiponectin levels failed to predict progression of cognitive dysfunction from normal to MCI and from MCI to AD (Teixeira et al., 2013). One larger study also reported low levels of plasma adiponectin to be associated with MCI, even though this association was observed in men, but not in women (Kamogawa et al., 2010). In line with these observations, it has been shown that, in diabetic patients, low plasma levels of adiponectin correlate with lower gray-matter volume and reduced glucose utilization in temporal regions of the brain, similarly to what is observed in AD (García-Casares et al., 2016). Finally, a recent study reports that levels of adiponectin are higher in blood but lower in CSF of AD and MCI patients.

Available data regarding a possible association between adiponectin levels in blood and CSF to MCI and AD are conflicting and inconclusive. Therefore, further studies are warranted to reveal the potential use of adiponectin measurement for diagnostic purposes and its clinical relevance for the physiopathology of these neurological conditions. Worth mentioning, some studies found that the association between adiponectin levels and dementia can be sex-specific (Kamogawa et al., 2010). This may be of particular relevance in the case of AD, where a considerable sexual dichotomy is observed with women being at a significantly higher risk to develop the disease.

CONCLUDING REMARKS

Obesity is pandemic in present days. Beyond its intrinsic complications, and the obvious social and psychological impact, obesity harms extend to a wide range of associated health conditions to which it represents a major risk factor. More recently, growing attention is being given to the impact of obesity on CNS function, as accumulating evidence indicate higher incidence of neurological disorders in the obese population. The mechanisms by which fat accumulation and adipose tissue dysfunction in obesity result in CNS pathology are poorly understood. It is widely accepted that dissection of such mechanisms will greatly improve our knowledge on the cross-talk between peripheral metabolism and brain physiology, and may provide novel targets for therapeutic intervention for prevention and/or treatment of neurological dysfunctions associated with obesity.

Adipokines are secreted factors which carry regulatory signals from adipose tissue through systemic circulation to control a wide range of physiological functions throughout the human body. Not surprisingly, adipokine dysregulation in obesity results in the disruption of homeostasis in a variety of organs and systems, and underlie obesity complications and risk for associated chronic conditions. In this context, adipokines emerged as strong candidates to represent the mediators of pathological signals from adipose tissue to CNS in metabolic disorders.

The studies reviewed here provide evidence supporting a role of leptin and adiponectin, two highly abundant and well characterized adipokines, as key mediators of obesity-related CNS dysfunctions (**Figure 1**). We found consistent evidence that leptin and adiponectin, as well as their receptors, are present in the brain and function as important regulators of different aspects of brain physiology. Importantly, leptin (**Table 1**) and adiponectin (**Table 2**) signaling have been shown to interfere with a range of neuropathological events covering those most commonly present in neurodegenerative diseases and, in particular, in AD. These include amyloidogenesis, tau hyperphosphorylation, neuroinflammation, oxidative stress, endoplasmic reticulum stress, insulin resistance, synaptic dysfunction and cognitive impairment. Remarkably, the phenotype of adiponectin- or adiponectin receptor-deficient mice recapitulates the majority of AD neuropathological hallmarks. Therefore, dysregulated adiponectin and leptin signaling may mediate the detrimental impact of obesity on CNS and raise the risk for cognitive decline and AD. Importantly, restoring proper leptin and adiponectin signaling in the brain may constitute beneficial, disease-modifying therapeutic interventions in such neurological conditions (**Figure 1**).

AUTHOR CONTRIBUTIONS

LF-G and MV wrote the manuscript. MV designed the figure. LF-G, FDF, and MV planned the scope and reviewed the final manuscript.

REFERENCES

Ahima, R. S. (2012). Adipose tissue as an endocrine organ. *Obesity* 14, 242S–249S. doi: 10.1038/oby.2006.317

Ahima, R. S., Blüher, M., Mantzoros, C. S., Dhar, M., Wayman, G. A., Zhu, M., et al. (2017). Adiposity and cognitive decline: underlying mechanisms. *Nature* 30, 203–217. doi: 10.3233/JAD-2012-120487

Ahima, R. S., Prabakaran, D., and Flier, J. S. (1998). Postnatal leptin surge and regulation of circadian rhythm of leptin by feeding. Implications for energy homeostasis and neuroendocrine function. *J. Clin. Invest.* 101, 1020–1027. doi: 10.1172/JCI1176

Ahuja, C. S., Wilson, J. R., Nori, S., Kotter, M. R. N., Druschel, C., Curt, A., et al. (2017). Traumatic spinal cord injury. *Nat. Rev. Dis. Primers* 3:17018.

Alhurani, R. E., Vassilaki, M., Aakre, J., Mielke, M. M., Kremers, W. K., Machulda, M. M., et al. (2016). Decline in weight and incident mild cognitive impairment: mayo clinic study of aging. *JAMA Neurol.* 73, 439–446. doi: 10.1001/jamaneurol.2015.4756

Ali, T., Yoon, G. H., Shah, S. A., Lee, H. Y., and Kim, M. O. (2015). Osmotin attenuates amyloid beta-induced memory impairment, tau phosphorylation and neurodegeneration in the mouse hippocampus. *Sci. Rep.* 5:11708. doi: 10.1038/srep11708

Allison, M. B., and Myers, M. G. (2014). Connecting leptin signaling to biological function. *J. Endocrinol.* 223, T25–T35. doi: 10.1530/JOE-14-0404

Angelidis, G., Dafopoulos, K., Messini, C. I., Valotassiou, V., Tsikouras, P., Vrachnis, N., et al. (2012). The emerging roles of adiponectin in female reproductive system-associated disorders and pregnancy. *Reprod. Sci.* 20, 872–881. doi: 10.1177/1933719112468954

Antoniades, C., Antonopoulos, A. S., Tousoulis, D., and Stefanadis, C. (2009). Adiponectin: from obesity to cardiovascular disease. *Obes. Rev.* 10, 269–279. doi: 10.1111/j.1467-789X.2009.00571.x

Arendt, T., Bigl, V., Arendt, A., and Tennstedt, A. (1983). Loss of neurons in the nucleus basalis of Meynert in Alzheimer's disease, paralysis agitans and Korsakoff's disease. *Acta Neuropathol.* 61, 101–108.

Arita, Y., Kihara, S., Ouchi, N., Takahashi, M., Maeda, K., Miyagawa, J., et al. (1999). Paradoxical decrease of an adipose-specific protein, adiponectin, in obesity. *Biochem. Biophys. Res. Commun.* 257, 79–83.

Arnold, S. E., Arvanitakis, Z., Macauley-Rambach, S. L., Koenig, A. M., Wang, H.-Y., Ahima, R. S., et al. (2018). Brain insulin resistance in type 2 diabetes and Alzheimer disease: concepts and conundrums. *Nat. Rev. Neurol.* 14, 168–181. doi: 10.1038/nrneurol.2017.185

Arshad, N., Lin, T. S., and Yahaya, M. F. (2018). Metabolic syndrome and its effect on the brain: possible mechanism. *CNS Neurol. Disord. Drug Targets* 17, 595–603. doi: 10.2174/1871527317666180724143258

Baker, L. D., Cross, D. J., Minoshima, S., Belongia, D., Watson, G. S., and Craft, S. (2011). Insulin resistance and Alzheimer-like reductions in regional cerebral glucose metabolism for cognitively normal adults with prediabetes or early type 2 diabetes. *Arch. Neurol.* 68, 51–57. doi: 10.1001/archneurol.2010.225

Balland, E., Dam, J., Langlet, F., Caron, E., Steculorum, S., Messina, A., et al. (2014). Hypothalamic tanycytes are an ERK-gated conduit for leptin into the brain. *Cell Metab.* 19, 293–301. doi: 10.1016/j.cmet.2013.12.015

Bamberger, M. E., Harris, M. E., McDonald, D. R., Husemann, J., and Landreth, G. E. (2003). A cell surface receptor complex for fibrillar beta-amyloid mediates microglial activation. *J. Neurosci.* 23, 2665–2674.

Banks, W. (2005). Blood-brain barrier transport of cytokines: a mechanism for neuropathology. *Curr. Pharm. Des.* 11, 973–984. doi: 10.2174/1381612053381684

Banks, W. A., Coon, A. B., Robinson, S. M., Moinuddin, A., Shultz, J. M., Nakaoke, R., et al. (2004). Triglycerides induce leptin resistance at the blood-brain barrier. *Diabetes* 53, 1253–1260.

Banks, W. A., Farr, S. A., Salameh, T. S., Niehoff, M. L., Rhea, E. M., Morley, J. E., et al. (2018). Triglycerides cross the blood-brain barrier and induce central leptin and insulin receptor resistance. *Int. J. Obes.* 42, 391–397. doi: 10.1038/ijo.2017.231

Banks, W. A., Kastin, A. J., Huang, W., Jaspan, J. B., and Maness, L. M. (1996). Leptin enters the brain by a saturable system independent of insulin. *Peptides* 17, 305–311. doi: 10.1016/0196-9781(96)00025-3

Bao, Y., Giovannucci, E. L., Kraft, P., Stampfer, M. J., Ogino, S., Ma, J., et al. (2013). A prospective study of plasma adiponectin and pancreatic cancer risk in five US cohorts. *J. Natl. Cancer Inst.* 105, 95–103. doi: 10.1093/jnci/djs474

Baranowska-Bik, A., Bik, W., Styczynska, M., Chodakowska-Zebrowska, M., Barcikowska, M., Wolinska-Witort, E., et al. (2015). Plasma leptin levels and free leptin index in women with Alzheimer's disease. *Neuropeptides* 52, 73–78. doi: 10.1016/j.npep.2015.05.006

Barrett-Connor, E., Edelstein, S. L., Corey-Bloom, J., and Wiederholt, W. C. (1996).

Weight loss precedes dementia in community-dwelling older adults. *J. Am. Geriatr. Soc.* 44, 1147–1152. doi: 10.1111/j.1532-5415.1996.tb01362.x

Bartolome, F., Antequera, D., Tavares, E., Pascual, C., Maldonado, R., Camins, A., et al. (2017). Obesity and neuroinflammatory phenotype in mice lacking endothelial megalin. *J. Neuroinflammation* 14:26. doi: 10.1186/s12974-017-0800-2

Batista, A. F., Forny-Germano, L., Clarke, J. R., Lyra e Silva, N. M., Brito-Moreira, J., Boehnke, S. E., et al. (2018). The diabetes drug liraglutide reverses cognitive impairment in mice and attenuates insulin receptor and synaptic pathology in a non-human primate model of Alzheimer's disease. *J. Pathol.* 245, 85–100. doi: 10.1002/path.5056

Beattie, E. C., Carroll, R. C., Yu, X., Morishita, W., Yasuda, H., von Zastrow, M., et al. (2000). Regulation of AMPA receptor endocytosis by a signaling mechanism shared with LTD. *Nat. Neurosci.* 3, 1291–1300. doi: 10.1038/81823

Bell, S. P., Liu, D., Samuels, L. R., Saraf, A. A., Gifford, K. A., Hohman, T. J., et al. (2017). Late-life body mass index, rapid weight loss, Apolipoprotein E ε4 and the risk of cognitive decline and incident dementia. *J. Nutr. Health Aging* 21, 1259–1267. doi: 10.1007/s12603-017-0906-3

Bhat, A. H., Dar, K. B., Anees, S., Zargar, M. A., Masood, A., Sofi, M. A., et al. (2015). Oxidative stress, mitochondrial dysfunction and neurodegenerative diseases; a mechanistic insight. *Biomed. Pharmacother.* 74, 101–110. doi: 10.1016/j.biopha.2015.07.025

Bigalke, B., Schreitmüller, B., Sopova, K., Paul, A., Stransky, E., Gawaz, M., et al. (2011). Adipocytokines and $CD34^+$ progenitor cells in Alzheimer's disease. *PLoS One* 6:e20286. doi: 10.1371/journal.pone.0020286

Bjørbaek, C., and Kahn, B. B. (2004). Leptin signaling in the central nervous system and the periphery. *Recent Prog. Horm. Res.* 59, 305–331.

Bliss, T. V. P., and Collingridge, G. L. (1993). A synaptic model of memory: long-term potentiation in the hippocampus. *Nature* 361, 31–39.

Bluher, M. (2016). Adipose tissue inflammation: a cause or consequence of obesity-related insulin resistance? *Clin. Sci.* 130, 1603–1614. doi: 10.1042/CS20160005

Bomfim, T. R., Forny-Germano, L., Sathler, L. B., Brito-Moreira, J., Houzel, J.-C., Decker, H., et al. (2012). An anti-diabetes agent protects the mouse brain from defective insulin signaling caused by Alzheimer's disease–associated Aβ oligomers. *J. Clin. Invest.* 122, 1339–1353. doi: 10.1172/JCI57256

Bonda, D. J., Stone, J. G., Torres, S. L., Siedlak, S. L., Perry, G., Kryscio, R., et al. (2014). Dysregulation of leptin signaling in Alzheimer disease: evidence for neuronal leptin resistance. *J. Neurochem.* 128, 162–172. doi: 10.1111/jnc.12380

Bouret, S. G. (2010). Neurodevelopmental actions of leptin. *Brain Res.* 1350, 2–9. doi: 10.1016/j.brainres.2010.04.011

Buchman, A. S., Wilson, R. S., Bienias, J. L., Shah, R. C., Evans, D. A., and Bennet, D. A. (2005). Change in body mass index and risk of incident Alzheimer disease. *Neurology* 65, 892–897. doi: 10.1212/01.wnl.0000176061.33817.90

Cao, B., Chen, Y., Brietzke, E., Cha, D., Shaukat, A., Pan, Z., et al. (2018). Leptin and adiponectin levels in major depressive disorder: a systematic review and meta-analysis. *J. Affect. Disord.* 238, 101–110. doi: 10.1016/j.jad.2018.05.008

Caprio, M., Fabbrini, E., Isidori, A. M., Aversa, A., and Fabbri, A. (2001). Leptin in reproduction. *Trends Endocrinol. Metab.* 12, 65–72. doi: 10.1016/S1043-2760(00)00352-0

Caron, A., Lee, S., Elmquist, J. K., and Gautron, L. (2018). Leptin and brain–adipose crosstalks. *Nat. Rev. Neurosci.* 19, 153–165. doi: 10.1038/nrn.2018.7

Carro, E., Spuch, C., Trejo, J. L., Antequera, D., and Torres-Aleman, I. (2005). Choroid plexus megalin is involved in neuroprotection by serum insulin-like growth factor I. *J. Neurosci.* 25, 10884–10893. doi: 10.1523/JNEUROSCI.2909-05.2005

Cezaretto, A., Suemoto, C. K., Bensenor, I., Lotufo, P. A., de Almeida-Pititto, B., Ferreira, S. R. G., et al. (2018). Association of adiponectin with cognitive function precedes overt diabetes in the Brazilian Longitudinal Study of Adult Health: ELSA. *Diabetol. Metab. Syndr.* 10:54. doi: 10.1186/s13098-018-0354-1

Chabry, J., Nicolas, S., Cazareth, J., Murris, E., Guyon, A., Glaichenhaus, N., et al. (2015). Enriched environment decreases microglia and brain macrophages inflammatory phenotypes through adiponectin-dependent mechanisms: relevance to depressive-like behavior. *Brain Behav. Immun.* 50, 275–287. doi: 10.1016/j.bbi.2015.07.018

Chakrabarti, S. (2014). Altered serum levels of adipokines and insulin in probable Alzheimer's disease. *J. Alzheimers Dis.* 41, 525–533. doi: 10.3233/JAD-140006

Chan, J. S. M., Li, A., Ng, S.-M., Ho, R. T. H., Xu, A., Yao, T.-J., et al. (2017). Adiponectin potentially contributes to the antidepressive effects of baduanjin qigong exercise in women with chronic fatigue syndrome-like illness. *Cell Transplant.* 26, 493–501. doi: 10.3727/096368916X694238

Chan, K.-H., Lam, K. S.-L., Cheng, O.-Y., Kwan, J. S.-C., Ho, P. W.-L., Cheng, K. K.-Y., et al. (2012). Adiponectin is protective against oxidative stress induced cytotoxicity in amyloid-beta neurotoxicity. *PLoS One* 7:e52354. doi: 10.1371/journal.pone.0052354

Chandrasekar, B., Boylston, W. H., Venkatachalam, K., Webster, N. J. G., Prabhu, S. D., and Valente, A. J. (2008). Adiponectin blocks interleukin-18-mediated endothelial cell death via APPL1-dependent AMP-activated protein kinase (AMPK) activation and IKK/NF-κB/PTEN suppression. *J. Biol. Chem.* 283, 24889–24898. doi: 10.1074/jbc.M804236200

Chehab, F. F. (2014). Leptin and reproduction: past milestones, present undertakings and future endeavors. *J. Endocrinol.* 223, T37–T48. doi: 10.1530/JOE-14-0413

Chen, B., Liao, W.-Q., Xu, N., Xu, H., Wen, J.-Y., Yu, C.-A., et al. (2009). Adiponectin protects against cerebral ischemia–reperfusion injury through anti-inflammatory action. *Brain Res.* 1273, 129–137. doi: 10.1016/j.brainres.2009.04.002

Cheng, A., Uetani, N., Simoncic, P. D., Chaubey, V. P., Lee-Loy, A., McGlade, C. J., et al. (2002). Attenuation of leptin action and regulation of obesity by protein tyrosine phosphatase 1B. *Dev. Cell* 2, 497–503. doi: 10.1016/S1534-5807(02)00149-1

Cheng, K. K. Y., Lam, K. S. L., Wang, Y., Huang, Y., Carling, D., Wu, D., et al. (2007). Adiponectin-induced endothelial nitric oxide synthase activation and nitric oxide production are mediated by APPL1 in endothelial cells. *Diabetes* 56, 1387–1394. doi: 10.2337/db06-1580

Cisternas, P., Martinez, M., Ahima, R. S., William Wong, G., and Inestrosa, N. C. (2018). Modulation of glucose metabolism in hippocampal neurons by adiponectin and resistin. *Mol. Neurobiol.* doi: 10.1007/s12035-018-1271-x [Epub ahead of print].

Coope, A., Milanski, M., Araújo, E. P., Tambascia, M., Saad, M. J. A., Geloneze, B., et al. (2008). AdipoR1 mediates the anorexigenic and insulin/leptin-like actions of adiponectin in the hypothalamus. *FEBS Lett.* 582, 1471–1476. doi: 10.1016/j.febslet.2008.03.037

De Felice, F. G. (2013). Alzheimer's disease and insulin resistance: translating basic science into clinical applications. *J. Clin. Invest.* 123, 531–539. doi: 10.1172/JCI64595

De Felice, F. G., and Ferreira, S. T. (2014). Inflammation, defective insulin signaling, and mitochondrial dysfunction as common molecular denominators connecting type 2 diabetes to Alzheimer disease. *Diabetes* 63, 2262–2272. doi: 10.2337/db13-1954

De Felice, F. G., and Lourenco, M. V. (2015). Brain metabolic stress and neuroinflammation at the basis of cognitive impairment in Alzheimer's disease. *Front. Aging Neurosci.* 7:94. doi: 10.3389/fnagi.2015.00094

De Felice, F. G., Vieira, M. N. N., Bomfim, T. R., Decker, H., Velasco, P. T., Lambert, M. P., et al. (2009). Protection of synapses against Alzheimer's-linked toxins: insulin signaling prevents the pathogenic binding of Aβ oligomers. *Proc. Natl. Acad. Sci. U.S.A.* 106, 1971–1976. doi: 10.1073/pnas.0809158106

de Git, K. C. G., and Adan, R. A. H. (2015). Leptin resistance in diet-induced obesity: the role of hypothalamic inflammation. *Obes. Rev.* 16, 207–224. doi: 10.1111/obr.12243

de la Monte, S. M. (2017). Insulin resistance and neurodegeneration: progress towards the development of new therapeutics for Alzheimer's disease. *Drugs* 77, 47–65. doi: 10.1007/s40265-016-0674-0

de la Monte, S. M., Longato, L., Tong, M., and Wands, J. R. (2009). Insulin resistance and neurodegeneration: roles of obesity, type 2 diabetes mellitus and non-alcoholic steatohepatitis. *Curr. Opin. Investig. Drugs* 10, 1049–1060.

DeKosky, S. T., and Scheff, S. W. (1990). Synapse loss in frontal cortex biopsies in Alzheimer's disease: correlation with cognitive severity. *Ann. Neurol.* 27, 457–464. doi: 10.1002/ana.410270502

Denver, R. J., Bonett, R. M., and Boorse, G. C. (2011). Evolution of leptin structure and function. *Neuroendocrinology* 94, 21–38. doi: 10.1159/000328435

Di Spiezio, A., Sandin, E. S., Dore, R., Müller-Fielitz, H., Storck, S. E., Bernau, M., et al. (2018). The LepR-mediated leptin transport across brain barriers controls food reward. *Mol. Metab.* 8, 13–22. doi: 10.1016/j.molmet.2017.12.001

Dietrich, M. O., Spuch, C., Antequera, D., Rodal, I., de Yébenes, J. G., Molina, J. A., et al. (2008). Megalin mediates the transport of leptin across the blood-CSF barrier. *Neurobiol. Aging* 29, 902–912. doi: 10.1016/j.neurobiolaging.2007.01.008

Doherty, G. H., Beccano-Kelly, D., Yan, S. D., Gunn-Moore, F. J., and Harvey, J. (2013). Leptin prevents hippocampal synaptic disruption and neuronal cell death induced by amyloid β. *Neurobiol. Aging* 34, 226–237. doi: 10.1016/J.NEUROBIOLAGING.2012.08.003

Dong, X., Wang, Y., and Qin, Z. (2009). Molecular mechanisms of excitotoxicity and their relevance to pathogenesis of neurodegenerative diseases. *Acta Pharmacol. Sin.* 30, 379–387. doi: 10.1038/aps.2009.24

Elfeky, M., Kaede, R., Okamatsu-Ogura, Y., and Kimura, K. (2016). Adiponectin inhibits LPS-induced HMGB1 release through an AMP kinase and Heme Oxygenase-1-dependent pathway in RAW 264 macrophage cells. *Mediators Inflamm.* 2016:5701959. doi: 10.1155/2016/5701959

Elfeky, M., Yoneshiro, T., Okamatsu-Ogura, Y., and Kimura, K. (2018). Adiponectin suppression of late inflammatory mediator, HMGB1-induced cytokine expression in RAW264 macrophage cells. *J. Biochem.* 163, 143–153. doi: 10.1093/jb/mvx069

Elias, M. F., Elias, P. K., Sullivan, L. M., Wolf, P. A., and D'Agostino, R. B. (2005). Obesity, diabetes and cognitive deficit: the Framingham Heart Study. *Neurobiol. Aging* 26, 11–16. doi: 10.1016/j.neurobiolaging.2005.08.019

Elmquist, J. K., Bjørbæk, C., Ahima, R. S., Flier, J. S., and Saper, C. B. (1998). Distributions of leptin receptor mRNA isoforms in the rat brain. *J. Comp. Neurol.* 395, 535–547.

Elmquist, J. K., Coppari, R., Balthasar, N., Ichinose, M., and Lowell, B. B. (2005). Identifying hypothalamic pathways controlling food intake, body weight, and glucose homeostasis. *J. Comp. Neurol.* 493, 63–71. doi: 10.1002/cne.20786

Emmerzaal, T. L., Kiliaan, A. J., and Gustafson, D. R. (2014). 2003-2013: a decade of body mass index, Alzheimer's disease, and dementia. *J. Alzheimers Dis.* 43, 739–755. doi: 10.3233/JAD-141086

Engin, A. (2017). Diet-induced obesity and the mechanism of leptin resistance. *Adv. Exp. Med. Biol.* 960, 381–397. doi: 10.1007/978-3-319-48382-5_16

Espeland, M. A., Luchsinger, J. A., Baker, L. D., Neiberg, R., Kahn, S. E., Arnold, S. E., et al. (2017). Effect of a long-term intensive lifestyle intervention on prevalence of cognitive impairment. *Neurology* 88, 2026–2035. doi: 10.1212/WNL.0000000000003955

Farr, S. A., Banks, W. A., and Morley, J. E. (2006). Effects of leptin on memory processing. *Peptides* 27, 1420–1425. doi: 10.1016/j.peptides.2005.10.006

Fasshauer, M., and Blüher, M. (2015). Adipokines in health and disease. *Trends Pharmacol. Sci.* 36, 461–470. doi: 10.1016/j.tips.2015.04.014

Ferreira, S. T., Clarke, J. R., Bomfim, T. R., and De Felice, F. G. (2014). Inflammation, defective insulin signaling, and neuronal dysfunction in Alzheimer's disease. *Alzheimers Dement.* 10, S76–S83. doi: 10.1016/j.jalz.2013.12.010

Ferreira, S. T., and Klein, W. L. (2011). The Aβ oligomer hypothesis for synapse failure and memory loss in Alzheimer's disease. *Neurobiol. Learn. Mem.* 96, 529–543. doi: 10.1016/j.nlm.2011.08.003

Fewlass, D. C., Noboa, K., Pi-Sunyer, F. X., Johnston, J. M., Yan, S. D., and Tezapsidis, N. (2004). Obesity-related leptin regulates Alzheimer's Abeta. *FASEB J.* 18, 1870–1878. doi: 10.1096/fj.04-2572com

Forny-Germano, L., Lyra e Silva, N. M., Batista, A. F., Brito-Moreira, J., Gralle, M., Boehnke, S. E., et al. (2014). Alzheimer's disease-like pathology induced by amyloid-β oligomers in nonhuman primates. *J. Neurosci.* 34, 13629–13643. doi: 10.1523/JNEUROSCI.1353-14.2014

Friedemann, C., Heneghan, C., Mahtani, K., Thompson, M., Perera, R., and Ward, A. M. (2012). Cardiovascular disease risk in healthy children and its association with body mass index: systematic review and meta-analysis. *BMJ* 345:e4759. doi: 10.1136/bmj.e4759

Friedman, J. (2016). The long road to leptin. *J. Clin. Invest.* 126, 4727–4734. doi: 10.1172/JCI91578

Frisardi, V., Solfrizzi, V., Seripa, D., Capurso, C., Santamato, A., Sancarlo, D., et al. (2010). Metabolic-cognitive syndrome: a cross-talk between metabolic syndrome and Alzheimer's disease. *Ageing Res. Rev.* 9, 399–417. doi: 10.1016/j.arr.2010.04.007

Fruebis, J., Tsao, T.-S., Javorschi, S., Ebbets-Reed, D., Erickson, M. R. S., Yen, F. T., et al. (2001). Proteolytic cleavage product of 30-kDa adipocyte complement-related protein increases fatty acid oxidation in muscle and causes weight loss in mice. *Proc. Natl. Acad. Sci. U.S.A.* 98, 2005–2010. doi: 10.1073/PNAS.98.4.2005

Furigo, I. C., Melo, H. M., Lyra, E., Silva, N. M., Ramos-Lobo, A. M., Teixeira, P. D. S., et al. (2018). Brain STAT5 signaling modulates learning and memory formation. *Brain Struct. Funct.* 223, 2229–2241. doi: 10.1007/s00429-018-1627-z

Gallo, V., Wark, P. A., Jenab, M., Pearce, N., Brayne, C., Vermeulen, R., et al. (2013). Prediagnostic body fat and risk of death from amyotrophic lateral sclerosis: the EPIC cohort. *Neurology* 80, 829–838. doi: 10.1212/WNL.0b013e3182840689

Gao, S., Nguyen, J. T., Hendrie, H. C., Unverzagt, F. W., Hake, A., Smith-Gamble, V., et al. (2011). Accelerated weight loss and incident dementia in an elderly African-American cohort. *J. Am. Geriatr. Soc.* 59, 18–25. doi: 10.1111/j.1532-5415.2010.03169.x

García-Casares, N., García-Arnés, J. A., Rioja, J., Ariza, M. J., Gutiérrez, A., Alfaro, F., et al. (2016). Alzheimer's like brain changes correlate with low adiponectin plasma levels in type 2 diabetic patients. *J. Diabetes Complications* 30, 281–286. doi: 10.1016/j.jdiacomp.2015.12.001

García-García, I., Michaud, A., Dadar, M., Zeighami, Y., Neseliler, S., Collins, D. L., et al. (2018). Neuroanatomical differences in obesity: meta-analytic findings and their validation in an independent dataset. *Int. J. Obes.* doi: 10.1038/s41366-018-0164-4 [Epub ahead of print].

Garza, J. C., Guo, M., Zhang, W., and Lu, X.-Y. (2008). Leptin increases adult hippocampal neurogenesis *in Vivo* and *in Vitro*. *J. Biol. Chem.* 283, 18238–18247. doi: 10.1074/jbc.M800053200

Gong, Y., Ishida-Takahashi, R., Villanueva, E. C., Fingar, D. C., Münzberg, H., and Myers, M. G. (2007). The long form of the leptin receptor regulates STAT5 and ribosomal protein S6 via alternate mechanisms. *J. Biol. Chem.* 282, 31019–31027. doi: 10.1074/jbc.M702838200

Greco, S. J., Bryan, K. J., Sarkar, S., Zhu, X., Smith, M. A., Ashford, J. W., et al. (2010). Leptin reduces pathology and improves memory in a transgenic mouse model of Alzheimer's disease. *J. Alzheimers Dis.* 19, 1155–1167. doi: 10.3233/JAD-2010-1308

Greco, S. J., Sarkar, S., Johnston, J. M., Zhu, X., Su, B., Casadesus, G., et al. (2008). Leptin reduces Alzheimer's disease-related tau phosphorylation in neuronal cells. *Biochem. Biophys. Res. Commun.* 376, 536–541. doi: 10.1016/j.bbrc.2008.09.026

Gruol, D. L. (2015). IL-6 regulation of synaptic function in the CNS. *Neuropharmacology* 96, 42–54. doi: 10.1016/j.neuropharm.2014.10.023

Gunstad, J., Paul, R. H., Cohen, R. A., Tate, D. F., Spitznagel, M. B., and Gordon, E. (2007). Elevated body mass index is associated with executive dysfunction in otherwise healthy adults. *Compr. Psychiatry* 48, 57–61. doi: 10.1016/j.comppsych.2006.05.001

Guo, F., Jiang, T., Song, W., Wei, H., Wang, F., Liu, L., et al. (2015). Electroacupuncture attenuates cerebral ischemia-reperfusion injury in diabetic mice through adiponectin receptor 1-mediated phosphorylation of GSK-3β. *Mol. Neurobiol.* 51, 685–695. doi: 10.1007/s12035-014-8765-y

Gustafson, D. R., Bäckman, K., Lissner, L., Carlsson, L., Waern, M., Östling, S., et al. (2012). Leptin and dementia over 32 years-The Prospective Population Study of Women. *Alzheimers Dement.* 8, 272–277. doi: 10.1016/j.jalz.2011.05.2411

Harvey, J. (2015). "Leptin and Alzheimer's disease," in *Diet and Nutrition in Dementia and Cognitive Decline*, eds C. Martin and V. Preedy (San Diego, CA: Academic Press), 457–467.

Haslam, D. W., and James, W. P. T. (2005). Obesity. *Lancet* 366, 1197–1209. doi: 10.1016/S0140-6736(05)67483-1

Hassing, L. B., Dahl, A. K., Thorvaldsson, V., Berg, S., Gatz, M., Pedersen, N. L., et al. (2009). Overweight in midlife and risk of dementia: a 40-year follow-up study. *Int. J. Obes.* 33, 893–898. doi: 10.1038/ijo.2009.104

Hendrickx, H., McEwen, B. S., and van der Ouderaa, F. (2005). Metabolism, mood and cognition in aging: the importance of lifestyle and dietary intervention. *Neurobiol. Aging* 26, 1–5. doi: 10.1016/j.neurobiolaging.2005.10.005

Heneka, M. T., Carson, M. J., El Khoury, J., Landreth, G. E., Brosseron, F., Feinstein, D. L., et al. (2015). Neuroinflammation in Alzheimer's disease. *Lancet Neurol.* 14, 388–405. doi: 10.1016/S1474-4422(15)70016-5

Hileman, S. M., Pierroz, D. D., Masuzaki, H., Bjørbæk, C., El-Haschimi, K., Banks, W. A., et al. (2002). Characterization of short isoforms of the leptin receptor in rat cerebral microvessels and of brain uptake of leptin in mouse models of obesity. *Endocrinology* 143, 775–783.

Hill, J. O., Wyatt, H. R., and Peters, J. C. (2012). Energy balance and obesity. *Circulation* 126, 126–132. doi: 10.1161/CIRCULATIONAHA.111.087213

Holden, K. F., Lindquist, K., Tylavsky, F. A., Rosano, C., Harris, T. B., and Yaffe, K. (2009). Serum leptin level and cognition in the elderly: findings from the Health ABC Study. *Neurobiol. Aging* 30, 1483–1489. doi: 10.1016/j.neurobiolaging.2007.11.024

Hong, F., Xu, P., and Zhai, Y. (2018). The opportunities and challenges of peroxisome proliferator-activated receptors ligands in clinical drug discovery and development. *Int. J. Mol. Sci.* 19:E2189. doi: 10.3390/ijms19082189

Hotamisligil, G. S. (2017). Foundations of immunometabolism and implications for metabolic health and disease. *Immunity* 47, 406–420. doi: 10.1016/j.immuni.2017.08.009

Hotta, K., Funahashi, T., Bodkin, N. L., Ortmeyer, H. K., Arita, Y., Hansen, B. C., et al. (2001). Circulating concentrations of the adipocyte protein adiponectin are decreased in parallel with reduced insulin sensitivity during the progression to type 2 diabetes in rhesus monkeys. *Diabetes* 50, 1126–1133.

Hoyda, T. D., Fry, M., Ahima, R. S., and Ferguson, A. V. (2007). Adiponectin selectively inhibits oxytocin neurons of the paraventricular nucleus of the hypothalamus. *J. Physiol.* 585, 805–816. doi: 10.1113/jphysiol.2007.144519

Hube, F., Lietz, U., Igel, M., Jensen, P. B., Tornqvist, H., Joost, H. G., et al. (1996). Difference in leptin mRNA levels between omental and subcutaneous abdominal adipose tissue from obese humans. *Horm. Metab. Res.* 28, 690–693. doi: 10.1055/s-2007-979879

Hughes, T. F., and Ganguli, M. (2009). Modifiable midlife risk factors for late-life cognitive impairment and dementia. *Curr. Psychiatry Rev.* 5, 73–92.

Iraizoz, I., Guijarro, J. L., Gonzalo, L. M., and de Lacalle, S. (1999). Neuropathological changes in the nucleus basalis correlate with clinical measures of dementia. *Acta Neuropathol.* 98, 186–196.

Irving, A. J., and Harvey, J. (2013). Leptin regulation of hippocampal synaptic function in health and disease. *Philos. Trans. R. Soc. B Biol. Sci.* 369:20130155. doi: 10.1098/rstb.2013.0155

Iwahara, N., Hisahara, S., Kawamata, J., Matsumura, A., Yokokawa, K., Saito, T., et al. (2017). Role of suppressor of cytokine signaling 3 (SOCS3) in altering activated microglia phenotype in APPswe/PS1dE9 mice. *J. Alzheimers Dis.* 55, 1235–1247. doi: 10.3233/JAD-160887

Jeon, B. T., Shin, H. J., Kim, J. B., Kim, Y. K., Lee, D. H., Kim, K. H., et al. (2009). Adiponectin protects hippocampal neurons against kainic acid-induced excitotoxicity. *Brain Res. Rev.* 61, 81–88. doi: 10.1016/j.brainresrev.2009.05.002

Jeong, H.-G., Min, B. J., Lim, S., Kim, T. H., Lee, J. J., Park, J. H., et al. (2012). Plasma adiponectin elevation in elderly individuals with subsyndromal depression. *Psychoneuroendocrinology* 37, 948–955. doi: 10.1016/j.psyneuen.2011.11.002

Johnson, D., Wilkins, C., and Morris, J. (2006). Accelerated weight loss may precede diagnosis in alzheimer disease. *Arch. Neurol.* 63, 1312–1317.

Johnston, J. M., Hu, W. T., Fardo, D. W., Greco, S. J., Perry, G., Montine, T. J., et al. (2014). Low plasma leptin in cognitively impaired ADNI subjects: gender differences and diagnostic and therapeutic potential. *Curr. Alzheimer Res.* 11, 165–174.

Joo, S. H., Yun, S. H., Kang, D. W., Hahn, C. T., Lim, H. K., and Lee, C. U. (2018). Body mass index in mild cognitive impairment according to age, sex, cognitive intervention, and hypertension and risk of progression to Alzheimer's disease. *Front. Psychiatry* 9:142. doi: 10.3389/fpsyt.2018.00142

Jung, T. W., Lee, J. Y., Shim, W. S., Kang, E. S., Kim, J. S., Ahn, C. W., et al. (2006). Adiponectin protects human neuroblastoma SH-SY5Y cells against MPP+-induced cytotoxicity. *Biochem. Biophys. Res. Commun.* 343, 564–570. doi: 10.1016/j.bbrc.2006.02.186

Jürgensen, S., Antonio, L. L., Mussi, G. E. A., Brito-Moreira, J., Bomfim, T. R., De Felice, F. G., et al. (2011). Activation of D1/D5 dopamine receptors protects neurons from synapse dysfunction induced by amyloid-β oligomers. *J. Biol. Chem.* 286, 3270–3276. doi: 10.1074/jbc.M110.177790

Kaminski, T., Smolinska, N., Maleszka, A., Kiezun, M., Dobrzyn, K., Czerwinska, J., et al. (2014). Expression of adiponectin and its receptors in the porcine hypothalamus during the oestrous cycle. *Reprod. Domest. Anim.* 49, 378–386. doi: 10.1111/rda.12282

Kamogawa, K., Kohara, K., Tabara, Y., Uetani, E., Nagai, T., Yamamoto, M., et al. (2010). Abdominal fat, adipose-derived hormones and mild cognitive impairment: the J-SHIPP study. *Dement. Geriatr. Cogn. Disord.* 30, 432–439. doi: 10.1159/000321985

Kerwin, D. R., Gaussoin, S. A., Chlebowski, R. T., Kuller, L. H., Vitolins, M., Coker, L. H., et al. (2011). Interaction between body mass index and central adiposity and risk of incident cognitive impairment and dementia: results from the women's health initiative memory study. *J. Am. Geriatr. Soc.* 59, 107–112. doi: 10.1111/j.1532-5415.2010.03219.x

Khemka, V. K., Bagchi, D., Bandyopadhyay, K., Bir, A., Chattopadhyay, M., Biswas, A., et al. (2014a). Altered serum levels of adipokines and insulin in probable Alzheimer's disease. *J. Alzheimers Dis.* 41, 525–533. doi: 10.3233/JAD-140006

Khemka, V. K., Ganguly, A., Bagchi, D., Ghosh, A., Bir, A., Biswas, A., et al. (2014b). Raised serum proinflammatory cytokines in Alzheimer's disease with depression. *Aging Dis.* 5, 170–176. doi: 10.14336/AD.2014.0500170

Kiliaan, A. J., Arnoldussen, I. A. C., and Gustafson, D. R. (2014). Adipokines: a link between obesity and dementia? *Lancet Neurol.* 13, 913–923. doi: 10.1016/S1474-4422(14)70085-7

Kim, B., and Feldman, E. L. (2015). Insulin resistance as a key link for the increased risk of cognitive impairment in the metabolic syndrome. *Exp. Mol. Med.* 47:e149. doi: 10.1038/emm.2015.3

Kim, M. W., Abid, N. B., Jo, M. H., Jo, M. G., Yoon, G. H., and Kim, M. O. (2017). Suppression of adiponectin receptor 1 promotes memory dysfunction and Alzheimer's disease-like pathologies. *Sci. Rep.* 7:12435. doi: 10.1038/s41598-017-12632-9

King, A., Brain, A., Hanson, K., Dittmann, J., Vickers, J., and Fernandez-Martos, C. (2018). Disruption of leptin signalling in a mouse model of Alzheimer's disease. *Metab. Brain Dis.* 33, 1097–1110. doi: 10.1007/s11011-018-0203-9

Kivipelto, M., Ngandu, T., Fratiglioni, L., Viitanen, M., Kåreholt, I., Winblad, B., et al. (2005). Obesity and vascular risk factors at midlife and the risk of dementia and Alzheimer disease. *Arch. Neurol.* 62, 1556–1560. doi: 10.1001/archneur.62.10.1556

Kleinert, M., Clemmensen, C., Hofmann, S. M., Moore, M. C., Renner, S., Woods, S. C., et al. (2018). Animal models of obesity and diabetes mellitus. *Nat. Rev. Endocrinol.* 14, 140–162.

Komatsu, M., Ohfusa, H., Sato, Y., Yajima, H., Yamauchi, K., Aizawa, T., et al. (2004). Strong inverse correlation between serum adiponectin level and heart rate-corrected QT interval in an apparently healthy population: a suggestion for a direct antiatherogenic effect of adiponectin. *Diabetes Care* 27, 1237–1238.

Kubota, N., Yano, W., Kubota, T., Yamauchi, T., Itoh, S., Kumagai, H., et al. (2007). Adiponectin stimulates AMP-activated protein kinase in the hypothalamus and increases food intake. *Cell Metab.* 6, 55–68. doi: 10.1016/j.cmet.2007.06.003

Kusminski, C. M., McTernan, P. G., Schraw, T., Kos, K., O'Hare, J. P., Ahima, R., et al. (2007). Adiponectin complexes in human cerebrospinal fluid: distinct complex distribution from serum. *Diabetologia* 50, 634–642. doi: 10.1007/s00125-006-0577-9

Lambert, M. P., Barlow, A. K., Chromy, B. A., Edwards, C., Freed, R., Liosatos, M., et al. (1998). Diffusible, nonfibrillar ligands derived from Abeta1-42 are potent central nervous system neurotoxins. *Proc. Natl. Acad. Sci. U.S.A.* 95, 6448–6453.

Lee, B. C., and Lee, J. (2014). Cellular and molecular players in adipose tissue inflammation in the development of obesity-induced insulin resistance. *Biochim. Biophys. Acta* 1842, 446–462. doi: 10.1016/j.bbadis.2013.05.017

Lee, G. H., Proenca, R., Montez, J. M., Carroll, K. M., Darvishzadeh, J. G., Lee, J. I., et al. (1996). Abnormal splicing of the leptin receptor in diabetic mice. *Nature* 379, 632–635. doi: 10.1038/379632a0

Lee, M.-H., Klein, R. L., El-Shewy, H. M., Luttrell, D. K., and Luttrell, L. M. (2008). The adiponectin receptors AdipoR1 and AdipoR2 activate ERK1/2 through a Src/Ras-dependent pathway and stimulate cell growth †. *Biochemistry* 47, 11682–11692. doi: 10.1021/bi801451f

Lehr, S., Hartwig, S., Lamers, D., Famulla, S., Müller, S., Hanisch, F.-G., et al. (2012). Identification and validation of novel adipokines released from primary human adipocytes. *Mol. Cell. Proteomics* 11:M111.010504. doi: 10.1074/mcp.M111.010504

Lehtisalo, J., Lindström, J., Ngandu, T., Kivipelto, M., Ahtiluoto, S., Ilanne-Parikka, P., et al. (2016). Association of long-term dietary fat intake, exercise, and weight with later cognitive function in the Finnish Diabetes Prevention Study. *J. Nutr. Health Aging* 20, 146–154. doi: 10.1007/s12603-015-0565-1

Lengyel, E., Makowski, L., DiGiovanni, J., and Kolonin, M. G. (2018). Cancer as a matter of fat: the crosstalk between adipose tissue and tumors. *Trends Cancer* 4, 374–384. doi: 10.1016/j.trecan.2018.03.004

Li, A., Yau, S., Machado, S., Yuan, T.-F., and So, K.-F. (2015). Adult neurogenic and antidepressant effects of adiponectin: a potential replacement for exercise? *CNS Neurol. Disord. Drug Targets* 14, 1129–1144. doi: 10.2174/1871527315666151111125533

Li, S., Hong, S., Shepardson, N. E., Walsh, D. M., Shankar, G. M., and Selkoe, D. (2009). Soluble oligomers of amyloid β protein facilitate hippocampal long-term depression by disrupting neuronal glutamate uptake. *Neuron* 62, 788–801. doi: 10.1016/j.neuron.2009.05.012

Li, S., and Stys, P. K. (2000). Mechanisms of ionotropic glutamate receptor-mediated excitotoxicity in isolated spinal cord white matter. *J. Neurosci.* 20, 1190–1198.

Li, X.-L., Aou, S., Oomura, Y., Hori, N., Fukunaga, K., and Hori, T. (2002). Impairment of long-term potentiation and spatial memory in leptin receptor-deficient rodents. *Neuroscience* 113, 607–615.

Licinio, J., Mantzoros, C., Negrão, A. B., Cizza, G., Wong, M.-L., Bongiorno, P. B., et al. (1997). Human leptin levels are pulsatile and inversely related to pituitary–adrenal function. *Nat. Med.* 3, 575–579.

Lieb, W., Beiser, A. S., Vasan, R. S., Tan, Z. S., Au, R., Harris, T. B., et al. (2009). Association of plasma leptin levels with incident Alzheimer's disease and MRI measures of brain aging: the Framingham study. *JAMA* 302, 2565–2572. doi: 10.1001/jama.2009.1836

Liu, A. K., Chang, R. C.-C., Pearce, R. K. B., and Gentleman, S. M. (2015). Nucleus basalis of Meynert revisited: anatomy, history and differential involvement in Alzheimer's and Parkinson's disease. *Acta Neuropathol.* 129, 527–540. doi: 10.1007/s00401-015-1392-5

Liu, Y., Palanivel, R., Rai, E., Park, M., Gabor, T. V., Scheid, M. P., et al. (2015). Adiponectin stimulates autophagy and reduces oxidative stress to enhance insulin sensitivity during high-fat diet feeding in mice. *Diabetes* 64, 36–48. doi: 10.2337/db14-0267

Liu, C., Feng, X., Li, Q., Wang, Y., Li, Q., and Hua, M. (2016). Adiponectin, TNF-α and inflammatory cytokines and risk of type 2 diabetes: a systematic review and meta-analysis. *Cytokine* 86, 100–109. doi: 10.1016/j.cyto.2016.06.028

Liu, M., and Liu, F. (2014). Regulation of adiponectin multimerization, signaling and function. *Best Pract. Res. Clin. Endocrinol. Metab.* 28, 25–31. doi: 10.1016/j.beem.2013.06.003

Lourenco, M. V., Clarke, J. R., Frozza, R. L., Bomfim, T. R., Forny-Germano, L., Batista, A. F., et al. (2013). TNF-α mediates PKR-dependent memory impairment and brain IRS-1 inhibition induced by Alzheimer's β-amyloid oligomers in mice and monkeys. *Cell Metab.* 18, 831–843. doi: 10.1016/j.cmet.2013.11.002

Lu, X.-Y., Kim, C. S., Frazer, A., and Zhang, W. (2006). Leptin: a potential novel antidepressant. *Proc. Natl. Acad. Sci. U.S.A.* 103, 1593–1598. doi: 10.1073/pnas.0508901103

Luo, X., McGregor, G., Irving, A. J., and Harvey, J. (2015). Leptin induces a novel form of NMDA receptor-dependent LTP at hippocampal temporoammonic-CA1 synapses. *eNeuro* 2:ENEURO.0007-ENEURO.15. doi: 10.1523/ENEURO.0007-15.2015

Luppino, F., de Wit, L., Bouvy, P., and Et, A. (2010). Overweight, obesity, and depression: a systematic review and meta-analysis of longitudinal studies. *Arch. Gen. Psychiatry* 67, 220–229. doi: 10.1001/archgenpsychiatry.2010.2

Ma, J.-J., Shang, J., Wang, H., Sui, J.-R., Liu, K., and Du, J.-X. (2016). Serum adiponectin levels are inversely correlated with leukemia: a meta-analysis. *J. Cancer Res. Ther.* 12, 897–902. doi: 10.4103/0973-1482.186695

Ma, L., Wang, R., Dong, W., and Zhao, Z. (2018). Caloric restriction can improve learning and memory in C57/BL mice probably via regulation of the AMPK signaling pathway. *Exp. Gerontol.* 102, 28–35. doi: 10.1016/j.exger.2017.11.013

Maddineni, S., Metzger, S., Ocón, O., Hendricks, G., and Ramachandran, R. (2005). Adiponectin gene is expressed in multiple tissues in the chicken: food deprivation influences adiponectin messenger ribonucleic acid expression. *Endocrinology* 146, 4250–4256. doi: 10.1210/en.2005-0254

Maioli, S., Lodeiro, M., Merino-Serrais, P., Falahati, F., Khan, W., Puerta, E., et al. (2015). Alterations in brain leptin signalling in spite of unchanged CSF leptin levels in Alzheimer's disease. *Aging Cell* 14, 122–129. doi: 10.1111/acel.12281

Malenka, R. C., and Bear, M. F. (2004). LTP and LTD. *Neuron* 44, 5–21. doi: 10.1016/j.neuron.2004.09.012

Malinowski, J. M., and Bolesta, S. (2000). Rosiglitazone in the treatment of type 2 diabetes mellitus: a critical review. *Clin. Ther.* 22, 1151–1168. doi: 10.1016/S0149-2918(00)83060-X

Man, H. Y., Ju, W., Ahmadian, G., and Wang, Y. T. (2000). Intracellular trafficking of AMPA receptors in synaptic plasticity. *Cell. Mol. Life Sci.* 57, 1526–1534.

Mansur, R. B., Brietzke, E., and McIntyre, R. S. (2015). Is there a "metabolic-mood syndrome"? A review of the relationship between obesity and mood disorders. *Neurosci. Biobehav. Rev.* 52, 89–104. doi: 10.1016/j.neubiorev.2014.12.017

Mao, X., Kikani, C. K., Riojas, R. A., Langlais, P., Wang, L., Ramos, F. J., et al. (2006). APPL1 binds to adiponectin receptors and mediates adiponectin signalling and function. *Nat. Cell Biol.* 8, 516–523. doi: 10.1038/ncb1404

Marqués-Iturria, I., Pueyo, R., Garolera, M., Segura, B., Junqué, C., García-García, I., et al. (2013). Frontal cortical thinning and subcortical volume reductions in early adulthood obesity. *Psychiatry Res. Neuroimaging* 214, 109–115. doi: 10.1016/j.pscychresns.2013.06.004

Marwarha, G., Dasari, B., Jaya Prasanthi, R. P., Schommer, J., and Ghribi, O. (2010). β-amyloid regulates leptin expression and tau phosphorylation through the mTORC1 signaling pathway. *J. Neurochem.* 115, 373–384. doi: 10.1111/j.1471-4159.2010.06929.x

Mather, A. A., Cox, B. J., Enns, M. W., and Sareen, J. (2009). Associations of obesity with psychiatric disorders and suicidal behaviors in a nationally representative sample. *J. Psychosom. Res.* 66, 277–285. doi: 10.1016/j.jpsychores.2008.09.008

McCrimmon, R. J., Ryan, C. M., and Frier, B. M. (2012). Diabetes and cognitive dysfunction. *Lancet* 379, 2291–2299. doi: 10.1016/S0140-6736(12)60360-2

McGregor, G., Clements, L., Farah, A., Irving, A. J., and Harvey, J. (2018). Age-dependent regulation of excitatory synaptic transmission at hippocampal temporoammonic-CA1 synapses by leptin. *Neurobiol. Aging* 69, 76–93. doi: 10.1016/j.neurobiolaging.2018.05.007

McGregor, G., and Harvey, J. (2017). Leptin regulation of synaptic function at hippocampal TA-CA1 and SC-CA1 synapses: implications for health and disease. *Neurochem. Res.* doi: 10.1007/s11064-017-2362-1 [Epub ahead of print].

McGregor, G., Irving, A. J., and Harvey, J. (2017). Canonical JAK-STAT signaling is pivotal for long-term depression at adult hippocampal temporoammonic-CA1 synapses. *FASEB J.* 31, 3449–3466. doi: 10.1096/fj.201601293RR

Mcguire, M. J., and Ishii, M. (2016). Leptin dysfunction and Alzheimer's disease: evidence from cellular, animal, and human studies. *Cell. Mol. Neurobiol.* 36, 203–217. doi: 10.1007/s10571-015-0282-7.Leptin

McLean, F. H., Grant, C., Morris, A. C., Horgan, G. W., Polanski, A. J., Allan, K., et al. (2018). Rapid and reversible impairment of episodic memory by a high-fat diet in mice. *Sci. Rep.* 8:11976. doi: 10.1038/s41598-018-30265-4

Mercer, J. G., Hoggard, N., Williams, L. M., Lawrence, C. B., Hannah, L. T., and Trayhurn, P. (2018). Localization of leptin receptor mRNA and the long form splice variant (Ob-Rb) in mouse hypothalamus and adjacent brain regions by in situ hybridization. *FEBS Lett.* 387, 113–116. doi: 10.1016/0014-5793(96)00473-5

Miyatake, Y., Shiuchi, T., Ueta, T., Taniguchi, Y., Futami, A., Sato, F., et al. (2015). Intracerebroventricular injection of adiponectin regulates locomotor activity in rats. *J. Med. Investig.* 62, 199–203. doi: 10.2152/jmi.62.199

Miyoshi, Y., Funahashi, T., Kihara, S., Taguchi, T., Tamaki, Y., Matsuzawa, Y., et al. (2003). Association of serum adiponectin levels with breast cancer risk. *Clin. Cancer Res.* 9, 5699–5704.

Mody, N., Agouni, A., Mcilroy, G. D., Platt, B., and Delibegovic, M. (2011). Susceptibility to diet-induced obesity and glucose intolerance in the APPSWE/PSEN1A246E mouse model of Alzheimer's disease is associated with increased brain levels of protein tyrosine phosphatase 1B (PTP1B) and retinol-binding protein 4 (RBP4), and basal. *Diabetologia* 54, 2143–2151. doi: 10.1007/s00125-011-2160-2

Morash, B., Li, A., Murphy, P. R., Wilkinson, M., and Ur, E. (1999). Leptin gene expression in the brain and pituitary gland. *Endocrinology* 140, 5995–5998. doi: 10.1210/endo.140.12.7288

Morrison, C. D., White, C. L., Wang, Z., Lee, S.-Y., Lawrence, D. S., Cefalu, W. T., et al. (2007). Increased hypothalamic protein tyrosine phosphatase 1B contributes to leptin resistance with age. *Endocrinology* 148, 433–440. doi: 10.1210/en.2006-0672

Moult, P., and Harvey, J. (2009). Regulation of glutamate receptor trafficking by leptin. *Biochem. Soc. Trans.* 37, 1364–1368. doi: 10.1042/BST0371364

Moult, P. R., Cross, A., Santos, S. D., Carvalho, A.-L., Lindsay, Y., Connolly, C. N., et al. (2010). Leptin regulates AMPA receptor trafficking via PTEN inhibition. *J. Neurosci.* 30, 4088–4101. doi: 10.1523/JNEUROSCI.3614-09.2010

Moult, P. R., and Harvey, J. (2011). NMDA receptor subunit composition determines the polarity of leptin-induced synaptic plasticity.

Neuropharmacology 61, 924–936. doi: 10.1016/j.neuropharm.2011.06.021

Moult, P. R., Milojkovic, B., and Harvey, J. (2009). Leptin reverses long-term potentiation at hippocampal CA1 synapses. *J. Neurochem.* 108, 685–696. doi: 10.1111/j.1471-4159.2008.05810.x

Myers, M. G., Cowley, M. A., and Münzberg, H. (2008). Mechanisms of leptin action and leptin resistance. *Annu. Rev. Physiol.* 70, 537–556. doi: 10.1146/annurev.physiol.70.113006.100707

Myers, M. G., Heymsfield, S. B., Haft, C., Kahn, B. B., Laughlin, M., Leibel, R. L., et al. (2012). Defining clinical leptin resistance - challenges and opportunities. *Cell Metab.* 15, 150–156. doi: 10.1016/j.cmet.2012.01.002

Myers, M. G., Leibel, R. L., Seeley, R. J., and Schwartz, M. W. (2010). Obesity and leptin resistance: distinguishing cause from effect. *Trends Endocrinol. Metab.* 21, 643–651. doi: 10.1016/j.tem.2010.08.002

Nägga, K., Gustavsson, A.-M., Stomrud, E., Lindqvist, D., van Westen, D., Blennow, K., et al. (2018). Increased midlife triglycerides predict brain β-amyloid and tau pathology 20 years later. *Neurology* 90, e73–e81. doi: 10.1212/WNL.0000000000004749

Nelson, T. E., Engberink, A. O., Hernandez, R., Puro, A., Huitron-Resendiz, S., Hao, C., et al. (2012). Altered synaptic transmission in the hippocampus of transgenic mice with enhanced central nervous systems expression of interleukin-6. *Brain Behav. Immun.* 26, 959–971. doi: 10.1016/j.bbi.2012.05.005

Neumeier, M., Weigert, J., Buettner, R., Wanninger, J., Schäffler, A., Müller, A. M., et al. (2007). Detection of adiponectin in cerebrospinal fluid in humans. *Am. J. Physiol. Endocrinol. Metab.* 293, E965–E969. doi: 10.1152/ajpendo.00119.2007

Ng, R. C. L., and Chan, K. H. (2017). Potential neuroprotective effects of adiponectin in Alzheimer's disease. *Int. J. Mol. Sci.* 18, 1–13. doi: 10.3390/ijms18030592

Ng, R. C.-L., Cheng, O.-Y., Jian, M., Kwan, J. S.-C., Ho, P. W.-L., Cheng, K. K.-Y., et al. (2016). Chronic adiponectin deficiency leads to Alzheimer's disease-like cognitive impairments and pathologies through AMPK inactivation and cerebral insulin resistance in aged mice. *Mol. Neurodegener.* 11:71. doi: 10.1186/s13024-016-0136-x

Nguyen, J. C. D., Killcross, A. S., and Jenkins, T. A. (2014). Obesity and cognitive decline: role of inflammation and vascular changes. *Front. Neurosci.* 8:375 doi: 10.3389/fnins.2014.00375

Nicolas, S., Cazareth, J., Zarif, H., Guyon, A., Heurteaux, C., Chabry, J., et al. (2017). Globular adiponectin limits microglia pro-inflammatory phenotype through an AdipoR1/NF-κB signaling pathway. *Front. Cell. Neurosci.* 11:352. doi: 10.3389/fncel.2017.00352

Nicolas, S., Debayle, D., Béchade, C., Maroteaux, L., Gay, A.-S., Bayer, P., et al. (2018). Adiporon, an adiponectin receptor agonist acts as an antidepressant and metabolic regulator in a mouse model of depression. *Transl. Psychiatry* 8:159. doi: 10.1038/s41398-018-0210-y

Nicolas, S., Veyssière, J., Gandin, C., Zsürger, N., Pietri, M., Heurteaux, C., et al. (2015). Neurogenesis-independent antidepressant-like effects of enriched environment is dependent on adiponectin. *Psychoneuroendocrinology* 57, 72–83. doi: 10.1016/j.psyneuen.2015.03.017

Nie, J.-M., and Li, H.-F. (2017). Metformin in combination with rosiglitazone contribute to the increased serum adiponectin levels in people with type 2 diabetes mellitus. *Exp. Ther. Med.* 14, 2521–2526. doi: 10.3892/etm.2017.4823

Oania, R., and McEvoy, L. K. (2015). Plasma leptin levels are not predictive of dementia in patients with mild cognitive impairment. *Age Ageing* 44, 53–58. doi: 10.1093/ageing/afu160

Odegaard, J. I., and Chawla, A. (2013). Pleiotropic actions of insulin resistance and inflammation in metabolic homeostasis. *Science* 339, 172–177. doi: 10.1126/science.1230721

Ohashi, K., Yuasa, D., Shibata, R., Murohara, T., and Ouchi, N. (2015). Adiponectin as a target in obesity-related inflammatory state. *Endocr. Metab. Immune Disord. Drug Targets* 15, 145–150.

Okada-Iwabu, M., Yamauchi, T., Iwabu, M., Honma, T., Hamagami, K., Matsuda, K., et al. (2013). A small-molecule AdipoR agonist for type 2 diabetes and short life in obesity. *Nature* 503, 493–499. doi: 10.1038/nature12656

Oomura, Y., Hori, N., Shiraishi, T., Fukunaga, K., Takeda, H., Tsuji, M., et al. (2006). Leptin facilitates learning and memory performance and enhances hippocampal CA1 long-term potentiation and CaMK II phosphorylation in rats. *Peptides* 27, 2738–2749. doi: 10.1016/j.peptides.2006.07.001

Paganoni, S., Deng, J., Jaffa, M., Cudkowicz, M. E., and Wills, A.-M. (2011). Body mass index, not dyslipidemia, is an independent predictor of survival in amyotrophic lateral sclerosis. *Muscle Nerve* 44, 20–24. doi: 10.1002/mus.22114

Pákáski, M., Fehér, A., Juhász, A., Drótos, G., Fazekas, O. C., Kovács, J., et al. (2013). Serum adipokine levels modified by donepezil treatment in Alzheimer's disease. *J. Alzheimers Dis.* 38, 371–377. doi: 10.3233/JAD-131139

Pal, K., Mukadam, N., Petersen, I., and Cooper, C. (2018). Mild cognitive impairment and progression to dementia in people with diabetes, prediabetes and metabolic syndrome: a systematic review and meta-analysis. *Soc. Psychiatry Psychiatr. Epidemiol.* 53, 1149–1160. doi: 10.1007/s00127-018-1581-3

Palta, P., Carlson, M. C., Crum, R. M., Colantuoni, E., Sharrett, A. R., Yasar, S., et al. (2018). Diabetes and cognitive decline in older adults: the ginkgo evaluation of memory study. *J. Gerontol. Ser. A* 73, 123–130. doi: 10.1093/gerona/glx076

Pan, W., Tu, H., and Kastin, A. J. (2006). Differential BBB interactions of three ingestive peptides: obestatin, ghrelin, and adiponectin. *Peptides* 27, 911–916. doi: 10.1016/j.peptides.2005.12.014

Pan, W. W., and Myers, M. G. Jr. (2018). Leptin and the maintenance of elevated body weight. *Nat. Rev. Neurosci.* 19, 95–105. doi: 10.1038/nrn.2017.168

Pannacciulli, N., Del Parigi, A., Chen, K., Le, D. S. N. T., Reiman, E. M., and Tataranni, P. A. (2006). Brain abnormalities in human obesity: a voxel-based morphometric study. *Neuroimage* 31, 1419–1425. doi: 10.1016/j.neuroimage.2006.01.047

Park, H.-K., and Ahima, R. S. (2015). Physiology of leptin: energy homeostasis, neuroendocrine function and metabolism. *Metabolism* 64, 24–34. doi: 10.1016/j.metabol.2014.08.004

Patterson, C. M., Leshan, R. L., Jones, J. C., and Myers, M. G. (2011). Molecular mapping of mouse brain regions innervated by leptin receptor-expressing cells. *Brain Res.* 1378, 18–28. doi: 10.1016/j.brainres.2011.01.010

Paula-Lima, A. C., Brito-Moreira, J., and Ferreira, S. T. (2013). Deregulation of excitatory neurotransmission underlying synapse failure in Alzheimer's disease. *J. Neurochem.* 126, 191–202. doi: 10.1111/jnc.12304

Paz-Filho, G., Wong, M.-L., and Licinio, J. (2010). The procognitive effects of leptin in the brain and their clinical implications. *Int. J. Clin. Pract.* 64, 1808–1812. doi: 10.1111/j.1742-1241.2010.02536.x

Pei, J.-J., Sersen, E., Iqbal, K., and Grundke-Iqbal, I. (1994). Expression of protein phosphatases (PP-1, PP-2A, PP-2B and PTP-1B) and protein kinases (MAP kinase and P34cdc2) in the hippocampus of patients with Alzheimer disease and normal aged individuals. *Brain Res.* 655, 70–76. doi: 10.1016/0006-8993(94)91598-9

Pérez-González, R., Alvira-Botero, M. X., Robayo, O., Antequera, D., Garzón, M., Martín-Moreno, A. M., et al. (2014). Leptin gene therapy attenuates neuronal damages evoked by amyloid-β and rescues memory deficits in APP/PS1 mice. *Gene Ther.* 21, 298–308. doi: 10.1038/gt.2013.85

Pérez-González, R., Antequera, D., Vargas, T., Spuch, C., Bolós, M., and Carro, E. (2011). Leptin induces proliferation of neuronal progenitors and neuroprotection in a mouse model of Alzheimer's disease. *J. Alzheimers Dis.* 24, 17–25. doi: 10.3233/JAD-2011-102070

Platzer, M., Fellendorf, F. T., Bengesser, S. A., Birner, A., Dalkner, N., Hamm, C., et al. (2018). Adiponectin is decreased in bipolar depression. *World J. Biol. Psychiatry* doi: 10.1080/15622975.2018.1500033 [Epub ahead of print].

Pousti, F., Ahmadi, R., Mirahmadi, F., Hosseinmardi, N., and Rohampour, K. (2018). Adiponectin modulates synaptic plasticity in hippocampal dentate gyrus. *Neurosci. Lett.* 662, 227–232. doi: 10.1016/j.neulet.2017.10.042

Psilopanagioti, A., Papadaki, H., Kranioti, E. F., Alexandrides, T. K., and Varakis, J. N. (2009). Expression of adiponectin and adiponectin receptors in human pituitary gland and brain. *Neuroendocrinology* 89, 38–47. doi: 10.1159/000151396

Qi, Y., Takahashi, N., Hileman, S. M., Patel, H. R., Berg, A. H., Pajvani, U. B., et al. (2004). Adiponectin acts in the brain to decrease body weight. *Nat. Med.* 10, 524–529. doi: 10.1038/nm1029

Qiu, G., Wan, R., Hu, J., Mattson, M. P., Spangler, E., Liu, S., et al. (2011). Adiponectin protects rat hippocampal neurons against excitotoxicity. *Age* 33, 155–165. doi: 10.1007/s11357-010-9173-5

Raji, C. A., Ho, A. J., Parikshak, N., Becker, J. T., Lopez, O. L., Kuller, L. H., et al. (2010). Brain structure and obesity. *Hum. Brain Mapp.* 31, 353–364. doi: 10.1002/hbm.20870

Ramos-Lobo, A. M., and Donato, J. (2017). The role of leptin in health and disease. *Temperature* 4, 258–291. doi: 10.1080/23328940.2017.1327003

Rizzo, F. R., Musella, A., De Vito, F., Fresegna, D., Bullitta, S., Vanni, V., et al. (2018). Tumor necrosis factor and interleukin-1 β modulate synaptic plasticity during neuroinflammation. *Neural Plast.* 2018, 1–12. doi: 10.1155/2018/8430123

Rosengren, A., Skoog, I., Gustafson, D., and Wilhelmsen, L. (2005). Body mass index, other cardiovascular risk factors, and hospitalization for dementia. *Arch. Intern. Med.* 165, 321–326.

Ryu, J., Galan, A. K., Xin, X., Dong, F., Abdul-Ghani, M. A., Zhou, L., et al. (2014). APPL1 potentiates insulin sensitivity by facilitating the binding of IRS1/2 to the Insulin Receptor. *Cell Rep.* 7, 1227–1238. doi: 10.1016/j.celrep.2014.04.006

Saad, M. F., Damani, S., Gingerich, R. L., Riad-Gabriel, M. G., Khan, A., Boyadjian, R., et al. (1997). Sexual dimorphism in plasma leptin concentration. *J. Clin. Endocrinol. Metab.* 82, 579–584.

Saltiel, A. R., and Olefsky, J. M. (1996). Thiazolidinediones in the treatment of insulin resistance and type II diabetes. *Diabetes* 45, 1661–1669.

Saltiel, A. R., and Olefsky, J. M. (2017). Inflammatory mechanisms linking obesity and metabolic disease. *J. Clin. Invest.* 127, 1–4. doi: 10.1172/JCI92035

Sarlus, H., and Heneka, M. T. (2017). Microglia in Alzheimer's disease. *J. Clin. Invest.* 127, 3240–3249. doi: 10.1172/JCI90606

Schwartz, M. W., Seeley, R. J., Campfield, L. A., Burn, P., and Baskin, D. G. (1996). Identification of targets of leptin action in rat hypothalamus. *J. Clin. Invest.* 98, 1101–1106. doi: 10.1172/JCI118891

Scott, M. M., Lachey, J. L., Sternson, S. M., Lee, C. E., Elias, C. F., Friedman, J. M., et al. (2009). Leptin targets in the mouse brain. *J. Comp. Neurol.* 514, 518–532. doi: 10.1002/cne.22025

Seixas da Silva, G. S., Melo, H. M., Lourenco, M. V., Lyra e Silva, N. M., de Carvalho, M. B., Alves-Leon, S., et al. (2017). Amyloid-β oligomers transiently inhibit AMP-activated kinase and cause metabolic defects in hippocampal neurons. *J. Biol. Chem.* 292, 7395–7406. doi: 10.1074/jbc.M116.753525

Shah, S. A., Yoon, G. H., Chung, S. S., Abid, M. N., Kim, T. H., Lee, H. Y., et al. (2017). Novel osmotin inhibits SREBP2 via the AdipoR1/AMPK/SIRT1 pathway to improve Alzheimer's disease neuropathological deficits. *Mol. Psychiatry* 22, 407–416. doi: 10.1038/mp.2016.23

Shankar, G. M., Li, S., Mehta, T. H., Garcia-Munoz, A., Shepardson, N. E., Smith, I., et al. (2008). Amyloid-β protein dimers isolated directly from Alzheimer's brains impair synaptic plasticity and memory. *Nat. Med.* 14, 837–842. doi: 10.1038/nm1782

Shanley, L. J., Irving, A. J., and Harvey, J. (2001). Leptin enhances NMDA receptor function and modulates hippocampal synaptic plasticity. *J. Neurosci.* 21:RC186.

Sharkey, R. J., Karama, S., and Dagher, A. (2015). Overweight is not associated with cortical thickness alterations in children. *Front. Neurosci.* 9:24. doi: 10.3389/fnins.2015.00024

Shen, L.-H., Miao, J., Zhao, Y.-J., Zhao, Y.-J., and Liang, W. (2014). Expression of brain adiponectin in a murine model of transient cerebral ischemia. *Int. J. Clin. Exp. Med.* 7, 4590–4596.

Skeberdis, V. A., Lan, J.-Y., Zheng, X., Zukin, R. S., and Bennett, M. V. L. (2001). Insulin promotes rapid delivery of N-methyl-D- aspartate receptors to the cell surface by exocytosis. *Proc. Natl. Acad. Sci. U.S.A.* 98, 3561–3566. doi: 10.1073/pnas.051634698

Song, J., Choi, S.-M., and Kim, B. C. (2017). Adiponectin regulates the polarization and function of microglia via PPAR-γ signaling under amyloid β toxicity. *Front. Cell. Neurosci.* 11:64. doi: 10.3389/fncel.2017.00064

Song, W., Guo, F., Zhong, H., Liu, L., Yang, R., Wang, Q., et al. (2015). Therapeutic window of globular adiponectin against cerebral ischemia in diabetic mice: the role of dynamic alteration of adiponectin/adiponectin receptor expression. *Sci. Rep.* 5:17310. doi: 10.1038/srep17310

Song, W., Huo, T., Guo, F., Wang, H., Wei, H., Yang, Q., et al. (2013). Globular adiponectin elicits neuroprotection by inhibiting NADPH oxidase-mediated oxidative damage in ischemic stroke. *Neuroscience* 248, 136–144. doi: 10.1016/j.neuroscience.2013.05.063

Spranger, J., Verma, S., Göhring, I., Bobbert, T., Seifert, J., Sindler, A. L., et al. (2006). Adiponectin does not cross the blood-brain barrier but modifies cytokine expression of brain endothelial cells. *Diabetes* 55, 141–147.

Steen, E., Terry, B. M., Rivera, E. J., Cannon, J. L., Neely, T. R., Tavares, R., et al. (2005). Impaired insulin and insulin-like growth factor expression and signaling mechanisms in Alzheimer's disease–is this type 3 diabetes? *J. Alzheimers Dis.* 7, 63–80.

Stewart, R., and Liolitsa, D. (1999). Type 2 diabetes mellitus, cognitive impairment and dementia. *Diabet. Med.* 16, 93–112.

Stewart, R., Masaki, K., Xue, Q., Peila, R., Petrovitch, H., White, L. R., et al. (2005). A 32-year prospective study of change in body weight and incident dementia: the honolulu-asia aging study. *Arch. Neurol.* 62, 55–60.

Sun, F., Lei, Y., You, J., Li, C., Sun, L., Garza, J., et al. (2018). Adiponectin modulates ventral tegmental area dopamine neuron activity and anxiety-related behavior through AdipoR1. *Mol. Psychiatry* doi: 10.1038/s41380-018-0102-9 [Epub ahead of print].

Suyama, S., Maekawa, F., Maejima, Y., Kubota, N., Kadowaki, T., and Yada, T. (2016). Glucose level determines excitatory or inhibitory effects of adiponectin on arcuate POMC neuron activity and feeding. *Sci. Rep.* 6:30796. doi: 10.1038/srep30796

Takemura, Y., Ouchi, N., Shibata, R., Aprahamian, T., Kirber, M. T., Summer, R. S., et al. (2007). Adiponectin modulates inflammatory reactions via calreticulin receptor-dependent clearance of early apoptotic bodies. *J. Clin. Invest.* 117, 375–386. doi: 10.1172/JCI29709

Talbot, K., Wang, H.-Y., Kazi, H., Han, L.-Y., Bakshi, K. P., Stucky, A., et al. (2012). Demonstrated brain insulin resistance in Alzheimer's disease patients is associated with IGF-1 resistance, IRS-1 dysregulation, and cognitive decline. *J. Clin. Invest.* 122, 1316–1338. doi: 10.1172/JCI59903

Tartaglia, L. A., Dembski, M., Weng, X., Deng, N., Culpepper, J., Devos, R., et al. (1995). Identification and expression cloning of a leptin receptor, OB-R. *Cell* 83, 1263–1271. doi: 10.1016/0092-8674(95)90151-5

Teixeira, A. L., Diniz, B. S., Campos, A. C., Miranda, A. S., Rocha, N. P., Talib, L. L., et al. (2013). Decreased levels of circulating adiponectin in mild cognitive impairment and Alzheimer's disease. *Neuromolecular Med.* 15, 115–121. doi: 10.1007/s12017-012-8201-2

Terry, R. D., Masliah, E., Salmon, D. P., Butters, N., DeTeresa, R., Hill, R., et al. (1991). Physical basis of cognitive alterations in Alzheimer's disease: synapse loss is the major correlate of cognitive impairment. *Ann. Neurol.* 30, 572–580. doi: 10.1002/ana.410300410

Thundyil, J., Pavlovski, D., Sobey, C. G., and Arumugam, T. V. (2012). Adiponectin receptor signalling in the brain. *Br. J. Pharmacol.* 165, 313–327. doi: 10.1111/j.1476-5381.2011.01560.x

Tong, J.-Q., Zhang, J., Hao, M., Yang, J., Han, Y.-F., Liu, X.-J., et al. (2015). Leptin attenuates the detrimental effects of β-amyloid on spatial memory and hippocampal later-phase long term potentiation in rats. *Horm. Behav.* 73, 125–130. doi: 10.1016/j.yhbeh.2015.06.013

Trayhurn, P., Thomas, M. E., Duncan, J. S., and Rayner, D. V. (1995). Effects of fasting and refeeding on ob gene expression in white adipose tissue of lean and obese (OBlob) mice. *FEBS Lett.* 368, 488–490.

Tsuchida, A., Yamauchi, T., Takekawa, S., Hada, Y., Ito, Y., Maki, T., et al. (2005). Peroxisome proliferator-activated receptor (PPAR)α activation increases adiponectin receptors and reduces obesity-related inflammation in adipose tissue. *Diabetes* 54, 3358–3370.

Une, K., Takei, Y. A., Tomita, N., Asamura, T., Ohrui, T., Furukawa, K., et al. (2010). Adiponectin in plasma and cerebrospinal fluid in MCI and Alzheimer's disease. *Eur. J. Neurol.* 18, 1006–1009. doi: 10.1111/j.1468-1331.2010.03194.x

van Boxtel, M. P. J., Baars, L., and Jolles, J. (2007). Obesity, blood pressure and cognitive function: a reply to Waldstein and Katzel. *Int. J. Obes.* 31:1186.

van Himbergen, T. M., Beiser, A. S., Ai, M., Seshadri, S., Otokozawa, S., Au, R., et al. (2012). Biomarkers for insulin resistance and inflammation and the risk for all-cause dementia and Alzheimer disease: results from the Framingham heart study. *Arch. Neurol.* 69, 594–600.

Vannucchi, G., Toni, C., Maremmani, I., and Perugi, G. (2014). Does obesity predict bipolarity in major depressive patients? *J. Affect. Disord.* 155, 118–122. doi: 10.1016/j.jad.2013.10.035

Várhelyi, Z. P., Kálmán, J., Oláh, Z., Ivitz, E. V., Fodor, E. K., Sántha, M., et al. (2017). Adiponectin receptors are less sensitive to stress in a transgenic mouse model of Alzheimer's disease. *Front. Neurosci.* 11:199. doi: 10.3389/fnins.2017.00199

Veit, R., Kullmann, S., Heni, M., Machann, J., Häring, H.-U., Fritsche, A., et al. (2014). Reduced cortical thickness associated with visceral fat and BMI. *Neuroimage* 6, 307–311. doi: 10.1016/j.nicl.2014.09.013

Vemuri, P., Knopman, D. S., Lesnick, T. G., Przybelski, S. A., Mielke, M. M., Graff-Radford, J., et al. (2017). Evaluation of amyloid protective factors and Alzheimer disease neurodegeneration protective factors in elderly individuals. *JAMA Neurol.* 74, 718–726. doi: 10.1001/jamaneurol.2017.0244

Vieira, M. N. N., and Beckman, D. (2017). Training microglia to resist Alzheimer's disease. *J. Neurosci.* 37, 477–479.

Vieira, M. N. N., Lima-Filho, R. A. S., and De Felice, F. G. (2018). Connecting Alzheimer's disease to diabetes: underlying mechanisms and potential therapeutic targets. *Neuropharmacology* 136, 160–171. doi: 10.1016/j.neuropharm.2017.11.014

Vieira, M. N. N., Lyra e Silva, N. M., Ferreira, S. T., and De Felice, F. G. (2017). Protein tyrosine phosphatase 1B (PTP1B): a potential target for Alzheimer's therapy? *Front. Aging Neurosci.* 9:7. doi: 10.3389/fnagi.2017.00007

Vogelzangs, N., Kritchevsky, S. B., Beekman, A. T. F., Brenes, G. A., Newman, A. B., Satterfield, S., et al. (2010). Obesity and onset of significant depressive symptoms: results from a community-based cohort of older men and women. *J. Clin. Psychiatry* 71, 391–399. doi: 10.4088/JCP.08m04743blu

Waki, H., Yamauchi, T., Kamon, J., Ito, Y., Uchida, S., Kita, S., et al. (2003). Impaired multimerization of human adiponectin mutants associated with diabetes. Molecular structure and multimer formation of adiponectin. *J. Biol. Chem.* 278, 40352–40363. doi: 10.1074/jbc.M300365200

Walker, D. G., Whetzel, A. M., and Lue, L.-F. (2015). Expression of suppressor of cytokine signaling (SOCS) genes in human elderly and Alzheimer's disease brains and human microglia. *Neuroscience* 302, 121–137. doi: 10.1016/j.neuroscience.2014.09.052

Wang, H.-W., Pasternak, J. F., Kuo, H., Ristic, H., Lambert, M. P., Chromy, B., et al. (2002). Soluble oligomers of β amyloid (1-42) inhibit long-term potentiation but not long-term depression in rat dentate gyrus. *Brain Res.* 924, 133–140. doi: 10.1016/S0006-8993(01)03058-X

Wang, M. Y., Zhou, Y. T., Newgard, C. B., and Unger, R. H. (1996). A novel leptin receptor isoform in rat. *FEBS Lett.* 392, 87–90. doi: 10.1016/0014-5793(96)00790-9

Wang, R., and Reddy, P. H. (2017). Role of glutamate and NMDA receptors in Alzheimer's disease. *J. Alzheimers Dis.* 57, 1041–1048. doi: 10.3233/JAD-160763

Wang, S., Zhou, Y., Yang, B., Li, L., Yu, S., Chen, Y., et al. (2016). C1q/tumor necrosis factor-related protein-3 attenuates brain injury after intracerebral hemorrhage via AMPK-dependent pathway in rat. *Front. Cell. Neurosci.* 10:237. doi: 10.3389/fncel.2016.00237

Wang, Y., Lam, K. S. L., Yau, M., and Xu, A. (2008). Post-translational modifications of adiponectin: mechanisms and functional implications. *Biochem. J.* 409, 623–633. doi: 10.1042/BJ20071492

Waterson, M. J., and Horvath, T. L. (2015). Neuronal regulation of energy homeostasis: beyond the hypothalamus and feeding. *Cell Metab.* 22, 962–970. doi: 10.1016/j.cmet.2015.09.026

Wauman, J., and Tavernier, J. (2011). Leptin receptor signaling: pathways to leptin resistance. *Front. Biosci.* 16, 2771–2793.

White, C. L., Whittington, A., Barnes, M. J., Wang, Z., Bray, G. A., and Morrison, C. D. (2009). HF diets increase hypothalamic PTP1B and induce leptin resistance through both leptin-dependent and -independent mechanisms. *Am. J. Physiol. Endocrinol. Metab.* 296, E291–E299. doi: 10.1152/ajpendo.90513.2008

Whitehouse, P. J., Martino, A. M., Antuono, P. G., Lowenstein, P. R., Coyle, J. T., Price, D. L., et al. (1986). Nicotinic acetylcholine binding sites in Alzheimer's disease. *Brain Res.* 371, 146–151. doi: 10.1016/0006-8993(86)90819-X

Whitmer, R. A., Gunderson, E. P., Barrett-Connor, E., Quesenberry, C. P., and Yaffe, K. (2005). Obesity in middle age and future risk of dementia: a 27 year longitudinal population based study. *BMJ* 330:1360.

Whitmer, R. A., Gustafson, D. R., Barrett-Connor, E., Haan, M. N., Gunderson, E. P., and Yaffe, K. (2008). Central obesity and increased risk of dementia more than three decades later. *Neurology* 71, 1057–1064. doi: 10.1212/01.wnl.0000306313.89165.ef

Winocur, G., Greenwood, C. E., Piroli, G. G., Grillo, C. A., Reznikov, L. R., Reagan, L. P., et al. (2005). Memory impairment in obese Zucker rats: an investigation of cognitive function in an animal model of insulin resistance and obesity. *Behav. Neurosci.* 119, 1389–1395. doi: 10.1037/0735-7044.119.5.1389

Xu, H., Gelyana, E., Rajsombath, M., Yang, T., Li, S., and Selkoe, D. (2016). Environmental enrichment potently prevents microglia-mediated neuroinflammation by human amyloid β-protein oligomers. *J. Neurosci.* 36, 9041–9056. doi: 10.1523/JNEUROSCI.1023-16.2016

Xu, L., Rensing, N., Yang, X.-F., Zhang, H. X., Thio, L. L., Rothman, S. M., et al. (2008). Leptin inhibits 4-aminopyridine-and pentylenetetrazole-induced seizures and AMPAR-mediated synaptic transmission in rodents. *J. Clin. Invest.* 118, 272–280. doi: 10.1172/JCI33009

Xu, W. L., Atti, A. R., Gatz, M., Pedersen, N. L., Johansson, B., and Fratiglioni, L. (2011). Midlife overweight and obesity increase late-life dementia risk: a population-based twin study. *Neurology* 76, 1568–1574. doi: 10.1212/WNL.0b013e3182190d09

Xu, Z. P., Gan, G. S., Liu, Y. M., Xiao, J. S., Liu, H. X., Mei, B., et al. (2018). Adiponectin attenuates streptozotocin-induced tau hyperphosphorylation and cognitive deficits by rescuing PI3K/Akt/GSK-3β pathway. *Neurochem. Res.* 43, 316–323. doi: 10.1007/s11064-017-2426-2

Yamauchi, T., Hara, K., Kubota, N., Terauchi, Y., Tobe, K., Froguel, P., et al. (2003a). Dual roles of adiponectin/Acrp30 in vivo as an anti-diabetic and anti-atherogenic adipokine. *Curr. Drug Targets Immune Endocr. Metabol. Disord.* 3, 243–254.

Yamauchi, T., Kamon, J., Ito, Y., Tsuchida, A., Yokomizo, T., Kita, S., et al. (2003b). Cloning of adiponectin receptors that mediate antidiabetic metabolic effects. *Nature* 423, 762–769. doi: 10.1038/nature01705

Yamauchi, T., Kamon, J., Minokoshi, Y., Ito, Y., Waki, H., Uchida, S., et al. (2002). Adiponectin stimulates glucose utilization and fatty-acid oxidation by activating AMP-activated protein kinase. *Nat. Med.* 8, 1288–1295. doi: 10.1038/nm788

Yamauchi, T., Kamon, J., Waki, H., Terauchi, Y., Kubota, N., Hara, K., et al. (2001). The fat-derived hormone adiponectin reverses insulin resistance associated with both lipoatrophy and obesity. *Nat. Med.* 7, 941–946. doi: 10.1038/90984

Yamauchi, T., Nio, Y., Maki, T., Kobayashi, M., Takazawa, T., Iwabu, M., et al. (2007). Targeted disruption of AdipoR1 and AdipoR2 causes abrogation of adiponectin binding and metabolic actions. *Nat. Med.* 13, 332–339. doi: 10.1038/nm1557

Yang, B., Wang, S., Yu, S., Chen, Y., Li, L., Zhang, H., et al. (2017). C1q/tumor necrosis factor-related protein 3 inhibits oxidative stress during intracerebral hemorrhage via PKA signaling. *Brain Res.* 1657, 176–184. doi: 10.1016/j.brainres.2016.11.016

Yang, W.-S., Lee, W.-J., Funahashi, T., Tanaka, S., Matsuzawa, Y., Chao, C.-L., et al. (2001). Weight reduction increases plasma levels of an adipose-derived anti-inflammatory protein, adiponectin. *J. Clin. Endocrinol. Metab.* 86, 3815–3819. doi: 10.1210/jcem.86.8.7741

Yarchoan, M., and Arnold, S. E. (2014). Repurposing diabetes drugs for brain insulin resistance in Alzheimer disease. *Diabetes* 63, 2253–2261. doi: 10.2337/db14-0287

Yau, S. Y., Li, A., Hoo, R. L. C., Ching, Y. P., Christie, B. R., Lee, T. M. C., et al. (2014). Physical exercise-induced hippocampal neurogenesis and antidepressant effects are mediated by the adipocyte hormone adiponectin. *Proc. Natl. Acad. Sci. U.S.A.* 111, 15810–15815. doi: 10.1073/pnas.1415219111

Yin, H., Tian, S., Huang, R., Cai, R., Guo, D., Lin, H., et al. (2018). Low plasma leptin and high soluble leptin receptor levels are associated with mild cognitive impairment in type 2 diabetic patients. *Front. Aging Neurosci.* 10:132. doi: 10.3389/fnagi.2018.00132

Yokota, T., Oritani, K., Takahashi, I., Ishikawa, J., Matsuyama, A., Ouchi, N., et al. (2000). Adiponectin, a new member of the family of soluble defense collagens, negatively regulates the growth of myelomonocytic progenitors and the functions of macrophages. *Blood* 96, 1723–1732.

Yokum, S., Ng, J., and Stice, E. (2011). Relation of regional gray and white matter volumes to current BMI and future increases in BMI: a prospective MRI study. *Int. J. Obes.* 36, 656–664. doi: 10.1038/ijo.2011.175

Yoon, G., Shah, S. A., Ali, T., and Kim, M. O. (2018). The adiponectin homolog osmotin enhances neurite outgrowth and synaptic complexity via AdipoR1/NgR1 signaling in Alzheimer's disease. *Mol. Neurobiol.* 55, 6673–6686. doi: 10.1007/s12035-017-0847-1

Yu, J. G., Javorschi, S., Hevener, A. L., Kruszynska, Y. T., Norman, R. A., Sinha, M., et al. (2002). The effect of thiazolidinediones on plasma adiponectin levels in normal, obese, and type 2 diabetic subjects. *Diabetes* 51, 2968–2974.

Zabolotny, J. M., Bence-Hanulec, K. K., Stricker-Krongrad, A., Haj, F., Wang, Y., Minokoshi, Y., et al. (2002). PTP1B regulates leptin signal transduction in vivo. *Dev. Cell* 2, 489–495.

Zhang, D., Wang, X., and Lu, X.-Y. (2016). Adiponectin exerts neurotrophic effects on dendritic arborization, spinogenesis, and neurogenesis of the dentate gyrus of male mice. *Endocrinology* 157, 2853–2869. doi: 10.1210/en.2015-2078

Zhang, D., Wang, X., Wang, B., Garza, J. C., Fang, X., Wang, J., et al. (2017). Adiponectin regulates contextual fear extinction and intrinsic excitability of dentate gyrus granule neurons through AdipoR2 receptors. *Mol. Psychiatry* 22, 1044–1055. doi: 10.1038/mp.2016.58

Zhang, Y., Proenca, R., Maffei, M., Barone, M., Leopold, L., and Friedman, J. M.

(1994). Positional cloning of the mouse obese gene and its human homologue. *Nature* 372, 425–432.

Zhao, L., Chen, S., Sherchan, P., Ding, Y., Zhao, W., Guo, Z., et al. (2018). Recombinant CTRP9 administration attenuates neuroinflammation via activating adiponectin receptor 1 after intracerebral hemorrhage in mice. *J. Neuroinflammation* 15:215. doi: 10.1186/s12974-018-1256-8

Zhao, W.-Q., Chen, H., Quon, M. J., and Alkon, D. L. (2004). Insulin and the insulin receptor in experimental models of learning and memory. *Eur. J. Pharmacol.* 490, 71–81. doi: 10.1016/j.ejphar.2004.02.045

Zhou, Q., Xiang, H., Li, A., Lin, W., Huang, Z., Guo, J., et al. (2018). Activating adiponectin signaling with exogenous AdipoRon reduces myelin lipid accumulation and suppresses macrophage recruitment after spinal cord injury. *J. Neurotrauma* doi: 10.1089/neu.2018.5783 [Epub ahead of print].

5

Inflammation and Gut-Brain Axis During Type 2 Diabetes: Focus on the Crosstalk Between Intestinal Immune Cells and Enteric Nervous System

Arnaud Bessac[1,2], *Patrice D. Cani*[1,3], *Etienne Meunier*[4], *Gilles Dietrich*[1,2] *and Claude Knauf*[1,2]*

[1] NeuroMicrobiota, European Associated Laboratory INSERM/UCLouvain, Brussels, Belgium, [2] Institut National de la Santé et de la Recherche Médicale, U1220, Université Paul Sabatier, Institut de Recherche en Santé Digestive et Nutrition, Toulouse, France, [3] Metabolism and Nutrition Research Group, Walloon Excellence in Life Sciences and Biotechnology, Louvain Drug Research Institute, UCLouvain, Université catholique de Louvain, Brussels, Belgium, [4] Institut de Pharmacologie et de Biologie Structurale, UMR 5089, Université Paul Sabatier, Toulouse, France

***Correspondence:**
Claude Knauf
claude.knauf@inserm.fr

The gut-brain axis is now considered as a major actor in the control of glycemia. Recent discoveries show that the enteric nervous system (ENS) informs the hypothalamus of the nutritional state in order to control glucose entry in tissues. During type 2 diabetes (T2D), this way of communication is completely disturbed leading to the establishment of hyperglycemia and insulin-resistance. Indeed, the ENS neurons are largely targeted by nutrients (e.g., lipids, peptides) but also by inflammatory factors from different origin (i.e., host cells and gut microbiota). Inflammation, and more particularly in the intestine, contributes to the development of numerous pathologies such as intestinal bowel diseases, Parkinson diseases and T2D. Therefore, targeting the couple ENS/inflammation could represent an attractive therapeutic solution to treat metabolic diseases. In this review, we focus on the role of the crosstalk between intestinal immune cells and ENS neurons in the control of glycemia. In addition, given the growing evidence showing the key role of the gut microbiota in physiology, we will also briefly discuss its potential contribution and role on the immune and neuronal systems.

Keywords: enteric nervous system, immune cells, microbiota, gut-brain axis, diabetes

OVERVIEW OF THE DIFFERENT TYPES OF IMMUNE CELLS IN THE INTESTINE: THE EXAMPLE OF ITS RELATION WITH THE GUT MICROBIOTA

The population of gut microbiota is estimated to 100 trillion microorganisms. Thus, our body is composed of 50% of bacteria and 50% of human cells (Cani, 2016). Precisely, the human body encloses approximatively 4.10^{13} bacteria cells with the largest amount inside the large intestine (10^{11} bacteria cells/g of wet stools) (Sender et al., 2016a). In the last estimation, almost 10 million non-redundant microbial genes have been identified in the human gut (Li et al., 2014). The intestinal tract is subjected to an environmental pressure due to the high microbial load of the luminal content (Sender et al., 2016b). Regarding microbial load, one recent article shows that it is the absolute quantity of microbes and not the proportions of microbes that really matters

(Vandeputte et al., 2017). Depending of the mode of analysis of gut microbiota population (classical relative abundance-based profiling vs. quantitative microbiome profiling), the interpretation of data could be completely different, and maybe falsely interpreted. The study of gut microbiota impacts in physiology is also complicated due to the controversial data present in the literature. In fact, results could differ depending of numerous factors that we have to take into account such as for example dietary environments, but also the composition and the activity of the gut microbes (Cani, 2018a). To illustrate this controversy, *Prevotella copri* and its metabolites could be considered as pro- or anti-diabetic actions depending on the diet or the model used (Cani, 2018a). Therefore, these few examples clearly highlight the fact that we are still at the beginning of the story, and we will need more time to better understand the gut microbiota and its importance in human health.

Nowadays, the impact of gut microbiota in the control of various physiological functions is proposed (Cani, 2018a). Abnormal composition and/or activity of the gut microbiota are associated with the development of numerous pathologies such as cancer, obesity and type 2 diabetes (T2D) (Cani, 2018a; Cani and Jordan, 2018b; Rastelli et al., 2018). Despite the complexity of the crosstalk, a clear link is established between inflammation and modification of the gut microbiota (Stecher, 2015; Cani, 2018a). Here, we will mainly introduce how gut bacteria could modulate the function of intestinal immune cells, and describe the molecular actors involved.

Intestinal bacteria are physically separated from mucosal immune system by a single epithelial cell layer, which the primary function is to absorb nutrients (small intestine) and water (colon). Mucosal immune system prevent microbial invasion and is tightly regulated. One of its major role is to avoid the development of chronic inflammation and the subsequent loss of the intestinal epithelium integrity. Microfold cells or M cells, in the specialized follicle-associated epithelium overlying Peyer Patches (PP), and isolated lymphoid follicles (ILF) are the major cell types that sample bacteria and associated antigens. Processed bacterial-derived antigens are presented locally (i.e., into the PP or ILF) or within the mesenteric lymph nodes that drain dendritic cells to initiate an adaptive immune response (Wells et al., 2017). Both effector- and regulatory-T lymphocytes scattered within the intestinal mucosa are generated in response to commensal bacterial antigens. At steady state, the number and the spectrum of effector-T lymphocytes subsets that are present within the intestinal mucosa are dependent on the host's microbiota. Any pathogen invasion, disruptions of the mucus barrier or of the intestinal epithelium integrity, and/or failure in the regulatory mechanisms of the immune response may result in mucosal inflammation (Barreau and Hugot, 2014; Al Nabhani et al., 2017). Immune mediators released upon inflammation are largely dependent on the nature of the microbes triggering the immune system (Maloy and Powrie, 2011). Intestinal epithelial cells and resident innate immune cells sense pathogens locally. The interactions between the pathogens and the pattern-recognition receptors (PRRs) expressed both by stromal and immune cells trigger rapid production of immune and microbicide mediators (e.g., cytokines, chemokines, bioactive lipids, and cell-autonomous immune effectors), which restrict pathogen growth. In parallel, dendritic cells will mature upon contact with microbe-associated molecular patterns (MAMPs) or when some factors are released by injured tissues, namely the damage associated molecular patterns (DAMPs) (i.e., a process allowing antigen presentation to T cells) (Maloy and Powrie, 2011; Geginat et al., 2015). Regarding the intrinsic properties of mature dendritic cells and their soluble (e.g., cytokines, chemokines) and cellular (stromal, myeloid and lymphoid cells) immune environment, antigen-primed $CD4^+$ T lymphocytes may acquire different effector functions. Indeed, viral or intracellular bacterial infections drive T lymphocyte commitment toward the Th1 phenotype, a process that relies both on the production of IL-12 and IL-18 by myeloid cells and the subsequent IFNγ released by innate lymphoid cells (ILC)1 (Trinchieri, 2003; Bernink et al., 2013). Th1 $CD4^+$ lymphocytes produce high levels of IFNγ but also TNF-α. The clearance of extracellular bacteria and fungi mainly depends on Th17-polarized lymphocytes that produce IL-17, IL-22, IL-21, TNF-α and GMCSF. The differentiation of naïve $CD4^+$ T lymphocytes into Th17 involves an environment enriched in TGFβ, IL-1β and STAT3-inducing cytokines including IL-6 and IL-23 produced by myeloid cells (e.g., dendritic cells and macrophages). IL-23 plays a key role by reinforcing Th17 functional activity and inducing production of GMCSF and TNF-α. The immune polarization of ILCs from group 2 by IL-25, IL-33 and thymic stromal lymphopoietin is a process specific to helminth parasites. This leads to a potent IL-13 release, crucial immune mediator of the anti-parasitic response (Neill et al., 2010). This frontline type 2 cytokine signaling drives the differentiation of T lymphocytes toward the Th2 phenotype, which is characterized by the synthesis of IL4, IL-5 and IL-13 cytokines, that are key to restrict helminth infections. In addition to cytokines, $CD4^+$ T lymphocytes may also produce neuropeptides including opioids, serotonin and vasoactive intestinal peptide (O'Connell et al., 2006; Boue et al., 2011; Souza-Moreira et al., 2011). Within the site of inflammation, most of these neuropeptides as well as chemokines, proteases and bioactive lipids are also produced by endothelial and epithelial cells, migrant and resident innate immune cells.

How make the link between gut microbiota, immunity and metabolic diseases? The development of metabolic disorders is clearly linked with modification of the gut microbiota population, but there are many other factors in the intestine (e.g., bioactive molecules, metabolites, endocrine cells) that are disturbed in pathological state. The diversity of the gut microbiota may not fully explain the pathologic phenotype. In fact, recent data show the importance of specific alterations that may arise at the level of the crosstalk occurring between gut microbes but also luminal and intestinal factors during metabolic disorders (Aron-Wisnewsky et al., 2018; Cani, 2018). One may also mention the controversy regarding microbial diversity and its potential link with the onset of inflammation. This important topic has been recently reviewed and clearly described the potential interaction between microbes and host cells *via* immune factors (Cani, 2018a). Modifications of the balance (i.e., gut microbiota and immunity) between healthy and pathological situations participate to the establishment of a type 2 diabetic state. For example in this review (Cani, 2018a), it is discussed that the production of the short-chain fatty acids propionate is altered during diabetes. In physiological condition, propionate can bind to GPR-43 located on intestinal lymphocytes. In pathological situations, the decrease of propionate may lead to the lower abundance of specific T cells (mucosal-associated invariant T cells and Treg) in the lamina propria of the gut. Consequently, the gut barrier function could be altered, and some pathogen-associated molecular patterns (PAMPs) can reach the circulation. This is for instance the case for the levels of lipopolysaccharides (LPS) that are significantly increased in the blood, and trigger systemic low-grade inflammation (Cani et al., 2007; Chu et al., 2018) observed in the whole body and can generate the insulin resistance state observed during diabetes (Cani et al., 2012).

INTESTINAL INFLAMMATION AND TYPE 2 DIABETES

Obesity and associated metabolic disorders such as T2D are closely related to a « low-grade » inflammation state as described above (Wellen and Hotamisligil, 2005). In addition to well-described tissues (liver, adipose tissue,...) (Hotamisligil, 2006), the intestine may presents an alteration of the gut barrier function thereby leading hyper-permeability, which is associated with a dysbiosis and in some cases with a certain degree of inflammation at the level of the gut (for review see Slyepchenko et al., 2016). Indeed, in response to a high-fat diet (HFD) that induces insulin resistance, it has been proposed that the intestinal tract may develop an inflammatory response characterized by an increase in pro-inflammatory cytokines expression such as TNF-α, IL-1β, IL-6 (Ding et al., 2010; Kim et al., 2012). Some studies have also reported an increase in myeloperoxidase activity (de La Serre et al., 2010) and/or a decrease in IL-18 and IL-22 expression (Everard et al., 2014a; Wang et al., 2014), two cytokines involved in the intestinal barrier homeostasis and the defense against pathogens. However, it is important to note that the degree of inflammation observed during obesity and diabetes does not reach the same magnitude as the one observed during intestinal inflammatory bowel diseases or severe infection. Nevertheless, besides HFD, data also support that the genetic deletion of leptin (ob/ob) or leptin receptors (db/db) in mice leads to the development of obesity and T2D with a significant increase in pro-inflammatory cytokines (TNF-α, IL-1β, IFNγ, IL-6) in the portal vein, as well as an altered gut barrier (Brun et al., 2007). In addition to metabolic consequences, deletion of leptin receptors also alters immunological response against *Entamoeba histolytica* in mice (Guo et al., 2011) as well as in humans (Duggal et al., 2011). The direct link between intestinal inflammation and metabolic disorders is observed in mice knocked-out for TLR5, a component of the innate immune system. TLR5-deficient mice exhibit a diabetic phenotype associated with intestinal inflammation including increase in pro-inflammatory cytokines (IL-1β, TNF-α) and reduction of the length of the colon, one hallmark of intestinal inflammation (Vijay-Kumar et al., 2010; Chassaing et al., 2014).

What are the "local" consequences of this gut inflammation? All mice models above display alterations of the intestinal homeostasis suggesting as close interrelation between "inflammation, microbiota and metabolism" (Geurts et al., 2014). Because of this inflammatory environment, diabetic mice exhibit modifications of intestinal absorptive capacity characterized by an increase of glucose and/or lipids absorption (Ferraris and Vinnakota, 1995; Petit et al., 2007; Mao et al., 2013) that alters the energetic metabolism. Indeed, HFD diabetic mice develop hyperglycemia and hyperinsulinemia (Ding et al., 2010), glucose intolerance and insulin resistance correlated with a decrease in mucus thickness and increased intestinal permeability (Cani et al., 2008; Everard et al., 2013). This is associated with alteration of the gut microbiota composition and activity (Everard et al., 2011, 2014b; Kim et al., 2012; Molinaro et al., 2017) have shown that gut colonization of germ-free mice induces a bi-phasic inflammation that participates to a bi-phasic impairment of glucose metabolism. Interestingly, recent data have also shown in humans a link between gut microbiota and the accumulation of T cells in the gut of obese people following the ingestion of a high-fat diet (Monteiro-Sepulveda et al., 2015). Both the blunted insulin signaling in enterocytes and the altered localization of the glucose transporter GLUT2 in the enterocytes of obese subjects were linked to the nature of cytokines produced by mucosal T cells (Monteiro-Sepulveda et al., 2015). Conversely, in obese and type 2 diabetic patients another study has shown a decreased number of mucosal-associated invariant T cells (MAIT) producing high levels of Th1 and Th17 cytokines (Magalhaes et al., 2015).

Therefore, the molecular partners linking inflammation, gut microbiota and metabolic disorders could be multiple, but the incretin hormones may represent a real potential of interest. The intestinal tract has also the capacity to produce incretins such as Glucagon-Like Peptide-1 (GLP-1) or Gastric Inhibitory Polypeptide (GIP) in response to nutrients and/or bacterial factors (Cani et al., 2013; Rastelli et al., 2018). HFD and ob/ob mice display an alteration of gut endocrine system including the reduction of GIP- and GLP-1-producing cells and a decrease in proglucagon and GIP expression associated with the alteration of incretins secretion in response to an oral glucose load (Morgan et al., 1988; Anini and Brubaker, 2003; Richards et al., 2016; Shimazu-Kuwahara et al., 2017).

In line with these observations, we have demonstrated that prebiotic treatment in diabetic mice restores the level of GLP-1 to improve glucose metabolism (Cani et al., 2006). Moreover, a chronic exposure to TNF-α alters the release of GLP-1 in HFD mice by acting directly on GLP-1-producing cells (Gagnon et al., 2015). Conversely, a 2 weeks treatment with etanercept, an anti-TNF-α drug, reduces hyperglycemia and hyperinsulinemia of HFD mice. Nowadays, this tripartite concept developed in mice is considered as a potential target to treat metabolic disorders (Geurts et al., 2014).

GUT-BRAIN AXIS AND TYPE 2 DIABETES

The gut-brain axis is shown as a major signaling pathway controlling glucose homeostasis, and its disturbance is associated with a T2D phenotype (Abot et al., 2018a,b). In normal conditions, glucose is detected by intestinal glucose sensors (such as SGLT1, GLUT2, TASR1/2) present on intestinal cells (enteroendocrine and brush cells, enteric glial cells and neurons) which inform the whole body from the presence of glucose *via* the release of various factors (i.e., gut hormones, neurotransmitters, metabolites) (Fournel et al., 2016). Then, intestinal glucose detection generates an afferent nervous message that provokes an increase of hypothalamic nitric oxide (NO) release (Fournel et al., 2017). In turn, this increase of hypothalamic NO release favors the entry of glucose in tissues *via* an activation of the autonomic nervous system (Fournel et al., 2017). In db/db mice, intestinal inflammation perturbs the detection of glucose by enteric glucose sensors (Duparc et al., 2011). In this case, the intestine sends an aberrant nervous message that fails to increase hypothalamic NO release (Duparc et al., 2011). Accordingly, the insulin resistance state observed during T2D is linked to alteration of gut-brain axis. Recently, we have discovered that the enteric nervous system (ENS) is implicated in the maintenance of glycemia in the whole body *via* the brain. One of the main functions of ENS is to regulate contractions of intestinal smooth muscle cells. In physiological conditions, the reduction of intestinal contractions provokes a decreased fed hyperglycemia (Fournel et al., 2017; Abot et al., 2018b). The modifications of mechanical contractions are detected by the hypothalamus, which controls glucose utilization (Fournel et al., 2017). During T2D, intestinal inflammation is clearly associated with a dysfunction of ENS neurons (Gonzalez-Correa et al., 2017), which could favor duodenal hyper-contractility (Abot et al., 2018b). Our group has demonstrated that duodenal hyper-contractility participates to the establishment of hyperglycemia of HFD mice by modulating the hypothalamic NO release (Fournel et al., 2017).

Numerous pathologies that link inflammation, gut microbiota and ENS have been described (Greenwood-Van Meerveld et al., 2017). Along those lines, recent data have shown that specific neurodegenerative diseases (i.e., multiple sclerosis, Parkinson disease) were also characterized by gastrointestinal comorbidities. In these patients, the specific alterations in gut motility and other pre-motor symptoms are linked with changes in the gut microbiota composition and activity (Endres and Schafer, 2018). Whether the couple microbiota and metabolites influencing the intestinal neuronal system may explain the onset of the disease remains to be proven, but it is becoming clear that the ENS can be considered as a cellular target to treat inflammatory diseases (T2D, inflammatory bowel diseases and ulcers).

Therefore, targeting the intestinal inflammation and/or the gut microbiota to restore the glucose and mechano-sensors in type 2 diabetic patients presents a real potential of scientific interest, but remains to be determined.

HOW THE INFLAMMATION MODULATES THE ENTERIC NERVOUS SYSTEM?

Environmental changes related to the inflammatory processes that include a large spectrum of innate and adaptive immune responses, may affect ENS including myenteric plexus controlling gut motility (Cani et al., 2006).

Intestinal motility is regulated by ENS that includes intrinsic primary afferent neurons (IPAN), interneurons and choline acetyltransferase (ChAT)-producing excitatory and NO synthase (NOS)-producing inhibitory motor neurons (Abot et al., 2018a). In the context of immune-mediated regulation of intestinal motility, *muscularis* macrophages residing in the myenteric plexus have been largely studied (Mikkelsen, 2010; Muller et al., 2014; De Schepper et al., 2017). However, cytokines, proteases or neuropeptides produced by mucosal immune cells may also modulate the activity of sensory neurons.

IPANs with their axons extending throughout intestinal mucosa and their cell bodies connected with interneurons which synapse with motor neurons may thus constitute central players in the immune-modulation of the intestinal motility. Accordingly, inflammatory cytokines including TNF-α, IL-1β or IL-6 as well as neuromediators released by innate and adaptive immune cells upon intestinal inflammation alter intrinsic and extrinsic enteric sensory neuron activities (Kindt et al., 2010; Basso et al., 2014; Boue et al., 2014; Brierley and Linden, 2014; Buckley et al., 2014; Hughes Moretta et al., 2014; Mawe, 2015). A slower small-bowel transit and reduced smooth muscle contractility have been reported in patients with inflammatory bowel diseases (Rao et al., 1987; Mawe, 2015). In experimental colitis, intestinal motility is either enhanced or reduced depending on the Th1 or Th2 types of inflammation. Th2-driven colitis induces smooth muscle hyper-contractility and augments intestinal transit while Th1-driven colitis is rather associated with hypo-contractility and reduced intestinal transit (Zhao et al., 2003; Shea-Donohue et al., 2012). Moreover, chronic intestinal inflammation often results in increased innervation together with a reduction of the neuronal activation threshold (Villanacci et al., 2008; Brierley and Linden, 2014). The expression of TNF-α receptors (TNFR1, TNFR2) on enteric neurons also suggest that the neuronal activity maybe modulated directly by the inflammatory environment (Chandrasekharan et al., 2013; Gougeon et al., 2013). Actually, TNF-α has the capacity to modulate electrophysiologic properties of neurons *via* a potentiating effect by increasing the action of cholinergic agonists (carbachol) on gut motility (Rehn et al., 2004). This property of TNF-α could explain the negative impact of cytokines on gut motility. In a molecular point of view, the effect of TNF-α is mediated by an upregulation of the Cyclo-Oxygenase

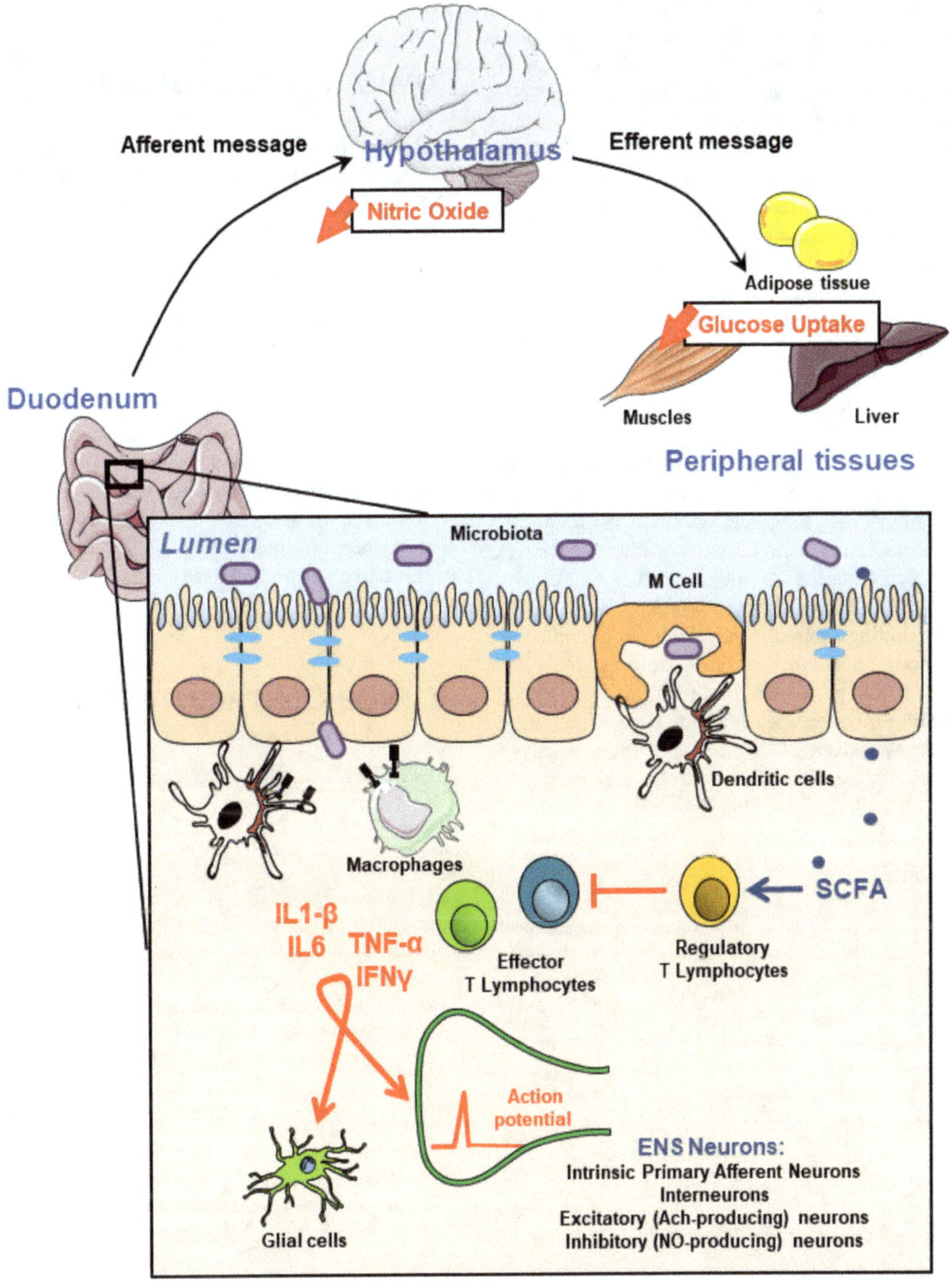

FIGURE 1 | Modulation of the enteric nervous system activity by intestinal immune system may impact on glycemia regulation. Most microbiota-derived products activate both epithelial cells and innate immune cells through pathogen recognition receptors such as toll-like receptors. They also initiate, mainly *via* microbe sampling through M(icrofold) cells, an adaptive immune response. This physiological immune response against intestinal flora generating pro-inflammatory effector T lymhocytes is tighly regulated by regulatory T lymphocytes which induction is associated with the production of short chain fatty acids (SCFAs) by commensal bacteria. Failure of the immune homeostasis may result in the release of higher amounts of proinflammatory cytokines including TNFα, IL1-β, IL6, IFNγ which, in turn, modulate either directly or through glial cells, enteric nervous system (ENS) activity. These alterations of the ENS contribute to impair gut-brain-peripheral axis leading to hyperglycemia and insulin-resistance.

(COX-2), which in turn increases the production of an arachidonic acid derived-molecule, Thromboxane A2 (TXA_2) (Rehn et al., 2005). In experimental colitis, Chandrasekharan et al. (2013) have also demonstrated that TNF-α has an effect on the apoptosis rate of enteric neurons. Treatment with TNF inhibitors provokes a significant decrease of inflammatory markers expression such as inducible NOS (iNOS). IL-1β is another cytokine that has its receptors on ENS neurons (Gougeon et al., 2013). Similarly to TNF-α, IL-1β may increase iNOS mRNA expression in myenteric neurons (Valentine et al., 1996). IL-1β could increase excitability of neurons by directly acting through its receptors expressed on cell surface. Mechanisms of IL-1β including depolarization of the membrane potential, decreased membrane conductance, and increased discharge of action potentials could explain the diarrhea phase, which appears in obese/diabetic patient (Acosta and Camilleri, 2014) or during intestinal inflammation (Xia et al., 1999).

In addition to neurons, the ENS is composed of glial cells that exert a crucial role in intestinal physiology. Suppression of glial cells alters the function of ENS neurons with an increase in excitatory ChAT neurons and a decrease in inhibitory NOS neurons (Aube et al., 2006). Glial cells are exposed to various molecules depending on the environment including immune factors. Proinflammatory cytokines such as IL-1β and/or low IL-10 concentrations have the capacity to block glial cells proliferation (Ruhl et al., 2001a), highlighting links between immune system and enteric nervous system. Moreover, IL-1β has also the capacity to regulate secretory functions of glial cells by increasing IL-6 synthesis and secretion (Ruhl et al., 2001b). In turn, IL-6 may modulate T cell apoptosis or control gut motility to delay gastric emptying (Atreya et al., 2000; Lang Lehrskov et al., 2018).

SUMMARY/CONCLUSION

T2D is associated with modification of the gut physiology including alterations of the function of immune cells and ENS. The crosstalk between the two partners is under the influence of the gut bacteria, which release bioactive factors that could participate as intermediate signaling molecules. Some evidence suggests that the establishment of T2D phenotypes (i.e., hyperglycemia, insulin resistance) may have a potential enteric origin; this is also the case of some neurological disorders (e.g., multiple sclerosis, Parkinson disease, autism). Deciphering the impact of "immune cells-ENS" communication and its impact on "gut-brain" axis could represent a new therapeutic perspective for diabetic patients (**Figure 1**). Therapeutic strategies have to take into account the importance of intestinal inflammation and its consequence on integrity of ENS. The gut microbiota and its bioactive releasing factors could represent one potential solution.

AUTHOR CONTRIBUTIONS

AB, PDC, EM, GD, and CK have wrote the manuscript.

REFERENCES

Abot, A., Cani, P. D., and Knauf, C. (2018a). Impact of intestinal peptides on the enteric nervous system: novel approaches to control glucose metabolism and food intake. *Front. Endocrinol.* 9:328. doi: 10.3389/fendo.2018.00328

Abot, A., Lucas, A., Bautzova, T., Bessac, A., Fournel, A., Le-Gonidec, S., et al. (2018b). Galanin enhances systemic glucose metabolism through enteric nitric oxide synthase-expressed neurons. *Mol. Metab.* 10, 100–108. doi: 10.1016/j.molmet.2018.01.020

Acosta, A., and Camilleri, M. (2014). Gastrointestinal morbidity in obesity. *Ann. N. Y. Acad. Sci.* 1311, 42–56. doi: 10.1111/nyas.12385

Al Nabhani, Z., Dietrich, G., Hugot, J. P., and Barreau, F. (2017). Nod2: the intestinal gate keeper. *PLoS Pathog.* 13:e1006177. doi: 10.1371/journal.ppat.1006177

Anini, Y., and Brubaker, P. L. (2003). Role of leptin in the regulation of glucagon-like peptide-1 secretion. *Diabetes Metab. Res. Rev.* 52, 252–259.

Aron-Wisnewsky, J., Prifti, E., Belda, E., Ichou, F., Kayser, B. D., Dao, M. C., et al. (2018). Major microbiota dysbiosis in severe obesity: fate after bariatric surgery. *Gut* doi: 10.1136/gutjnl-2018-316103 [Epub ahead of print].

Atreya, R., Mudter, J., Finotto, S., Mullberg, J., Jostock, T., Wirtz, S., et al. (2000). Blockade of interleukin 6 trans signaling suppresses T-cell resistance against apoptosis in chronic intestinal inflammation: evidence in crohn disease and experimental colitis in vivo. *Nat. Med.* 6, 583–588. doi: 10.1038/75068

Aube, A. C., Cabarrocas, J., Bauer, J., Philippe, D., Aubert, P., Doulay, F., et al. (2006). Changes in enteric neurone phenotype and intestinal functions in a transgenic mouse model of enteric glia disruption. *Gut* 55, 630–637. doi: 10.1136/gut.2005.067595

Barreau, F., and Hugot, J. P. (2014). Intestinal barrier dysfunction triggered by invasive bacteria. *Curr. Opin. Microbiol.* 17, 91–98. doi: 10.1016/j.mib.2013.12.003

Basso, L., Boue, J., Bourreille, A., and Dietrich, G. (2014). Endogenous regulation of inflammatory pain by T-cell-derived opioids: when friend turns to foe. *Inflamm. Bowel Dis.* 20, 1870–1877. doi: 10.1097/MIB.0000000000000073

Bernink, J. H., Peters, C. P., Munneke, M., te Velde, A. A., Meijer, S. L., Weijer, K., et al. (2013). Human type 1 innate lymphoid cells accumulate in inflamed mucosal tissues. *Nat. Immunol.* 14, 221–229. doi: 10.1038/ni.2534

Boue, J., Basso, L., Cenac, N., Blanpied, C., Rolli-Derkinderen, M., Neunlist, M., et al. (2014). Endogenous regulation of visceral pain via production of opioids by colitogenic CD4(+) T cells in mice. *Gastroenterology* 146, 166–175. doi: 10.1053/j.gastro.2013.09.020

Boue, J., Blanpied, C., Brousset, P., Vergnolle, N., and Dietrich, G. (2011). Endogenous opioid-mediated analgesia is dependent on adaptive T cell response in mice. *J. Immunol.* 186, 5078–5084. doi: 10.4049/jimmunol.1003335

Brierley, S. M., and Linden, D. R. (2014). Neuroplasticity and dysfunction after gastrointestinal inflammation. *Nat. Rev. Gastroenterol. Hepatol.* 11, 611–627. doi: 10.1038/nrgastro.2014.103

Brun, P., Castagliuolo, I., Di Leo, V., Buda, A., Pinzani, M., Palu, G., et al. (2007). Increased intestinal permeability in obese mice: new evidence in the pathogenesis of nonalcoholic steatohepatitis. *Am. J. Physiol. Gastrointest. Liver Physiol.* 292, G518–G525. doi: 10.1152/ajpgi.00024.2006

Buckley, M. M., O'Halloran, K. D., Rae, M. G., Dinan, T. G., and O'Malley, D. (2014). Modulation of enteric neurons by interleukin-6 and corticotropin-releasing factor contributes to visceral hypersensitivity and altered colonic motility in a rat model of irritable bowel syndrome. *J. Physiol.* 592, 5235–5250. doi: 10.1113/jphysiol.2014.279968

Cani, P. D. (2016). Interactions between gut microbes and host cells control gut barrier and metabolism. *Int. J. Obes. Suppl.* 6(Suppl. 1), S28–S31. doi: 10.1038/ijosup.2016.6

Cani, P. D. (2018). Severe obesity and gut microbiota: does bariatric surgery really reset the system? *Gut* doi: 10.1136/gutjnl-2018-316815 [Epub ahead of print].

Cani, P. D. (2018a). Human gut microbiome: hopes, threats and promises. *Gut* 67, 1716–1725. doi: 10.1136/gutjnl-2018-316723

Cani, P. D., Amar, J., Iglesias, M. A., Poggi, M., Knauf, C., Bastelica, D., et al. (2007). Metabolic endotoxemia initiates obesity and insulin resistance. *Diabetes Metab. Res. Rev.* 56, 1761–1772.

Cani, P. D., Bibiloni, R., Knauf, C., Waget, A., Neyrinck, A. M., Delzenne, N. M., et al. (2008). Changes in gut microbiota control metabolic endotoxemia-induced inflammation in high-fat diet-induced obesity and diabetes in mice. *Diabetes Metab. Res. Rev.* 57, 1470–1481. doi: 10.2337/db07-1403

Cani, P. D., Everard, A., and Duparc, T. (2013). Gut microbiota, enteroendocrine functions and metabolism. *Curr. Opin. Pharmacol.* 13, 935–940. doi: 10.1016/j.coph.2013.09.008

Cani, P. D., and Jordan, B. F. (2018b). Gut microbiota-mediated inflammation in obesity: a link with gastrointestinal cancer. *Nat. Rev. Gastroenterol. Hepatol.* doi: 10.1038/s41575-018-0025-6 [Epub ahead of print].

Cani, P. D., Knauf, C., Iglesias, M., Drucker, D., Delzenne, N., and Burcelin, R. (2006). Improvement of glucose tolerance and hepatic insulin sensitivity by oligofructose requires a functional GLP-1 receptor. *Diabetes Metab. Res. Rev.* 55, 1484–1490.

Cani, P. D., Osto, M., Geurts, L., and Everard, A. (2012). Involvement of gut microbiota in the development of low-grade inflammation and type 2 diabetes associated with obesity. *Gut Microbes* 3, 279–288. doi: 10.4161/gmic.19625

Chandrasekharan, B., Jeppsson, S., Pienkowski, S., Belsham, D. D., Sitaraman, S. V., Merlin, D., et al. (2013). Tumor necrosis factor-neuropeptide Y cross talk regulates inflammation, epithelial barrier functions, and colonic motility. *Inflamm. Bowel Dis.* 19, 2535–2546. doi: 10.1097/01.MIB.0000437042.59208.9f

Chassaing, B., Ley, R. E., and Gewirtz, A. T. (2014). Intestinal epithelial cell toll-like receptor 5 regulates the intestinal microbiota to prevent low-grade inflammation and metabolic syndrome in mice. *Gastroenterology* 147, 1363.e17–1377.e17. doi: 10.1053/j.gastro.2014.08.033

Chu, H., Duan, Y., Yang, L., and Schnabl, B. (2018). Small metabolites, possible big changes: a microbiota-centered view of non-alcoholic fatty liver disease. *Gut* doi: 10.1136/gutjnl-2018-316307 [Epub ahead of print].

de La Serre, C. B., Ellis, C. L., Lee, J., Hartman, A. L., Rutledge, J. C., and Raybould, H. E. (2010). Propensity to high-fat diet-induced obesity in rats is associated with changes in the gut microbiota and gut inflammation. *Am. J. Physiol. Gastrointest. Liver Physiol.* 299, G440–G448. doi: 10.1152/ajpgi.00098.2010

De Schepper, S., Stakenborg, N., Matteoli, G., Verheijden, S., and Boeckxstaens, G. E. (2017). Muscularis macrophages: key players in intestinal homeostasis and disease. *Cell. Immunol.* 330, 142–150. doi: 10.1016/j.cellimm.2017.12.009

Ding, S., Chi, M. M., Scull, B. P., Rigby, R., Schwerbrock, N. M., Magness, S., et al. (2010). High-fat diet: bacteria interactions promote intestinal inflammation which precedes and correlates with obesity and insulin resistance in mouse. *PLoS One* 5:e12191. doi: 10.1371/journal.pone.0012191

Duggal, P., Guo, X., Haque, R., Peterson, K. M., Ricklefs, S., Mondal, D., et al. (2011). A mutation in the leptin receptor is associated with *Entamoeba histolytica* infection in children. *J. Clin. Invest.* 121, 1191–1198. doi: 10.1172/JCI45294

Duparc, T., Naslain, D., Colom, A., Muccioli, G. G., Massaly, N., Delzenne, N. M., et al. (2011). Jejunum inflammation in obese and diabetic mice impairs enteric glucose detection and modifies nitric oxide release in the hypothalamus. *Antioxid. Redox. Signal.* 14, 415–423. doi: 10.1089/ars.2010.3330

Endres, K., and Schafer, K. H. (2018). Influence of commensal microbiota on the enteric nervous system and its role in neurodegenerative diseases. *J. Innate. Immun.* 10, 172–180. doi: 10.1159/000488629

Everard, A., Belzer, C., Geurts, L., Ouwerkerk, J. P., Druart, C., Bindels, L. B., et al. (2013). Cross-talk between *Akkermansia muciniphila* and intestinal epithelium controls diet-induced obesity. *Proc. Natl. Acad. Sci. U.S.A.* 110, 9066–9071. doi: 10.1073/pnas.1219451110

Everard, A., Geurts, L., Caesar, R., Van Hul, M., Matamoros, S., Duparc, T., et al. (2014a). Intestinal epithelial MyD88 is a sensor switching host metabolism towards obesity according to nutritional status. *Nat. Commun.* 5:5648. doi: 10.1038/ncomms6648

Everard, A., Lazarevic, V., Gaia, N., Johansson, M., Stahlman, M., Backhed, F., et al. (2014b). Microbiome of prebiotic-treated mice reveals novel targets involved in host response during obesity. *ISME J.* 8, 2116–2130. doi: 10.1038/ismej.2014.45

Everard, A., Lazarevic, V., Derrien, M., Girard, M., Muccioli, G. G., Neyrinck, A. M., et al. (2011). Responses of gut microbiota and glucose and lipid metabolism to prebiotics in genetic obese and diet-induced leptin-resistant mice. *Diabetes Metab. Res. Rev.* 60, 2775–2786. doi: 10.2337/db11-0227

Ferraris, R. P., and Vinnakota, R. R. (1995). Intestinal nutrient transport in genetically obese mice. *Am. J. Clin. Nutr.* 62, 540–546. doi: 10.1093/ajcn/62.3.540

Fournel, A., Drougard, A., Duparc, T., Marlin, A., Brierley, S. M., Castro, J., et al. (2017). Apelin targets gut contraction to control glucose metabolism via the brain. *Gut* 66, 258–269. doi: 10.1136/gutjnl-2015-310230

Fournel, A., Marlin, A., Abot, A., Pasquio, C., Cirillo, C., Cani, P. D., et al. (2016). Glucosensing in the gastrointestinal tract: impact on glucose metabolism. *Am. J. Physiol. Gastrointest. Liver Physiol.* 310, G645–G658. doi: 10.1152/ajpgi.00015.2016

Gagnon, J., Sauve, M., Zhao, W., Stacey, H. M., Wiber, S. C., Bolz, S. S., et al. (2015). Chronic exposure to TNFalpha impairs secretion of glucagon-like peptide-1. *Endocrinology* 156, 3950–3960. doi: 10.1210/en.2015-1361

Geginat, J., Nizzoli, G., Paroni, M., Maglie, S., Larghi, P., Pascolo, S., et al. (2015). Immunity to pathogens taught by specialized human dendritic cell subsets. *Front. Immunol.* 6:527. doi: 10.3389/fimmu.2015.00527

Geurts, L., Neyrinck, A. M., Delzenne, N. M., Knauf, C., and Cani, P. D. (2014). Gut microbiota controls adipose tissue expansion, gut barrier and glucose metabolism: novel insights into molecular targets and interventions using prebiotics. *Benef. Microbes* 5, 3–17. doi: 10.3920/BM2012.0065

Gonzalez-Correa, C. A., Mulett-Vasquez, E., Miranda, D. A., Gonzalez-Correa, C. H., and Gomez-Buitrago, P. A. (2017). The colon revisited or the key to wellness, health and disease. *Med. Hypotheses* 108, 133–143. doi: 10.1016/j.mehy.2017.07.032

Gougeon, P. Y., Lourenssen, S., Han, T. Y., Nair, D. G., Ropeleski, M. J., and Blennerhassett, M. G. (2013). The pro-inflammatory cytokines IL-1beta and TNFalpha are neurotrophic for enteric neurons. *J. Neurosci.* 33, 3339–3351. doi: 10.1523/JNEUROSCI.3564-12.2013

Greenwood-Van Meerveld, B., Johnson, A. C., and Grundy, D. (2017). Gastrointestinal physiology and function. *Handb. Exp. Pharmacol.* 239, 1–16. doi: 10.1007/164_2016_118

Guo, X., Roberts, M. R., Becker, S. M., Podd, B., Zhang, Y., Chua, S. C. Jr., et al. (2011). Leptin signaling in intestinal epithelium mediates resistance to enteric infection by *Entamoeba histolytica*. *Mucosal Immunol.* 4, 294–303. doi: 10.1038/mi.2010.76

Hotamisligil, G. S. (2006). Inflammation and metabolic disorders. *Nature* 444, 860–867. doi: 10.1038/nature05485

Hughes, P. A., Moretta, M., Lim, A., Grasby, D. J., Bird, D., Brierley, S. M., et al. (2014). Immune derived opioidergic inhibition of viscerosensory afferents is decreased in irritable bowel syndrome patients. *Brain Behav. Immun.* 42, 191–203. doi: 10.1016/j.bbi.2014.07.001

Kim, K. A., Gu, W., Lee, I. A., Joh, E. H., and Kim, D. H. (2012). High fat diet-induced gut microbiota exacerbates inflammation and obesity in mice via the TLR4 signaling pathway. *PLoS One* 7:e47713. doi: 10.1371/journal.pone.0047713

Kindt, S., Vanden Berghe, P., Boesmans, W., Roosen, L., and Tack, J. (2010). Prolonged IL-1beta exposure alters neurotransmitter and electrically induced

Ca(2 +) responses in the myenteric plexus. *Neurogastroenterol. Motil.* 22:321-e85. doi: 10.1111/j.1365-2982.2009.01414.x

Lang Lehrskov, L., Lyngbaek, M. P., Soederlund, L., Legaard, J., Ehses, A., Heywood, S. E., et al. (2018). Interleukin-6 delays gastric emptying in humans with direct effects on glycemic control. *Cell Metab.* 27, 1201.e3–1211.e3. doi: 10.1016/j.cmet.2018.04.008

Li, J., Jia, H., Cai, X., Zhong, H., Feng, Q., Sunagawa, S., et al. (2014). An integrated catalog of reference genes in the human gut microbiome. *Nat. Biotechnol.* 32, 834–841. doi: 10.1038/nbt.2942

Magalhaes, I., Pingris, K., Poitou, C., Bessoles, S., Venteclef, N., Kiaf, B., et al. (2015). Mucosal-associated invariant T cell alterations in obese and type 2 diabetic patients. *J. Clin. Invest.* 125, 1752–1762. doi: 10.1172/JCI78941

Maloy, K. J., and Powrie, F. (2011). Intestinal homeostasis and its breakdown in inflammatory bowel disease. *Nature* 474, 298–306. doi: 10.1038/nature10208

Mao, J., Hu, X., Xiao, Y., Yang, C., Ding, Y., Hou, N., et al. (2013). Overnutrition stimulates intestinal epithelium proliferation through beta-catenin signaling in obese mice. *Diabetes Metab. Res. Rev.* 62, 3736–3746. doi: 10.2337/db13-0035

Mawe, G. M. (2015). Colitis-induced neuroplasticity disrupts motility in the inflamed and post-inflamed colon. *J. Clin. Invest.* 125, 949–955. doi: 10.1172/JCI76306

Mikkelsen, H. B. (2010). Interstitial cells of Cajal, macrophages and mast cells in the gut musculature: morphology, distribution, spatial and possible functional interactions. *J. Cell Mol. Med.* 14, 818–832. doi: 10.1111/j.1582-4934.2010.01025.x

Molinaro, A., Caesar, R., Holm, L. M., Tremaroli, V., Cani, P. D., and Backhed, F. (2017). Host-microbiota interaction induces bi-phasic inflammation and glucose intolerance in mice. *Mol. Metab.* 6, 1371–1380. doi: 10.1016/j.molmet.2017.08.016

Monteiro-Sepulveda, M., Touch, S., Mendes-Sa, C., Andre, S., Poitou, C., Allatif, O., et al. (2015). Jejunal T Cell inflammation in human obesity correlates with decreased enterocyte insulin signaling. *Cell Metab.* 22, 113–124. doi: 10.1016/j.cmet.2015.05.020

Morgan, L. M., Hampton, S. M., Tredger, J. A., Cramb, R., and Marks, V. (1988). Modifications of gastric inhibitory polypeptide (GIP) secretion in man by a high-fat diet. *Br. J. Nutr.* 59, 373–380. doi: 10.1079/BJN19880046

Muller, P. A., Koscso, B., Rajani, G. M., Stevanovic, K., Berres, M. L., Hashimoto, D., et al. (2014). Crosstalk between muscularis macrophages and enteric neurons regulates gastrointestinal motility. *Cell* 158:1210. doi: 10.1016/j.cell.2014.08.002

Neill, D. R., Wong, S. H., Bellosi, A., Flynn, R. J., Daly, M., Langford, T. K., et al. (2010). Nuocytes represent a new innate effector leukocyte that mediates type-2 immunity. *Nature* 464, 1367–1370. doi: 10.1038/nature08900

O'Connell, P. J., Wang, X., Leon-Ponte, M., Griffiths, C., Pingle, S. C., and Ahern, G. P. (2006). A novel form of immune signaling revealed by transmission of the inflammatory mediator serotonin between dendritic cells and T cells. *Blood* 107, 1010–1017. doi: 10.1182/blood-2005-07-2903

Petit, V., Arnould, L., Martin, P., Monnot, M. C., Pineau, T., Besnard, P., et al. (2007). Chronic high-fat diet affects intestinal fat absorption and postprandial triglyceride levels in the mouse. *J. Lipid Res.* 48, 278–287. doi: 10.1194/jlr.M600283-JLR200

Rao, S. S., Read, N. W., Davison, P. A., Bannister, J. J., and Holdsworth, C. D. (1987). Anorectal sensitivity and responses to rectal distention in patients with ulcerative colitis. *Gastroenterology* 93, 1270–1275. doi: 10.1016/0016-5085(87)90255-1

Rastelli, M., Knauf, C., and Cani, P. D. (2018). Gut microbes and health: a focus on the mechanisms linking microbes, obesity, and related disorders. *Obesity* 26, 792–800. doi: 10.1002/oby.22175

Rehn, M., Hild, D., and Diener, M. (2005). Upregulation of cyclooxygenase-2 and thromboxane A2 production mediate the action of tumor necrosis factor-alpha in isolated rat myenteric ganglia. *Am. J. Physiol. Gastrointest. Liver Physiol.* 289, G586–G591. doi: 10.1152/ajpgi.00020.2005

Rehn, M., Hubschle, T., and Diener, M. (2004). TNF-alpha hyperpolarizes membrane potential and potentiates the response to nicotinic receptor stimulation in cultured rat myenteric neurones. *Acta Physiol. Scand.* 181, 13–22. doi: 10.1111/j.1365-201X.2004.01269.x

Richards, P., Pais, R., Habib, A. M., Brighton, C. A., Yeo, G. S., Reimann, F., et al. (2016). High fat diet impairs the function of glucagon-like peptide-1 producing L-cells. *Peptides* 77, 21–27. doi: 10.1016/j.peptides.2015.06.006

Ruhl, A., Franzke, S., and Stremmel, W. (2001a). IL-1beta and IL-10 have dual effects on enteric glial cell proliferation. *Neurogastroenterol. Motil.* 13, 89–94.

Ruhl, A., Franzke, S., Collins, S. M., and Stremmel, W. (2001b). Interleukin-6 expression and regulation in rat enteric glial cells. *Am. J. Physiol. Gastrointest. Liver Physiol.* 280, G1163–G1171.

Sender, R., Fuchs, S., and Milo, R. (2016a). Are we really vastly outnumbered? Revisiting the ratio of bacterial to host cells in humans. *Cell* 164, 337–340. doi: 10.1016/j.cell.2016.01.013

Sender, R., Fuchs, S., and Milo, R. (2016b). Revised estimates for the number of human and bacteria cells in the body. *PLoS Biol.* 14:e1002533. doi: 10.1371/journal.pbio.1002533

Shea-Donohue, T., Notari, L., Sun, R., and Zhao, A. (2012). Mechanisms of smooth muscle responses to inflammation. *Neurogastroenterol. Motil.* 24, 802–811. doi: 10.1111/j.1365-2982.2012.01986.x

Shimazu-Kuwahara, S., Harada, N., Yamane, S., Joo, E., Sankoda, A., Kieffer, T. J., et al. (2017). Attenuated secretion of glucose-dependent insulinotropic polypeptide (GIP) does not alleviate hyperphagic obesity and insulin resistance in ob/ob mice. *Mol. Metab.* 6, 288–294. doi: 10.1016/j.molmet.2017.01.006

Slyepchenko, A., Maes, M., Machado-Vieira, R., Anderson, G., Solmi, M., Sanz, Y., et al. (2016). Intestinal dysbiosis, gut hyperpermeability and bacterial translocation: missing links between depression, obesity and type 2 diabetes. *Curr. Pharm. Des.* 22, 6087–6106. doi: 10.2174/1381612822666160922165706

Souza-Moreira, L., Campos-Salinas, J., Caro, M., and Gonzalez-Rey, E. (2011). Neuropeptides as pleiotropic modulators of the immune response. *Neuroendocrinology* 94, 89–100. doi: 10.1159/000328636

Stecher, B. (2015). The roles of inflammation, nutrient availability and the commensal microbiota in enteric pathogen infection. *Microbiol. Spectr.* 3, 1–17. doi: 10.1128/microbiolspec.MBP-0008-2014

Trinchieri, G. (2003). Interleukin-12 and the regulation of innate resistance and adaptive immunity. *Nat. Rev. Immunol.* 3, 133–146. doi: 10.1038/nri1001

Valentine, J. F., Tannahill, C. L., Stevenot, S. A., Sallustio, J. E., Nick, H. S., and Eaker, E. Y. (1996). Colitis and interleukin 1beta up-regulate inducible nitric oxide synthase and superoxide dismutase in rat myenteric neurons. *Gastroenterology* 111, 56–64. doi: 10.1053/gast.1996.v111.pm8698225

Vandeputte, D., Kathagen, G., D'Hoe, K., Vieira-Silva, S., Valles-Colomer, M., Sabino, J., et al. (2017). Quantitative microbiome profiling links gut community variation to microbial load. *Nature* 551, 507–511. doi: 10.1038/nature24460

Vijay-Kumar, M., Aitken, J. D., Carvalho, F. A., Cullender, T. C., Mwangi, S., Srinivasan, S., et al. (2010). Metabolic syndrome and altered gut microbiota in mice lacking Toll-like receptor 5. *Science* 328, 228–231. doi: 10.1126/science.1179721

Villanacci, V., Bassotti, G., Nascimbeni, R., Antonelli, E., Cadei, M., Fisogni, S., et al. (2008). Enteric nervous system abnormalities in inflammatory bowel diseases. *Neurogastroenterol. Motil.* 20, 1009–1016. doi: 10.1111/j.1365-2982.2008.01146.x

Wang, X., Ota, N., Manzanillo, P., Kates, L., Zavala-Solorio, J., Eidenschenk, C., et al. (2014). Interleukin-22 alleviates metabolic disorders and restores mucosal immunity in diabetes. *Nature* 514, 237–241. doi: 10.1038/nature13564

Wellen, K. E., and Hotamisligil, G. S. (2005). Inflammation, stress, and diabetes. *J. Clin. Invest.* 115, 1111–1119. doi: 10.1172/JCI25102

Wells, J. M., Brummer, R. J., Derrien, M., MacDonald, T. T., Troost, F., Cani, P. D., et al. (2017). Homeostasis of the gut barrier and potential biomarkers. *Am. J. Physiol. Gastrointest. Liver Physiol.* 312, G171–G193. doi: 10.1152/ajpgi.00048.2015

Xia, Y., Hu, H. Z., Liu, S., Ren, J., Zafirov, D. H., and Wood, J. D. (1999). IL-1beta and IL-6 excite neurons and suppress nicotinic and noradrenergic neurotransmission in guinea pig enteric nervous system. *J. Clin. Invest.* 103,

1309–1316. doi: 10.1172/JCI5823
Zhao, A., McDermott, J., Urban, J. F. Jr., Gause, W., Madden, K. B., Yeung, K. A., et al. (2003). Dependence of IL-4, IL-13, and nematode-induced alterations in murine small intestinal smooth muscle contractility on Stat6 and enteric nerves. *J. Immunol.* 171, 948–954. doi: 10.4049/jimmunol.171.2.948

6

Cholinergic Control of Inflammation, Metabolic Dysfunction and Cognitive Impairment in Obesity-Associated Disorders: Mechanisms and Novel Therapeutic Opportunities

Eric H. Chang[1,2], Sangeeta S. Chavan[1,2*] and Valentin A. Pavlov[1,2*]*

[1] Center for Bioelectronic Medicine and Biomedical Sciences, Feinstein Institute for Medical Research, Northwell Health, Manhasset, NY, United States, [2] Donald and Barbara Zucker School of Medicine at Hofstra/Northwell, Hempstead, NY, United States

***Correspondence:**
Eric H. Chang
echang1@northwell.edu
Sangeeta S. Chavan
schavan@northwell.edu
Valentin A. Pavlov
vpavlov@northwell.edu

Obesity and obesity-associated disorders have become world-wide epidemics, substantially increasing the risk of debilitating morbidity and mortality. A characteristic feature of these disorders, which include the metabolic syndrome (MetS) and type 2 diabetes, is chronic low-grade inflammation stemming from metabolic and immune dysregulation. Inflammation in the CNS (neuroinflammation) and cognitive impairment have also been associated with obesity-driven disorders. The nervous system has a documented role in the regulation of metabolic homeostasis and immune function, and recent studies have indicated the important role of vagus nerve and brain cholinergic signaling in this context. In this review, we outline relevant aspects of this regulation with a specific focus on obesity-associated conditions. We outline accumulating preclinical evidence for the therapeutic efficacy of cholinergic stimulation in alleviating obesity-associated inflammation, neuroinflammation, and metabolic derangements. Recently demonstrated beneficial effects of galantamine, a centrally acting cholinergic drug and cognitive enhancer, in patients with MetS are also summarized. These studies provide a rationale for further therapeutic developments using pharmacological and bioelectronic cholinergic modulation for clinical benefit in obesity-associated disorders.

Keywords: cholinergic, brain, vagus nerve, obesity, metabolic syndrome, inflammation, neuroinflammation, cognition

INTRODUCTION

Obesity and obesity-related disorders have become prevalent conditions in our modern society, impacting over 1 billion people worldwide (Zimmet et al., 2001; Grundy, 2008; Aguilar et al., 2015; Kim et al., 2019). Obesity and the closely related metabolic syndrome (MetS) generate a substantial risk of developing type 2 diabetes, cardiovascular disease, and other debilitating and life-threatening diseases (Eckel et al., 2005; Grundy, 2008; van Dieren et al., 2010). Therefore, treating these conditions is of primary importance. Diet and exercise are key approaches, but in many cases these lifestyle modifications are either not sustainable or difficult to implement. Clearly, there is a considerable need for better understanding of the complex pathology underlying obesity-driven disorders and for strategizing novel therapeutic approaches. Obesity-related chronic low-grade inflammation provides an important link to metabolic derangements including insulin resistance in these disorders (Shoelson et al., 2007). In addition to peripheral inflammation, inflammation in the CNS (neuroinflammation), affecting the hypothalamus and other brain regions, has also been described and associated with cognitive impairment in the context of obesity (Guillemot-Legris and Muccioli, 2017). Multiple links between peripheral and brain alterations, involving inflammatory, metabolic, and neural components, have been identified in obesity-associated conditions (Schwartz and Porte, 2005; Pavlov and Tracey, 2012). Of note, the role of the nervous system in this relationship has been a specific focus of ongoing research. The nervous system and the brain regulate feeding behavior, energy intake and expenditure, and metabolic homeostasis (Pavlov and Tracey, 2012; Kaelberer et al., 2018). The vagus nerve (the tenth cranial nerve), which contains fibers carrying ascending sensory signals to the brain and descending motor signals to the visceral organs, is importantly involved in these regulatory processes (Pavlov et al., 2018).

The nervous system also communicates with the immune system (Dantzer, 2018; Pavlov et al., 2018), and research during the last 20 years has revealed the important role of the vagus nerve in this communication. A body of preclinical evidence has demonstrated that the vagus nerve regulates inflammatory responses within a physiological mechanism termed *the inflammatory reflex* (Tracey, 2002; Pavlov et al., 2003). Accordingly, electrical vagus nerve stimulation (VNS) has been shown to control the release of pro-inflammatory cytokines and aberrant inflammation in many conditions (Chavan et al., 2017; Pavlov and Tracey, 2017). The mechanisms of the inflammatory reflex, which will be discussed in more detail later, involve alpha7 nicotinic acetylcholine receptor (α7nAChR)-mediated signaling in its efferent arm. Cholinergic compounds, including α7nAChR agonists and centrally acting acetylcholinesterase inhibitors (AChE), have also been shown to alleviate inflammation and metabolic derangements in obesity and MetS (Pavlov and Tracey, 2012). One of these drugs, the centrally acting AChE inhibitor galantamine is in clinical use for counteracting cognitive impairment in Alzheimer's disease (Hampel et al., 2018). A recent clinical trial revealed the anti-inflammatory and beneficial metabolic effects of galantamine in patients with MetS (Consolim-Colombo et al., 2017). Recent clinical studies also demonstrated the utility of bioelectronic VNS in rheumatoid arthritis and inflammatory bowel disease (IBD) – conditions characterized by immune and metabolic dysregulation (Bonaz et al., 2016; Koopman et al., 2016). Future applications of VNS in the arena of MetS and other obesity-driven disorders are feasible and of significant interest.

In this review, we briefly summarize the role of brain and the vagus nerve cholinergic signaling in the regulation of metabolic homeostasis and the role of the vagus nerve-based inflammatory reflex in controlling inflammation. We further point to important aspects of the relationship between inflammation, metabolic deterioration, neuroinflammation, and cognitive impairment in obesity-driven disorders. In this context, we elaborate on accumulating pre-clinical and clinical evidence for therapeutic benefit of stimulating brain and vagus nerve cholinergic signaling. We also consider the potential benefit of enhancing cholinergic signaling by centrally acting AChE inhibitors and VNS for counteracting cognitive deterioration in obesity-driven conditions.

THE BRAIN AND VAGUS NERVE IN METABOLIC REGULATION AND A ROLE FOR CHOLINERGIC SIGNALING

One of the first indications that the brain regulates body metabolism came from studies performed by the 19th century French physiologist Claude Bernard. He reported that electrically stimulating the floor of the fourth ventricle in the brain increased circulating blood glucose and induced a type of transient diabetes, thus connecting the brain with glucose and diabetes (Bernard, 1855). This intriguing brain-to-body metabolism and diabetes link was not intensely studied as the discovery of insulin in 1923 subsequently dominated the diabetes field. However, recent studies have provided important new insights into the role of the brain in the control of peripheral metabolic function and in the context of obesity-driven disorders, including type 2 diabetes. Accumulating evidence indicates that the brain closely monitors peripheral metabolic processes and plays a key role in regulating energy intake and metabolic homeostasis (Morton et al., 2006). The mechanisms involved in this regulation are complex, involving cholecystokinin, leptin, and insulin signaling, and several adiposity-related feedback loops (Morton et al., 2006; van Dijk et al., 2011).

Extensive research has characterized the hypothalamus as an important forebrain region in the regulation of metabolic homeostasis (van Dijk et al., 2011). Neuronal circuitry in the arcuate nucleus within the mediobasal hypothalamus plays a major regulatory role in food intake and metabolism mediating brain effects of leptin, insulin, melanocortins, and other metabolic molecules (Morton et al., 2006; Andermann and Lowell, 2017). For instance, the complex action of leptin on feeding behavior importantly involves activation of an appetite-suppressing population of pro-opiomelanocortin neurons and inhibition of neurons that express agouti-related protein and neuropeptide Y in the arcuate nucleus. Through a circuitry involving other proximal hypothalamic nuclei, such as the paraventricular nucleus and lateral hypothalamic area, these neurons communicate with the brainstem nucleus tractus solitarius (NTS) and promote afferent vagus nerve-mediated satiety and meal termination (Morton et al., 2006). Insulin also stimulates pro-opiomelanocortin neurons, which in turn causes suppression of appetite-promoting population of agouti-related protein neurons (Guilherme et al., 2019). In addition, insulin action in the arcuate nucleus is importantly implicated in the regulation of hepatic glucose production and adipose lipolysis (Konner et al., 2007; Shin et al., 2017). Specific insulin signaling in agouti-related peptide-expressing neurons mediates the suppression of hepatic glucose production by this molecule (Konner et al., 2007) while insulin action on pro-opiomelanocortin neurons is linked to restraining adipose tissue lipolysis (Shin et al., 2017).

The pro-opiomelanocortin neuronal circuit in the hypothalamic arcuate nucleus was also identified as a major mediator of the appetite-suppressing effect of nicotine, thus providing a mechanistic insight into the apparent link between smoking and suppressed appetite (Mineur et al., 2011). α3β4nAChRs on these neurons have an essential role in mediating the suppressive effects of nicotine and other more selective agonists on food intake and weight gain in mice (Andermann and Lowell, 2017). These and other studies implicated brain α3β4 and other nAChRs, and the brain cholinergic system in the regulation of feeding behavior (Jo et al., 2002; Picciotto et al., 2012). As shown in **Figure 1**, major components of this system are the basal forebrain cholinergic system, comprised by several nuclei and the mesopontine/brainstem cholinergic system represented by the pedunculopontine and laterodorsal tegmental nuclei (Woolf and Butcher, 2011; Ballinger et al., 2016; Hampel et al., 2018). Basal forebrain cholinergic neurons innervate different cortex areas, the hippocampus, amygdala, and other regions (**Figure 1**). Among others, major projections of the cholinergic neurons in the mesopontine nuclei include the thalamus and hypothalamus (**Figure 1**). Cholinergic neurons residing in the brainstem dorsal motor nucleus of the vagus (DMN) and nucleus ambiguus (NA) provide peripheral axonal projections within the vagus nerve (**Figure 1**). Recently, basal forebrain cholinergic signaling was importantly implicated in the regulation of feeding behavior using selective optogenetic modulation (Herman et al., 2016; **Figure 1**). Both acute and chronic inactivation of cholinergic neurons in the basal forebrain diagonal band of Broca increases food intake while their stimulation results in decreased food intake (Herman et al., 2016). It was proposed that an extended brain network that regulates targets in the hypothalamic arcuate nucleus may mediate these cholinergic effects (Herman et al., 2016). In addition to nAChRs, muscarinic acetylcholine receptors (mAChRs) importantly mediate brain cholinergic neurotransmission and have also been associated with peripheral metabolic regulation. For instance, cholinergic mAChR-mediated activation in the hypothalamus results in increased hepatic glycogen synthesis and this effect is vagus nerve mediated (Shimazu et al., 1976; Matsushita et al., 1979). In addition, cholinergic M1 mAChR-mediated hypothalamic activation has also been shown to result in increased pancreatic exocrine secretion through the vagus nerve (Li et al., 2003; **Figure 1**).

The vagus nerve is a major conduit linking the brain and periphery in the regulation of metabolism (Berthoud, 2008; Andermann and Lowell, 2017; Metz and Pavlov, 2018). Sensory (afferent) fibers within the vagus nerve with cell bodies in the nodose ganglia communicate signals for alterations in nutrients and metabolic molecules, including cholecystokinin, leptin, and glucose from the gastrointestinal tract and the hepatic portal system to the brainstem (Pavlov and Tracey, 2012; Kaelberer et al., 2018; **Figure 2**). This communication involves neural synaptic transmission that occurs on the timescale of milliseconds, and slower humoral communication on the order of minutes. These signals arrive at NTS in the brainstem medulla oblongata, which is anatomically and functionally linked to DMN. Efferent (motor) vagus nerve cholinergic neurons originating from DMN and NA provide preganglionic innervations to visceral organs and regulate a range of vital cardiovascular, respiratory, and gastrointestinal functions, mediated through mAChRs on the effector cardiac myocytes, smooth muscle cells, and glandular cells (**Figure 1**). The

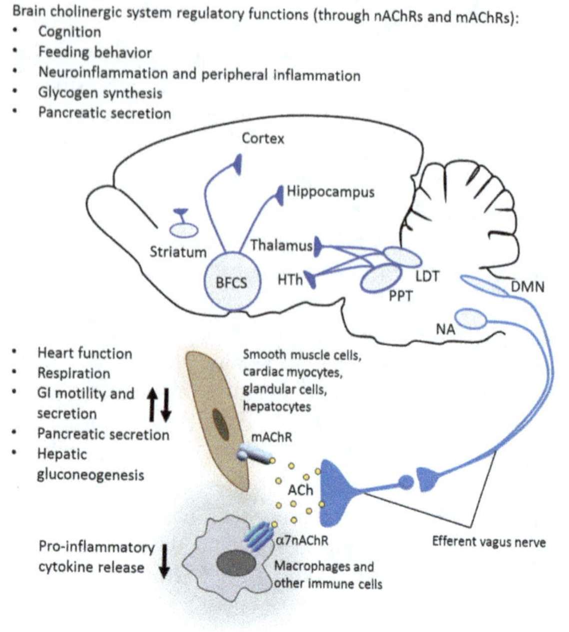

FIGURE 1 | Brain cholinergic system: anatomy and functional control. Important constituents of the brain cholinergic system are the basal forebrain cholinergic system (BFCS) comprised of several nuclei, the mesopontine pedunculopontine and laterodorsal tegmental nuclei (PPT and LDT), and intraneurons in the striatum. Cholinergic neurons provide innervations to different cortex areas, hippocampus, amygdala, olfactory bulb, hypothalamus (HTh), thalamus, and other regions. In addition to its well-documented role in the regulation of cognition, brain cholinergic signaling is implicated in the regulation of appetite and feeding behavior, local brain inflammatory responses (neuroinflammation), hepatic glycogen synthesis, pancreatic secretion, and control of peripheral inflammation (through vagus nerve-mediated mechanisms). Cholinergic neurons in the brainstem dorsal motor nucleus of the vagus (DMN) and nucleus ambiguus (NA) provide axonal projections within preganglionic efferent vagus nerve fibers. These long fibers interact with short postganglionic neurons in proximity or within the innervated organs, including the heart, lungs, gastrointestinal tract, liver, and pancreas. Acetylcholine (ACh) released from these neurons interacts with muscarinic acetylcholine receptors (mAChRs) on targeted cells and regulates several metabolic functions. ACh also regulates (inhibits) the release of pro-inflammatory cytokines and inflammation via alpha 7 nicotinic acetylcholine receptors (α7nAChRs) on immune cells (see the text for more details). (A rodent brain is shown as a substantial part of the information summarized is based on preclinical studies.)

efferent vagus nerve also regulates hepatic gluconeogenesis and pancreatic exocrine and endocrine secretion (Schwartz, 1983; Pocai et al., 2005; Pavlov and Tracey, 2012). For instance, efferent vagus nerve cholinergic signaling stimulates insulin release in the pancreas through M3 mAChR-mediated mechanism (Ruiz de Azua et al., 2011). In addition, mice with selective pancreatic β cells deficiency of the M3 mAChR have lower insulin secretion and impaired glucose tolerance (Gautam et al., 2006). NTS, DMN, and the closely located area postrema (a circumventricular organ) form the dorsal vagal complex, with reciprocal neuronal connectivity with hypothalamic nuclei and other forebrain regions, thus providing an extended brain network in the control of metabolic homeostasis (Pavlov and Tracey, 2012). The vagus nerve through its afferent fibers is a major mediator of satiety and a regulator of feeding behavior (Smith et al., 1981; Berthoud, 2008; Owyang and Heldsinger, 2011; **Figure 2**). Accordingly, a recent study demonstrated the substantial efficacy of implanted battery-free device-generated stimulation of afferent vagus nerve fibers (associated with stomach peristalsis) in achieving and maintaining weight loss in rats (Yao et al., 2018). This finding suggests the possibility of specifically targeting abdominal afferent vagus nerve fibers by bioelectronic devices as a therapeutic approach in obesity.

VAGUS NERVE AND BRAIN CHOLINERGIC SIGNALING IN CONTROLLING INFLAMMATION

Inflammation is a vital physiological response to harmful stimuli, including pathogen invasion and tissue injury through a number of processes and pathways, including the activation of specific immune cell types (e.g., neutrophils and macrophages) and the release of inflammatory mediators (e.g., cytokines and chemokines) (Chen and Nunez, 2010; Olofsson et al., 2017). Inflammation is generally a localized event, which resolves and then the body returns to homeostasis (Chen and Nunez, 2010; Serhan and Levy, 2018). However, different forms of non-resolved, exacerbated, or chronic inflammation cause secondary tissue injury and mediate pathogenesis in sepsis, IBD, rheumatoid arthritis, and many other diseases (Firestein, 2003; Tracey, 2007; Chavan and Tracey, 2017). Therefore, controlling inflammation is critically important in disease prevention and a useful therapeutic strategy in disease treatment. In addition to immune and hormonal regulation, research during the last 20 years has demonstrated an important role of vagus nerve-mediated neural mechanisms in controlling inflammation (Chavan and Tracey, 2017). Several studies have shown that sensory vagus neurons can be activated by cytokines, including IL-1β, TNF, and other inflammatory molecules (Goehler et al., 2000; Steinberg et al., 2016; Zanos et al., 2018). These peripheral inflammatory alterations are communicated to the brainstem and in a reflex arc, vagus nerve cholinergic anti-inflammatory output is generated (Tracey, 2002).

These studies led to the concept of a physiological immunoregulatory mechanism termed the inflammatory reflex (Tracey, 2002). The efferent arm of this mechanism was termed *the cholinergic anti-inflammatory pathway* (Borovikova et al., 2000; Pavlov et al., 2003). Electrical VNS has been instrumental in revealing the anti-inflammatory role of the vagus nerve innervating the liver, gastrointestinal tract, pancreas, and other organs in animal models (Borovikova et al., 2000; de Jonge et al., 2005; Bonaz et al., 2018; Metz and Pavlov, 2018). Cholinergic signaling is translated into suppression of pro-inflammatory cytokine release via α7nAChR-mediated signaling (Wang et al., 2003; Olofsson et al., 2012) and intracellular mechanisms, including suppression of NF-κB nuclear translocation, and JAK2/STAT3 activation (**Figure 3**) (Guarini et al., 2004; de Jonge et al., 2005; Parrish et al., 2008). In addition, recent studies have shown a mediating role for inflammasome inhibition and cAMP signaling (Tarnawski et al., 2018). Substantial advance in our understanding of the inflammatory reflex was achieved by revealing the functional cooperation between the vagus nerve and the splenic nerve and identifying a subset of splenic T cells, containing the enzyme choline acetyltransferase, as a source of acetylcholine in this circuit (Rosas-Ballina et al., 2011; **Figure 3**). Identifying the mediating role of the α7nAChR in the inflammatory reflex generated a line of research demonstrating the anti-inflammatory and disease-alleviating efficacy of α7nAChR agonists in numerous murine models of inflammatory diseases (Pavlov et al., 2007; Parrish et al., 2008; Pavlov and Tracey, 2015). Several studies have also shown that the inflammatory reflex and its efferent arm – the cholinergic anti-inflammatory pathway – can be activated through brain mAChR signaling. The anti-inflammatory and beneficial metabolic effects of centrally acting mAChR ligands and the AChE inhibitor galantamine have been demonstrated in murine models of endotoxemia, IBD, hemorrhagic shock, lupus, and other disorders and linked to the inflammatory reflex (Pavlov et al., 2006, 2009; Lee et al., 2010; Ji et al., 2014; Munyaka et al., 2014; Rosas-Ballina et al., 2015; Pham et al., 2018). In addition to galantamine, the anti-inflammatory effects of other AChE inhibitors and cholinergic drugs clinically approved for the treatment of Alzheimer's disease, such as donepezil and rivastigmine, have also been demonstrated (Lataro et al., 2015; Pavlov and Tracey, 2015; Zhang et al., 2016).

In addition to inflammation in the periphery, inflammation in the CNS and specifically in the brain also occurs in response to tissue damage and pathogens. Persistent neuroinflammation is a characteristic feature of traumatic brain injury, sepsis, multiple sclerosis, other neurodegenerative diseases, and other disorders (Amor et al., 2014; Borst et al., 2018; Pavlov et al., 2018). A link between inflammation, neuroinflammation, and cognitive deterioration has also been identified (Nizri et al., 2008; Terrando et al., 2011; Miller and Spencer, 2014; McManus and Heneka, 2017; Borst et al., 2018). Of note, galantamine, rivastigmine, and donepezil have been shown to alleviate neuroinflammation and improve cognition in preclinical studies (Nizri et al., 2008; Dasuri et al., 2016; Wang et al., 2018; **Figure 2**). In addition, a very recent study demonstrated that in addition to suppressing peripheral inflammation, VNS also alleviates neuroinflammation and cognitive dysfunction in murine endotoxemia (Huffman et al., 2019).

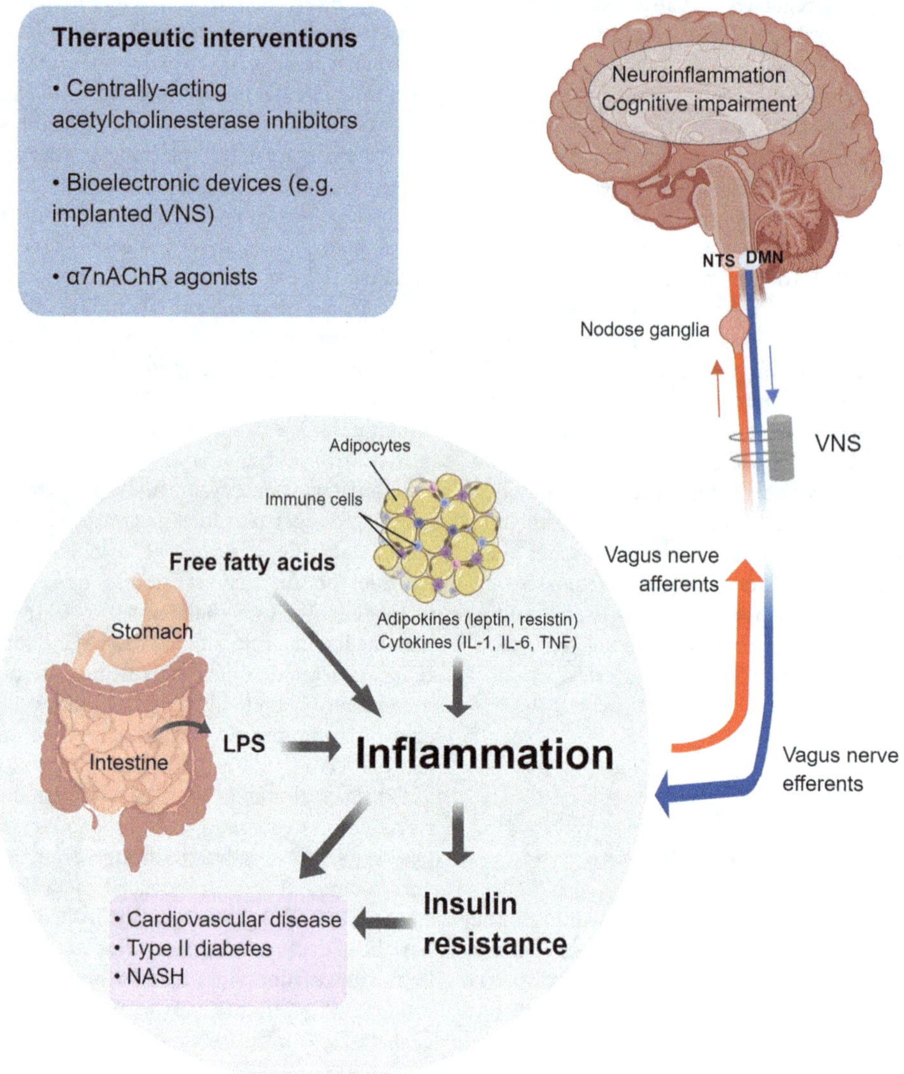

FIGURE 2 | Cholinergic control of inflammation and metabolic derangements in obesity-driven disorders. Inflammation in obesity is a major driver of insulin resistance and other metabolic derangements linked to an increased risk of cardiovascular disease, type 2 diabetes, NASH, and other disorders. Main factors that contribute to this low-grade chronic inflammation are: adipokines and cytokines released from enlarged adipocytes and immune cells infiltrating the expanded white adipose tissue; LPS as a result of microbiota alterations and increased intestinal permeability; and increased levels of free fatty acids. Inflammation and neuroinflammation in obesity are also linked to cognitive impairment. The vagus nerve provides a major conduit for communication between the brain and the periphery. Afferent (sensory) neurons residing in the nodose ganglia and terminating in the NTS detect alterations in peripheral inflammatory and metabolic molecules and communicate this information to the brain. Signaling through efferent cholinergic fibers that originate in the dorsal motor nucleus (DMN) plays an important role in controlling inflammation and metabolic derangements. Brain cholinergic signaling also is implicated in the regulation of cognition and controlling neuroinflammation. Brain and peripheral (vagus nerve) cholinergic signaling can be explored for therapeutic benefit in obesity and obesity-driven conditions. Preclinical and clinical studies have shown the efficacy of galantamine and other centrally acting acetylcholinesterase inhibitors, bioelectronic VNS, and α7nAChRs agonists in alleviating inflammation, metabolic derangements, neuroinflammation, and in improving cognition (See text for details). (This figure was created with BioRender.)

CHOLINERGIC CONTROL OF OBESITY-ASSOCIATED INFLAMMATION AND METABOLIC DERANGEMENTS

Chronic low-grade inflammation is a characteristic pathological feature of obesity and MetS (Eckel et al., 2005; Tilg and Moschen, 2006; Nathan, 2008; Gregor and Hotamisligil, 2011; Lumeng and Saltiel, 2011; Pavlov and Tracey, 2012). Inflammation in obesity is manifested by increased circulating levels of classical pro-inflammatory cytokines, such as TNF and altered levels of adipokines, including leptin, resistin, and adiponectin (Tilg and Moschen, 2006; Lumeng and Saltiel, 2011; Pavlov and Tracey, 2012). Expanded abdominal white adipose tissue in obesity and the crosstalk between metabolically active adipocytes and immune cells infiltrating the adipose tissue, including macrophages, neutrophils, and T lymphocytes, have been identified as a major source of cytokines and adipokines and contributors to this characteristic inflammation (Tilg and Moschen, 2006; Nishimura et al., 2009; Pavlov and Tracey, 2012; Engin, 2017; **Figure 2**). Both enlarged adipocytes and infiltrating immune cells release pro-inflammatory cytokines such as TNF, interleukin-1 (IL-1β), and IL-6 (Pavlov and Tracey, 2012; Engin, 2017). Increased circulating levels of lipopolysaccharide (LPS, endotoxin) have been also detected in obesity (Cani et al., 2007). Microbiota alterations in the gut (increased LPS-containing microbiota) as a result of high-fat diet intake and increased body weight, and the consequent increased intestinal permeability have been associated with this "metabolic endotoxemia," which is another major contributor to inflammation in obesity (Cani et al., 2007; Cani and Delzenne, 2009; Delzenne et al., 2011). LPS, acting through a toll-like receptor 4 (TLR4)-mediated mechanism, triggers the release of TNF and other pro-inflammatory cytokines, mediating pro-inflammatory signals in liver, skeletal muscle, and adipose tissue (Cani et al., 2007; Castanon et al., 2014). Another important contributor to inflammation and other metabolic derangements in obesity is the high levels of free fatty acids (Lumeng and Saltiel, 2011). Acting through TLR4-mediated mechanisms on adipocytes, macrophages, and hepatocytes, free fatty acids trigger intracellular signaling resulting in NF-κB activation and increased TNF and other pro-inflammatory cytokine release (Shi et al., 2006; Baker et al., 2011; Lumeng and Saltiel, 2011; Pavlov and Tracey, 2012). Inflammation in obesity is linked to insulin resistance (Cani et al., 2007; Shoelson et al., 2007; Olefsky and Glass, 2010; Vandanmagsar et al., 2011). For instance, TNF has been shown to directly induce insulin resistance (Hotamisligil et al., 1993; Hotamisligil et al., 1996). In addition, obesity-related inflammation and insulin resistance are linked to fatty liver disease and the development of non-alcoholic steatohepatitis (NASH) (Shoelson et al., 2007; Carter-Kent et al., 2008; Lumeng and Saltiel, 2011; Schuppan and Schattenberg, 2013; **Figure 2**).

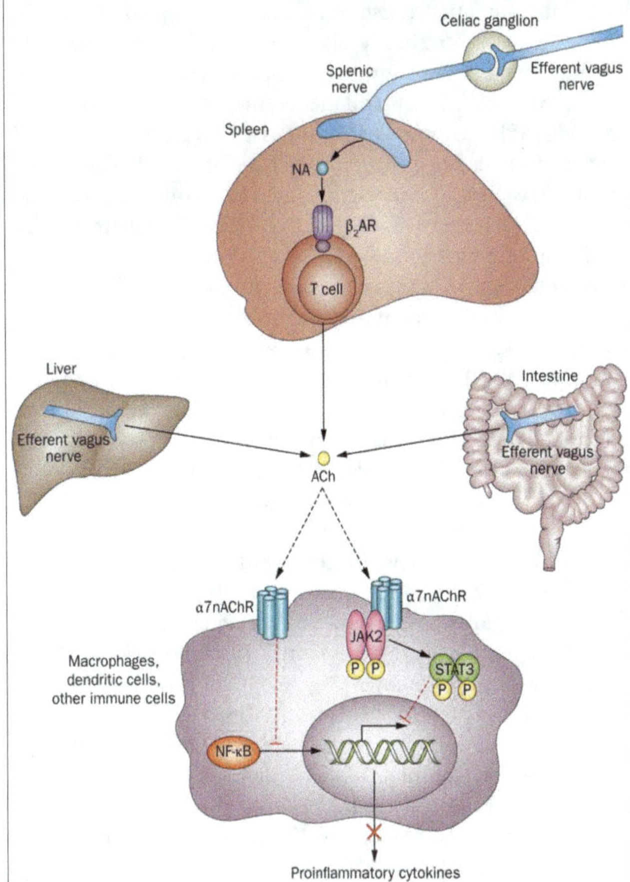

FIGURE 3 | Molecular mechanisms of cholinergic control of inflammation. Efferent vagus nerve activity is translated into catecholamine-mediated activation of T-cell-derived ACh release in the spleen and into direct ACh release from efferent vagus nerve endings in other organs. Inhibition of NF-κB nuclear translocation and activation of a JAK2-STAT3-mediated signaling cascade in macrophages and other immune cells are implicated in cholinergic α7nAChR-mediated control of pro-inflammatory cytokine production. ACh, acetylcholine; β_2AR, β_2 adrenergic receptor; JAK2, Janus kinase 2; α7nAChR, α 7 nicotinic acetylcholine receptor; NA, noradrenaline; NF-κB, nuclear factor κB; STAT3, signal transducer and activator of transcription 3.

Approaches based on electrical VNS have been successfully explored in the treatment of obesity (Val-Laillet et al., 2010; Malbert et al., 2017; Masi et al., 2018). Several studies have also indicated the efficacy of targeting the inflammatory reflex using pharmacological modalities in alleviating inflammation and metabolic derangements interrelated in obesity-driven conditions (Pavlov and Tracey, 2012; **Figure 2**). Administration of nicotine (an α7nAChR agonist) to genetically obese *db/db* mice lacking the leptin receptor and mice with high-fat diet-induced obesity suppresses adipose tissue and systemic TNF levels (Wang et al., 2011). Nicotine also decreases adipose tissue expression of *CCL2* and the macrophage marker *F4/80*, pointing to alleviation of adipose tissue macrophage infiltration. In addition, α7nAChR KO mice on a high-fat diet have increased M1 macrophage infiltration and upregulated expression of TNF and CCL2 in adipose tissue compared to WT controls (Wang et al., 2011). Oral administration of the selective α7nAChR agonist TC-7020 to *db/db* mice significantly lowers systemic TNF and this effect is abrogated by co-administering methyllycaconitine – a selective α7nAChR antagonist (Marrero et al., 2010). TC-7020 administration to *db/db* mice also reduces weight gain, food intake and blood glucose, HbA1c, and triglyceride levels and these beneficial effects are also abrogated by methyllycaconitine (Marrero et al., 2010). Importantly, administration of a JAK2 inhibitor significantly diminishes the TC-7020 effects on body weight, food intake, and blood glucose levels, a finding that suggests a link between α7nAChR- and JAK2-mediated signaling (Marrero et al., 2010). An important role for vagus nerve α7nAChR-mediated cholinergic signaling in experimental NASH was also demonstrated (Nishio et al., 2017). In a murine model of diet-induced NASH, α7nAChR KO chimeric mice (produced by transplanting α7nAChR bone marrow cells into γ-irradiated and Kupffer cell-depleted wild-type recipients) develop an accelerated form of disease (Nishio et al., 2017). These mice have significantly upregulated pro-inflammatory cytokine expression and altered/abnormal lipid metabolic pattern. Selective hepatic vagotomy in this model also results in increased TNF, IL-12, and CCL2 (MCP-1) levels indicative for increased hepatic inflammation (Nishio et al., 2017). Using α7nAChR KO mice, another recent study also demonstrated the tonic anti-inflammatory and anti-fibrotic role of this receptor in models of atherogenic high-fat diet- and methionine/choline-deficient diet-induced NASH (Kimura et al., 2018). In these models, α7nAChR deficiency resulted in exacerbated hepatic fibrosis, higher plasma transaminase levels, and significantly increased Col1a1 gene-encoding alpha-1 type I collagen (mediating liver fibrosis) *Ccl2* and *Tnf* gene expression (Kimura et al., 2018).

As noted above, the inflammatory reflex can be activated by the centrally acting cholinergic drug, the AChE inhibitor galantamine (Pavlov et al., 2009; Ji et al., 2014; Pham et al., 2018). Galantamine alleviates inflammation and metabolic derangements in a high-fat diet-induced model of obesity and MetS (Satapathy et al., 2011). Galantamine treatment of mice with established obesity (after 8 weeks on a high-fat diet) significantly lowers plasma IL-6, CCL2, leptin, and resistin levels, and reduces body weight, food intake, and abdominal white adipose depots (Satapathy et al., 2011). Galantamine also decreases blood glucose, plasma insulin, and cholesterol levels, and alleviates insulin resistance and fatty liver disease in these mice (Satapathy et al., 2011). Recent work has also shown that galantamine has anti-diabetic effects in murine models (Ali et al., 2015; Hanes et al., 2015). Of note, the anti-diabetic effects of galantamine treatment of rats with established n5-STZ diabetes are greater than the effects of the anti-diabetic drug vildagliptin also used in the study (Ali et al., 2015). These and other preclinical studies indicate that neural cholinergic modulation, either pharmacologically or through bioelectronic VNS, can be further explored to treat obesity-related inflammatory and metabolic derangements.

NEUROINFLAMMATION AND COGNITIVE IMPAIRMENT IN OBESITY-DRIVEN DISORDERS: A CHOLINERGIC LINK TO TREATMENT

In addition to inflammation in the periphery, obesity is associated with neuroinflammation (Miller and Spencer, 2014; Guillemot-Legris and Muccioli, 2017; Lainez et al., 2018; **Figure 2**). This neuroinflammation occurs in multiple brain structures, including the hypothalamus, hippocampus, amygdala, neocortex, and cerebellum, and there is evidence that it is sex-specific (Miller and Spencer, 2014; Guillemot-Legris and Muccioli, 2017; Lainez et al., 2018). In these brain regions, diet-induced obesity is associated with increased levels of pro-inflammatory cytokines along with higher expression of NF-κB and TLR4, two important molecular mediators of innate immune responses (Biessels et al., 2014). This type of neuroinflammation may involve recruitment of peripheral immune cells (Miller and Spencer, 2014; Lainez et al., 2018) and there is evidence that peripheral inflammation precipitates brain inflammation (Miller and Spencer, 2014; Guillemot-Legris and Muccioli, 2017). Studies have linked obesity with cognitive impairment and both inflammation and neuroinflammation may play a mediating role in this context (Pistell et al., 2010; Sellbom and Gunstad, 2012; Miller and Spencer, 2014). Association between obesity and diabetes derangements, and increased risk of developing dementia has also been indicated (Whitmer et al., 2005; Strachan et al., 2011; Biessels et al., 2014).

The brain cholinergic system (**Figure 1**) plays a major role in the regulation of memory, attention, and learning (Ballinger et al., 2016; Hampel et al., 2018). Cholinergic neurodegeneration predominantly affecting the basal forebrain neurons and neuroinflammation are hallmarks of brain pathology in Alzheimer's disease (Heneka et al., 2015; Hampel et al., 2018). As mentioned earlier, centrally acting AChE inhibitors, including galantamine, donepezil, and rivastigmine, are clinically approved cholinergic drugs for treating cognitive impairment in Alzheimer's disease (Hampel et al., 2018). There is accumulating experimental evidence that brain cholinergic dysfunction is implicated in cognitive impairment in obesity as recently reviewed (Martinelli et al., 2017). High-fat diet-induced obesity in mice results in increased brain AChE expression and neuroinflammation manifested by microglial activation (Dasuri et al., 2016). Of note, donepezil treatment suppresses brain microglial activation and neuroinflammation in this model (Dasuri et al., 2016). There is also experimental evidence that enhancing cholinergic signaling by galantamine and rivastigmine also results in anti-inflammatory effects in the brain and improved cognition (Nizri et al., 2008; Wang et al., 2018). It is interesting and important that many brain regions affected by neuroinflammation in obesity, including the hypothalamus, hippocampus, amygdala, and cortex receive cholinergic innervations (**Figure 1**). Whether cholinergic dysfunction facilitates neuroinflammation in obesity is a question that remains to be further addressed.

Together these findings paint a picture of peripheral inflammation and neuroinflammation interrelated with cognitive impairment and cholinergic dysfunction in obesity. An improved understanding of the relationship between these elements of pathology in obesity would provide a solid rationale for designing new therapeutic approaches.

CLINICAL TRANSLATION OF CHOLINERGIC MODULATION IN OBESITY-DRIVEN DISORDERS

Obesity and obesity-related conditions, including MetS, type 2 diabetes, NASH, and cardiovascular disease, present a substantial health burden. Current treatment options are limited to lifestyle modifications, non-specific drugs, or insulin injections for those with type 2 diabetes. Unfortunately, lifestyle changes and dietary modifications are only temporarily effective for durable weight loss. For instance, a study with obese women subjected to caloric restrictions and behavioral therapy showed that nearly 50% of lost weight is regained within 1 year and almost all of it is regained within 5 years (Wadden et al., 1989). Non-specific weight loss medications have a blemished track record and are also often ineffective as long-term solutions. Obesity-related type 2 diabetes is a progressive disorder and most patients eventually require treatment with insulin to control blood glucose levels as β cells in the pancreas lose their ability to produce insulin (Kahn and Hull, 2006). While generally effective, injectable insulin can produce side effects such as hypoglycemia, hunger, weakness, irritability, and requires frequent monitoring of blood glucose levels. The current studies on closed-loop control systems in diabetes known as "the artificial pancreas" may provide a significant advance in overcoming these disadvantages (Kovatchev, 2018). Other treatment options for obesity-driven disorders include surgical interventions with bariatric surgery which can result in long-term weight loss, but surgical treatments come with significant risks and are only recommended for the morbidly obese (Chang et al., 2014). Thus, the limitations of currently available treatments for obesity-driven disorders invite an exploration of new targets and pathways. In this context, targeting inflammation remains an attractive area for further exploration (Goldfine et al., 2011; Esser et al., 2015).

Based on preclinical evidence for beneficial anti-inflammatory and metabolic efficacy, cholinergic modulation in treating obesity-driven disorders is of specific interest (**Figure 2**). An additional advantage is that cholinergic drugs such as centrally acting AChE inhibitors and bioelectronics, including implanted devices for VNS are already clinically approved for other indications. Galantamine is a centrally acting AChE inhibitor that has been FDA approved to treat the cognitive impairment in patients with Alzheimer's disease in the United States for more than a decade (Hampel et al., 2018). There is a large amount of safety information available, making galantamine an attractive candidate to be clinically repurposed. A major obesity-driven disorder is MetS, a cluster of conditions that includes high blood pressure, high blood glucose levels, abdominal obesity, and dyslipidemia (Eckel et al., 2005; Grundy, 2008). The combination of these conditions within MetS generates a significantly higher risk of developing type 2 diabetes, cardiovascular disease, cancer, and other life-threatening and debilitating diseases, compared to the individual condition-related risk (Eckel et al., 2005). Apart from lifestyle modifications, treating MetS as a whole presents a significant challenge, and usually several medications targeting the separate risk factors are prescribed. Inflammation as a driver of insulin resistance and other pathogenesis in MetS provides an attractive therapeutic target (Esser et al., 2015). Based on preclinical findings, the efficacy of galantamine in alleviating inflammation and insulin resistance alongside other metabolic indices in people with MetS was recently studied in a randomized, placebo-controlled, double blind trial (Consolim-Colombo et al., 2017). Relatively short treatment (for 12 weeks) with galantamine in doses clinically approved for Alzheimer's disease, significantly decreased plasma TNF and leptin levels and increased IL-10 and adiponectin levels (Consolim-Colombo et al., 2017). Galantamine treatment vs. placebo also modulated the autonomic neural regulation, as determined by heart rate variability analysis, toward parasympathetic (vagal) predominance (Consolim-Colombo et al., 2017).

Another approach of cholinergic neuromodulation to explore in treating obesity-driven diseases is VNS. The feasibility of this approach for treating immune and metabolic derangements in humans was recently demonstrated in clinical trials with patients with IBD and rheumatoid arthritis (Bonaz et al., 2016; Koopman et al., 2016). Interestingly, humans with obesity have reduced vagal tone (Karason et al., 1999; Carnethon et al., 2003), coexisting with inflammation and metabolic deterioration. Since activation of vagal efferents attenuates immune and metabolic dysfunction, it is possible that reduced vagal cholinergic output plays a causative role in immune and metabolic dysregulation. VNS is clinically approved for epilepsy and depression (Ben-Menachem, 2001; Bonaz, 2018). Of note, patients receiving VNS for medication-refractory epilepsy or depression have also reported weight loss, in as high as 60% of the patients tested (Burneo et al., 2002; Pardo et al., 2007). While these patients were receiving VNS for other non-metabolic indications, these weight loss effects suggest the possible therapeutic utility of VNS in obesity-associated conditions. VNS implants for epilepsy and depression have been routinely used and the therapy is well-tolerated (Ben-Menachem, 2001). The risks associated with VNS implantation surgery are low and side effects of the stimulation itself are minor, typically limited to cough and hoarseness (Sackeim et al., 2001; O'Reardon et al., 2006). A recent study demonstrated that specific vagus nerve signals in response to alterations in cytokine levels can be recorded (Zanos et al., 2018). Therefore, in the future, an advanced version of bioelectronic vagus nerve modulation could potentially provide the additional advantage of enabling "closed-loop" control of immune and metabolic dysfunctions. Preclinical research has also indicated the possibility to use α7nAChR agonists in treating inflammatory and metabolic derangements in human obesity. This is also supported by demonstrating α7nAChR expression in human adipocytes and its role in controlling pro-inflammatory gene expression (Cancello et al., 2012). Furthermore, obesity is associated with significant decrease in human adipocyte α7nAChR and weight loss partially restores its expression (Cancello et al., 2012).

Cognitive deterioration and an increased risk of developing dementia are documented in obesity, MetS, and type 2 diabetes (Strachan et al., 2011; Biessels et al., 2014). This cognitive dysfunction is interrelated with inflammatory and metabolic derangements and treating these conditions is challenging (Strachan et al., 2011; Guillemot-Legris and Muccioli, 2017). An important point is that while designing new approaches for treating obesity and related conditions, one should account for their effects on the brain in relation to cognitive impairment (Strachan et al., 2011). The cholinergic system in the brain has a key role in the regulation of cognition (Picciotto et al., 2012; Ballinger et al., 2016). Numerous studies have evaluated galantamine, donepezil, and rivastigmine as cognitive enhancers and these drugs are in current clinical use for the symptomatic treatment of Alzheimer's disease. As recently demonstrated, galantamine has beneficial anti-inflammatory and metabolic effects in patients with MetS (Consolim-Colombo et al., 2017).

Therefore, future developments with galantamine and other centrally acting AChE inhibitors in the treatment of patients with obesity-associated disorders may include assessing the potential benefit of these drugs on cognition. VNS has been also associated with pro-cognitive effects especially in the domains of verbal recognition, memory, and executive function (Groves and Brown, 2005; Vonck et al., 2014). The precise mechanisms of these VNS pro-cognitive effects are largely unknown and one possibility that remains to be explored is a mediating role of brain cholinergic signaling. Recent findings have indicated that NTS afferent vagus nerve signaling reaches basal forebrain cholinergic nuclei innervating the hippocampus and cortex and implicated in cognitive regulation (Suarez et al., 2018). These studies and other clinical trials currently underway (ClinicalTrials.gov Identifier: NCT02365285) generate a growing platform for further studies on the therapeutic utility of cholinergic modulation in obesity-associated disorders.

CONCLUDING REMARKS

In obesity and obesity-associated conditions, immune and metabolic dysregulation result in chronic systemic inflammation, neuroinflammation, exacerbated insulin resistance, fatty liver disease, cognitive impairment, and other pathological manifestations. An improved understanding of this complex pathology requires providing new insight into the regulatory role of the nervous system. Neural circuitry, including vagus nerve cholinergic signaling, plays a major role in controlling metabolic and immune homeostasis (**Figures 1–3**). Vagus nerve cholinergic signaling within the inflammatory reflex has an important regulatory role in the crosstalk between immune and metabolic alterations in obesity-driven disorders. Activation of cholinergic signaling by VNS, α7nAChR agonists, and centrally acting drugs such as galantamine results in anti-inflammatory effects, alleviation of insulin resistance and hepatic steatosis, and other beneficial effects in murine models of obesity, MetS, NASH, and type 2 diabetes. This large body of preclinical evidence and the fact that both centrally acting AChE inhibitors and VNS are already in clinical use provide a rationale for expanding these approaches into clinical settings of obesity. A recent clinical trial with galantamine in MetS demonstrated the translational applicability of this research and the anti-inflammatory and beneficial metabolic effects of AChE inhibitors (Consolim-Colombo et al., 2017). Enhancing brain cholinergic signaling by these drugs and the use of VNS to alleviate obesity-associated brain pathology, including neuroinflammation and cognitive deterioration in humans, are feasible approaches that remain to be studied. Recent discoveries of gut–brain neural circuits that involve the vagus nerve (Han et al., 2018; Kaelberer et al., 2018) and future preclinical research using advances in molecular genetics within the growing field of bioelectronic medicine (Olofsson and Tracey, 2017; Pavlov and Tracey, 2019) will improve our understanding of neural regulation of immunity and metabolism and its implications in obesity. This research holds the potential to identify new therapeutic avenues for alleviation of the obesity disease burden.

AUTHOR CONTRIBUTIONS

EHC, SSC, and VAP wrote, edited, and finalized the manuscript.

ACKNOWLEDGMENTS

The authors thank Kevin J. Tracey for his comments on the manuscript.

REFERENCES

Aguilar, M., Bhuket, T., Torres, S., Liu, B., and Wong, R. J. (2015). Prevalence of the metabolic syndrome in the United States, 2003-2012. *JAMA* 313, 1973–1974. doi: 10.1001/jama.2015.4260

Ali, M. A., El-Abhar, H. S., Kamel, M. A., and Attia, A. S. (2015). Antidiabetic effect of galantamine: novel effect for a known centrally acting drug. *PLoS One* 10:e0134648. doi: 10.1371/journal.pone.0134648

Amor, S., Peferoen, L. A., Vogel, D. Y., Breur, M., van der Valk, P., Baker, D., et al. (2014). Inflammation in neurodegenerative diseases–an update. *Immunology* 142, 151–166. doi: 10.1111/imm.12233

Andermann, M. L., and Lowell, B. B. (2017). Toward a wiring diagram understanding of appetite control. *Neuron* 95, 757–778. doi: 10.1016/j.neuron.2017.06.014

Baker, R. G., Hayden, M. S., and Ghosh, S. (2011). NF-kappaB, inflammation, and metabolic disease. *Cell Metab.* 13, 11–22. doi: 10.1016/j.cmet.2010.12.008

Ballinger, E. C., Ananth, M., Talmage, D. A., and Role, L. W. (2016). Basal forebrain cholinergic circuits and signaling in cognition and cognitive decline. *Neuron* 91, 1199–1218. doi: 10.1016/j.neuron.2016.09.006

Ben-Menachem, E. (2001). Vagus nerve stimulation, side effects, and long-term safety. *J. Clin. Neurophysiol.* 18, 415–418. doi: 10.1097/00004691-200109000-00005

Bernard, C. (1855). *Leçons de Physiologie Expérimentale Appliquée à la Médecine: Faites au Collège de France*. Paris: Hachette Livre. doi: 10.5962/bhl.title.1818

Berthoud, H. R. (2008). The vagus nerve, food intake and obesity. *Regul. Pept.* 149, 15–25. doi: 10.1016/j.regpep.2007.08.024

Biessels, G. J., Strachan, M. W., Visseren, F. L., Kappelle, L. J., and Whitmer, R. A. (2014). Dementia and cognitive decline in type 2 diabetes and prediabetic stages: towards targeted interventions. *Lancet Diabetes Endocrinol.* 2, 246–255. doi: 10.1016/S2213-8587(13)70088-3

Bonaz, B. (2018). Is-there a place for vagus nerve stimulation in inflammatory bowel diseases? *Bioelectron. Med.* 4:4. doi: 10.1186/s42234-018-0004-9

Bonaz, B., Bazin, T., and Pellissier, S. (2018). The vagus nerve at the interface of the microbiota-gut-brain axis. *Front. Neurosci.* 12:49. doi: 10.3389/fnins.2018.00049

Bonaz, B., Sinniger, V., Hoffmann, D., Clarencon, D., Mathieu, N., Dantzer, C., et al. (2016). Chronic vagus nerve stimulation in Crohn's disease: a 6-month follow-up pilot study. *Neurogastroenterol. Motil.* 28, 948–953. doi: 10.1111/nmo.12792

Borovikova, L. V., Ivanova, S., Zhang, M., Yang, H., Botchkina, G. I., Watkins, L. R., et al. (2000). Vagus nerve stimulation attenuates the systemic inflammatory response to endotoxin. *Nature* 405, 458–462. doi: 10.1038/35013070

Borst, K., Schwabenland, M., and Prinz, M. (2018). Microglia metabolism in health and disease. *Neurochem. Int.* doi: 10.1016/j.neuint.2018.11.006 [Epub ahead of print].

Burneo, J. G., Faught, E., Knowlton, R., Morawetz, R., and Kuzniecky, R. (2002). Weight loss associated with vagus nerve stimulation. *Neurology* 59, 463–464. doi: 10.1212/WNL.59.3.463

Cancello, R., Zulian, A., Maestrini, S., Mencarelli, M., Della Barba, A., Invitti, C., et al. (2012). The nicotinic acetylcholine receptor alpha7 in subcutaneous mature adipocytes: downregulation in human obesity and modulation by diet-induced weight loss. *Int. J. Obes.* 36, 1552–1557. doi: 10.1038/ijo.2011.275

Cani, P. D., Amar, J., Iglesias, M. A., Poggi, M., Knauf, C., Bastelica, D., et al. (2007). Metabolic endotoxemia initiates obesity and insulin resistance. *Diabetes* 56, 1761–1772. doi: 10.2337/db06-1491

Cani, P. D., and Delzenne, N. M. (2009). The role of the gut microbiota in energy metabolism and metabolic disease. *Curr. Pharm. Des.* 15, 1546–1558. doi: 10.2174/138161209788168164

Carnethon, M. R., Jacobs, D. R. Jr., Sidney, S., and Liu, K. (2003). Influence of autonomic nervous system dysfunction on the development of type 2 diabetes: the CARDIA study. *Diabetes Care* 26, 3035–3041. doi: 10.2337/diacare.26.11.3035

Carter-Kent, C., Zein, N. N., and Feldstein, A. E. (2008). Cytokines in the pathogenesis of fatty liver and disease progression to steatohepatitis: implications for treatment. *Am. J. Gastroenterol.* 103, 1036–1042. doi: 10.1111/j.1572-0241.2007.01709.x

Castanon, N., Lasselin, J., and Capuron, L. (2014). Neuropsychiatric comorbidity in obesity: role of inflammatory processes. *Front. Endocrinol.* 5:74. doi: 10.3389/fendo.2014.00074

Chang, S. H., Stoll, C. R., Song, J., Varela, J. E., Eagon, C. J., and Colditz, G. A. (2014). The effectiveness and risks of bariatric surgery: an updated systematic review and meta-analysis, 2003-2012. *JAMA Surg.* 149, 275–287. doi: 10.1001/jamasurg.2013.3654

Chavan, S. S., Pavlov, V. A., and Tracey, K. J. (2017). Mechanisms and therapeutic relevance of neuro-immune communication. *Immunity* 46, 927–942. doi: 10.1016/j.immuni.2017.06.008

Chavan, S. S., and Tracey, K. J. (2017). Essential neuroscience in immunology. *J. Immunol.* 198, 3389–3397. doi: 10.4049/jimmunol.1601613

Chen, G. Y., and Nunez, G. (2010). Sterile inflammation: sensing and reacting to damage. *Nat. Rev. Immunol.* 10, 826–837. doi: 10.1038/nri2873

Consolim-Colombo, F. M., Sangaleti, C. T., Costa, F. O., Morais, T. L., Lopes, H. F., Motta, J. M., et al. (2017). Galantamine alleviates inflammation and insulin resistance in patients with metabolic syndrome in a randomized trial. *JCI Insight* 2:93340. doi: 10.1172/jci.insight.93340

Dantzer, R. (2018). Neuroimmune interactions: from the brain to the immune system and vice versa. *Physiol. Rev.* 98, 477–504. doi: 10.1152/physrev.00039.2016

Dasuri, K., Zhang, L., Kim, S. O., Bruce-Keller, A. J., and Keller, J. N. (2016). Dietary and donepezil modulation of mTOR signaling and neuroinflammation in the brain. *Biochim. Biophys. Acta* 1862, 274–283. doi: 10.1016/j.bbadis.2015.11.002

de Jonge, W. J., van der Zanden, E. P., The, F. O., Bijlsma, M. F., van Westerloo, D. J., Bennink, R. J., et al. (2005). Stimulation of the vagus nerve attenuates macrophage activation by activating the Jak2-STAT3 signaling pathway. *Nat. Immunol.* 6, 844–851. doi: 10.1038/ni1229

Delzenne, N. M., Neyrinck, A. M., Backhed, F., and Cani, P. D. (2011). Targeting gut microbiota in obesity: effects of prebiotics and probiotics. *Nat. Rev. Endocrinol.* 7, 639–646. doi: 10.1038/nrendo.2011.126

Eckel, R. H., Grundy, S. M., and Zimmet, P. Z. (2005). The metabolic syndrome. *Lancet* 365, 1415–1428. doi: 10.1016/S0140-6736(05)66378-7

Engin, A. (2017). The pathogenesis of obesity-associated adipose tissue inflammation. *Adv. Exp. Med. Biol.* 960, 221–245. doi: 10.1007/978-3-319-48382-5_9

Esser, N., Paquot, N., and Scheen, A. J. (2015). Anti-inflammatory agents to treat or prevent type 2 diabetes, metabolic syndrome and cardiovascular disease. *Expert Opin. Investig. Drugs* 24, 283–307. doi: 10.1517/13543784.2015.974804

Firestein, G. S. (2003). Evolving concepts of rheumatoid arthritis. *Nature* 423, 356–361. doi: 10.1038/nature01661

Gautam, D., Han, S. J., Hamdan, F. F., Jeon, J., Li, B., Li, J. H., et al. (2006). A critical role for beta cell M3 muscarinic acetylcholine receptors in regulating insulin release and blood glucose homeostasis in vivo. *Cell Metab.* 3, 449–461. doi: 10.1016/j.cmet.2006.04.009

Goehler, L. E., Gaykema, R. P., Hansen, M. K., Anderson, K., Maier, S. F., and Watkins, L. R. (2000). Vagal immune-to-brain communication: a visceral chemosensory pathway. *Auton. Neurosci.* 85, 49–59. doi: 10.1016/S1566-0702(00)00219-8

Goldfine, A. B., Fonseca, V., and Shoelson, S. E. (2011). Therapeutic approaches to target inflammation in type 2 diabetes. *Clin. Chem.* 57, 162–167. doi: 10.1373/clinchem.2010.148833

Gregor, M. F., and Hotamisligil, G. S. (2011). Inflammatory mechanisms in obesity. *Annu. Rev. Immunol.* 29, 415–445. doi: 10.1146/annurev-immunol-031210-101322

Groves, D. A., and Brown, V. J. (2005). Vagal nerve stimulation: a review of its applications and potential mechanisms that mediate its clinical effects. *Neurosci. Biobehav. Rev.* 29, 493–500. doi: 10.1016/j.neubiorev.2005.01.004

Grundy, S. M. (2008). Metabolic syndrome pandemic. *Arterioscler. Thromb. Vasc. Biol.* 28, 629–636. doi: 10.1161/ATVBAHA.107.151092

Guarini, S., Cainazzo, M. M., Giuliani, D., Mioni, C., Altavilla, D., Marini, H., et al. (2004). Adrenocorticotropin reverses hemorrhagic shock in anesthetized rats through the rapid activation of a vagal anti-inflammatory pathway. *Cardiovasc. Res.* 63, 357–365. doi: 10.1016/j.cardiores.2004.03.029

Guilherme, A., Henriques, F., Bedard, A. H., and Czech, M. P. (2019). Molecular pathways linking adipose innervation to insulin action in obesity and diabetes mellitus. *Nat. Rev. Endocrinol.* doi: 10.1038/s41574-019-0165-y [Epub ahead of print].

Guillemot-Legris, O., and Muccioli, G. G. (2017). Obesity-induced neuroinflammation: beyond the hypothalamus. *Trends Neurosci.* 40, 237–253. doi: 10.1016/j.tins.2017.02.005

Hampel, H., Mesulam, M. M., Cuello, A. C., Farlow, M. R., Giacobini, E., Grossberg, G. T., et al. (2018). The cholinergic system in the pathophysiology and treatment of Alzheimer's disease. *Brain* 141, 1917–1933. doi: 10.1093/brain/awy132

Han, W., Tellez, L. A., Perkins, M. H., Perez, I. O., Qu, T., Ferreira, J., et al. (2018). A neural circuit for gut-induced reward. *Cell* 175, 665–678.e23. doi: 10.1016/j.cell.2018.08.049

Hanes, W. M., Olofsson, P. S., Kwan, K., Hudson, L. K., Chavan, S. S., Pavlov, V. A., et al. (2015). Galantamine attenuates type 1 diabetes and inhibits anti-insulin antibodies in non-obese diabetic mice. *Mol. Med.* 21, 702–708. doi: 10.2119/molmed.2015.00142

Heneka, M. T., Carson, M. J., El Khoury, J., Landreth, G. E., Brosseron, F., Feinstein, D. L., et al. (2015). Neuroinflammation in Alzheimer's disease. *Lancet Neurol.* 14, 388–405. doi: 10.1016/S1474-4422(15)70016-5

Herman, A. M., Ortiz-Guzman, J., Kochukov, M., Herman, I., Quast, K. B., Patel, J. M., et al. (2016). A cholinergic basal forebrain feeding circuit modulates appetite suppression. *Nature* 538, 253–256. doi: 10.1038/nature19789

Hotamisligil, G. S., Peraldi, P., Budavari, A., Ellis, R., White, M. F., and Spiegelman, B. M. (1996). IRS-1-mediated inhibition of insulin receptor tyrosine kinase activity in TNF-alpha- and obesity-induced insulin resistance. *Science* 271, 665–668. doi: 10.1126/science.271.5249.665

Hotamisligil, G. S., Shargill, N. S., and Spiegelman, B. M. (1993). Adipose expression of tumor necrosis factor-alpha: direct role in obesity-linked insulin resistance. *Science* 259, 87–91. doi: 10.1126/science.7678183

Huffman, W. J., Subramaniyan, S., Rodriguiz, R. M., Wetsel, W. C., Grill, W. M., and Terrando, N. (2019). Modulation of neuroinflammation and memory dysfunction using percutaneous vagus nerve stimulation in mice. *Brain Stimul.* 12, 19–29. doi: 10.1016/j.brs.2018.10.005

Ji, H., Rabbi, M. F., Labis, B., Pavlov, V. A., Tracey, K. J., and Ghia, J. E. (2014). Central cholinergic activation of a vagus nerve-to-spleen circuit alleviates experimental colitis. *Mucosal Immunol.* 7, 335–347. doi: 10.1038/mi.2013.52

Jo, Y. H., Talmage, D. A., and Role, L. W. (2002). Nicotinic receptor-mediated effects on appetite and food intake. *J. Neurobiol.* 53, 618–632. doi: 10.1002/neu.10147

Kaelberer, M. M., Buchanan, K. L., Klein, M. E., Barth, B. B., Montoya, M. M., Shen, X., et al. (2018). A gut-brain neural circuit for nutrient sensory transduction. *Science* 361:eaat5236. doi: 10.1126/science.aat5236

Kahn, S. E., and Hull, R. L. (2006). Utzschneider KM. Mechanisms linking obesity to insulin resistance and type 2 diabetes. *Nature* 444, 840–846. doi: 10.1038/nature05482

Karason, K., Molgaard, H., Wikstrand, J., and Sjostrom, L. (1999). Heart rate variability in obesity and the effect of weight loss. *Am. J. Cardiol.* 83, 1242–1247. doi: 10.1016/S0002-9149(99)00066-1

Kim, M., Basharat, A., Santosh, R., Mehdi, S. F., Razvi, Z., Yoo, S. K., et al. (2019). Reuniting overnutrition and undernutrition, macronutrients, and micronutrients. *Diabetes Metab. Res. Rev.* 35:e3072. doi: 10.1002/dmrr.3072

Kimura, K., Inaba, Y., Watanabe, H., Matsukawa, T., Matsumoto, M., and Hiroshi, I. (2018). Nicotinic alpha 7 acetylcholine receptor deficiency exacerbates hepatic inflammation and fibrosis in a mouse model of nonalcoholic steatohepatitis. *J. Diabetes Investig.* doi: 10.1111/jdi.12964 [Epub ahead of print].

Konner, A. C., Janoschek, R., Plum, L., Jordan, S. D., Rother, E., Ma, X., et al. (2007). Insulin action in AgRP-expressing neurons is required for suppression of hepatic glucose production. *Cell Metab.* 5, 438–449. doi: 10.1016/j.cmet.2007.05.004

Koopman, F. A., Chavan, S. S., Miljko, S., Grazio, S., Sokolovic, S., Schuurman, P. R., et al. (2016). Vagus nerve stimulation inhibits cytokine production and attenuates disease severity in rheumatoid arthritis. *Proc. Natl. Acad. Sci. U.S.A.* 113, 8284–8289. doi: 10.1073/pnas.1605635113

Kovatchev, B. (2018). Automated closed-loop control of diabetes: the artificial pancreas. *Bioelectron. Med.* 4:14. doi: 10.1186/s42234-018-0015-6

Lainez, N. M., Jonak, C. R., Nair, M. G., Ethell, I. M., Wilson, E. H., Carson, M. J., et al. (2018). Diet-induced obesity elicits macrophage infiltration and reduction in spine density in the hypothalami of male but not female mice. *Front. Immunol.* 9:1992. doi: 10.3389/fimmu.2018.01992

Lataro, R. M., Silva, C. A., Tefe-Silva, C., Prado, C. M., and Salgado, H. C. (2015). Acetylcholinesterase inhibition attenuates the development of hypertension and inflammation in spontaneously hypertensive rats. *Am. J. Hypertens.* 28, 1201–1208. doi: 10.1093/ajh/hpv017

Lee, S. T., Chu, K., Jung, K. H., Kang, K. M., Kim, J. H., Bahn, J. J., et al. (2010). Cholinergic anti-inflammatory pathway in intracerebral hemorrhage. *Brain Res.* 1309, 164–171. doi: 10.1016/j.brainres.2009.10.076

Li, Y., Wu, X., Zhu, J., Yan, J., and Owyang, C. (2003). Hypothalamic regulation of pancreatic secretion is mediated by central cholinergic pathways in the rat. *J. Physiol.* 552, 571–587. doi: 10.1113/jphysiol.2003.049122

Lumeng, C. N., and Saltiel, A. R. (2011). Inflammatory links between obesity and metabolic disease. *J. Clin. Investig.* 121, 2111–2117. doi: 10.1172/JCI57132

Malbert, C. H., Picq, C., Divoux, J. L., Henry, C., and Horowitz, M. (2017). Obesity-associated alterations in glucose metabolism are reversed by chronic bilateral stimulation of the abdominal vagus nerve. *Diabetes* 66, 848–857. doi: 10.2337/db16-0847

Marrero, M. B., Lucas, R., Salet, C., Hauser, T. A., Mazurov, A., Lippiello, P. M., et al. (2010). An alpha7 nicotinic acetylcholine receptor-selective agonist reduces weight gain and metabolic changes in a mouse model of diabetes. *J. Pharmacol. Exp. Ther.* 332, 173–180. doi: 10.1124/jpet.109.154633

Martinelli, I., Tomassoni, D., Moruzzi, M., Traini, E., Amenta, F., and Tayebati, S. K. (2017). Obesity and metabolic syndrome affect the cholinergic transmission and cognitive functions. *CNS Neurol. Disord. Drug Targets* 16, 664–676. doi: 10.2174/1871527316666170428123853

Masi, E. B., Valdes-Ferrer, S. I., and Steinberg, B. E. (2018). The vagus neurometabolic interface and clinical disease. *Int. J. Obes.* 42, 1101–1111. doi: 10.1038/s41366-018-0086-1

Matsushita, H., Ishikawa, K., and Shimazu, T. (1979). Chemical coding of the hypothalamic neurones in metabolic control. I. Acetylcholine-sensitive neurones and glycogen synthesis in liver. *Brain Res.* 163, 253–261. doi: 10.1016/0006-8993(79)90353-6

McManus, R. M., and Heneka, M. T. (2017). Role of neuroinflammation in neurodegeneration: new insights. *Alzheimers Res. Ther.* 9:14. doi: 10.1186/s13195-017-0241-2

Metz, C. N., and Pavlov, V. A. (2018). Vagus nerve cholinergic circuitry to the liver and the gastrointestinal tract in the neuroimmune communicatome. *Am. J. Physiol. Gastrointest. Liver Physiol.* 315, G651–G658. doi: 10.1152/ajpgi.00195.2018

Miller, A. A., and Spencer, S. J. (2014). Obesity and neuroinflammation: a pathway to cognitive impairment. *Brain Behav. Immun.* 42, 10–21. doi: 10.1016/j.bbi.2014.04.001

Mineur, Y. S., Abizaid, A., Rao, Y., Salas, R., DiLeone, R. J., Gundisch, D., et al. (2011). Nicotine decreases food intake through activation of POMC neurons. *Science* 332, 1330–1332. doi: 10.1126/science.1201889

Morton, G. J., Cummings, D. E., Baskin, D. G., Barsh, G. S., and Schwartz, M. W. (2006). Central nervous system control of food intake and body weight. *Nature* 443, 289–295. doi: 10.1038/nature05026

Munyaka, P., Rabbi, M. F., Pavlov, V. A., Tracey, K. J., Khafipour, E., and Ghia, J. E. (2014). Central muscarinic cholinergic activation alters interaction between splenic dendritic cell and CD4+CD25- T cells in experimental colitis. *PLoS One* 9:e109272. doi: 10.1371/journal.pone.0109272

Nathan, C. (2008). Epidemic inflammation: pondering obesity. *Mol. Med.* 14, 485–492. doi: 10.2119/2008-00038.Nathan

Nishimura, S., Manabe, I., Nagasaki, M., Eto, K., Yamashita, H., Ohsugi, M., et al. (2009). CD8+ effector T cells contribute to macrophage recruitment and adipose tissue inflammation in obesity. *Nat. Med.* 15, 914–920. doi: 10.1038/nm.1964

Nishio, T., Taura, K., Iwaisako, K., Koyama, Y., Tanabe, K., Yamamoto, G., et al. (2017). Hepatic vagus nerve regulates Kupffer cell activation via alpha7 nicotinic acetylcholine receptor in nonalcoholic steatohepatitis. *J. Gastroenterol.* 52, 965–976. doi: 10.1007/s00535-016-1304-z

Nizri, E., Irony-Tur-Sinai, M., Faranesh, N., Lavon, I., Lavi, E., Weinstock, M., et al. (2008). Suppression of neuroinflammation and immunomodulation by the acetylcholinesterase inhibitor rivastigmine. *J. Neuroimmunol.* 203, 12–22. doi: 10.1016/j.jneuroim.2008.06.018

Olefsky, J. M., and Glass, C. K. (2010). Macrophages, inflammation, and insulin resistance. *Annu. Rev. Physiol.* 72, 219–246. doi: 10.1146/annurev-physiol-021909-135846

Olofsson, P. S., Katz, D. A., Rosas-Ballina, M., Levine, Y. A., Ochani, M., Valdes-Ferrer, S. I., et al. (2012). alpha7 nicotinic acetylcholine receptor (alpha 7 nAChR) expression in bone marrow-derived non-T cells is required for the inflammatory reflex. *Mol. Med.* 18, 539–543. doi: 10.2119/molmed.2011.00405

Olofsson, P. S., Metz, C. N., and Pavlov, V. A. (2017). "The neuroimmune communicatome in inflammation," in *Inflammation: from Molecular and Cellular Mechanisms to the Clinic*, eds J. Cavaillon and M. Singer (Weinheim: Wiley-VCH Verlag GmbH & Co), 1485–1516. doi: 10.1002/9783527692156.ch59

Olofsson, P. S., and Tracey, K. J. (2017). Bioelectronic medicine: technology targeting molecular mechanisms for therapy. *J. Intern. Med.* 282, 3–4. doi: 10.1111/joim.12624

O'Reardon, J. P., Cristancho, P., and Peshek, A. D. (2006). Vagus Nerve Stimulation (VNS) and treatment of depression: to the brainstem and beyond. *Psychiatry* 3, 54–63.

Owyang, C., and Heldsinger, A. (2011). Vagal control of satiety and hormonal regulation of appetite. *J. Neurogastroenterol. Motil.* 17, 338–348. doi: 10.5056/jnm.2011.17.4.338

Pardo, J. V., Sheikh, S. A., Kuskowski, M. A., Surerus-Johnson, C., Hagen, M. C., Lee, J. T., et al. (2007). Weight loss during chronic, cervical vagus nerve stimulation in depressed patients with obesity: an observation. *Int. J. Obes.* 31, 1756–1759. doi: 10.1038/sj.ijo.0803666

Parrish, W. R., Rosas-Ballina, M., Gallowitsch-Puerta, M., Ochani, M., Ochani, K., Yang, L. H., et al. (2008). Modulation of TNF release by choline requires alpha7 subunit nicotinic acetylcholine receptor-mediated signaling. *Mol. Med.* 14, 567–574. doi: 10.2119/2008-00079.Parrish

Pavlov, V. A., Chavan, S. S., and Tracey, K. J. (2018). Molecular and functional neuroscience in immunity. *Annu. Rev. Immunol.* 36, 783–812. doi: 10.1146/annurev-immunol-042617-053158

Pavlov, V. A., Ochani, M., Gallowitsch-Puerta, M., Ochani, K., Huston, J. M., Czura, C. J., et al. (2006). Central muscarinic cholinergic regulation of the systemic inflammatory response during endotoxemia. *Proc. Natl. Acad. Sci. U.S.A.* 103, 5219–5223. doi: 10.1073/pnas.0600506103

Pavlov, V. A., Ochani, M., Yang, L. H., Gallowitsch-Puerta, M., Ochani, K., Lin, X., et al. (2007). Selective alpha7-nicotinic acetylcholine receptor agonist GTS-21 improves survival in murine endotoxemia and severe sepsis. *Crit. Care Med.* 35, 1139–1144. doi: 10.1097/01.CCM.0000259381.56526.96

Pavlov, V. A., Parrish, W. R., Rosas-Ballina, M., Ochani, M., Puerta, M., Ochani, K., et al. (2009). Brain acetylcholinesterase activity controls systemic cytokine levels through the cholinergic anti-inflammatory pathway. *Brain Behav. Immun.* 23, 41–45. doi: 10.1016/j.bbi.2008.06.011

Pavlov, V. A., and Tracey, K. J. (2012). The vagus nerve and the inflammatory reflex–linking immunity and metabolism. *Nat. Rev. Endocrinol.* 8, 743–754. doi: 10.1038/nrendo.2012.189

Pavlov, V. A., and Tracey, K. J. (2015). Neural circuitry and immunity. *Immunol. Res.* 63, 38–57. doi: 10.1007/s12026-015-8718-1

Pavlov, V. A., and Tracey, K. J. (2017). Neural regulation of immunity: molecular mechanisms and clinical translation. *Nat. Neurosci.* 20, 156–166. doi: 10.1038/nn.4477

Pavlov, V. A., and Tracey, K. J. (2019). Bioelectronic medicine: updates, challenges and paths forward. *Bioelectron. Med.* 5:1. doi: 10.1186/s42234-019-0018-y

Pavlov, V. A., Wang, H., Czura, C. J., Friedman, S. G., and Tracey, K. J. (2003). The cholinergic anti-inflammatory pathway: a missing link in neuroimmunomodulation. *Mol. Med.* 9, 125–134. doi: 10.1007/BF03402177

Pham, G. S., Wang, L. A., and Mathis, K. W. (2018). Pharmacological potentiation of the efferent vagus nerve attenuates blood pressure and renal injury in a murine model of systemic lupus erythematosus. *Am. J. Physiol. Regul. Integr. Comp. Physiol.* 315, R1261–R1271. doi: 10.1152/ajpregu.00362.2017

Picciotto, M. R., Higley, M. J., and Mineur, Y. S. (2012). Acetylcholine as a neuromodulator: cholinergic signaling shapes nervous system function and behavior. *Neuron* 76, 116–129. doi: 10.1016/j.neuron.2012.08.036

Pistell, P. J., Morrison, C. D., Gupta, S., Knight, A. G., Keller, J. N., Ingram, D. K., et al. (2010). Cognitive impairment following high fat diet consumption is associated with brain inflammation. *J. Neuroimmunol.* 219, 25–32. doi: 10.1016/j.jneuroim.2009.11.010

Pocai, A., Lam, T. K., Gutierrez-Juarez, R., Obici, S., Schwartz, G. J., Bryan, J., et al. (2005). Hypothalamic K(ATP) channels control hepatic glucose production. *Nature* 434, 1026–1031. doi: 10.1038/nature03439

Rosas-Ballina, M., Olofsson, P. S., Ochani, M., Valdes-Ferrer, S. I., Levine, Y. A., Reardon, C., et al. (2011). Acetylcholine-synthesizing T cells relay neural signals in a vagus nerve circuit. *Science* 334, 98–101. doi: 10.1126/science.1209985

Rosas-Ballina, M., Valdes-Ferrer, S. I., Dancho, M. E., Ochani, M., Katz, D., Cheng, K. F., et al. (2015). Xanomeline suppresses excessive pro-inflammatory cytokine responses through neural signal-mediated pathways and improves survival in lethal inflammation. *Brain Behav. Immun.* 44, 19–27. doi: 10.1016/j.bbi.2014.07.010

Ruiz de Azua, I., Gautam, D., Guettier, J. M., and Wess, J. (2011). Novel insights into the function of beta-cell M3 muscarinic acetylcholine receptors: therapeutic implications. *Trends Endocrinol. Metab.* 22, 74–80. doi: 10.1016/j.tem.2010.10.004

Sackeim, H. A., Rush, A. J., George, M. S., Marangell, L. B., Husain, M. M., Nahas, Z., et al. (2001). Vagus nerve stimulation (VNS) for treatment-resistant depression: efficacy, side effects, and predictors of outcome. *Neuropsychopharmacology* 25, 713–728. doi: 10.1016/S0893-133X(01)00271-8

Satapathy, S. K., Ochani, M., Dancho, M., Hudson, L. K., Rosas-Ballina, M., Valdes-Ferrer, S. I., et al. (2011). Galantamine alleviates inflammation and other obesity-associated complications in high-fat diet-fed mice. *Mol. Med.* 17, 599–606. doi: 10.2119/molmed.2011.00083

Schuppan, D., and Schattenberg, J. M. (2013). Non-alcoholic steatohepatitis: pathogenesis and novel therapeutic approaches. *J. Gastroenterol. Hepatol.* 28(Suppl. 1), 68–76. doi: 10.1111/jgh.12212

Schwartz, M. W., and Porte, D. Jr. (2005). Diabetes, obesity, and the brain. *Science* 307, 375–379. doi: 10.1126/science.1104344

Schwartz, T. W. (1983). Pancreatic polypeptide: a unique model for vagal control of endocrine systems. *J. Auton. Nerv. Syst.* 9, 99–111. doi: 10.1016/0165-1838(83)90134-0

Sellbom, K. S., and Gunstad, J. (2012). Cognitive function and decline in obesity. *J. Alzheimers Dis.* 30(Suppl. 2), S89–S95. doi: 10.3233/JAD-2011-111073

Serhan, C. N., and Levy, B. D. (2018). Resolvins in inflammation: emergence of the pro-resolving superfamily of mediators. *J. Clin. Investig.* 128, 2657–2669. doi: 10.1172/JCI97943

Shi, H., Kokoeva, M. V., Inouye, K., Tzameli, I., Yin, H., and Flier, J. S. (2006). TLR4 links innate immunity and fatty acid-induced insulin resistance. *J. Clin. Investig.* 116, 3015–3025. doi: 10.1172/JCI28898

Shimazu, T., Matsushita, H., and Ishikawa, K. (1976). Cholinergic stimulation of the rat hypothalamus: effects of liver glycogen synthesis. *Science* 194, 535–536. doi: 10.1126/science.9692

Shin, A. C., Filatova, N., Lindtner, C., Chi, T., Degann, S., Oberlin, D., et al. (2017). Insulin receptor signaling in POMC, but Not AgRP, neurons controls adipose tissue insulin action. *Diabetes* 66, 1560–1571. doi: 10.2337/db16-1238

Shoelson, S. E., Herrero, L., and Naaz, A. (2007). Obesity, inflammation, and insulin resistance. *Gastroenterology* 132, 2169–2180. doi: 10.1053/j.gastro.2007.03.059

Smith, G. P., Jerome, C., Cushin, B. J., Eterno, R., and Simansky, K. J. (1981). Abdominal vagotomy blocks the satiety effect of cholecystokinin in the rat. *Science* 213, 1036–1037. doi: 10.1126/science.7268408

Steinberg, B. E., Silverman, H. A., Robbiati, S., Gunasekaran, M. K., Tsaava, T., Battinelli, E., et al. (2016). Cytokine-specific neurograms in the sensory vagus nerve. *Bioelectron. Med.* 3, 7–17.

Strachan, M. W., Reynolds, R. M., Marioni, R. E., and Price, J. F. (2011). Cognitive function, dementia and type 2 diabetes mellitus in the elderly. *Nat. Rev. Endocrinol.* 7, 108–114. doi: 10.1038/nrendo.2010.228

Suarez, A. N., Hsu, T. M., Liu, C. M., Noble, E. E., Cortella, A. M., Nakamoto, E. M., et al. (2018). Gut vagal sensory signaling regulates hippocampus function through multi-order pathways. *Nat. Commun.* 9:2181. doi: 10.1038/s41467-018-04639-1

Tarnawski, L., Reardon, C., Caravaca, A. S., Rosas-Ballina, M., Tusche, M. W., Drake, A. R., et al. (2018) Adenylyl Cyclase 6 Mediates Inhibition of TNF in the Inflammatory Reflex. *Front. Immunol.* 9:2648. doi: 10.3389/fimmu.2018.02648

Terrando, N., Eriksson, L. I., Ryu, J. K., Yang, T., Monaco, C., Feldmann, M., et al. (2011). Resolving postoperative neuroinflammation and cognitive decline. *Ann. Neurol.* 70, 986–995. doi: 10.1002/ana.22664

Tilg, H., and Moschen, A. R. (2006). Adipocytokines: mediators linking adipose tissue, inflammation and immunity. *Nat. Rev. Immunol.* 6, 772–783. doi: 10.1038/nri1937

Tracey, K. J. (2002). The inflammatory reflex. *Nature* 420, 853–859. doi: 10.1038/nature01321

Tracey, K. J. (2007). Physiology and immunology of the cholinergic antiinflammatory pathway. *J. Clin. Investig.* 117, 289–296. doi: 10.1172/JCI30555

Val-Laillet, D., Biraben, A., Randuineau, G., and Malbert, C. H. (2010). Chronic vagus nerve stimulation decreased weight gain, food consumption and sweet craving in adult obese minipigs. *Appetite* 55, 245–252. doi: 10.1016/j.appet.2010.06.008

van Dieren, S., Beulens, J. W., van der Schouw, Y. T., Grobbee, D. E., and Neal, B. (2010). The global burden of diabetes and its complications: an emerging pandemic. *Eur. J. Cardiovasc. Prev. Rehabil.* 17(Suppl. 1), S3–S8. doi: 10.1097/01.hjr.0000368191.86614.5a

van Dijk, G., Evers, S. S., Guidotti, S., Thornton, S. N., Scheurink, A. J., and Nyakas, C. (2011). The lateral hypothalamus: a site for integration of nutrient and fluid balance. *Behav. Brain Res.* 221, 481–487. doi: 10.1016/j.bbr.2011.01.047

Vandanmagsar, B., Youm, Y. H., Ravussin, A., Galgani, J. E., Stadler, K., Mynatt, R. L., et al. (2011). The NLRP3 inflammasome instigates obesity-induced inflammation and insulin resistance. *Nat. Med.* 17, 179–188. doi: 10.1038/nm.2279

Vonck, K., Raedt, R., Naulaerts, J., De Vogelaere, F., Thiery, E., Van Roost, D., et al. (2014). Vagus nerve stimulation..25 years later! What do we know about the effects on cognition? *Neurosci. Biobehav. Rev.* 45, 63–71. doi: 10.1016/j.neubiorev.2014.05.005

Wadden, T. A., Sternberg, J. A., Letizia, K. A., Stunkard, A. J., and Foster, G. D. (1989). Treatment of obesity by very low calorie diet, behavior therapy, and their combination: a five-year perspective. *Int. J. Obes.* 13(Suppl. 2), 39–46.

Wang, H., Yu, M., Ochani, M., Amella, C. A., Tanovic, M., Susarla, S., et al. (2003). Nicotinic acetylcholine receptor alpha7 subunit is an essential regulator of inflammation. *Nature* 421, 384–388. doi: 10.1038/nature01339

Wang, T., Zhu, H., Hou, Y., Gu, W., Wu, H., Luan, Y., et al. (2018). Galantamine reversed early postoperative cognitive deficit via alleviating inflammation and enhancing synaptic transmission in mouse hippocampus. *Eur. J. Pharmacol.* 846, 63–72. doi: 10.1016/j.ejphar.2018.12.034

Wang, X., Yang, Z., Xue, B., and Shi, H. (2011). Activation of the cholinergic antiinflammatory pathway ameliorates obesity-induced inflammation and insulin resistance. *Endocrinology* 152, 836–846. doi: 10.1210/en.2010-0855

Whitmer, R. A., Gunderson, E. P., Barrett-Connor, E., Quesenberry, C. P. Jr., and Yaffe, K. (2005). Obesity in middle age and future risk of dementia: a 27 year longitudinal population based study. *BMJ* 330:1360. doi: 10.1136/bmj.38446.466238.E0

Woolf, N. J., and Butcher, L. L. (2011). Cholinergic systems mediate action from movement to higher consciousness. *Behav. Brain Res.* 221, 488–498. doi: 10.1016/j.bbr.2009.12.046

Yao, G., Kang, L., Li, J., Long, Y., Wei, H., Ferreira, C. A., et al. (2018). Effective weight control via an implanted self-powered vagus nerve stimulation device. *Nat. Commun.* 9:5349. doi: 10.1038/s41467-018-07764-z

Zanos, T. P., Silverman, H. A., Levy, T., Tsaava, T., Battinelli, E., Lorraine, P. W., et al. (2018). Identification of cytokine-specific sensory neural signals by decoding murine vagus nerve activity. *Proc. Natl. Acad. Sci. U.S.A.* 115, E4843–E4852. doi: 10.1073/pnas.1719083115

Zhang, J., Zhang, L., Sun, X., Yang, Y., Kong, L., Lu, C., et al. (2016). Acetylcholinesterase inhibitors for Alzheimer's disease treatment ameliorate acetaminophen-induced liver injury in mice via central cholinergic system regulation. *J. Pharmacol. Exp. Ther.* 359, 374–382. doi: 10.1124/jpet.116.233841

Zimmet, P., Alberti, K. G., and Shaw, J. (2001). Global and societal implications of the diabetes epidemic. *Nature* 414, 782–787. doi: 10.1038/414782a

7

Insulin and Autophagy in Neurodegeneration

Natália Prudente de Mello[1†], Ana Maria Orellana[2†], Caio Henrique Mazucanti[2†], Geovanni de Morais Lima[1], Cristoforo Scavone[2] and Elisa Mitiko Kawamoto[1]*

[1] Laboratory of Molecular and Functional Neurobiology, Department of Pharmacology, Institute of Biomedical Sciences, University of São Paulo, São Paulo, Brazil, [2] Laboratory of Molecular Neuropharmacology, Department of Pharmacology, Institute of Biomedical Sciences, University of São Paulo, São Paulo, Brazil

***Correspondence:**
Cristoforo Scavone
cristoforo.scavone@gmail.com

† These authors have contributed equally to this work

Crosstalk in the pathophysiological processes underpinning metabolic diseases and neurodegenerative disorders have been the subject of extensive investigation, in which insulin signaling and autophagy impairment demonstrate to be a common factor in both conditions. Although it is still somewhat conflicting, pharmacological and genetic strategies that regulate these pathways may be a promising approach for aggregate protein clearancing and consequently the delaying of onset or progression of the disease. However, as the response due to this modulation seems to be time-dependent, finding the right regulation of autophagy may be a potential target for drug development for neurodegenerative diseases. In this way, this review focuses on the role of insulin signaling/resistance and autophagy in some neurodegenerative diseases, discussing pharmacological and non-pharmacological interventions in these diseases.

Keywords: obesity, type 2 diabetes, insulin, autophagy, neurodegenerative diseases

INTRODUCTION

Metabolic disorders such as obesity and type 2 diabetes (T2D) are a worldwide epidemic challenge of the 21st century that, besides resulting in reduced life expectancy and increased medical comorbidities, have been said to be risk factors for the development of neurodegenerative diseases (El Sayed et al., 2012). According to literature, both obesity and T2D contribute to an increased prevalence of dementia and cognitive decline (Arvanitakis et al., 2004; Kopf and Frölich, 2009; Nameni et al., 2017; Zhang et al., 2017), as well as to the onset of insulin resistance (Schneeberger et al., 2015), which is proposed to play a critical role in the link between metabolic disorders and central nervous system (CNS) impairment (Schneeberger et al., 2015; Nameni et al., 2017). Nowadays, it is known that insulin receptor (IR) is widely expressed in the CNS, and, although the exact link between brain insulin and neurodegenerative diseases remains still unknown, a plethora of studies have demonstrated that an optimal insulin signaling homeostasis is important to the maintenance of brain health.

The maintenance of cellular homeostasis is a complex process, which includes an interesting crosstalk between autophagy and apoptosis, involving, among other processes, the regulation of the phosphatidylinositol (3,4,5)-trisphosphate kinase (PI3K)-protein kinase B (AKT)-mammalian target of rapamycin (mTOR) and AMP-dependent protein kinase (AMPK) pathways. The mTOR is a serine/threonine kinase that is ubiquitously expressed, modulating cell proliferation, protein synthesis, and death or survival signalings. Localized mainly in the cytoplasm, mTOR is composed of two different protein complexes, mTOR complex 1 (mTORC1) and mTOR complex 2 (mTORC2), which differ in many respects, including protein complex components, and responsiveness to rapamycin, as well as activators or downstream signaling pathways. However, crosstalk between both complexes is mediated by AKT (Perluigi et al., 2015). The AKT signaling pathway can be triggered by insulin-like growth factor 1 (IGF-1) and insulin, which bind to transmembrane receptors and activate insulin receptor substrate 1 (IRS-1), leading to PI3K activation and subsequent phosphatidylinositol (3,4,5)-trisphosphate (PIP_3) generation. AKT is responsible for the inhibition of negative regulators of mTOR, such as tuberous sclerosis complex (TSC1/2), whilst pyruvate dehydrogenase kinase 1(PDK1) induces the mTOR activator Rheb (Ras homolog enriched in brain), thereby releasing the mTOR complex to phosphorylate its targets (Perluigi et al., 2015). Interestingly, the chronically hyperactivation of mTOR by hyperinsulinemia is proposed to contribute to insulin resistance (Ueno et al., 2005).

Autophagy is an important cellular process, whereby cell debris, including proteins and organelles, are degraded and recycled in order to prevent the build up of protein clusters and aggregates (Klionsky and Emr, 2000; Rubinsztein et al., 2005). During this process, portions of cytoplasm or organelles are engulfed by double membrane structures called autophagosomes, which fuse with lysosomes or vacuoles allowing the degradation of their cargo material (organelles and macromolecules) and its subsequent release into the cytosol for recycling (Kundu and Thompson, 2005). This complex process is regulated by more than 30 autophagy-related proteins (ATGs), as well as by the PI3K, the Unc-51-like kinase 1 (ULK1) and the microtubule-associated protein 1 light chain 3 (LC3) pathways. Under physiological condition, PI3K type I is activated by growth factors resulting in mTOR activation and consequently autophagy downregulation by phosphorylating and inactivating ULK1, which is an initiator of mammalian autophagy (Axe et al., 2008). Besides mTOR, AMPK also suppresses autophagy through the phosphorylation of different amino acid residues of ULK1 (Nishida et al., 2009). However, under some stress condition such as nutrient starvation, ULK1 is dephosphorylated by protein phosphatase 2A (PP2A), resulting in phosphorylation of multiple substrates and initiation of the conventional autophagy (Axe et al., 2008; Nishida et al., 2009; Mizushima and Komatsu, 2011). After that, together with other components, the Beclin1-containing class-III PI3K complex (Beclin 1, VPS15 and ATG14, class III VPS34) induces the formation of phagophore, an initial membrane component of the isolation membrane, which then expands, curves and closes due to two conjugation pathways, the ATG5-ATG12 and the LC3, turning into a completed autophagosome (Mizushima and Komatsu, 2011; **Figure 1**).

In this way, this review summarizes the origin and the role of insulin in the CNS, and discusses the relationship between insulin and autophagy in some neurodegenerative diseases, such as Alzheimer's disease (AD), Parkinson's disease (PD), Huntington's disease (HD), amyotrophic lateral sclerosis (ALS) and frontotemporal dementia (FTD), as well as in spinocerebellar ataxia type 3 (SCA3) and Lafora disease (LD). Although there are at least three well-known distinct autophagic pathways, such as chaperone-mediated autophagy, microautophagy and macroautophagy, this review focuses on macroautophagy, hereafter referred to as autophagy.

INSULIN RESISTANCE IN THE CENTRAL NERVOUS SYSTEM AND NEURODEGENERATION

The sugar lowering properties of the endocrine secretion of the pancreas were described by Banting and Best (1922), and insulin itself was crystallized shortly after, in 1926 (Abel, 1926). The number of scientific publications describing insulin and its functions exploded in the 1940s and, until the 1960s, most of the scientific community considered the brain to be an organ insensitive to insulin. The first half of 60s, however, was punctuated with compelling work done by separate groups that forced this discussion to be reopened. Work published in 1961 by Rafaelsen showed glucose uptake modulation by insulin in isolated rat spinal cord (Rafaelsen, 1961a) as well as rat cortical brain slices and cerebellum (Rafaelsen, 1961b). Butterfield et al. (1966), after measuring brain glucose uptake in 5 healthy male volunteers with insulin infusions, suggested that the human brain could be, after all, sensitive to insulin (Butterfield et al., 1966).

Recent work has confirmed insulin effects in the brain, although these can be quite distinct from its effects in the periphery, although the idea that insulin has exclusively neurotrophic effects in the brain has been contested by a few recent publications. In 2016, García-Cáceres et al. (2016) showed that signaling through the IR in hypothalamic astrocytes may affect the activity of glucose-sensing pro-opiomelanocortin neurons, suggesting the importance of insulin in the regulation of brain glucose uptake (García-Cáceres et al., 2016). Insulin-like growth factor I (IGF-I) is another important endogenous ligand of the IR, and works alongside insulin binding to the astrocytic IR in order to activate a non-canonical pathway, the mitogen-activated protein kinases (MAPK)/protein kinase D (PKD) pathway, which ultimately leads to the membrane translocation of glucose transporter (GLUT)1, a glucose transporter previously known to be insulin-insensitive. The combined effects of insulin and IGF-1 therefore modulate brain glucose (Fernandez et al., 2017). The following sections focus on the neurotrophic effects of insulin.

ORIGINS OF BRAIN INSULIN

Insulin was first successfully identified in dog cerebrospinal fluid (CSF) in 1967 by Margolis and Altszuler (1967). Through a continuous intravenous insulin infusion and periodic CSF and blood sampling, Margolis & Altszuler showed, for the first time, that fasted levels of insulin in the CSF were, on average, 27% of the insulin concentration found in plasma. Furthermore, it was the first report proving that insulin could cross the brain barriers, albeit in a very limited way. The concept that insulin can cross the blood-brain and the blood-CSF through a saturable transport system, and not by passive diffusion, would then become a significant milestone that is still regarded as the most accepted hypothesis describing insulin within the brain.

Although pancreas is, undoubtedly, the body's primary source of insulin, the idea that insulin found in brain tissues and CSF is exclusively derived from the blood was first challenged in

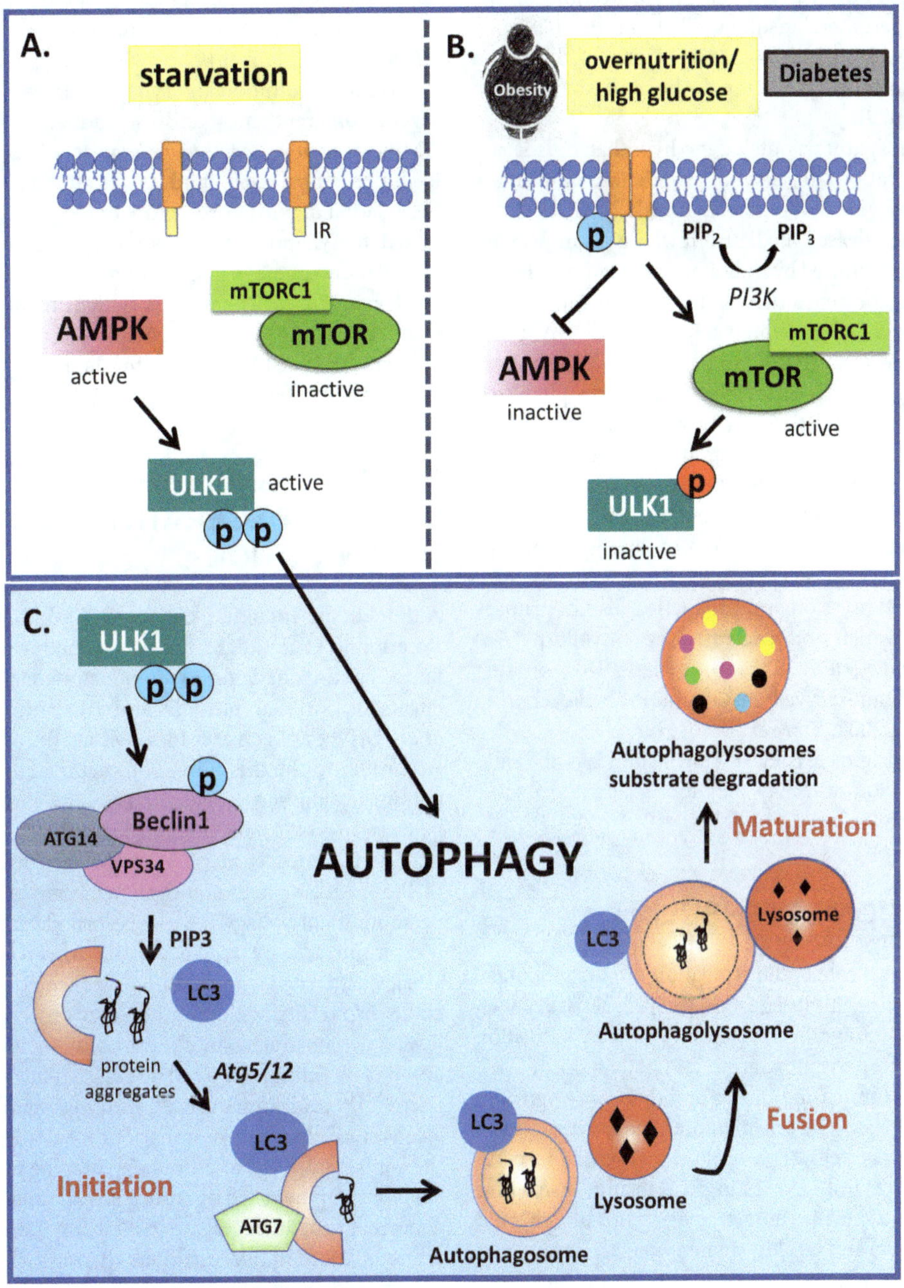

FIGURE 1 | Autophagy modulation by starvation and insulin signaling. **(A)** Autophagy is classically activated in starvation conditions through ULK1 activity. In low nutrient conditions, AMPK signaling is activated, phosphorylating ULK1 in two different activation sites. Opposite to starvation, **(B)** in overnutrition condition or diabetes, PI3K type I is activated by growth factor receptors resulting in mTOR activation and AMPK inactivation. mTOR complex TORC1 phosphorylates and inactivates ULK1 (red circles), which is an initiator of mammalian autophagy. **(C)** During this process, protein-prone aggregates or damaged organelles are engulfed by double membrane structures called autophagosomes, which fuse with lysosomes or vacuoles allowing the degradation of their cargo material in the autophagolysosomes. This complex process starts with ULK1 phosphorylation in 2 different activation residues (indicated by blue circles). Active ULK1 phosphorylates Beclin 1, that together with other components induces the formation of phagophore, an initial membrane component of the isolation membrane, which then expands, curves and closes due to two conjugation pathways dependent of ATG5-ATG12 action to LC3 lipidation, turning into a completed autophagosome.

1978 by Havrankova et al. (1978), in a paper showing high levels of insulin extracted from different brain regions, with the highest concentrations being found in the olfactory bulb and hypothalamus. Following this observation, the same group confirmed their findings in models of obese hyperinsulinemic and diabetic insulinopenic rats. In contrast to what was observed (and expected) in the liver, IR levels throughout the brain did not change in either experimental group, suggesting the participation of the brain barriers in the protection of the CNS from dramatic peripheral insulin oscillations. Furthermore, central insulin levels also did not change in any of the tested models, suggesting *de novo* synthesis of the hormone in the brain (Havrankova et al., 1979).

Central insulin biosynthesis outside the hypothalamus is still controversial. Observations of insulin production in primary neuronal cell cultures were first reported in 1986 by Clarke et al. (1986). Analyzing the released media from whole-brain primary neuronal cultures, they showed by radioimmunoassay and HPLC analysis not only the presence of secreted insulin but also its positive regulation by depolarization, via K^+ and Ca^{2+}. As proof that these observations were specific to neuronal depolarization, Clarke showed that no such effect was possible in glial cells in culture. Preproinsulin mRNA and protein was reported in pyramidal neuronal cells of the hippocampus and olfactory bulb (Kuwabara et al., 2011), with further studies showing extensive distribution of insulin expression throughout the brain, with higher levels in the hippocampus, striatum, thalamus, entorhinal and prefrontal cortices (Mehran et al., 2012). Interestingly, recent reports show insulin expression and production also in primary cultured astrocytes, which was decreased by amyloid-β (Aβ) and lipopolysaccharide (LPS) (Takano et al., 2018). Another putative source of brain-derived insulin may be the choroid plexus (Lamotte et al., 2004; Yong et al., 2011).

Regardless of its origin, it is clear that insulin has different effects on brain function and may play a crucial role in some pathological conditions.

CENTRAL ACTIONS OF INSULIN

Insulin primarily plays a role in the regulation of glucose uptake of insulin-sensitive cells, with its effect on peripheral tissues such as muscle, adipose tissue, and liver, being very similar. Activation of its receptor leads to phosphorylation and activation of AKT and ERK pathways, culminating in the mobilization of glucose transporter 4 (GLUT4) to the cell membrane, allowing greater glucose uptake by these cells. The brain, however, behaves in a very different way, mainly expressing the insulin-insensitive glucose transporters GLUT1 (in astrocytes and blood-brain barrier endothelial cells) and GLUT3 (in neurons). Consequently, classical modeling of glucose uptake by cells in the brain considers this to be an insulin-insensitive process, although this is subject to some controversy, as indicated above. In contrast, central insulin effects are primarily regarded as neurotrophic, affecting synaptic physiology and, hence, memory and learning.

Insulin and its receptor have been implicated in neurite outgrowth and axon guidance, through activation of the PI3K/AKT pathway, as demonstrated in Drosophila (Song et al., 2003; Gu et al., 2014), murine (Grote et al., 2011) and human neuronal cells (Liu et al., 2013; Roloff et al., 2015). IRS p53 seems to play an essential role in dendritic arborization. IRSp53 is expressed in the post-synaptic membrane of neurons, where it co-localizes with the post-synaptic density and interacts with proteins that constitute the cytoskeleton (Abbott et al., 1999; Chiu and Cline, 2010). Overexpression of IRSp53 in neuronal cultures had been shown to correlate with higher levels of arborization (Govind et al., 2001), while its inhibition reduces the density and size of dendritic spines (Choi, 2005).

Insulin can modulate synaptic activity and plasticity by several different mechanisms, inducing the endocytosis of AMPA receptors for the generation of long-term depression in hippocampal cell cultures (Beattie et al., 2000) and the modulation of NMDA receptors in the post-synaptic membrane, linked to synaptic strengthening (Skeberdis et al., 2001). The modulation of these glutamatergic receptors allows insulin to participate in neuronal activity-dependent synaptic plasticity (Van Der Heide et al., 2005). Overall, such data clearly links central insulin effects to neuronal plasticity processes underpinning cognitive functioning.

INSULIN SIGNALLING AND AUTOPHAGY IN NEURODEGERATIVE DISEASES: AN INTRODUCTION

Although the literature data is still conflicting, as revised by Rotermund et al. (2018), the use of Metformin, one of the most famous anti-diabetic drugs, demonstrated to have some positive effects in, for example, PD and AD animal models (Lennox et al., 2014; Patil et al., 2014; Lu et al., 2016; Katila et al., 2017). According to the literature, both acute and chronic Metformin administration showed to increase the levels of glucagon-like peptide-1 (GLP-1), an incretin known as an inducer of insulin secretion (Maida et al., 2011), that may lead to the activation of PI3K/AKT signaling and higher brain ATG7 levels, thereby promoting autophagy (Candeias et al., 2017). Besides that, Metformin acts by regulating the AMPK signaling, which is already associated with insulin resistance in T2D (Xu et al., 2012) and is also related with the autophagy process (**Figure 2**).

As demonstrated by Yamamoto et al. (2018), transient autophagy inhibition can rescue glucose intolerance in $Becn1^{F121A}$ knocking mice fed with high-fat diet, which presents a constitutively active autophagy process, suggesting that finding the right regulation of autophagy may be a potential target for drug development for neurodegenerative diseases. Besides that, abnormal protein aggregates, which have been classically linked to neurodegenerative disorders (Lasagna-Reeves et al., 2011; Larson and Lesné, 2012; Lashuel et al., 2013) are known to be substrates of the ubiquitin-proteasome and macroautophagy systems (Filimonenko et al., 2010) that are less active along aging (Shibata et al., 2006). However, the relationship between these aggregates and cellular toxicity as well as between total plaque load and cognitive status remains a point of debate (Koss et al., 2016). Thus, this section summarizes and discusses the relationship between insulin signaling and autophagy in each of the neurodegenerative diseases.

ALZHEIMER'S DISEASE (AD)

Some research associating cerebral insulin resistance and neurodegeneration indicates that alterations in cerebral insulin

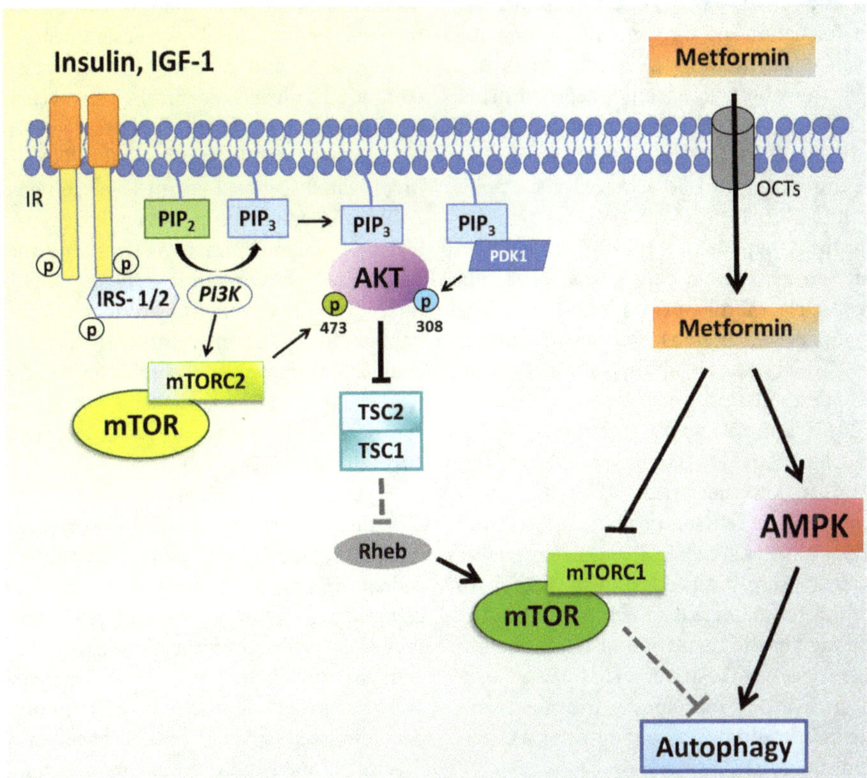

FIGURE 2 | PI3K-AKT-mTOR signaling and Metformin targets. The AKT signaling pathway can be triggered by insulin-like growth factor 1 (IGF-1) and insulin, which bind to transmembrane receptors tirosine kinase (RTK) leading to IRS-1/2 phosphorylation, PI3K activation and subsequent phosphatidylinositol-4,5-bisphosphate (PIP_2) to phosphatidylinositol-3,4,5-trisphosphate (PIP_3) conversion. AKT and PDK1 bind to PIP_3 at the plasma membrane, and PDK1 phosphorylates the activation loop of AKT at T308. RTK signaling also activates mTOR complex 2 (mTORC2) through an unknown mechanism, and mTORC2 phosphorylates AKT on S473. Active AKT is responsible for the inhibition of negative regulators of mTOR, such as tuberous sclerosis complex (TSC1/2), which induces the mTOR activator Rheb, thereby releasing the mTOR complex to phosphorylate its targets. mTORC1 activity inhibits autophagy. The Metformin enters the cell through organic cation transporters (OCTs) and is able to inhibit mTORC1 complex, while also activating AMPK thus leading to autophagy activation.

signaling may be a different and more complex process than processes derived from classical type I and II diabetes pathophysiology (Rivera et al., 2005; Steen et al., 2005). As indicated above, both *in vitro* and *in vivo* studies show insulin effects in neuronal cells, specifically on synaptic plasticity as well as its positive regulation of memory and learning. The positive effects of insulin in learning were first shown in 1976 when insulin administration attenuated memory impairment in rats subjected to hippocampal lesions (de Castro and Balagura, 1976). This was followed by similar work showing insulin to positively regulate spatial learning and memory post-ischemia, while also reducing neuronal necrotic tissue in the hippocampal CA1 region (Voll et al., 1989). Insulin signaling through its receptor in the pyramidal neurons of the CA1 is also implicated in spatial learning in the water maze test (Zhao et al., 1999, 2004). Intracerebroventricular injection of insulin also improves memory, as tested by a passive-avoidance test (Park et al., 2000).

In recent decades, insulin effects on human cognition have been described, including effects on selective attention and verbal memory in healthy participants within hours of insulin infusion (Kern et al., 2001). Given that intravenous infusions of insulin produce a range of unwanted effects, such as hypoglycemia and blood ionic imbalance, different routes of administration had to be used in order to achieve a brain-specific action. It was known for more than a decade that peptides and small proteins could access the CSF from the nasal mucosa through the intercellular spaces in the olfactory nerve and olfactory bulb (Balin et al., 1986; Sakane et al., 1991; Illum, 2000). This prompted Benedict et al. (2004) to investigate the effects of intranasal insulin on the memory of 38 healthy participants over an 8-week period (Benedict et al., 2004), with results showing improved word-recall memory scores, mood assessments, and self-confidence. Importantly, these effects were achieved without any disturbances in blood glucose or insulin levels. Hence, intranasal insulin has become the preferred route of insulin administration for studies investigating insulin effects in the brain.

Data in recent years have suggested a direct relationship between autophagic processes and the development of type II diabetes. In 2013, He et al. (2013) showed that Beclin 2, like Beclin 1, is an important modulator of autophagy. Beclin 2 heterozygous-deficient mice (beclin$2^{+/-}$) were fed for 8 weeks with a regular or high-fat diet (60% fat) with results in either condition showing an increase in body weight, food intake and in insulin resistance (He et al., 2013). Another study performed in diabetic and non-diabetic C57BL/6 mice observed an increase in autophagic vacuole formation in the presence of insulin resistance. The selectively inactivation of ATG7 in pancreatic β-cells showed that in the absence of autophagic process, ubiquitinated proteins and damaged organelles accumulate over time leading to pancreatic β-cell toxicity (Ebato et al., 2008).

Constitutively active autophagy can be achieved via a point mutation in Becn 1/Beclin 1 ($Becn1^{F121A/F121A}$). With a high-fat-diet challenge, such autophagy-hyperactive mice show improved insulin sensitivity dispite an increase in degradation of insulin granules in pancreatic β-cells (Yamamoto et al., 2018). The crossing of $Becn1^{F121A}$ mice with a transgenic murine model of AD, (5 × FAD), showed autophagy hyperactivation to significantly decrease Aβ accumulation, and to prevent cognitive decline (Rocchi et al., 2017). Autophagy hyperactivation in the 5 × FAD $Becn1^{F121A}$ murine model leads to lower levels of both soluble and insoluble Aβ42 in both the cortex and hippocampus, whilst no changes in amyloid precursor protein (APP) levels were observed. In a cellular model using HEK293 cells expressing $Becn1^{F121A}$ and APP, cells were transfected with siRNA to knockdown ATG7, leading to an increase in Aβ42, indicating the importance of autophagy in the regulation of Aβ formation (Rocchi et al., 2017). This suggests that strategies to hyperactivate the autophagic process, such as pharmacological treatment with ML246 or voluntary exercise, could decrease the risk of AD and cognitive decline (Rocchi et al., 2017).

In rodents, Caccamo et al. (2010) observed that 3 × Tg-AD mice fed for 10 weeks with rapamycin-containing food, versus a control diet, had a better performance in the Morris Water Maze task, suggesting a role for rapamycin in rescuing mice from early learning and memory deficits. 8 months of chronic rapamycin administration decreases mTOR activity in association with a decrease in hippocampal Aβ accumulation and tau hyperphosphorylation. Interestingly, this produced an autophagy gain of function, as indicated by raised levels of ATG7, ATG5/ATG12 complex and LC3-II (necessary of autophagy induction) in rapamycin-treated versus control 3 × Tg-AD mice. This effect was prevented by an autophagy inhibitor, 3-methyladenine (Caccamo et al., 2010).

Analyzing and comparing postmortem brain inferior parietal lobule tissue from patients diagnosed with mild cognitive impairment (MCI), AD, and healthy matched controls, Tramutola et al. (2015) showed that an increase in AKT and PI3K (p85 subunit) phosphorylation occurs in MCI and AD patients, coupled with mTOR hyperactivation. This increase in PI3K-AKT-mTOR signaling pathway was observed in early stage MCI as well as increased phosphorylation in the inhibitory site of IRS-1, coupled to a decrease in the autophagy markers, Beclin 1 and LC3, suggesting that such changes underpin the association of insulin resistance to early dementia. Importantly, the decrease in autophagy markers directly correlated with an increased Aβ levels. In a group of pre-clinical AD patients, with normal cognitive function ante-mortem coupled to AD neuropathology at autopsy, there was evidence of autophagy impairment although no changes in the PI3K-AKT-mTOR pathway were found, suggesting that disrupted autophagy may be an early event in Aβ deposition (Tramutola et al., 2015).

In a postmortem analysis of the midfrontal cortex gray matter, Beclin 1 levels were significantly decreased in severe AD (−30%) and mild-cognitive impairment (MCI) (−70%), compared to healthy controls. However, no significant decrease was observed in Huntington's disease (HD) or the LB variant of AD patients (Pickford et al., 2008). The same study also investigated cortical Beclin 1 levels in two different lines of aging APP transgenic mice expressing extensive Aβ deposits and high levels of mutant human APP, finding that Beclin 1 expression was the same as in nontransgenic, age-matched littermate control mice. Such data would suggest that autophagy impairment could happen in upstream events before APP pathology (Pickford et al., 2008). However, it should be noted that direct evidence of APP degradation by autophagic processes is the subject of some controversy (Boland et al., 2010; Jaeger et al., 2010; Tian et al., 2013; Rocchi et al., 2017).

Several processes and behaviors can regulate autophagy, including calorie restriction and exercise, which all improve insulin signaling and slow neurodegenerative processes. In rodents and primates maintained for several months on alternate day fasting, neurons are protected from neurodegenerative processes, in association with higher levels of brain derived neurotrophic factor (BDNF), CREB, and autophagy, as well as lower mTOR levels, improved mitochondrial function and decreased oxidative stress (reviewed in Mattson et al., 2017). Preclinical data indicate that intermittent fasting and alternate day fasting, which increase autophagy-promoting sirtuins, afford neuronal protection even in the presence of Aβ aggregates and tau accumulation, resulting in protection against cognitive impairment in 3 × TgAD mice (Halagappa et al., 2007). The mechanisms underlying the autophagy-promoting benefits of such calorie restriction diets require clarification, as these mechanisms are likely to afford some protection against neurodegenerative processes, especially in their early stages. Of note, a 24-hour fasting has been shown to increase autophagosomes and decrease mTOR signaling (Alirezaei et al., 2010). In the 5 × FAD transgenic mice that express mutant human APP770 and develop high levels of Aβ deposition at 3 months age, 48 hours of fasting was able to increase autophagy, although insufficient to clear the high levels of Aβ present in this model (Chen et al., 2015). As indicated previously, exercise is a significant positive regulator of autophagy, Aβ clearance, and improved cognition (Rocchi et al., 2017), with aerobic exercise, as well as food restriction, having a positive impact on cognitive performance of healthy participants (reviewed in Camandola and Mattson, 2017) and in animal models of AD (García-Mesa et al., 2011; **Figure 3**).

PARKINSON'S DISEASE

PD is a neurodegenerative disease with a slow progress that seems to begin many years before diagnosis with non-motor features such as olfactory and autonomic dysfunction, intestinal dysregulation, sleep disorders, fatigue, cognitive impairment and psychiatric symptoms. With disease progression classical motor symptoms appear, including bradykinesia, rest tremor, muscular

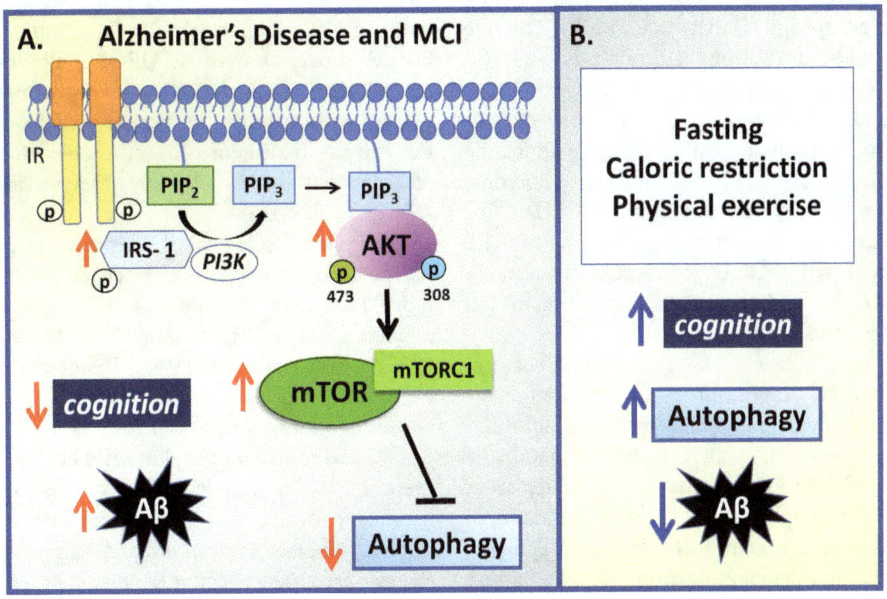

FIGURE 3 | Summary of insulin –autophagy signaling changes in Alzheimer's disease. **(A)** In mild cognitive impairment (MCI) and Alzheimer's Disease, an inverse correlation between cognition levels, insulin sensitivity, autophagy and amyloid-β (Aβ) aggregates is observed. An increase in IRS-1, PI3K and AKT phosphorylation coupled to mTORC1 hyperactivation downregulates autophagy activity, impairing Aβ degradation, which results in increased Aβ deposition and decreased cognition performance. **(B)** However, some non-pharmacological strategies have been presented to modulate some changes observed in AD and MCI such as fasting protocols, caloric restriction and physical exercise that can improve cognitive performance, increase autophagy and thus decrease Aβ aggregates. Red arrows represent changes in pathophysiology and blue arrows represent changes promoted by non-pharmacological strategies.

rigidity and postural impairment. Risk factors include genetic and environmental factors with classical symptomatology mediated by the loss of dopaminergic neurons within the substantia nigra pars compacta (Snpc), although other neuroanatomical regions can be also affected (Kalia and Lang, 2015).

In PD, as in many other neurodegenerative diseases, an increase in intracellular protein aggregates, LB, composed of abnormal aggregates αSynuclein protein (αSyn), is evident. Although the relationship between LB pathology and PD pathoetiology still requires clarification, there is epidemiological evidence to indicate that insulin signaling impairment is a relevant modulator (Driver et al., 2008; Schernhammer et al., 2011).

A study of 110 PD patients (53 with PD and dementia (PD/D) and 57 PD without dementia evaluated glucose and insulin levels after a 2 hours oral glucose tolerance-test (Bosco et al., 2012). These authors found that PD/D patients had higher prevalence of insulin resistance, with abnormal glucose metabolism (Bosco et al., 2012), although it should be noted that the association of diabetes with PD is complex and controversial (reviewed in Santiago and Potashkin, 2013). However, recent conceptualizations of type 2 diabetes have placed an emphasis on the importance of the gut-liver-pancreas axis, with alterations in the gut long appreciated as an early pathophysiological symptom in PD (Parkinson, 2002) as well as a possible site for the vagal transport of αSyn to the brain (Anderson et al., 2016). Clearly such systemic changes require further investigation.

In a postmortem study of four PD patients' brains homogenates from the substantia nigra and their age-matched controls, Sekar and Taghibiglou (2018) observed a significant decrease in PI3K p85, AKT, PIP_3, IRS-1 and IR levels, as well as an increase in glycogen synthase kinase (GSK)3β and nuclear translocation of tumor suppressor phosphatase and tensin homolog deleted on chromosome ten (PTEN), strongly suggesting an association between PD and insulin resistance (Sekar and Taghibiglou, 2018). Elevated levels of phosphorylated IRS-1 on serine residues block insulin/IGF-1 binding to the IR and so down-regulate downstream effectors such as AKT, which in turn blocks GSK3β phosphorylation. Once dephosphorylated, GSK3β becomes active and phosphorylates tau protein leading to hyperphosphorylation and neurofibrillary tangles deposition (Athauda and Foltynie, 2016). In advanced stages of AD and PD, protein aggregates of tau, Aβ and αSyn coexist (Yang et al., 2018).

In PD disruption of autophagy seems to be a process that is at least partially independent of alterations in the PI3K/AKT/mTOR pathway (Heras-Sandoval et al., 2014). Data from literature have been shown that overexpression of αSyn inhibits autophagy in cell culture and *in vivo* leading to accumulation of aggregate-prone proteins (Winslow et al., 2010). The αSyn aggregates can be alleviated by increased expression of Beclin 1, as observed in brain of transgenic mice model of αSyn overexpression, causing increased autophagy and neuronal protection (Spencer et al., 2010). Furthermore, work by Dehay et al. (2010) on a human neuroblastoma cell line as well as in the 1-methyl-4-phenyl-1, 2, 3, 6- tetrahydropyridine (MPTP) mouse model of PD led the authors to propose that the increased mitochondrial reactive oxygen species (ROS) evident in PD leads to abnormal permeabilization of lysosomal membranes, thereby causing lysosomal depletion and the accumulation of autophagosomes, resulting in inefficient autophagy (Dehay et al., 2010). The role of oxidative stress-induced disruption in autophagy was also confirmed by other studies (Lin and Kuang, 2014; Navarro-Yepes et al., 2014; Filomeni et al., 2015; Teves et al., 2018). An increase in autophagic flux was also measured in lysates from a dopaminergic neuroblastoma cell line (SH-SY5Y) and mouse embryonic fibroblast cells treated with 6-hydroxydopamine (6-OHDA) for 3 hours, which was coupled to a reduction in glutathione content, indicating that treatment with 6-OHDA leads to an increase in ROS levels, and AMPK/ULK1 activating autophagy, in an mTOR independent pathway (Urano et al., 2018).

Furthermore, increasing evidence has implicated lysosomal dysfunction in PD as an important factor in autophagy disruption. It should be noted that a new type of nonfibrillar phosphorylated αSyn (pαSyn*), which is conformationally distinct, has been identified in PD patients' brains, which seem to be the result of an incomplete autophagic degradation of pαSyn. The pαSyn* associates with mitochondria and is highly mitotoxic, causing structural damage. According to the author, pαSyn* may be the missing link between LB and mitochondrial impairment (Grassi et al., 2018). Furthermore, Grassi et al. (2018) propose that preformed pαSyn fibrils activate autophagy but the incomplete and/or abnormal autophagolysosomal degradation observed in PD is responsible for generation of pαSyn* that should migrate away from the fibrils and associate with mitochondria. The incomplete autophagic degradation can also be caused by mutations in ATP13A2 gene and SYT11, both observed in PD (Bento et al., 2016). This is an area clearly requiring further research.

Regarding insulin signaling in humans, a recent PD trial tested the effect of Exenatide, the first synthetic agonist of glucagon like peptide 1 (GLP-1), indicated to restore insulin pathway in type II diabetes (Sandoval and Sisley, 2015), and previously known to preserve mitochondrial function in dopaminergic neurons, reducing apoptotic death and lysosomal depletion as well as decreasing tau hyperphosphorylation and plaque load (reviewed in Athauda and Foltynie, 2018). The Exanatide-PD trial analyzed 60 idiopathic PD patients (both genders) who received exenatide or placebo, once weekly for 48 weeks, followed by a withdrawal of 12 weeks for analysis. Extracellular vesicles isolated from blood samples were used to indicate the brain insulin signaling pathway. Results showed Exenatide-treated patients to have a sustained increase in IRS-1 phosphorylation levels, total AKT and pAKT S473 after 24 weeks treatment and an increase in total and p-mTOR (S2448-mTORC1) at 48 weeks of treatment, compared to placebo. Increased levels of total mTOR (mTORC1/2) were associated with sustained clinical improvement on motor scores at 60 weeks (Athauda et al., 2019).

On the other hand, effects of rapamycin, a specific inhibitor of mTOR, require further clarification in PD models. In the 6-OHDA rat model of PD, Jiang et al. (2013), observed that rapamycin treatment with three different doses was able to decrease oxidative stress and mitochondrial injury consequently avoiding apoptotic dopaminergic neuronal loss (Jiang et al., 2013). These effects involved modulation of the mTORC1 complex, as mTORC2 is unresponsive to acute rapamycin treatment (Perluigi et al., 2015). Another study using the 6-OHDA model showed mTORC1 inhibition by rapamycin, or the selective blockade of its downstream target, S6K (by PF-4708671), to improve the memory deficit evident in this model. Rapamycin treatment was also able to reduce the anxiety and depression-like behavior observed in the rat PD model (Masini et al., 2018).

Non-pharmacological strategies to improve PD symptoms indicate exercise to have beneficial effects. In the 6-OHDA model, 8 weeks of 4 days/week treadmill running protected animals from 6-OHDA-induced oxidative stress (Tuon et al., 2012), whilst in the MPTP murine model, 8 weeks of treadmill running, 5 days/week, reduced αSyn levels in the striatum, and dopaminergic neuronal loss, as well as improving motor deficits and recovery of Beclin-1 and LC3-II levels, indicating that exercise could up-regulate autophagy (Koo and Cho, 2017). It is important to note that exercise duration seems to be a critical factor for the benefits observed in animals, as shorter periods of exercise are not so effective (Aguiar et al., 2014).

However, in human studies the effects of exercise in PD patients are much less conclusive (Ebersbach, 2015), although a large cohort study published by National Parkinson Foundation Quality Improvement Initiative Database in 2014 showed that a higher frequency on exercise leads to lower levels of disease severity and slows cognitive decline. The study analyzed data from 4,866 PD patients who were at different disease stages, although all were receiving treatment in United States centers of excellence (Oguh et al., 2014). Whether any exercise benefits are evident at later stages of PD still requires determination (Petzinger et al., 2013).

Other factors known to modulate autophagy, including dietary restriction, may also slow PD progression, as indicated in the MPTP rhesus monkey model, as indicated by the numbers of nigro-striatal dopaminergic neurons (Maswood et al., 2004). Any strategy that inhibits the insulin-AKT-mTORC1 signaling pathway is associated with increased longevity via autophagy activation (Ntsapi and Loos, 2016), and therefore would be expected to positively modulate PD incidence and pathophysiology (reviewed in Mattson, 2010). The benefits of dietary restriction in PD patients remain to be determined.

In summary, correlations of insulin resistance with abnormal autophagy seem important processes in the pathogenesis of AD and PD. However, there are some important differences across these disorders that future research should clarify. Clearly, increasing autophagic processes is beneficial in AD, whilst this requires further studies in PD patients, including as to how concurrent dementia interacts with wider PD processes, given that PD patients with dementia are more prone to develop insulin resistance. PD patients also have lower levels of the IR and its downstream proteins, although the origin of autophagy abnormalities remains undetermined. The roles of autophagy and mTOR in PD are still highly controversial, which considerably complicates treatment aimed at such processes and pathways (**Figure 4**).

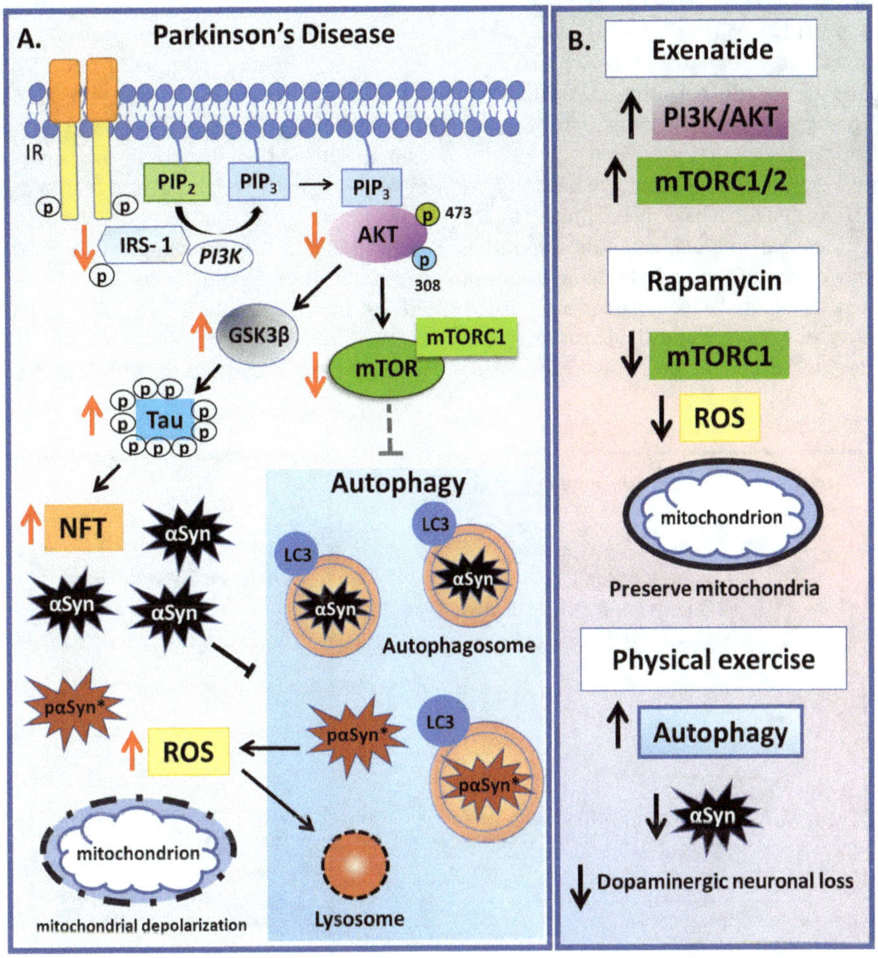

FIGURE 4 | Summary of changes related to insulin-autophagy pathway observed in Parkinson's Disease. **(A)** In Parkinson's disease, a decrease in PI3K-AKT-mTOR signaling is observed, which leads to GSK3β activation. GSK3β hyperphosphorylates tau protein leading to neurofibrillary tangles deposition. mTORC1 complex is inactive which causes autophagy to become activated. Otherwise, high levels of α-Synuclein (αSyn) impair the autophagic process together with increased mitochondrial reactive oxygen species (ROS). ROS leads to abnormal permeabilization of lysosomal membranes, thereby causing lysosomal depletion and the accumulation of autophagosomes, resulting in inefficient autophagy. As a result of an incomplete αSyn autophagic degradation, a new reactive specie called pαSyn* is generated inside autophagosomes and when released in cytosol it associates with mitochondrion being highly mitotoxic. Damaged mitochondrion is indicated by dashed line. **(B)** Some pharmacological and non-pharmacological strategies that act in PI3K-AKT-mTOR-autophagy signaling are presented. Exenatide-treated patients have a sustained increase in IRS-1 phosphorylation levels, total AKT and pAKT as well as increased levels of mTOR, reverting the impaired signaling observed in PD pathophysiology. Rapamycin, which specifically blocks mTORC1 activity, was able to decrease oxidative stress and mitochondrial injury in animal models, whereas physical exercise is associated with an increase in autophagy and a decrease in both αSyn aggregates and dopaminergic neuronal loss.

HUNTINGTON'S DISEASE

Huntington's disease is an autosomal dominant disorder characterized by severe motor and cognitive dysfunction, psychiatric disturbances and, ultimately, death. HD has long been appreciated to arise from a mutation in the Huntington (Htt) gene, which has a cytosine-adenine-guanine (CAG) expansion that encodes a polyQ repeat at the N-terminus in HD, resulting in impairments in protein functions and in protein aggregates (MacDonald et al., 1993). There is still no specific treatment for this condition, although studies in HD murine models show that the abolition of the expression of mutant Htt (mHtt) can rescue some of the symptoms and decrease protein aggregation in the brain (Yamamoto et al., 2000; Harper et al., 2005; Kordasiewicz et al., 2012). However, as functional Htt protein plays an important role in several physiological processes, such as mitochondrial dynamics, vesicle trafficking, axonal transport, synaptic function, and anti-apoptotic activity as well as autophagy, there are major problems in trying to suppress the activity of this gene (Choi et al., 2014; Ismailoglu et al., 2014; Wong and Holzbaur, 2014; Weiss and Littleton, 2016).

The loss of Htt functioning results in autophagy dysregulation, leading to protein accumulation and is likely to contribute to HD pathogenesis (Gelman et al., 2015). In contrast to other protein aggregation diseases, human and rodent HD samples show an upregulation of autophagosomes (Kegel et al., 2000; Petersen, 2001). However, these autophagosomes show some deficits in cargo recognition, resulting in inadequate degradation of aggregate proteins and damaged organelles (Boland et al., 2008; Martinez-Vicente et al., 2010). Besides that, it is also known that the silencing of either Htt or its interactor, Htt-associated protein 1 (HAP1), impairs the transport of autophagosome along the axon (Wong and Holzbaur, 2014), indicating that mHtt also modulates endocytic trafficking.

According with the literature, HD patients present higher basal plasma levels of IGF-1, which have been linked to the cognitive decline seen in these patients, leading to the hypothesis that IGF-1 resistance may be one of the underlying mechanisms involved in this pathology (Saleh et al., 2010; Salem et al., 2016). IGF-1, an upstream activator of the AKT-mTOR pathway, can inhibit mHtt-induced neuronal death and decrease the formation of intranuclear mHtt inclusions, via AKT phosphorylation of Htt, thereby providing a neuroprotective effect in HD (Humbert et al., 2002). Besides that, data from HD animal model showed AKT to be up-regulated with the intranasal administration of recombinant human IGF-1, increasing phosphorylation of mutant Htt and leading to an improvement in motor activity, as well as in both peripheral and central metabolic abnormalities (Lopes et al., 2014). On the other hand, according to Yamamoto et al. (2006), the dose-dependent clearance of the protein aggregate after insulin and IGF-1 treatment involves IRS-2 activation, and not IRS-1 or AKT activity (Yamamoto et al., 2006). Interestingly, depletion of the IGF-1 receptor (IGF-1R) resulted in decreased autophagy and increased mHtt levels, which

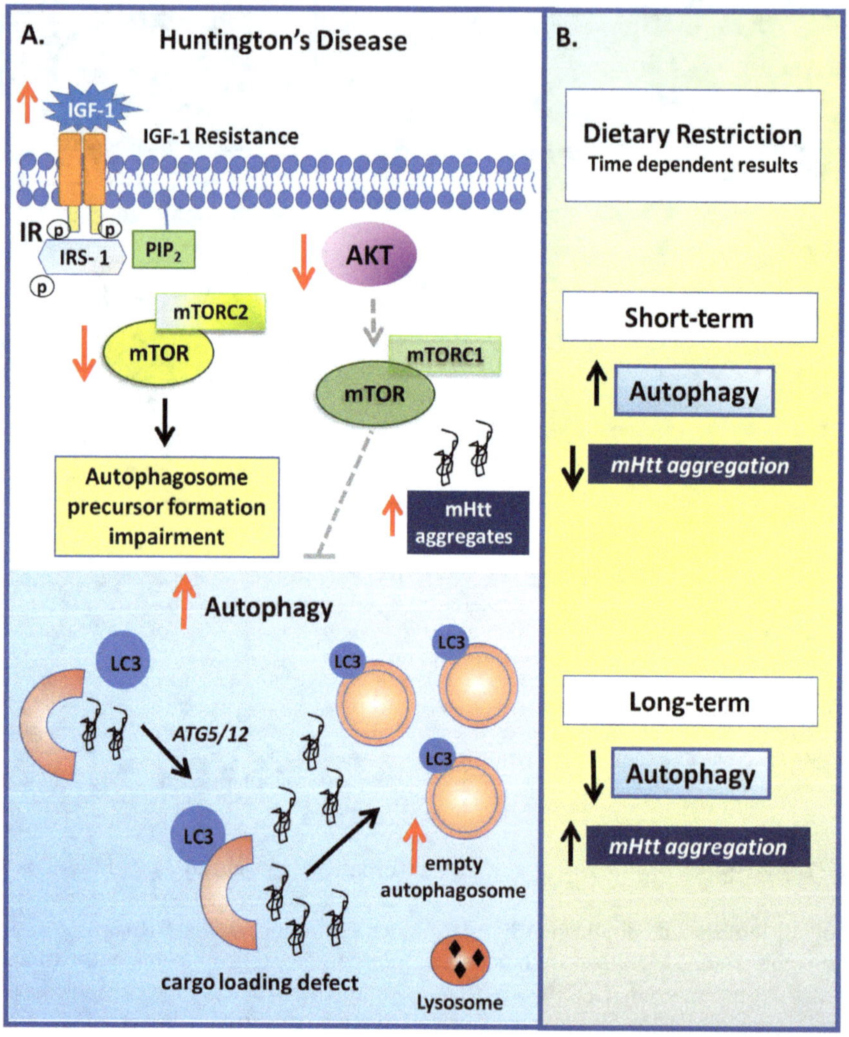

FIGURE 5 | Insulin and autophagy signaling modulation in Huntington's disease (HD). **(A)** Although the IGF-1 role on HD still seems paradoxical, it is clear that it develops an important role in this pathology. As observed in some studies, HD patients present higher basal plasma levels of IGF-1, which may be related with an IGF-1 resistance condition and a reduction in the insulin pathway. The reduction in IR activity results in reduced mTORC2 and AKT-mTORC1 activities, which leads to, respectively, a reduction in autophagosome precursor formation and an increase in the autophagy process, which may be related with the upregulation of autophagosomes with deficits in cargo recognition. However, long term IR down regulation, due to for example, receptor depletion or long term IR inhibition, results in reduced autophagy, which may be due to a lack of essential autophagosome precursor formation, and increased mHtt aggregates. **(B)** Non-pharmacological approaches such as dietary restriction also demonstrated to have a dual effect depending on the time. Short-term fasting resulted in increased autophagy and reduction on mHtt aggregation, while long-term serum deprivation resulted in reduced autophagosome formation.

was rescued only by prolonged (24 hours) IGF-1 treatment, in an AKT-independent pathway (Renna et al., 2013). Although another study demonstrated that IGF-1R deficiency affected only the size but not the mHtt levels in HD mice, it was observed that this deficiency had different consequences depending on the sex of the animal, causing some detrimental effects in the males, such as worsened rotarod performance and weight loss, but a delayed tremor onset in the females (Corrochano et al., 2014). Besides that, viral overexpression of the transcription factor EB (TFEB), a substrate of mTORC1 activity, resulted in increased autophagy and decreased levels of mHtt (Vodicka et al., 2016), indicating that the PI3K-AKT-mTOR pathway also plays an important role in this disease (Wu et al., 2009). As such, activation of the IGF-1/insulin pathway seems to have a dual and symptomatic utility, although the mechanisms involved require clarification.

Given that nutrient-rich or starvation diets can, respectively, suppress or increase autophagy via serine/threonine kinase phosphorylation of mTOR (Kim et al., 2008; Wong et al., 2015), a number of studies have investigated the utilization of dietary interventions in HD. Although the accumulation of mutant protein can lead to mTOR-independent autophagy with the degradation of accumulated proteins differing from the degradation under conditions of starvation (Yamamoto et al., 2006), dietary restriction in a HD mouse model resulted in an increase in autophagy and a reduction in mHtt aggregate formation and the normalization of blood glucose regulation, thereby contributing to a slower disease progression and an extended lifespan (Duan et al., 2003; Ehrnhoefer et al., 2018). However, although scheduled feeding demonstrates to increase autophagy, long-term serum deprivation, such as 8 to 24 hours, results in reduced autophagosome formation (Renna et al., 2013), suggesting that the autophagy regulation is influenced by the nutrient starvation time (**Figure 5**). Clearly, more studies are required on relevant processes in this area, including as to how dietary restriction may afford benefit in HD.

AMYOTROPHIC LATERAL SCLEROSIS AND FRONTOTEMPORAL DEMENTIA

Amyotrophic lateral sclerosis is a neurodegenerative disease that is characterized by the degeneration of upper and lower motor neurons of the primary motor cortex and spinal cord, resulting in muscle weakness and eventual paralysis, leading to death (Al-Chalabi and Hardiman, 2013). Although the pathoetiology of ALS is unknown, it has a not uncommon co-occurrence with FTD, which is marked by focal atrophy of both frontal and anterior temporal lobes (Van Langenhove et al., 2012). Moreover, as ALS and FTD share genetic risk factors, it has been proposed that they represent a continuum of neurodegenerative disorders (Van Langenhove et al., 2012).

ALS is associated with hypermetabolic and dyslipidemia states (Dupuis et al., 2008; Seelen et al., 2014), with an inverse risk factor association with obesity and type 2 diabetes (Gallo et al., 2013; Kioumourtzoglou et al., 2015). ALS patients with hyperlipidemia have an increased life expectancy, suggesting a neuroprotective role of lipids on ALS pathophysiology (Dupuis et al., 2008). Similar results are evident in the SOD1 mutant murine model of ALS, where high energy-diets prolong the lifespan (Dupuis et al., 2004). However, after adjusting for markers of disease severity, such as body mass index (BMI), forced vital capacity, and age, it was found that BMI, but not dyslipidemia, underlie this increased survival of ALS patients (Paganoni et al., 2011).

Although the role of lipids in ALS requires clarification, there is greater certainty as to the higher prevalence of hypermetabolism in ALS patients, which is linked with a faster rate of functional decline and shorter survival (Steyn et al., 2018).

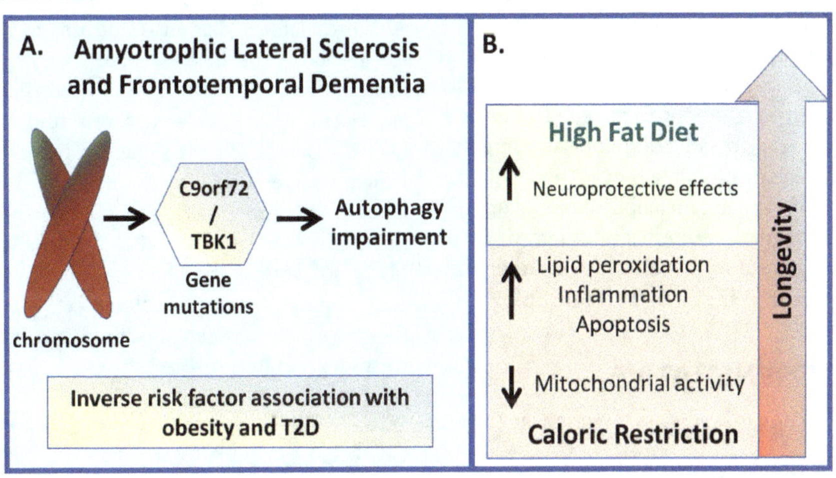

FIGURE 6 | Amyotrophic lateral sclerosis and Frontotemporal Dementia. **(A)** Genetic variations in genes such as C9orf72 and TBK1 are linked with both ALS and FTD disease development, which are associated with autophagy impairment. Besides that, since it is also associated with hypermetabolic and dyslipemia states, both conditions seem to present an inverse risk factor association with obesity and T2D. **(B)** Regarding the non-pharmacological inhibition, caloric restriction demonstrated to decrease lifespan due to an increase in lipid peroxidation, inflammation, and apoptosis, as well due to a reduction in mitochondrial activity, while high-energy diets resulted in increased lifespan.

Interestingly, hypermetabolism is associated with some genetic risk factors for ALS, although not for the C9ORf72 mutation (Steyn et al., 2018), which is the one most commonly associated with ALS-FTD (DeJesus-Hernandez et al., 2011). Remarkably, alterations in the C9ORf72 gene seem to have a dual function in autophagy regulation, with C9ORf72 positively regulating the initiation of autophagy by controlling the ULK1 complex, with its reduction resulting in autophagic dysfunction and protein aggregation (Webster et al., 2016). Other work shows the C9ORf72 gene to decrease autophagy through mTORC1 regulation (Ugolino et al., 2016). However, although Steyn et al. (2018) were not able to find any association between C9ORf72 and hypermetabolism, Liu et al. (2018) showed that loss of C9ORf72 gene function impairs lipid digestion and increases *de novo* fatty acid synthesis through dysregulated autophagic process under cell glucose starvation conditions (Liu et al., 2018). This could suggest that starvation or nutrient-rich conditions may play an important role in modulating C9ORf72 functions in autophagy.

Mutations leading to a loss-of-function in the TANK-binding kinase (TBK)1 phenotype also lead to an increased risk of developing ALS and FTD due to autophagy impairment (Cirulli et al., 2015; Freischmidt et al., 2015; Cui et al., 2018). Interestingly, a study performed on obese zucker rats provides evidence for the involvement of TBK1 in the mechanism of insulin resistance (Muñoz et al., 2009). This study shows that obese animals have increased hepatic TBK1 levels, leading to decreased IR activity due to Ser994 phosphorylation by TBK1 (Muñoz et al., 2009). Moreover, a high fat diet can positively modulate TBK1 gene expression in the liver and white adipose tissue (Chiang et al., 2009) whilst its accumulation in lipid rafts of hypothalamic neurons disrupts IR activation as well as AKT signaling, suggesting a potential role of TBK1 in brain insulin resistance (Delint-Ramirez et al., 2015). Overall, such data suggest that it is plausible that TBK1 may be one of the underlying mechanisms by which obesity is associated with a reduced risk of ALS and FTD.

An animal model of ALS under caloric restriction has a decreased lifespan due to an increase in lipid peroxidation, inflammation and apoptosis, as well a decrease in mitochondrial bioenergetic efficiency, when compared with mice fed *ad libitum* (Patel et al., 2010). Similarly, rapamycin treatment is detrimental, increasing motor neuron degeneration in a mouse model of ALS (Zhang et al., 2011). As autophagy and metabolism modulate ALS disease onset and progression, dietary interventions may prove of clinical utility in the management of this disorder, including the possibility of using a high-fat diet as treatment (**Figure 6**).

OTHER NEURODEGENERATIVE DISEASES

Spinocerebellar Ataxia Type 3

Spinocerebellar ataxia 3 (SCA3), a neurodegenerative disease characterized mainly by progressive ataxia affecting balance, gait and speech, is caused by a mutation in the C-terminus polyglutamine (PolyQ) region of the ataxin-3 protein, an ubiquitously expressed deubiquitinating enzyme with important functions in the proteasomal protein degradation pathway and regulation of transcription. According with the literature, the polyQ stretch in wild-type ataxin-3 induces autophagy by protecting Beclin-1 from proteasome-mediated degradation (Ashkenazi et al., 2017). As other neurodegenerative diseases, the only available treatments aim to reduce disease symptoms. However, although the underlying mechanisms are not completely understood, the regulation of autophagic process has demonstrated to be a potential target for ameliorating or stopping the progression of the disease (Menzies et al., 2010; Nascimento-Ferreira et al., 2011). As demonstrated by Menzies et al. (2010), the administration of rapamycin improved motor performance in an SCA3 animal model through mTOR inhibition and consequent autophagy upregulation. Besides that, according with Nascimento-Ferreira et al. (2011), Beclin-1 overexpression resulted in increased autophagic flux, mutant ataxin-3 clearance and other neuroprotective effects, rescuing the abnormal expression of endogenous autophagic markers, accumulation of autophagosomes and reduced levels of Beclin-1. In a similar way, another study observed decreased autophagosome production when comparing fibroblasts from SCA3 patients and healthy individuals. However, although Beclin-1 overexpression increased the autophagic flux, it did not result in higher levels of autophagosome production (Onofre et al., 2016). Taken together, this result supports the important role of autophagy in also regulating the SCA3 disease.

Lafora Disease

Lafora disease is a rare autosomal recessive, progressive and lethal neurodegenerative disease that is characterized by myoclonic epilepsy followed by continuous neurological decline. Reported in approximately 58% of the LD cases, mutation in the EPM2A gene, which encodes the glucan phosphatase laforin, is associated with the presence of intracellular inclusion bodies known as Lafora bodies (LB) in the brain, spinal cord and other peripheral tissues (Knecht et al., 2010). Although laforin demonstrated not to be absolutely necessary for autophagy, it was observed that it positively regulates this process (Knecht et al., 2010). According to this study, LD is associated with decreased levels and impaired formation of LC3-II, as well altered signaling in the AKT-mTOR pathway, which was rescued after laforin overexpression, reducing the amount of protein aggregates in an autophagy-dependent manner (Knecht et al., 2010). Moreover, besides autophagy, LD also seems to be associated with insulin resistance and hyperglycemia (Nicolescu et al., 2019), strengthening the crosstalk between insuling and autophagy signaling in neurodegenerative diseases.

CONCLUSION

Although it is clear that central insulin signaling and the regulation of autophagy are relevant to a host of diverse neurodegenerative disorders, which is supported by several studies including pharmacological inhibition, animal models, genetic strategies and patients, as well as by the link between metabolic disorders and the development of some neurodegenerative diseases, it is still hard to define statements as data from literature is controversial and the underlying mechanisms as well as the possible benefits of autophagy modulation seem to be specific for each disorder. As many key cellular processes are intimately associated with insulin signaling and autophagic process, pharmacological inhibition and/or stimulation may have some detrimental effects, especially considering long-term treatments, which may partly be responsible for the conflicting results in the literature. Besides that, it is important to consider that the onset of the disease, the age and also the sex can have a strong influence on the development and also on the treatment outcomes. In this context, genetic strategies that modulate metabolism and autophagy regulation can contribute to having a better understanding of the underlying mechanisms among these pathways and the neurodegenerative diseases. Besides that, as it seems that outcomes may vary according to stimulus duration, the study of the effects of non-pharmacological interventions such as physical exercise and intermittent fasting in the onset and progression of neurodegenerative diseases can also bring light to new information for the literature, as well as possible new approaches that may contribute to the conventional treatments. Thus, the understanding of how such processes are integrated in different central and systemic cells should provide better targeted treatment for these still poorly managed conditions.

AUTHOR CONTRIBUTIONS

CS and EK conceived the review idea, and edited final version of the text and figures. CM, NdM, and AO contributed equally writing the text. NdM and AO contributed equally conceiving the figures ideas. GdM contributed by drafiting the work and drawing the figures.

ACKNOWLEDGMENTS

We thank George Anderson, CRC Scotland and London for English editing.

REFERENCES

Abbott, M. A., Wells, D. G., and Fallon, J. R. (1999). The insulin receptor tyrosine kinase substrate p58/53 and the insulin receptor are components of CNS synapses. *J. Neurosci.* 19, 7300–7308. doi: 10.1523/JNEUROSCI.4306-08.2009

Abel, J. J. (1926). Crystalline insulin. *Proc. Natl. Acad. Sci. U.S.A.* 12, 132–136.

Aguiar, A. S., Tristão, F. S. M., Amar, M., Chevarin, C., Glaser, V., De Paula Martins, R., et al. (2014). Six weeks of voluntary exercise don't protect C57BL/6 mice against neurotoxicity of MPTP and MPP+. *Neurotox. Res.* 25, 147–152. doi: 10.1007/s12640-013-9412-5

Al-Chalabi, A., and Hardiman, O. (2013). The epidemiology of ALS: a conspiracy of genes, environment and time. *Nat. Rev. Neurol.* 9, 617–628. doi: 10.1038/nrneurol.2013.203

Alirezaei, M., Kemball, C. C., Flynn, C. T., Wood, M. R., Whitton, J. L., and Kiosses, W. B. (2010). Short-term fasting induces profound neuronal autophagy. *Autophagy* 6, 702–710. doi: 10.4161/auto.6.6.12376

Anderson, G., Seo, M., Berk, M., Carvalho, A. F., and Maes, M. (2016). Gut permeability and microbiota in Parkinson's disease: role of depression, tryptophan catabolites, oxidative and nitrosative stress and melatonergic pathways. *Curr. Pharm. Des.* 22, 6142–6151. doi: 10.2174/1381612822666160906161513

Arvanitakis, Z., Wilson, R. S., Bienias, J. L., Evans, D. A., and Bennett, D. A. (2004). Diabetes mellitus and risk of Alzheimer disease and decline in cognitive function. *Arch. Neurol.* 61, 661–666. doi: 10.1001/archneur.61.5.661

Ashkenazi, A., Bento, C. F., Ricketts, T., Vicinanza, M., Siddiqi, F., Pavel, M., et al. (2017). Polyglutamine tracts regulate beclin 1-dependent autophagy. *Nature* 545, 108–111. doi: 10.1038/nature22078

Athauda, D., and Foltynie, T. (2016). Insulin resistance and Parkinson's disease: a new target for disease modification? *Prog. Neurobiol.* 145–146, 98–120. doi: 10.1016/j.pneurobio.2016.10.001

Athauda, D., and Foltynie, T. (2018). Protective effects of the GLP-1 mimetic exendin-4 in Parkinson's disease. *Neuropharmacology* 136, 260–270. doi: 10.1016/j.neuropharm.2017.09.023

Athauda, D., Gulyani, S., Karnati, H., Li, Y., Tweedie, D., Mustapic, M., et al. (2019). Utility of neuronal-derived exosomes to examine molecular mechanisms that affect motor function in patients with Parkinson disease. *JAMA Neurol.* doi: 10.1001/jamaneurol.2018.4304 [Epub ahead of print].

Axe, E. L., Walker, S. A., Manifava, M., Chandra, P., Roderick, H. L., Habermann, A., et al. (2008). Autophagosome formation from membrane compartments enriched in phosphatidylinositol 3-phosphate and dynamically connected to the endoplasmic reticulum. *J. Cell Biol.* 182, 685–701. doi: 10.1083/jcb.200803137

Balin, B. J., Broadwell, R. D., Salcman, M., and El-Kalliny, M. (1986). Avenues for entry of peripherally administered protein to the central nervous system in mouse, rat, and squirrel monkey. *J. Comp. Neurol.* 251, 260–280. doi: 10.1002/cne.902510209

Banting, F. G., and Best, C. H. (1922). The internal secretion of the pancreas. *J. Lab. Clin. Med.* 7, 251–266.

Beattie, E. C., Carroll, R. C., Yu, X., Morishita, W., Yasuda, H., von Zastrow, M., et al. (2000). Regulation of AMPA receptor endocytosis by a signaling mechanism shared with LTD. *Nat. Neurosci.* 3, 1291–1300. doi: 10.1038/81823

Benedict, C., Hallschmid, M., Hatke, A., Schultes, B., Fehm, H. L., Born, J., et al. (2004). Intranasal insulin improves memory in humans. *Psychoneuroendocrinology* 29, 1326–1334. doi: 10.1016/j.psyneuen.2004.04.003

Bento, C. F., Ashkenazi, A., Jimenez-Sanchez, M., and Rubinsztein, D. C. (2016). The Parkinson's disease-associated genes ATP13A2 and SYT11 regulate autophagy via a common pathway. *Nat. Commun.* 7:11803. doi: 10.1038/ncomms11803

Boland, B., Kumar, A., Lee, S., Platt, F. M., Wegiel, J., Yu, W. H., et al. (2008). Autophagy induction and autophagosome clearance in neurons: relationship to autophagic pathology in Alzheimer's disease. *J. Neurosci.* 28, 6926–6937. doi: 10.1523/JNEUROSCI.0800-08.2008

Boland, B., Smith, D. A., Mooney, D., Jung, S. S., Walsh, D. M., and Platt, F. M. (2010). Macroautophagy is not directly involved in the metabolism of amyloid precursor protein. *J. Biol. Chem.* 285, 37415–37426. doi: 10.1074/jbc.M110.186411

Bosco, D., Plastino, M., Cristiano, D., Colica, C., Ermio, C., De Bartolo, M., et al. (2012). Dementia is associated with Insulin Resistance in patients with Parkinson's Disease. *J. Neurol. Sci.* 315, 39–43. doi: 10.1016/j.jns.2011.12.008

Butterfield, W. J. H., Abrams, M. E., Sells, R. A., Sterky, G., and Whichelow, M. J. (1966). Insulin sensitivity of the human brain. *Lancet* 287, 557–560. doi: 10.1016/s0140-6736(66)90757-4

Caccamo, A., Majumder, S., Richardson, A., Strong, R., and Oddo, S. (2010). Molecular interplay between mammalian target of rapamycin (mTOR), amyloid-β, and Tau: effects on cognitive impairments. *J. Biol. Chem.* 285, 13107–13120. doi: 10.1074/jbc.M110.100420

Camandola, S., and Mattson, M. P. (2017). Brain metabolism in health, aging, and neurodegeneration. *EMBO J.* 36, 1474–1492. doi: 10.15252/embj

Candeias, E., Sebastião, I., Cardoso, S., Carvalho, C., Santos, M. S., Oliveira, C. R., et al. (2017). Brain GLP-1/IGF-1 signaling and autophagy mediate exendin-4 protection against apoptosis in type 2 diabetic rats. *Mol. Neurobiol.* 55, 4030–4050. doi: 10.1007/s12035-017-0622-3

Chen, X., Kondo, K., Motoki, K., Homma, H., and Okazawa, H. (2015). Fasting activates macroautophagy in neurons of Alzheimer's disease mouse model but is insufficient to degrade amyloid-beta. *Sci. Rep.* 5:12115. doi: 10.1038/srep12115

Chiang, S.-H., Bazuine, M., Lumeng, C. N., Geletka, L. M., Mowers, J., White, N. M., et al. (2009). The protein kinase IKK? regulates energy balance in obese mice. *Cell* 138, 961–975. doi: 10.1016/j.cell.2009.06.046

Chiu, S.-L., and Cline, H. T. (2010). Insulin receptor signaling in the development of neuronal structure and function. *Neural Dev.* 5:7. doi: 10.1186/1749-8104-5-7

Choi, J. (2005). Regulation of dendritic spine morphogenesis by insulin receptor substrate 53, a downstream effector of Rac1 and Cdc42 small GTPases. *J. Neurosci.* 25, 869–879. doi: 10.1523/JNEUROSCI.3212-04.2005

Choi, Y.-B., Kadakkuzha, B. M., Liu, X.-A., Akhmedov, K., Kandel, E. R., and Puthanveettil, S. V. (2014). Huntingtin is critical both pre- and postsynaptically for long-term learning-related synaptic plasticity in aplysia. *PLoS One* 9:e103004. doi: 10.1371/journal.pone.0103004

Cirulli, E. T., Lasseigne, B. N., Petrovski, S., Sapp, P. C., Dion, P. A., Leblond, C. S., et al. (2015). Exome sequencing in amyotrophic lateral sclerosis identifies risk genes and pathways. *Science* 347, 1436–1441. doi: 10.1126/science.aaa3650

Clarke, D. W., Mudd, L., Boyd, F. T., Fields, M., and Raizada, M. K. (1986). Insulin is released from rat brain neuronal cells in culture. *J. Neurochem.* 47, 831–836. doi: 10.1111/j.1471-4159.1986.tb00686.x

Corrochano, S., Renna, M., Osborne, G., Carter, S., Stewart, M., May, J., et al. (2014). Reducing Igf-1r levels leads to paradoxical and sexually dimorphic effects in HD mice. *PLoS One* 9:e105595. doi: 10.1371/journal.pone.0105595

Cui, R., Tuo, M., Li, P., and Zhou, C. (2018). Association between TBK1 mutations and risk of amyotrophic lateral sclerosis/frontotemporal dementia spectrum: a meta-analysis. *Neurol. Sci.* 39, 811–820. doi: 10.1007/s10072-018-3246-0

de Castro, J. M., and Balagura, S. (1976). Insulin pretreatment facilitates recovery after dorsal hippocampal lesions. *Physiol. Behav.* 16, 517–520. doi: 10.1016/0031-9384(76)90208-0

Dehay, B., Bove, J., Rodriguez-Muela, N., Perier, C., Recasens, A., Boya, P., et al. (2010). Pathogenic lysosomal depletion in Parkinson's disease. *J. Neurosci.* 30, 12535–12544. doi: 10.1523/JNEUROSCI.1920-10.2010

DeJesus-Hernandez, M., Mackenzie, I. R., Boeve, B. F., Boxer, A. L., Baker, M., Rutherford, N. J., et al. (2011). Expanded GGGGCC hexanucleotide repeat in noncoding region of C9ORF72 causes chromosome 9p-linked FTD and ALS. *Neuron* 72, 245–256. doi: 10.1016/j.neuron.2011.09.011

Delint-Ramirez, I., Maldonado Ruiz, R., Torre-Villalvazo, I., Fuentes-Mera, L., Garza ñas, L., Tovar, A., et al. (2015). Genetic obesity alters recruitment of TANK-binding kinase 1 and AKT into hypothalamic lipid rafts domains. *Neurochem. Int.* 80, 23–32. doi: 10.1016/j.neuint.2014.11.002

Driver, J. A., Smith, A., Buring, J. E., Gaziano, J. M., Kurth, T., and Logroscino, G. (2008). Prospective cohort study of type 2 diabetes and the risk of Parkinson's disease. *Diabetes Care* 31, 2003–2005. doi: 10.2337/dc08-0688

Duan, W., Guo, Z., Jiang, H., Ware, M., Li, X.-J., and Mattson, M. P. (2003). Dietary restriction normalizes glucose metabolism and BDNF levels, slows disease progression, and increases survival in huntingtin mutant mice. *Proc. Natl. Acad. Sci. U.S.A.* 100, 2911–2916. doi: 10.1073/pnas.0536856100

Dupuis, L., Corcia, P., Fergani, A., Gonzalez De Aguilar, J.-L., Bonnefont-Rousselot, D., Bittar, R., et al. (2008). Dyslipidemia is a protective factor in amyotrophic lateral sclerosis. *Neurology* 70, 1004–1009. doi: 10.1212/01.wnl.0000285080.70324.27

Dupuis, L., Oudart, H., Rene, F., de Aguilar, J.-L. G., and Loeffler, J.-P. (2004). Evidence for defective energy homeostasis in amyotrophic lateral sclerosis: benefit of a high-energy diet in a transgenic mouse model. *Proc. Natl. Acad. Sci. U.S.A.* 101, 11159–11164. doi: 10.1073/pnas.0402026101

Ebato, C., Uchida, T., Arakawa, M., Komatsu, M., Ueno, T., Komiya, K., et al. (2008). Autophagy is important in islet homeostasis and compensatory increase of beta cell mass in response to high-fat diet. *Cell Metab.* 8, 325–332. doi: 10.1016/j.cmet.2008.08.009

Ebersbach, G. (2015). Exercise matters in patients with PD—another piece of evidence. *Nat. Rev. Neurol.* 11, 9–10. doi: 10.1038/nrneurol.2014.231

Ehrnhoefer, D. E., Martin, D. D. O., Schmidt, M. E., Qiu, X., Ladha, S., Caron, N. S., et al. (2018). Preventing mutant huntingtin proteolysis and intermittent fasting promote autophagy in models of Huntington disease. *Acta Neuropathol. Commun.* 6:16. doi: 10.1186/s40478-018-0518-0

El Sayed, L. A., Elattar, S., and Eltablawy, N. (2012). Nerve conduction velocity of sciatic nerve in high fat diet induced obesity in rats: effect of corn oil and omega 3 fatty acids supplement. *Life Sci. J.* 9, 458–471.

Fernandez, A. M., Hernandez-Garzón, E., Perez-Domper, P., Perez-Alvarez, A., Mederos, S., Matsui, T., et al. (2017). Insulin regulates astrocytic glucose handling through cooperation with IGF-I. *Diabetes* 66, 64–74. doi: 10.2337/db16-0861

Filimonenko, M., Isakson, P., Finley, K. D., Anderson, M., Jeong, H., Melia, T. J., et al. (2010). The selective macroautophagic degradation of aggregated proteins requires the PI3P-binding protein alfy. *Mol. Cell* 38, 265–279. doi: 10.1016/j.molcel.2010.04.007

Filomeni, G., De Zio, D., and Cecconi, F. (2015). Oxidative stress and autophagy: the clash between damage and metabolic needs. *Cell Death Differ.* 22, 377–388. doi: 10.1038/cdd.2014.150

Freischmidt, A., Wieland, T., Richter, B., Ruf, W., Schaeffer, V., Müller, K., et al. (2015). Haploinsufficiency of TBK1 causes familial ALS and fronto-temporal dementia. *Nat. Neurosci.* 18, 631–636. doi: 10.1038/nn.4000

Gallo, V., Wark, P. A., Jenab, M., Pearce, N., Brayne, C., Vermeulen, R., et al. (2013). Prediagnostic body fat and risk of death from amyotrophic lateral sclerosis: the EPIC cohort. *Neurology* 80, 829–838. doi: 10.1212/WNL.0b013e3182840689

García-Cáceres, C., Quarta, C., Varela, L., Gao, Y., Gruber, T., Legutko, B., et al. (2016). Astrocytic insulin signaling couples brain glucose uptake with nutrient availability. *Cell* 166, 867–880. doi: 10.1016/j.cell.2016.07.028

García-Mesa, Y., López-Ramos, J. C., Giménez-Llort, L., Revilla, S., Guerra, R., Gruart, A., et al. (2011). Physical exercise protects against Alzheimer's disease in 3xTg-AD mice. *J. Alzheimers Dis.* 24, 421–454. doi: 10.3233/JAD-2011-101635

Gelman, A., Rawet-Slobodkin, M., and Elazar, Z. (2015). Huntingtin facilitates selective autophagy. *Nat. Cell Biol.* 17, 214–215. doi: 10.1038/ncb3125

Govind, S., Kozma, R., Monfries, C., Lim, L., and Ahmed, S. (2001). Cdc42Hs facilitates cytoskeletal reorganization and neurite outgrowth by localizing the 58-kD insulin receptor substrate to filamentous actin. *J. Cell Biol.* 152, 579–594. doi: 10.1083/jcb.152.3.579

Grassi, D., Howard, S., Zhou, M., Diaz-Perez, N., Urban, N. T., Guerrero-Given, D., et al. (2018). Identification of a highly neurotoxic α-synuclein species inducing mitochondrial damage and mitophagy in Parkinson's disease. *Proc. Natl. Acad. Sci. U.S.A.* 115, E2634–E2643. doi: 10.1073/pnas.1713849115

Grote, C. W., Morris, J. K., Ryals, J. M., Geiger, P. C., and Wright, D. E. (2011). Insulin receptor substrate 2 expression and involvement in neuronal insulin resistance in diabetic neuropathy. *Exp. Diabetes Res.* 2011:212571. doi: 10.1155/2011/212571

Gu, T., Zhao, T., and Hewes, R. S. (2014). Insulin signaling regulates neurite growth during metamorphic neuronal remodeling. *Biol. Open* 3, 81–93. doi: 10.1242/bio.20136437

Halagappa, V. K. M., Guo, Z., Pearson, M., Matsuoka, Y., Cutler, R. G., LaFerla, F. M., et al. (2007). Intermittent fasting and caloric restriction ameliorate age-related behavioral deficits in the triple-transgenic mouse model of Alzheimer's disease. *Neurobiol. Dis.* 26, 212–220. doi: 10.1016/j.nbd.2006.12.019

Harper, S. Q., Staber, P. D., He, X., Eliason, S. L., Martins, I. H., Mao, Q., et al. (2005). RNA interference improves motor and neuropathological abnormalities in a Huntington's disease mouse model. *Proc. Natl. Acad. Sci. U.S.A.* 102, 5820–5825. doi: 10.1073/pnas.0501507102

Havrankova, J., Roth, J., and Brownstein, M. J. (1979). Concentrations of insulin and insulin receptors in the brain are independent of peripheral insulin levels. Studies of obese and streptozotocin-treated rodents. *J. Clin. Invest.* 64, 636–642. doi: 10.1172/JCI109504

Havrankova, J., Schmechelt, D., Roth, J., and Brownsteint, A. M. (1978). Identification of insulin in rat brain. *Neurobiology* 75, 5737–5741. doi: 10.1073/pnas.75.11.5737

He, C., Wei, Y., Sun, K., Li, B., Dong, X., Zou, Z., et al. (2013). Beclin 2 functions in autophagy, degradation of G protein-coupled receptors, and metabolism. *Cell* 154, 1085–1099. doi: 10.1016/j.cell.2013.07.035

Heras-Sandoval, D., Pérez-Rojas, J. M., Hernández-Damián, J., and Pedraza-Chaverri, J. (2014). The role of PI3K/AKT/mTOR pathway in the modulation of autophagy and the clearance of protein aggregates in neurodegeneration. *Cell. Signal.* 26, 2694–2701. doi: 10.1016/j.cellsig.2014.08.019

Humbert, S., Bryson, E. A., Cordelières, F. P., Connors, N. C., Datta, S. R., Finkbeiner, S., et al. (2002). The IGF-1/Akt pathway is neuroprotective in Huntington's disease and involves huntingtin phosphorylation by akt. *Dev. Cell* 2, 831–837. doi: 10.1016/s1534-5807(02)00188-0

Illum, L. (2000). Transport of drugs from the nasal cavity to the central nervous system. *Eur. J. Pharm. Sci.* 11, 1–18. doi: 10.1016/s0928-0987(00)00087-7

Ismailoglu, I., Chen, Q., Popowski, M., Yang, L., Gross, S. S., and Brivanlou, A. H. (2014). Huntingtin protein is essential for mitochondrial metabolism, bioenergetics and structure in murine embryonic stem cells. *Dev. Biol.* 391, 230–240. doi: 10.1016/j.ydbio.2014.04.005

Jaeger, P. A., Pickford, F., Sun, C.-H., Lucin, K. M., Masliah, E., and Wyss-Coray, T. (2010). Regulation of amyloid precursor protein processing by the beclin 1 complex. *PLoS One* 5:e11102. doi: 10.1371/journal.pone.0011102

Jiang, J., Jiang, J., Zuo, Y., and Gu, Z. (2013). Rapamycin protects the mitochondria against oxidative stress and apoptosis in a rat model of Parkinson's disease. *Int. J. Mol. Med.* 31, 825–832. doi: 10.3892/ijmm.2013.1280

Kalia, L. V., and Lang, A. E. (2015). Parkinson's disease. *Lancet* 386, 896–912.

Katila, N., Bhurtel, S., Shadfar, S., Srivastav, S., Neupane, S., Ojha, U., et al. (2017). Metformin lowers α-synuclein phosphorylation and upregulates neurotrophic factor in the MPTP mouse model of Parkinson's disease. *Neuropharmacology* 125, 396–407. doi: 10.1016/j.neuropharm.2017.08.015

Kegel, K. B., Kim, M., Sapp, E., McIntyre, C., Castaño, J. G., Aronin, N., et al. (2000). Huntingtin expression stimulates endosomal–lysosomal activity, endosome tubulation, and autophagy. *J. Neurosci.* 20, 7268–7278. doi: 10.1523/JNEUROSCI.20-19-07268.2000

Kern, W., Peters, A., Fruehwald-Schultes, B., Deininger, E., Born, J., and Fehm, H. L. (2001). Improving influence of insulin on cognitive functions in humans. *Neuroendocrinology* 74, 270–280. doi: 10.1159/000054694

Kim, E., Goraksha-Hicks, P., Li, L., Neufeld, T. P., and Guan, K.-L. (2008). Regulation of TORC1 by Rag GTPases in nutrient response. *Nat. Cell Biol.* 10, 935–945. doi: 10.1038/ncb1753

Kioumourtzoglou, M.-A., Rotem, R. S., Seals, R. M., Gredal, O., Hansen, J., and Weisskopf, M. G. (2015). Diabetes mellitus, obesity, and diagnosis of amyotrophic lateral sclerosis. *JAMA Neurol.* 72, 905–911. doi: 10.1001/jamaneurol.2015.0910

Klionsky, D. J., and Emr, S. D. (2000). Autophagy as a regulated pathway of cellular degradation. *Science* 290, 1717–1721. doi: 10.1126/science.290.5497.1717

Knecht, E., Aguado, C., Sarkar, S., Korolchuk, V. I., Criado-García, O., Vernia, S., et al. (2010). Impaired autophagy in Lafora disease. *Autophagy* 6, 991–993. doi: 10.4161/auto.6.7.13308

Koo, J.-H., and Cho, J.-Y. (2017). Treadmill exercise attenuates α-synuclein levels by promoting mitochondrial function and autophagy possibly via SIRT1 in the chronic MPTP/P-induced mouse model of Parkinson's disease. *Neurotox. Res.* 32, 473–486. doi: 10.1007/s12640-017-9770-5

Kopf, D., and Frölich, L. (2009). Risk of incident Alzheimer's disease in diabetic patients: a systematic review of prospective trials. *J. Alzheimers Dis.* 16, 677–685. doi: 10.3233/jad-2009-1011

Kordasiewicz, H. B., Stanek, L. M., Wancewicz, E. V., Mazur, C., McAlonis, M. M., Pytel, K. A., et al. (2012). Sustained therapeutic reversal of Huntington's disease by transient repression of huntingtin synthesis. *Neuron* 74, 1031–1044. doi: 10.1016/j.neuron.2012.05.009

Koss, D. J., Jones, G., Cranston, A., Gardner, H., Kanaan, N. M., and Platt, B. (2016). Soluble pre-fibrillar tau and β-amyloid species emerge in early human Alzheimer's disease and track disease progression and cognitive decline. *Acta Neuropathol.* 132, 875–895. doi: 10.1007/s00401-016-1632-3

Kundu, M., and Thompson, C. B. (2005). Macroautophagy versus mitochondrial autophagy: a question of fate? *Cell Death Differ.* 12, 1484–1489. doi: 10.1038/sj.cdd.4401780

Kuwabara, T., Kagalwala, M. N., Onuma, Y., Ito, Y., Warashina, M., Terashima, K., et al. (2011). Insulin biosynthesis in neuronal progenitors derived from adult hippocampus and the olfactory bulb. *EMBO Mol. Med.* 3, 742–754. doi: 10.1002/emmm.201100177

Lamotte, L., Jackerott, M., Bucchini, D., Jami, J., Joshi, R., and Deltour, L. (2004). Knock-in of diphteria toxin a chain gene at Ins2 locus: effects on islet development and localization of Ins2 expression in the brain. *Transgenic Res.* 13, 463–473. doi: 10.1007/s11248-004-9587-x

Larson, M. E., and Lesné, S. E. (2012). Soluble Aβ oligomer production and toxicity. *J. Neurochem.* 120, 125–139. doi: 10.1111/j.1471-4159.2011.07478.x

Lasagna-Reeves, C. A., Castillo-Carranza, D. L., Sengupta, U., Clos, A. L., Jackson, G. R., and Kayed, R. (2011). Tau oligomers impair memory and induce synaptic and mitochondrial dysfunction in wild-type mice. *Mol. Neurodegener.* 6:39. doi: 10.1186/1750-1326-6-39

Lashuel, H. A., Overk, C. R., Oueslati, A., and Masliah, E. (2013). The many faces of α-synuclein: from structure and toxicity to therapeutic target. *Nat. Rev. Neurosci.* 14, 38–48. doi: 10.1038/nrn3406

Lennox, R., Porter, D. W., Flatt, P. R., Holscher, C., Irwin, N., and Gault, V. A. (2014). Comparison of the independent and combined effects of sub-chronic therapy with metformin and a stable GLP-1 receptor agonist on cognitive function, hippocampal synaptic plasticity and metabolic control in high-fat fed mice. *Neuropharmacology* 86, 22–30. doi: 10.1016/j.neuropharm.2014.06.026

Lin, W., and Kuang, H. (2014). Oxidative stress induces autophagy in response to multiple noxious stimuli in retinal ganglion cells. *Autophagy* 10, 1692–1701. doi: 10.4161/auto.36076

Liu, Y., Wang, T., Ji, Y. J., Johnson, K., Liu, H., Johnson, K., et al. (2018). A C9orf72–CARM1 axis regulates lipid metabolism under glucose starvation-induced nutrient stress. *Genes Dev.* 32, 1380–1397. doi: 10.1101/gad.315564.118

Liu, Y., Yao, Z., Zhang, L., Zhu, H., Deng, W., and Qin, C. (2013). Insulin induces neurite outgrowth via SIRT1 in SH-SY5Y cells. *Neuroscience* 238, 371–380. doi: 10.1016/j.neuroscience.2013.01.034

Lopes, C., Ribeiro, M., Duarte, A. I., Humbert, S., Saudou, F., Pereira De Almeida, L., et al. (2014). IGF-1 intranasal administration rescues Huntington's disease phenotypes in YAC128 mice. *Mol. Neurobiol.* 49, 1126–1142. doi: 10.1007/s12035-013-8585-5

Lu, M., Su, C., Qiao, C., Bian, Y., Ding, J., and Hu, G. (2016). Metformin prevents dopaminergic neuron death in MPTP/P-induced mouse model of Parkinson's disease via autophagy and mitochondrial ROS clearance. *Int. J. Neuropsychopharmacol.* 19:yw047. doi: 10.1093/ijnp/pyw047

MacDonald, M. E., Bates, G. P., Buckler, A. J., Altherr, M., Tagle, D., and Snell, R. (1993). A novel gene containing a trinucleotide repeat that is expanded and unstable on Huntington's disease chromosomes. *Cell* 72, 971–983. doi: 10.1016/0092-8674(93)90585-E

Maida, A., Lamont, B. J., Cao, X., and Drucker, D. J. (2011). Metformin regulates the incretin receptor axis via a pathway dependent on peroxisome proliferator-activated receptor-α in mice. *Diabetologia* 54, 339–349. doi: 10.1007/s00125-010-1937-z

Margolis, R. U., and Altszuler, N. (1967). Insulin in the cerebrospinal fluid. *Nature* 215, 1375–1376.

Martinez-Vicente, M., Talloczy, Z., Wong, E., Tang, G., Koga, H., Kaushik, S., et al. (2010). Cargo recognition failure is responsible for inefficient autophagy in Huntington's disease. *Nat. Neurosci.* 13, 567–576. doi: 10.1038/nn.2528

Masini, D., Bonito-Oliva, A., Bertho, M., and Fisone, G. (2018). Inhibition of mTORC1 signaling reverts cognitive and affective deficits in a mouse model of Parkinson's disease. *Front. Neurol.* 9:208. doi: 10.3389/fneur.2018.00208

Maswood, N., Young, J., Tilmont, E., Zhang, Z., Gash, D. M., Gerhardt, G. A., et al. (2004). Caloric restriction increases neurotrophic factor levels and attenuates neurochemical and behavioral deficits in a primate model of Parkinson's disease. *Proc. Natl. Acad. Sci. U.S.A.* 101, 18171–18176. doi: 10.1073/pnas.0405831102

Mattson, M. P. (2010). The impact of dietary energy intake on cognitive aging. *Front. Aging Neurosci.* 2:5. doi: 10.3389/neuro.24.005.2010

Mattson, M. P., Longo, V. D., and Harvie, M. (2017). Impact of intermittent fasting on health and disease processes. *Ageing Res. Rev.* 39, 46–58. doi: 10.1016/j.arr.2016.10.005

Mehran, A. E., Templeman, N. M., Brigidi, G. S., Lim, G. E., Chu, K. Y., Hu, X., et al. (2012). Hyperinsulinemia drives diet-induced obesity independently of brain insulin production. *Cell Metab.* 16, 723–737. doi: 10.1016/j.cmet.2012.10.019

Menzies, F. M., Huebener, J., Renna, M., Bonin, M., Riess, O., and Rubinsztein, D. C. (2010). Autophagy induction reduces mutant ataxin-3 levels and toxicity in a mouse model of spinocerebellar ataxia type 3. *Brain* 133, 93–104. doi: 10.1093/brain/awp292

Mizushima, N., and Komatsu, M. (2011). Autophagy: renovation of cells and tissues. *Cell* 147, 728–741. doi: 10.1016/j.cell.2011.10.026

Muñoz, M. C., Giani, J. F., Mayer, M. A., Toblli, J. E., Turyn, D., and Dominici, F. P. (2009). TANK-binding kinase 1 mediates phosphorylation of insulin receptor at serine residue 994: a potential link between inflammation and insulin resistance. *J. Endocrinol.* 201, 185–197. doi: 10.1677/JOE-08-0276

Nameni, G., Farhangi, M. A., Hajilouian, G., Shahabi, P., and Abbasi, M. M. (2017). Insulin deficiency: a possible link between obesity and cognitive function. *Int. J. Dev. Neurosci.* 59, 15–20. doi: 10.1016/j.ijdevneu.2017.02.008

Nascimento-Ferreira, I., Santos-Ferreira, T., Sousa-Ferreira, L., Auregan, G., Onofre, I., Alves, S., et al. (2011). Overexpression of the autophagic beclin-1 protein clears mutant ataxin-3 and alleviates Machado–Joseph disease. *Brain* 134, 1400–1415. doi: 10.1093/brain/awr047

Navarro-Yepes, J., Burns, M., Anandhan, A., Khalimonchuk, O., del Razo, L. M., Quintanilla-Vega, B., et al. (2014). Oxidative stress, redox signaling, and autophagy: cell death versus survival. *Antioxid. Redox Signal.* 21, 66–85. doi: 10.1089/ars.2014.5837

Nicolescu, R. C., Al-Khawaga, S., Minassian, B. A., and Hussain, K. (2019). Diabetes mellitus in a patient with Lafora disease: possible links with pancreatic β-cell dysfunction and insulin resistance. *Front. Pediatr.* 6:424. doi: 10.3389/fped.2018.00424

Nishida, Y., Arakawa, S., Fujitani, K., Yamaguchi, H., Mizuta, T., Kanaseki, T., et al. (2009). Discovery of Atg5/Atg7-independent alternative macroautophagy. *Nature* 461, 654–658. doi: 10.1038/nature08455

Ntsapi, C., and Loos, B. (2016). Caloric restriction and the precision-control of autophagy: a strategy for delaying neurodegenerative disease progression. *Exp. Gerontol.* 83, 97–111. doi: 10.1016/j.exger.2016.07.014

Oguh, O., Eisenstein, A., Kwasny, M., and Simuni, T. (2014). Back to the basics: regular exercise matters in Parkinson's disease: results from the national Parkinson foundation QII registry study. *Parkinsonism Relat. Disord.* 20, 1221–1225. doi: 10.1016/j.parkreldis.2014.09.008

Onofre, I., Mendonça, N., Lopes, S., Nobre, R., de Melo, J. B., Carreira, I. M., et al. (2016). Fibroblasts of Machado Joseph Disease patients reveal autophagy impairment. *Sci. Rep.* 6:28220. doi: 10.1038/srep28220

Paganoni, S., Deng, J., Jaffa, M., Cudkowicz, M. E., and Wills, A.-M. (2011). Body mass index, not dyslipidemia, is an independent predictor of survival in amyotrophic lateral sclerosis. *Muscle Nerve* 44, 20–24. doi: 10.1002/mus.22114

Park, C. R., Seeley, R. J., Craft, S., and Woods, S. C. (2000). Intracerebroventricular insulin enhances memory in a passive-avoidance task. *Physiol. Behav.* 68, 509–514. doi: 10.1016/s0031-9384(99)00220-6

Parkinson, J. (2002). An essay on the shaking palsy. *J. Neuropsychiatry Clin. Neurosci.* 14, 223–236. doi: 10.1176/jnp.14.2.223

Patel, B. P., Safdar, A., Raha, S., Tarnopolsky, M. A., and Hamadeh, M. J. (2010). Caloric restriction shortens lifespan through an increase in lipid peroxidation, inflammation and apoptosis in the G93A mouse, an animal model of ALS. *PLoS One* 5:e9386. doi: 10.1371/journal.pone.0009386

Patil, S. P., Jain, P. D., Ghumatkar, P. J., Tambe, R., and Sathaye, S. (2014). Neuroprotective effect of metformin in MPTP-induced Parkinson's disease in mice. *Neuroscience* 277, 747–754. doi: 10.1016/j.neuroscience.2014.07.046

Perluigi, M., Di Domenico, F., and Butterfield, D. A. (2015). mTOR signaling in aging and neurodegeneration: at the crossroad between metabolism dysfunction and impairment of autophagy. *Neurobiol. Dis.* 84, 39–49. doi: 10.1016/j.nbd.2015.03.014

Petersen, A. (2001). Expanded CAG repeats in exon 1 of the Huntington's disease gene stimulate dopamine-mediated striatal neuron autophagy and degeneration. *Hum. Mol. Genet.* 10, 1243–1254. doi: 10.1093/hmg/10.12.1243

Petzinger, G. M., Fisher, B. E., McEwen, S., Beeler, J. A., Walsh, J. P., and Jakowec, M. W. (2013). Exercise-enhanced neuroplasticity targeting motor and cognitive circuitry in Parkinson's disease. *Lancet Neurol.* 12, 716–726. doi: 10.1016/s1474-4422(13)70123-6

Pickford, F., Masliah, E., Britschgi, M., Lucin, K., Narasimhan, R., Jaeger, P. A., et al. (2008). The autophagy-related protein beclin 1 shows reduced expression in early Alzheimer disease and regulates amyloid β accumulation in mice. *J. Clin. Invest.* 118, 2190–2199. doi: 10.1172/JCI33585

Rafaelsen, O. J. (1961a). Action of insulin on carbohydrate uptake of isolated rat spinal cord. *J. Neurochem.* 7, 33–44. doi: 10.1111/j.1471-4159.1961.tb13495.x

Rafaelsen, O. J. (1961b). Action of insulin on glucose uptake of rat brain slices and isolated rat cerebellum. *J. Neurochem.* 7, 45–51. doi: 10.1111/j.1471-4159.1961.tb13496.x

Renna, M., Bento, C. F., Fleming, A., Menzies, F. M., Siddiqi, F. H., Ravikumar, B., et al. (2013). IGF-1 receptor antagonism inhibits autophagy. *Hum. Mol. Genet.* 22, 4528–4544. doi: 10.1093/hmg/ddt300

Rivera, E. J., Goldin, A., Fulmer, N., Tavares, R., Wands, J. R., and de la Monte, S. M. (2005). Insulin and insulin-like growth factor expression and function deteriorate with progression of Alzheimer's disease: link to brain reductions in acetylcholine. *J. Alzheimers Dis.* 8, 247–268. doi: 10.3233/jad-2005-8304

Rocchi, A., Yamamoto, S., Ting, T., Fan, Y., Sadleir, K., Wang, Y., et al. (2017). A Becn1 mutation mediates hyperactive autophagic sequestration of amyloid oligomers and improved cognition in Alzheimer's disease. *PLoS Genet.* 13:e1006962. doi: 10.1371/journal.pgen.1006962

Roloff, F., Scheiblich, H., Dewitz, C., Dempewolf, S., Stern, M., and Bicker, G. (2015). Enhanced neurite outgrowth of human model (NT2) neurons by small-molecule inhibitors of Rho/ROCK signaling. *PLoS One* 10:e0118536. doi: 10.1371/journal.pone.0118536

Rotermund, C., Machetanz, G., and Fitzgerald, J. C. (2018). The therapeutic potential of metformin in neurodegenerative diseases. *Front. Endocrinol.* 9:400. doi: 10.3389/fendo.2018.00400

Rubinsztein, D. C., Difiglia, M., Heintz, N., Nixon, R. A., Qin, Z., Ravikumar, B., et al. (2005). Autophagy and its possible roles in nervous system diseases, KEY WORDS RIB. *Autophagy* 1, 11–22. doi: 10.4161/auto.1.1.1513

Sakane, T., Akizuki, M., Yamashita, S., Nadai, T., Hashida, M., and Sezaki, H. (1991). The transport of a drug to the cerebrospinal fluid directly from the nasal cavity: the relation to the lipophilicity of the drug. *Chem. Pharm. Bull.* 39, 2456–2458. doi: 10.1248/cpb.37.3229

Saleh, N., Moutereau, S., Azulay, J. P., Verny, C., Simonin, C., Tranchant, C., et al. (2010). High insulinlike growth factor I is associated with cognitive decline in Huntington disease. *Neurology* 76, 675–676; authorrely 675–676. doi: 10.1212/WNL.0b013e3181e62076

Salem, L., Saleh, N., Désaméricq, G., Youssov, K., Dolbeau, G., Cleret, L., et al. (2016). Insulin-like growth factor-1 but not insulin predicts cognitive decline in Huntington's disease. *PLoS One* 11:e0162890. doi: 10.1371/journal.pone.0162890

Sandoval, D., and Sisley, S. R. (2015). Brain GLP-1 and insulin sensitivity. *Mol. Cell. Endocrinol.* 418, 27–32. doi: 10.1016/j.mce.2015.02.017

Santiago, J. A., and Potashkin, J. A. (2013). Shared dysregulated pathways lead to Parkinson's disease and diabetes. *Trends Mol. Med.* 19, 176–186. doi: 10.1016/j.molmed.2013.01.002

Schernhammer, E., Hansen, J., Rugbjerg, K., Wermuth, L., and Ritz, B. (2011). Diabetes and the risk of developing Parkinson's disease in Denmark. *Diabetes Care* 34, 1102–1108. doi: 10.2337/dc10-1333

Schneeberger, M., Everard, A., Gómez-Valadés, A. G., Matamoros, S., Ramírez, S., Delzenne, N. M., et al. (2015). *Akkermansia muciniphila* inversely correlates with the onset of inflammation, altered adipose tissue metabolism and metabolic disorders during obesity in mice. *Sci. Rep.* 5:16643. doi: 10.1038/srep16643

Seelen, M., van Doormaal, P. T. C., Visser, A. E., Huisman, M. H. B., Roozekrans, M. H. J., de Jong, S. W., et al. (2014). Prior medical conditions and the risk of amyotrophic lateral sclerosis. *J. Neurol.* 261, 1949–1956. doi: 10.1007/s00415-014-7445-1

Sekar, S., and Taghibiglou, C. (2018). Elevated nuclear phosphatase and tensin homolog (PTEN) and altered insulin signaling in substantia nigral region of patients with Parkinson's disease. *Neurosci. Lett.* 666, 139–143. doi: 10.1016/j.neulet.2017.12.049

Shibata, M., Lu, T., Furuya, T., Degterev, A., Mizushima, N., Yoshimori, T., et al. (2006). Regulation of intracellular accumulation of mutant huntingtin by beclin 1. *J. Biol. Chem.* 281, 14474–14485. doi: 10.1074/jbc.M600364200

Skeberdis, V. A., Lan, J.-Y., Zheng, X., Zukin, R. S., and Bennett, M. V. L. (2001). Insulin promotes rapid delivery of N-methyl-D- aspartate receptors to the cell surface by exocytosis. *Proc. Natl. Acad. Sci. U.S.A.* 98, 3561–3566. doi: 10.1073/pnas.051634698

Song, J., Wu, L., Chen, Z., Kohanski, R. A., and Pick, L. (2003). Axons guided by insulin receptor in *Drosophila* visual system. *Science* 300, 502–505. doi: 10.1126/science.1081203

Spencer, B., Potkar, R., Trejo, M., Rockenstein, E., Gindi, R., Adame, A., et al. (2010). Ameliorates the neurodegenerative pathology in A-. *Pathology* 29, 13578–13588. doi: 10.1523/JNEUROSCI.4390-09.2009.BECLIN

Steen, E., Terry, B. M. J., Rivera, E., Cannon, J. L., Neely, T. R., Tavares, R., et al. (2005). Impaired insulin and insulin-like growth factor expression and signaling mechanisms in Alzheimer's disease – is this type 3 diabetes? *J. Alzheimers Dis.* 7, 63–80. doi: 10.3233/jad-2005-7107

Steyn, F. J., Ioannides, Z. A., van Eijk, R. P. A., Heggie, S., Thorpe, K. A., Ceslis, A., et al. (2018). Hypermetabolism in ALS is associated with greater functional decline and shorter survival. *J. Neurol. Neurosurg. Psychiatry* 89, 1016–1023. doi: 10.1136/jnnp-2017-317887

Takano, K., Koarashi, K., Kawabe, K., Itakura, M., Nakajima, H., Moriyama, M., et al. (2018). Insulin expression in cultured astrocytes and the decrease by amyloid β. *Neurochem. Int.* 119, 171–177. doi: 10.1016/j.neuint.2017.10.017

Teves, J. M. Y., Bhargava, V., Kirwan, K. R., Corenblum, M. J., Justiniano, R., Wondrak, G. T., et al. (2018). Parkinson's disease skin fibroblasts display signature alterations in growth, redox homeostasis, mitochondrial function, and autophagy. *Front. Neurosci.* 11:737. doi: 10.3389/fnins.2017.00737

Tian, Y., Chang, J. C., Fan, E. Y., Flajolet, M., and Greengard, P. (2013). Adaptor complex AP2/PICALM, through interaction with LC3, targets Alzheimer's APP-CTF for terminal degradation via autophagy. *Proc. Natl. Acad. Sci. U.S.A.* 110, 17071–17076. doi: 10.1073/pnas.1315110110

Tramutola, A., Triplett, J. C., Di Domenico, F., Niedowicz, D. M., Murphy, M. P., Coccia, R., et al. (2015). Alteration of mTOR signaling occurs early in the progression of Alzheimer disease (AD): analysis of brain from subjects with pre-clinical AD, amnestic mild cognitive impairment and late-stage AD. *J. Neurochem.* 133, 739–749. doi: 10.1111/jnc.13037

Tuon, T., Valvassori, S. S., Lopes-Borges, J., Luciano, T., Trom, C. B., Silva, L. A., et al. (2012). Physical training exerts neuroprotective effects in the regulation of neurochemical factors in an animal model of Parkinson's disease. *Neuroscience* 227, 305–312. doi: 10.1016/j.neuroscience.2012.09.063

Ueno, M., Carvalheira, J. B. C., Tambascia, R. C., Bezerra, R. M. N., Amaral, M. E., Carneiro, E. M., et al. (2005). Regulation of insulin signalling by hyperinsulinaemia: role of IRS-1/2 serine phosphorylation and the mTOR/p70 S6K pathway. *Diabetologia* 48, 506–518. doi: 10.1007/s00125-004-1662-6

Ugolino, J., Ji, Y. J., Conchina, K., Chu, J., Nirujogi, R. S., Pandey, A., et al. (2016). Loss of C9orf72 enhances autophagic activity via deregulated mTOR and TFEB signaling. *PLoS Genet.* 12:e1006443. doi: 10.1371/journal.pgen.1006443

Urano, Y., Mori, C., Fuji, A., Konno, K., Yamamoto, T., Yashirogi, S., et al. (2018). 6-hydroxydopamine induces secretion of PARK7/DJ-1 via autophagy-based unconventional secretory pathway. *Autophagy* 14, 1943–1958. doi: 10.1080/15548627.2018.1493043

Van Der Heide, L. P., Kamal, A., Artola, A., Gispen, W. H., and Ramakers, G. M. J. (2005). Insulin modulates hippocampal activity-dependent synaptic plasticity in a N-methyl-D-aspartate receptor and phosphatidyl-inositol-3-kinase-dependent manner. *J. Neurochem.* 94, 1158–1166. doi: 10.1111/j.1471-4159.2005.03269.x

Van Langenhove, T., Van Der Zee, J., and Van Broeckhoven, C. (2012). The molecular basis of the frontotemporal lobar degeneration-amyotrophic lateral sclerosis spectrum. *Ann. Med.* 44, 817–828. doi: 10.3109/07853890.2012.665471

Vodicka, P., Chase, K., Iuliano, M., Tousley, A., Valentine, D. T., Sapp, E., et al. (2016). Autophagy activation by transcription factor EB (TFEB) in striatum of HDQ175/Q7 mice. *J. Huntingtons Dis.* 5, 249–260. doi: 10.3233/JHD-160211

Voll, C. L., Whishaw, I. Q., and Auer, R. N. (1989). Postischemic insulin reduces spatial learning deficit following transient forebrain ischemia in rats. *Stroke* 20, 646–651. doi: 10.1161/01.STR.20.5.646

Webster, C. P., Smith, E. F., Bauer, C. S., Moller, A., Hautbergue, G. M., Ferraiuolo, L., et al. (2016). The C9orf72 protein interacts with Rab1a and the ULK1 complex to regulate initiation of autophagy. *EMBO J.* 35, 1656–1676. doi: 10.15252/embj.201694401

Weiss, K. R., and Littleton, J. T. (2016). Characterization of axonal transport defects in *Drosophila* Huntingtin mutants. *J. Neurogenet.* 30, 212–221. doi: 10.1080/01677063.2016.1202950

Winslow, A. R., Chen, C.-W., Corrochano, S., Acevedo-Arozena, A., Gordon, D. E., Peden, A. A., et al. (2010). α-Synuclein impairs macroautophagy: implications for Parkinson's disease. *J. Cell Biol.* 190, 1023–1037. doi: 10.1083/jcb.201003122

Wong, P.-M., Feng, Y., Wang, J., Shi, R., and Jiang, X. (2015). Regulation of autophagy by coordinated action of mTORC1 and protein phosphatase 2A. *Nat. Commun.* 6:8048. doi: 10.1038/ncomms9048

Wong, Y. C., and Holzbaur, E. L. F. (2014). The regulation of autophagosome dynamics by huntingtin and HAP1 is disrupted by expression of mutant huntingtin, leading to defective cargo degradation. *J. Neurosci.* 34, 1293–1305. doi: 10.1523/JNEUROSCI.1870-13.2014

Wu, Y.-T., Tan, H.-L., Huang, Q., Ong, C.-N., and Shen, H.-M. (2009). Activation of the PI3K-Akt-mTOR signaling pathway promotes necrotic cell death via suppression of autophagy. *Autophagy* 5, 824–834. doi: 10.4161/auto.9099

Xu, X. J., Gauthier, M.-S., Hess, D. T., Apovian, C. M., Cacicedo, J. M., Gokce, N., et al. (2012). Insulin sensitive and resistant obesity in humans: AMPK activity, oxidative stress, and depot-specific changes in gene expression in adipose tissue. *J. Lipid Res.* 53, 792–801. doi: 10.1194/jlr.p022905

Yamamoto, A., Cremona, M. L., and Rothman, J. E. (2006). Autophagy-mediated clearance of huntingtin aggregates triggered by the insulin-signaling pathway. *J. Cell Biol.* 172, 719–731. doi: 10.1083/jcb.200510065

Yamamoto, A., Lucas, J. J., and Hen, R. (2000). Reversal of neuropathology and motor dysfunction in a conditional model of Huntington's disease. *Cell* 101, 57–66. doi: 10.1016/s0092-8674(00)80623-6

Yamamoto, S., Kuramoto, K., Wang, N., Situ, X., Priyadarshini, M., Zhang, W., et al. (2018). Autophagy differentially regulates insulin production and insulin sensitivity. *Cell Rep.* 23, 3286–3299. doi: 10.1016/j.celrep.2018.05.032

Yang, L., Wang, H., Liu, L., and Xie, A. (2018). The role of insulin/IGF-1/PI3K/Akt/GSK3β signaling in Parkinson's disease dementia. *Front. Neurosci.* 12:73. doi: 10.3389/fnins.2018.00073

Yong, J., Rasooly, J., Dang, H., Lu, Y., Middleton, B., Zhang, Z., et al. (2011). Multimodality imaging of β-cells in mouse models of type 1 and 2 diabetes. *Diabetes* 60, 1383–1392. doi: 10.2337/db10-0907

Zhang, J., Chen, C., Hua, S., Liao, H., Wang, M., Xiong, Y., et al. (2017). An updated meta-analysis of cohort studies: diabetes and risk of Alzheimer's disease. *Diabetes Res. Clin. Pract.* 124, 41–47. doi: 10.1016/j.diabres.2016.10.024

Zhang, X., Li, L., Chen, S., Yang, D., Wang, Y., Zhang, X., et al. (2011). Rapamycin treatment augments motor neuron degeneration in SOD1 G93A mouse model of amyotrophic lateral sclerosis. *Autophagy* 7, 412–425. doi: 10.4161/auto.7.4.14541

Zhao, W., Chen, H., Xu, H., Moore, E., Meiri, N., Quon, M. J., et al. (1999). Brain insulin receptors and spatial memory. Correlated changes in gene expression, tyrosine phosphorylation, and signaling molecules in the hippocampus of water maze trained rats. *J. Biol. Chem.* 274, 34893–34902. doi: 10.3368/er.26.4.311

Zhao, W. Q., Chen, H., Quon, M. J., and Alkon, D. L. (2004). Insulin and the insulin receptor in experimental models of learning and memory. *Eur. J. Pharmacol.* 490, 71–81. doi: 10.1016/j.ejphar.2004.02.045

8

Hypothalamic Microglial Activation in Obesity

Natália F. Mendes[1,2,3], Young-Bum Kim[2], Lício A. Velloso[3,4] and Eliana P. Araújo[1,3]*

[1] School of Nursing, State University of Campinas, Campinas, Brazil, [2] Department of Medicine, Division of Endocrinology, Diabetes, and Metabolism – Beth Israel Deaconess Medical Center, Harvard Medical School, Boston, MA, United States, [3] Laboratory of Cell Signaling, Obesity and Comorbidities Research Center, State University of Campinas, Campinas, Brazil, [4] National Institute of Science and Technology on Neuroimmunomodulation, Rio de Janeiro, Brazil

***Correspondence:**
Eliana P. Araújo
earaujo@unicamp.br;
pa.eliana@gmail.com

Emerging data demonstrate that microglia activation plays a pivotal role in the development of hypothalamic inflammation in obesity. Early after the introduction of a high-fat diet, hypothalamic microglia undergo morphological, and functional changes in response to excessive dietary saturated fats. Initially the resident microglia are affected; however, as diet-induced obesity persists, bone marrow-derived myeloid cells gradually replace resident microglia. Genetic and pharmacological approaches aimed at dampening the inflammatory activity in the hypothalamus of experimental models of obesity have proven beneficial to correct the obese phenotype and improve metabolic abnormalities commonly associated with obesity. These approaches provide an experimental proof-of-concept that hypothalamic inflammation is central to the pathophysiology of obesity; understanding the details of the roles played by microglia in this process may help the development of preventive and therapeutic advances in the field. In this review, we discuss the potential mechanisms underlying hypothalamic microglial activation in high-fat induced obesity.

Keywords: inflammation, chemokine, cytokine, brain, metabolism

INTRODUCTION

The mediobasal hypothalamus (MBH) is a key brain region involved in the central control of caloric intake and energy expenditure. Its function relies on a complex neuronal network that senses the energy status of the body and coordinates responses aimed at maintaining energetic homeostasis. First-order neurons in this network are located in the arcuate nucleus (ARC), sitting close to the median eminence (ME), which is richly irrigated by fenestrated capillaries that secure special permeability to the blood/spinal fluid interface (BSFI) (Rodríguez et al., 2010). The partially leaky ME-BSFI facilitates ARC neuronal and glial cells to rapidly and directly sense minimal changes in peripheral signals, such as hormones (e.g., leptin and insulin) and nutrients, essential to the regulation of whole-body energy homeostasis (Lam et al., 2005; Schaeffer et al., 2013; Timper and Brüning, 2017). Under physiological conditions, feeding leads to the activation of ARC proopiomelanocortin (POMC) and cocaine- and amphetamine-regulated transcript (CART) neurons resulting in suppressed food intake and increased energy expenditure. Conversely, fasting leads to the activation of neuropeptide Y (NPY) and agouti-related protein (AgRP) neurons, which antagonize the function of POMC neurons (Schwartz et al., 2000). Over time, the correct function of these neuronal subpopulations leads to body-mass stability. However, the excessive consumption of saturated fatty acids (SFAs) can disrupt the physiological pattern of food intake and energy expenditure control by triggering an inflammatory response in the hypothalamus, which affects the MBH at the functional and structural levels (De Souza et al., 2005; Velloso and Schwartz, 2011). Leptin resistance emerges as an early functional outcome of hypothalamic inflammation (Dragano et al., 2017; Pan and Myers, 2018), which can be overcome by reducing local inflammatory activity with genetic or pharmacological approaches, or simply by reducing the amount of SFAs in the diet. With time, chronic structural abnormalities can develop, such as changes in neuronal projections, gliosis, and eventually, neuronal death (Moraes et al., 2009; Dorfman and Thaler, 2015). The extension and chronicity of the structural and functional losses of the hypothalamus may explain the relapsing nature of obesity that can resist behavioral, pharmacological, and even surgical therapeutic measures. Thus, understanding the mechanisms involved in the evolution and persistence of hypothalamic inflammation may offer new insights into the development of strategies for the prevention and treatment of obesity.

Studies have shown that diet-induced inflammation initially and preferentially affects the MBH (Thaler et al., 2012). One of the particularities that may explain the anatomical specificity of this process is the nature of the ME-BSFI and the presence of tanycytes in this region, what makes the MBH more sensitive to dietary fats than other circumventricular organs, undergoing a rapid structural, and functional disorganization in mice fed a high-fat diet (HFD) (Ramalho et al., 2018). About the same time that structural and functional changes are occurring in the ME-BSFI, resident microglia undergo morphological and physiological alterations in the ARC region that neighbors the ME (Valdearcos et al., 2014). However, upon persistence of a HFD, bone marrow-derived myeloid cells (BMDM) migrate into the MBH, which is an important condition to secure chronic inflammation (Valdearcos et al., 2017). Approaches that inhibit the migration of BMDM cells to the MBH can reduce hypothalamic inflammation and attenuate diet-induced obesity (DIO). Despite the fact that most studies in this field were performed employing experimental models, there is evidence supporting the presence of inflammation and gliosis in the hypothalamus of obese humans as well (van de Sande-Lee et al., 2011; Thaler et al., 2012), further supporting hypothalamic inflammation as a potential pharmacological target for the obesity treatment. Here, we review the studies that provided progress in the characterization of abnormalities of MBH microglia in obesity.

DIETARY FATS MODIFY HYPOTHALAMIC MICROGLIAL MORPHOLOGY, DISTRIBUTION, AND FUNCTION

Microglial cells are the most abundant brain innate immune cells and are relatively quiescent under baseline conditions. However, when exposed to injury signals, microglia undergo a rapid reaction characterized by morphological and functional changes aimed at enabling them to mount an inflammatory response against the potentially existing treat (Saijo and Glass, 2011).

Studies with rodents have shown that microglia of the MBH are sensitive to SFAs (lauric, palmitic, and stearic acids) (Valdearcos et al., 2014). In the hypothalamus of rodents, consumption of large portions of SFAs promotes a rapid microglial response characterized by the appearance of a number of prolonged processes emanating from a discreetly enlarged cell body (Baufeld et al., 2016). Initially, these morphological changes are restricted to the ARC region nearby the transition between the MBH and ME and are accompanied by increased expression of inflammatory cytokines and other markers of inflammation. The hypothalamic inflammatory response to SFAs occurs in a biphasic mode. During the first week of a HFD, the mRNA and protein levels of hypothalamic cytokines such as TNF-α, IL1-β, and IL-6 increase, as well as chemokines such as MCP-1 and fractalkine (Morari et al., 2014). Upon the persistence, for 2 weeks and longer, of the exposure to SFAs in diets that are particularly rich in stearate and palmitate, the levels of inflammatory markers decrease, only to return after 4 weeks, and then persist for as long as the content of SFAs in the diet is excessive (Thaler et al., 2012).

The biphasic nature of the inflammatory response in the hypothalamus of experimental models of obesity occurs similarly to the classical biphasic inflammatory response in other tissues. One reason behind the biphasic nature of obesity-associated hypothalamic inflammation is that the initial response is mounted by resident microglia; however, as dietary-fat consumption persists, bone marrow-derived myeloid cells gradually replace the MBH microglia (Valdearcos et al., 2017). Thus, at this point, it is important to understand the mechanisms that govern microglia activation, phenotype definition, and the recruitment of bone marrow-derived myeloid cells to the site of injury.

MECHANISMS OF HYPOTHALAMIC MICROGLIA ACTIVATION IN OBESITY

Similar to the resident macrophages of tissues outside the brain, microglia of rodents are capable of sensing and responding to the presence of pathogen-associated molecular patterns (PAMPs) (Kigerl et al., 2014). The systemic injection of a single high-dose of lipopolysaccharide (LPS) promotes activation-like changes in the morphology of hypothalamic microglia, which is detected as early as 8 h after injection, peaking after 24 h and recovering after 7 days (Buttini et al., 1996). This is accompanied by increased expression of MHC-I and inflammatory cytokines (TNF-α, IL-1, and IL-6), and also by the activation of COX-1 and NF-κB (García-Bueno et al., 2009). Interestingly, the same macrophage receptor that is activated in response to LPS, TLR4, can be activated in response to SFAs (Huang et al., 2012).

Under baseline conditions, TLR4 is expressed at low levels in the brain, including the hypothalamus of rodents; however, its expression increases considerably when rodents are fed a HFD (Milanski et al., 2009). In other brain regions, TLR4 expression is involved in medical conditions such as autoimmunity (Kerfoot et al., 2004), HIV infection (Cheung et al., 2017) and Alzheimer's disease (Ledo et al., 2016), illustrating its pleiotropic roles in brain immunity and defense. A detailed screening of dietary fats that could potentially promote the activation of hypothalamic TLR4 identified long-chain SFAs as the most potent inducers of its association with MyD88, resulting in the activation of NF-κB and JNK and leading to endoplasmic reticulum stress (Zhang et al., 2008). When dietary SFAs are substituted by similar amounts of unsaturated fatty acids (flax seed oil and olive oil), the hypothalamic inflammation is dampened in parallel to the reduced activity of JNK and NF-κB (Cintra et al., 2012). The pharmacological and the genetic inhibition of TLR4 reduce diet-induced hypothalamic inflammation and protect rodents from DIO and glucose intolerance (Milanski et al., 2012). Importantly, contact with large portions of SFAs, and not the presence of obesity *per se*, is required to induce hypothalamic microglial activation; this is evidenced by the fact that genetically obese mice, such as, ob/ob (leptin-deficient), db/db (leptin receptor-deficient) and MC4R-KO, do not present hypothalamic microglia activation when they are fed on chow, despite the evidence that even on this diet they become obese (Gao et al., 2014).

Cell culture approaches were used to investigate additional details involving the activation of microglia by fatty acids. Palmitate and stearate are each capable of inducing a rapid activation of BV2 microglial cells line through a mechanism dependent on TLR4 (Wang et al., 2012). Reactive morphological changes and increased production of inflammatory cytokines, nitric oxide, and reactive oxygen species (ROS) characterize the activation of microglia (Wang et al., 2012). In addition, upon exposure to palmitate, another microglial cell line, THP-1, is capable of producing inflammatory cytokines and inducing neurotoxicity (Little et al., 2012).

As a proof-of-concept for the central implication of microglia in the development of diet-induced hypothalamic inflammation, Valdearcos et al. (2014) used distinct strategies to modify the number of microglia in the hypothalamus. When microglia is increased, the intensity of hypothalamic inflammation induced by SFAs is boosted; conversely, when MBH microglia is reduced hypothalamic inflammation is abrogated. Importantly, a positive relationship exists between the number of hypothalamic microglia and the obese phenotype (Baufeld et al., 2016).

In addition to the direct effects of dietary fats to induce hypothalamic inflammation and microglial activation, some studies have shown that neural afferents from the gut can also trigger an inflammatory response in the hypothalamus (Mulders et al., 2018). The gut inflammatory signals resulting from the consumption of HFD can act through vagal connections to the nodose ganglion to increase hypothalamic microglial cells and trigger inflammation in a mechanism that can be inhibited by ghrelin (Waise et al., 2015). Furthermore, in at least one study, the gut microbial landscape changes promoted by consumption of a HFD was shown to play a role in the development of diet-induced hypothalamic microgliosis (Zhuang et al., 2017).

It is worthwhile mentioning that brain regions other than hypothalamus can also present microglial activation in response to excessive consumption of dietary fats (Erion et al., 2014; Spencer et al., 2017). However, differently of the hypothalamus, microgliosis in other regions is a late event, reinforcing the current concept that hypothalamus is the first brain region affected in response to the consumption of large amounts of dietary fats (Thaler et al., 2012; Carraro et al., 2018). Particularly, in the hippocampus, diet-induced microgliosis has been identified in both human and experimental models of Alzheimer's disease and provides a potential mechanistic link between obesity/type 2 diabetes and the accelerated cognitive and memory decline that is present in this highly prevalent medical condition (Cope et al., 2018).

INTRACELLULAR SIGNALING TARGETS FOR REDUCING MICROGLIA INFLAMMATORY ACTIVATION

Microglial cells express triggering receptor of myeloid cell-2 (TREM2), which is an important negative regulator of NF-κB. *In vitro* studies showed that TREM2 overexpression inhibits neuroinflammation by down-regulating PI3K/AKT and NF-κB signaling in BV2 microglia (Zhong et al., 2017; Li et al., 2018). Curiously, LPS downregulates the expression of TREM2 through the activation of JNK and NF-κB signaling pathways, resulting in a pro-inflammatory vicious cycle (Zhong et al., 2017).

Quercetin, a polyphenolic flavonoid found in many dietary sources, is a molecule studied due to its anti-inflammatory functional properties and also reduces inflammatory responses through inhibition of NF-κB activity. Quercetin can suppress the lipid content inside the palmitic acid-treated microglia through heme oxygenase (HO-1) induction (Kang et al., 2013; Yang et al., 2017a). HO-1 is an antioxidant enzyme that plays a key role in defense mechanisms against oxidative damage and inflammation. In addition, quercetin suppresses LPS-induced nitric oxide (NO) production and inducible NO synthase (iNOS) expression in BV2 cells (Kang et al., 2013).

Alpha-viniferin belongs to the same polyphenol group as quercetin and has anticancer and anti-inflammatory activity. In LPS-BV2 treated cells, α-viniferin suppresses the expression of the proinflammatory genes iNOS and COX-2 in the early stage of inflammation by inhibiting AKT/PI3K-dependent NF-κB activation and inhibits the production of proinflammatory mediators NO and PGE2 in the late stage by stimulating the Nrf2-mediated HO-1 signaling pathway (Dilshara et al., 2014). It is important to highlight that although many *in vivo* and *in vitro* studies have already shown these anti-inflammatory actions, the bioactive effects and bioavailability of these compounds in humans still need to be further investigated (Shanely et al., 2010; Pfeuffer et al., 2013; Lee et al., 2016).

Researchers have also studied other nutrients with functional properties in the context of HFD-induced microglial activation through modulation of NF-κB activity. Eicosapentaenoic acid (EPA) and docosahexaenoic acid (DHA) are the major ω-3 PUFAs of fish oil and have exhibited many anti-inflammatory effects in HFD-induced hypothalamic inflammation (Cintra et al., 2012; Nascimento et al., 2016). In the MG6 and BV2 microglial cell lines, EPA and DHA each suppressed the production of pro-inflammatory cytokines TNF-α and IL-6 throughout the inhibition of NF-κB activity and the activation of SIRT1 signaling (Inoue et al., 2017).

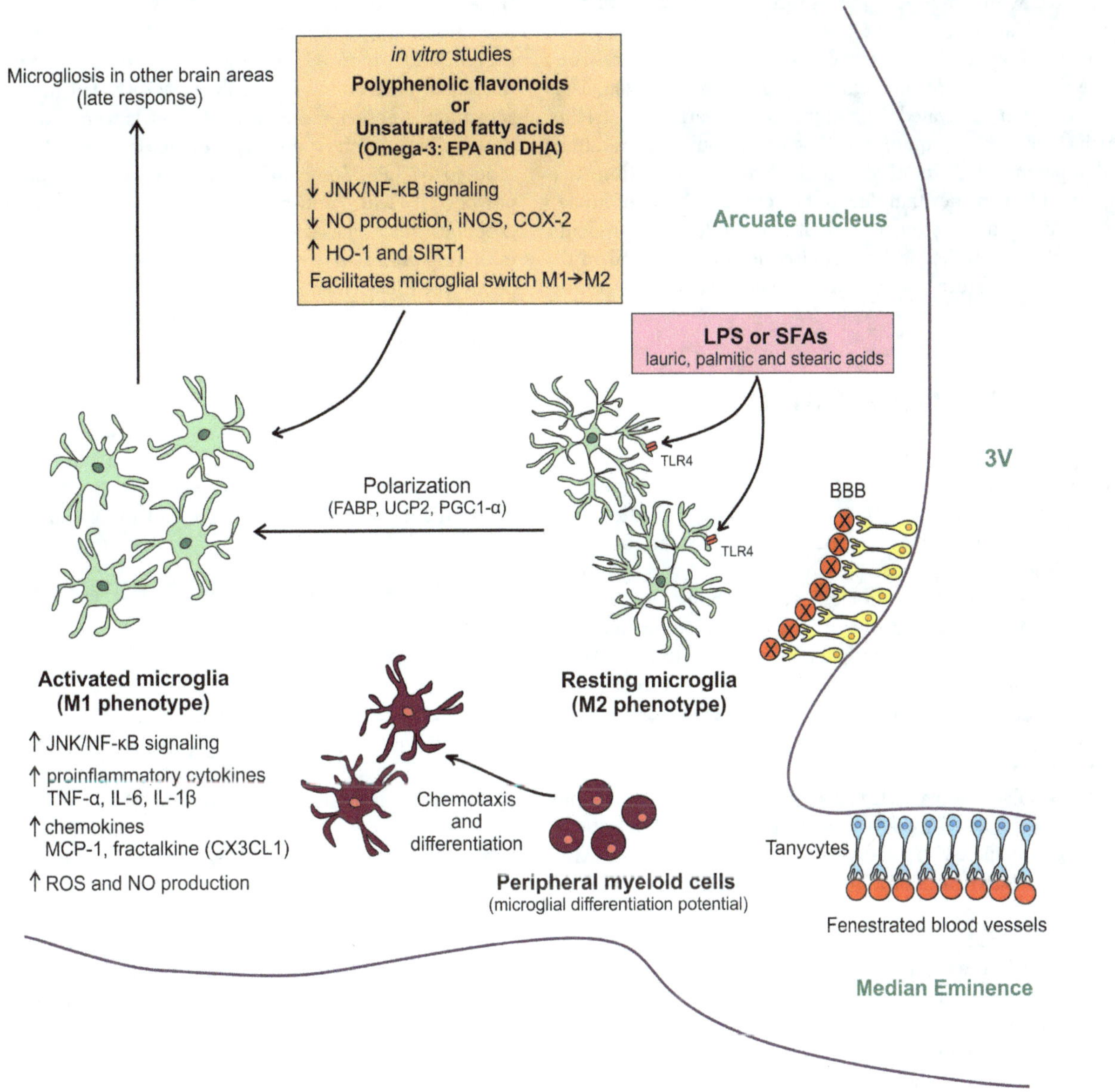

FIGURE 1 | Molecular mechanisms involved in the HFD-induced hypothalamic microgliosis. Diet-induced inflammation initially affects the MBH. Due to its anatomic location, microglial cells of arcuate nucleus are sensitive to LPS and SFAs from the diet. Both molecules activate TLR4 in the microglia membrane resulting in the switching to M1-like pro-inflammatory phenotype. This M2/M1 polarization has an energetic demand and depends on UCP2 activity, which is regulated by FABP, and on PGC-1α activation. The microglia activation results in an increased JNK/NF-kB activity, raised expression of pro-inflammatory cytokines and chemokines, as well as increased ROS and NO production. With the persistence of the high-fat feeding, peripheral myeloid cells are recruited to the neural tissue. These cells have a microglial differentiation potential and can quickly differentiate in activated cells helping resident microglia smother the hypothalamic inflammatory response. The chemotaxis of these peripheral cells is mainly controlled by MCP-1/CCR2 axis and fractalkine. As a late response, the microgliosis can also affect other non-hypothalamic brains areas. Some anti-inflammatory and antioxidants molecules, such as polyphenolic flavonoids and unsaturated fatty acids, have been tested *in vitro* for attenuating the microglial activation. The main benefits found in these studies were the reduction of JNK/NF-kB activity, decreased NO production, as well as iNOS and COX-2 expression, and increased HO-1 and SIRT-1 expression. Besides, these molecules also seem to facilitate the microglial switch M1/M2, reducing the inflammatory response. Further studies are still needed to further test these mechanisms in experimental models.

A few studies also investigated the potential involvement of ROS production as a mechanism of transducing inflammatory signals in microglia. Microglial inflammatory-response activation increases the production of oxidative-stress products. It is known that mitochondria constitute the major source of ROS generation in activated microglia (Park et al., 2015). ROS are capable of modifying microglial pro-inflammatory gene expression by modulating kinase cascades and activating some transcription factors, including MAPK and NF-κB (Pawate et al., 2004). LPS-treated BV2 cells show increased ROS production through NADPH oxidase, which raises the expression of TNF-α, activating NF-κB (Sumi et al., 2010). Otherwise, when these cells are treated with a NADPH oxidase inhibitor, ROS production decreases (Mander et al., 2006).

Thus, NF-κB and JNK signaling systems play central roles in the transduction of inflammatory signals in microglia. They can be either activated or inhibited by various nutrients, which make them important targets for approaches aimed at dampening HFD-induced hypothalamic inflammation. It is important to consider that due to the complex nature of human diet as compared to experimental diets offered to rodents, further clinical studies will be required in order to confirm the inflammatory nature of the hypothalamic damage in human obesity.

MICROGLIA POLARIZATION

Microglial cells are able to sense changes in the surrounding environment and become activated to either a pro-inflammatory (M1) or an anti-inflammatory (M2) phenotype (Kettenmann et al., 2011; Tang and Le, 2016). Polarized microglia are distinguished from polarized peripheral macrophages by protein expression, phagocytic capacity, and response to injuries (Durafourt et al., 2012; Girard et al., 2013). Considering that HFD leads to the recruitment of peripheral myeloid cells to the MBH, it is important to understand if some differences exist in the molecular mechanisms of polarization between microglial and infiltrated peripheral myeloid cells in the central nervous system (CNS).

Microglial cell polarization has an energetic demand and, thus, depends on uncoupling protein 2 (UCP2) activity, which is regulated by fatty-acid-binding proteins (FABP) (Hotamisligil and Bernlohr, 2015). Mice lacking FABP4 in the hypothalamus have increased UCP2 expression and reduced expression of TNF-α and ionized calcium-binding adapter molecule 1 (Iba1, a marker of microglial activation (Duffy et al., 2017). Pharmacological inhibition of FABP is an interesting therapeutic approach to reducing saturated-fat-induced pro-inflammatory response because it increases UCP2 expression. In addition, the inhibition of hypothalamic UCP2 increases the inflammatory damage inflicted by TNF-α, which places UCP2 as an important component in the polarization machinery of microglia (Degasperi et al., 2008).

Studies have identified a number of compounds that can reduce inflammation in the CNS by suppressing microglia M1 phenotype (Zhou et al., 2014; Orihuela et al., 2016). Conversely, only a few compounds, such as interleukin-4 and interleukin-13, can promote the polarization of microglia to the M2-like anti-inflammatory phenotype (Zhou et al., 2014). In this context, promoting an M1-M2 switch could be an interesting approach to attenuate inflammation of the neural tissue (Hu et al., 2015; Xu et al., 2015). In line, a recent study showed that betulinic acid (BA), a naturally pentacyclic triterpenoid with anti-inflammatory properties, promotes M2 polarization and inhibits M1 polarization in LPS-stimulated BV2 microglial cells and in the cerebral cortex of LPS-injected mice through calmodulin-dependent protein kinase kinase β (CaMKKβ)-dependent AMP-activated protein kinase (AMPK) activation (Li et al., 2018). In another study, Xu et al. (2015) showed that telmisartan, a potent angiotensin II receptor blocker, also prevents LPS-induced microglia activation throughout M2 microglia polarization through CaMKKβ-dependent AMPK activation. Another mechanism that leads to microglia M1/M2 polarization depends on PGC-1α inhibition, which can be induced by LPS. Some compounds, like resveratrol, a natural polyphenol with anti-inflammatory effects, has beneficial effects on microglia activation throughout PGC-1α activation, inhibiting the M1-like phenotype while stimulating the M2-like phenotype (Yang et al., 2017b).

Although a microglial switch offers a promising avenue for reducing HFD-induced microglial inflammation, further characterization of microglial phenotypic behavior, especially its temporal and spatial evolution, is critical in electing potential therapeutic approaches. Furthermore, it is important to consider that microglial polarization is a dynamic and natural reaction to saturated-fat overconsumption and its complete blockage could impair microglial activity in resolving inflammation.

THE RECRUITMENT OF PERIPHERAL MYELOID CELLS TO THE HYPOTHALAMUS IN DIO

Peripheral myeloid cells are recruited to MBH in mice fed a HFD and contribute to the development of obesity-associated hypothalamic microgliosis (Morari et al., 2014; Valdearcos et al., 2017). The fenestrated nature of the BSFI surrounding the MBH is regarded as an important factor involved in this process (Ramalho et al., 2018). Numerous studies showed that bone-marrow-derived microglia (BMDM) can infiltrate the brain parenchyma in distinct types of brain injury (Ajami et al., 2007; Davoust et al., 2008; Prinz and Mildner, 2011). Valdearcos et al. (2017) demonstrated that myeloid cells infiltrating the MBH in mice fed a HFD expressed neither typical microglial markers nor markers indicative of a bloodborne origin. Thus, it was initially suspected that these cells could represent a non-microglial population of brain-resident myeloid cells.

Under normal conditions, BMDM does not renew microglial cells, but under certain circumstances in which cells present in systemic circulation cross the BSFI, they can undergo differentiation into microglia. Thus, the adult bone marrow contains a subpopulation of cells displaying a microglial differentiation potential that can be mobilized promptly at any time (Davoust et al., 2008); however, which factors induce this specific type of monocyte chemotaxis into the MBH in the context of dietary excess is currently under investigation.

Fractalkine (CX3CL1), a chemokine that signals through the CX3CR1 receptor, is involved in this earlier activation of hypothalamic inflammation in HFD-fed mice (Morari et al., 2014). Another chemokine axis, MCP-1/CCR2, has also been described as an important potential mediator of the migration of monocytes into affected areas in brain diseases (Deshmane et al., 2009). Under chronic stress, e.g., a long period of high-fat feeding, the BMDM are recruited to the paraventricular nucleus of the hypothalamus (PVN) throughout, after the activation of the MCP-1/CCR2 axis (Ataka et al., 2013). In this study, the authors blocked the recruitment by peripheral administration of a CCR2 antagonist, which resulted in a reduction of local inflammation, providing evidence of an important role of the MCP-1/CCR2 axis in diet-induced hypothalamic inflammation.

Although the origin and identity of myeloid cells that migrate to the MBH after HFD consumption are unknown, these cells displayed morphological features of resident microglia (Valdearcos et al., 2017). The BMDM, as resident microglia, can be clearly distinguished from other CNS-infiltrating macrophages, based on its CD45 expression (Priller et al., 2001). In addition, BMDM can proliferate in the neural tissue when inflammation is induced, whereas infiltrating macrophages do not (Wirenfeldt et al., 2007).

Another important question still unanswered refers to the mechanism that induces the recruitment of BMDM into the peripheral circulation because it precedes recruitment to the CNS. SDF-1/CXCR4 interaction is required to recruit BMDM out of the bone marrow toward systemic circulation (Katayama et al., 2006). SDF-1 expression, in turn, is regulated by brain stimuli through sympathetic pathways, throughout β3-adrenergic receptors on bone marrow stromal cells (Lilly et al., 2011). Thus, it is possible that the signal that triggers the whole process is mediated by autonomic connections between the hypothalamus and the bone marrow; however, further studies are needed to clarify this important issue.

In conclusion, the current data are reshaping the concept that resident microglia constitutes a stable brain-cell population that is not affected by the recruitment of BMDM (Matsumoto and Fujiwara, 1987; Lassmann et al., 1993). Certain types of brain injury, including the damage caused in the hypothalamus by the excessive consumption of SFAs, can recruit BMDM, which seem to be an important event to modulate the inflammatory response. Particularly, after consumption of a HFD, it seems the recruitment of peripheral myeloid cells to the hypothalamus occurs in an attempt to help the resident microglia smother the inflammatory response. As this response happens at the beginning of HFD overconsumption, exploring which mechanisms are involved and how it alters hypothalamic neurocircuits involved in metabolic control represents a new frontier for proposing a viable therapeutic approach before the damage is established. **Figure 1** provides a summarized view of the mechanisms involved in the regulation of hypothalamic microglia in obesity.

OUTSTANDING QUESTIONS

(1) How do different subsets of microglia participate in the HFD-induced hypothalamic inflammation?
(2) Could microglia from other brain areas also migrate to the MBH contributing to the local inflammation?
(3) Is the recruitment of BMDM triggered by hypothalamic outputs? If so, which mechanisms are involved?
(4) Is there inflammation and microglial activation in the hypothalamus of obese humans? If so, is there any possibility of pharmacologically targeting this inflammation to treat human obesity?

AUTHOR CONTRIBUTIONS

All authors wrote the paper and approved the final version of the manuscript.

REFERENCES

Ajami, B., Bennett, J. L., Krieger, C., Tetzlaff, W., and Rossi, F. M. (2007). Local selfrenewal can sustain CNS microglia maintenance and function throughout adult life. *Nat. Neurosci.* 10, 1538–1543. doi: 10.1038/nn2014

Ataka, K., Asakawa, A., Nagaishi, K., Kaimoto, K., Sawada, A., Hayakawa, Y., et al. (2013). Bone marrow-derived microglia infiltrate into the paraventricular nucleus of chronic psychological stress-loaded mice. *PLoS One* 8:e81744. doi: 10.1371/journal.pone.0081744

Baufeld, C., Osterloh, A., Prokop, S., Miller, K. R., and Heppner, F. L. (2016). High-fat diet-induced brain region-specific phenotypic spectrum of CNS resident microglia. *Acta Neuropathol.* 132, 361–375. doi: 10.1007/s00401-016-1595-4

Buttini, M., Limonta, S., and Boddeke, H. W. (1996). Peripheral administration of lipopolysaccharide induces activation of microglial cells in rat brain. *Neurochem. Int.* 29, 25–35.

Carraro, R. S., Souza, G. F., Solon, C., Razolli, D. S., Chausse, B., Barbizan, R., et al. (2018). Hypothalamic mitochondrial abnormalities occur downstream of inflammation in diet-induced obesity. *Mol. Cell. Endocrinol.* 460, 238–245. doi: 10.1016/j.mce.2017.07.029

Cheung, A. K. L., Kwok, H. Y., Huang, Y., Chen, M., Mo, Y., Wu, X., et al. (2017). Gut-homing Δ42PD1+Vδ2 T cells promote innate mucosal damage via TLR4 during acute HIV type 1 infection. *Nat. Microbiol.* 2, 1389–1402. doi: 10.1038/s41564-017-0006-5

Cintra, D. E., Ropelle, E. R., Moraes, J. C., Pauli, J. R., Morari, J., and Souza, C. T. (2012). Unsaturated fatty acids revert diet-induced hypothalamic inflammation in obesity. *PLoS One* 7:e30571. doi: 10.1371/journal.pone.0030571

Cope, E. C., LaMarca, E. A., Monari, P. K., Olson, L. B., Martinez, S., Zych, A. D., et al. (2018). Microglia play an active role in obesity-associated cognitive decline. *J. Neurosci.* 38, 8889–8904. doi: 10.1523/JNEUROSCI.0789-18.2018

Davoust, N., Vuaillat, C., Androdias, G., and Nataf, S. (2008). From bone marrow to microglia: barriers and avenues. *Trends Immunol.* 29, 227–234. doi: 10.1016/j.it.2008.01.010

De Souza C. T., Araujo, E. P., Bordin, S., Ashimine, R., Zollner, R. L., Boschero, A. C., et al. (2005). Consumption of a fat-rich diet activates a proinflammatory response and induces insulin resistance in the hypothalamus. *Endocrinology* 146, 4192–4199. doi: 10.1210/en.2004-1520

Degasperi, G. R., Romanatto, T., Denis, R. G., Araújo, E. P., Moraes, J. C., Inada, N. M., et al. (2008). UCP2 protects hypothalamic cells from TNF-alpha-induced damage. *FEBS Lett.* 582, 3103–3110. doi: 10.1016/j.febslet.2008.08.006

Deshmane, S. L., Kremlev, S., Amini, S., and Sawaya, B. E. (2009). Monocyte chemoattractant protein-1 (MCP-1): an overview. *J. Interferon Cytokine Res.* 29, 313–326. doi: 10.1089/jir.2008.0027

Dilshara, M. G., Lee, K. T., Kim, H. J., Lee, H. J., Choi, Y. H., Lee, C. M., et al. (2014). Anti-inflammatory mechanism of α-viniferin regulates lipopolysaccharide-induced release of proinflammatory mediators in BV2 microglial cells. *Cell. Immunol.* 290, 21–29. doi: 10.1016/j.cellimm.2014.04.009

Dorfman, M. D., and Thaler, J. P. (2015). Hypothalamic inflammation and gliosis in obesity. *Curr. Opin. Endocrinol. Diabetes Obes.* 22, 325–330. doi: 10.1097/MED.0000000000000182

Dragano, N. R., Haddad-Tovolli, R., and Velloso, L. A. (2017). Leptin, neuroinflammation and obesity. *Front. Horm. Res.* 48, 84–96. doi: 10.1159/000452908

Duffy, C. M., Xu, H., Nixon, J. P., Bernlohr, D. A., and Butterick, T. A. (2017). Identification of a fatty acid binding protein4-UCP2 axis regulating microglial mediated neuroinflammation. *Mol. Cell. Neurosci.* 80, 52–57. doi: 10.1016/j.mcn.2017.02.004

Durafourt, B. A., Moore, C. S., Zammit, D. A., Johnson, T. A., Zaguia, F., and Guiot, M. C. (2012). Comparison of polarization properties of human adult microglia and blood-derived macrophages. *Glia* 60, 717–727. doi: 10.1002/glia.22298

Erion, J. R., Wosiski-Kuhn, M., Dey, A., Hao, S., Davis, C. L., Pollock, N. K., et al. (2014). Obesity elicits interleukin 1-mediated deficits in hippocampal synaptic plasticity. *J. Neurosci.* 34, 2618–2631. doi: 10.1523/JNEUROSCI.4200-13.2014

Gao, Y., Ottaway, N., Schriever, S. C., Legutko, B., García-Cáceres, C., de la Fuente, E., et al. (2014). Hormones and diet, but not body weight, control hypothalamic microglial activity. *Glia* 62, 17–25. doi: 10.1002/glia.22580

García-Bueno, B., Serrats, J., and Sawchenko, P. E. (2009). Cerebrovascular cyclooxygenase-1 expression, regulation, and role in hypothalamic-pituitary-adrenal axis activation by inflammatory stimuli. *J. Neurosci.* 29, 12970–12981. doi: 10.1523/JNEUROSCI.2373-09.2009

Girard, S., Brough, D., Lopez-Castejon, G., Giles, J., Rothwell, N. J., and Allan, S. M. (2013). Microglia and macrophages differentially modulate cell death after brain injury caused by oxygen-glucose deprivation in organotypic brain slices. *Glia* 61, 813–824. doi: 10.1002/glia.22478

Hotamisligil, G. S., and Bernlohr, D. A. (2015). Metabolic functions of FABPs–mechanisms and therapeutic implications. *Nat. Rev. Endocrinol.* 11, 592–605. doi: 10.1038/nrendo.2015.122

Hu, X., Leak, R. K., Shi, Y., Suenaga, J., Gao, Y., Zheng, P., et al. (2015). Microglial and macrophage polarization-new prospects for brain repair. *Nat. Rev. Neurol.* 11, 56–64. doi: 10.1038/nrneurol.2014.207

Huang, S., Rutkowsky, J. M., Snodgrass, R. G., Ono-Moore, K. D., Schneider, D. A., and Newman, J. W. (2012). Saturated fatty acids activate TLR-mediated proinflammatory signaling pathways. *J. Lipid Res.* 53, 2002–2013. doi: 10.1194/jlr.D029546

Inoue, T., Tanaka, M., Masuda, S., Ohue-Kitano, R., Yamakage, H., Muranaka, K., et al. (2017). Omega-3 polyunsaturated fatty acids suppress the inflammatory responses of lipopolysaccharide-stimulated mouse microglia by activating SIRT1 pathways. *Biochim. Biophys. Acta* 1862, 552–560. doi: 10.1016/j.bbalip.2017.02.010

Kang, C. H., Choi, Y. H., Moon, S. K., Kim, W. J., and Kim, G. Y. (2013). Quercetin inhibits lipopolysaccharide-induced nitric oxide production in BV2 microglial cells by suppressing the NF-κB pathway and activating the Nrf2-dependent HO-1 pathway. *Int. Immunopharmacol.* 17, 808–813. doi: 10.1016/j.intimp.2013.09.009

Katayama, Y., Battista, M., Kao, W. M., Hidalgo, A., Peired, A. J., Thomas, S. A., et al. (2006). Signals from the sympathetic nervous system regulate hematopoietic stem cell egress from bone marrow. *Cell* 124, 407–421. doi: 10.1016/j.cell.2005.10.041

Kerfoot, S. M., Long, E. M., Hickey, M. J., Andonegui, G., Lapointe, B. M., Zanardo, R. C., et al. (2004). TLR4 contributes to disease-inducing mechanisms resulting in central nervous system autoimmune disease. *J. Immunol.* 173, 7070–7077. doi: 10.4049/jimmunol.173.11.7070

Kettenmann, H., Hanisch, U. K., Noda, M., and Verkhratsky, A. (2011). Physiology of microglia. *Physiol. Rev.* 91, 461–553. doi: 10.1152/physrev.00011.2010

Kigerl, K. A., de Rivero Vaccari, J. P., Dietrich, W. D., Popovich, P. G., and Keane, R. W. (2014). Pattern recognition receptors and central nervous system repair. *Exp. Neurol.* 258, 5–16. doi: 10.1016/j.expneurol.2014.01.001

Lam, T. K., Schwartz, G. J., and Rossetti, L. (2005). Hypothalamic sensing of fatty acids. *Nat. Neurosci.* 8, 579–584. doi: 10.1038/nn1456

Lassmann, H., Schmied, M., Vass, K., and Hickey, W. F. (1993). Bone marrow derived elements and resident microglia in brain inflammation. *Glia* 7, 19–24.

Ledo, J. H., Azevedo, E. P., Beckman, D., Ribeiro, F. C., Santos, L. E., Razolli, D. S., et al. (2016). Cross talk between brain innate immunity and serotonin signaling underlies depressive-like behavior induced by Alzheimer's amyloid-β oligomers in mice. *J. Neurosci.* 36, 12106–12116. doi: 10.1523/JNEUROSCI.1269-16.2016

Lee, J., Cha, Y., Lee, K., and Yim, J. (2016). Onion peel extract reduces the percentage of body fat in overweight and obese subjects: a 12-week, randomized, double-blind, placebo-controlled study. *Nutr. Res. Pract.* 10, 175–181. doi: 10.4162/nrp.2016.10.2.175

Li, C., Zhang, C., Zhou, H., Feng, Y., Tang, F., Hoi, M. P. M., et al. (2018). Inhibitory effects of betulinic acid on LPS-induced neuroinflammation involve M2 microglial polarization via CaMKKβ-dependent AMPK activation. *Front. Mol. Neurosci.* 11:98. doi: 10.3389/fnmol.2018.00098

Lilly, A. J., Johnson, W. E., and Bunce, C. M. (2011). The haematopoietic stem cell niche: new insights into the mechanisms regulating haematopoietic stem cell behaviour. *Stem Cells Int.* 2011:274564. doi: 10.4061/2011/274564

Little, J. P., Madeira, J. M., and Klegeris, A. (2012). The saturated fatty acid palmitate induces human monocytic cell toxicity toward neuronal cells: exploring a possible link between obesity-related metabolic impairments and neuroinflammation. *J. Alzheimers Dis.* 2, S179–S183. doi: 10.3233/JAD-2011-111262

Mander, P. K., Jekabsone, A., and Brown, G. C. (2006). Microglia proliferation is regulated by hydrogen peroxide from NADPH oxidase. *J. Immunol.* 76, 1046–1052.

Matsumoto, Y., and Fujiwara, M. (1987). Absence of donor-type major histocompatibility complex class I antigen-bearing microglia in the rat central nervous system of radiation bone marrow chimeras. *J. Neuroimmunol.* 17, 71–82.

Milanski, M., Arruda, A. P., Coope, A., Ignacio-Souza, L. M., Nunez, C. E., Roman, E. A., et al. (2012). Inhibition of hypothalamic inflammation reverses diet-induced insulin resistance in the liver. *Diabetes* 61, 1455–1462. doi: 10.2337/db11-0390

Milanski, M., Degasperi, G., Coope, A., Morari, J., Denis, R., Cintra, D. E., et al. (2009). Saturated fatty acids produce an inflammatory response predominantly through the activation of TLR4 signaling in hypothalamus: implications for the pathogenesis of obesity. *J. Neurosci.* 29, 359–370. doi: 10.1523/JNEUROSCI.2760-08.2009

Moraes, J. C., Coope, A., Morari, J., Cintra, D. E., Roman, E. A., Pauli, J. R., et al. (2009). High-fat diet induces apoptosis of hypothalamic neurons. *PLoS One* 4:e5045. doi: 10.1371/journal.pone.0005045

Morari, J., Anhe, G. F., Nascimento, L. F., de Moura, R. F., Razolli, D., Solon, C., et al. (2014). Fractalkine (CX3CL1) is involved in the early activation of hypothalamic inflammation in experimental obesity. *Diabetes* 63, 3770–3784. doi: 10.2337/db13-1495

Mulders, R. J., de Git, K. C. G., Schéle, E., Dickson, S. L., Sanz, Y., and Adan, R. A. H. (2018). Microbiota in obesity: interactions with enteroendocrine, immune and central nervous systems. *Obes. Rev.* 19, 435–451. doi: 10.1111/obr.12661

Nascimento, L. F., Souza, G. F., Morari, J., Barbosa, G. O., Solon, C., Moura, R. F., et al. (2016). n-3 fatty acids induce neurogenesis of predominantly POMC-expressing cells in the hypothalamus. *Diabetes* 65, 673–686. doi: 10.2337/db15-0008

Orihuela, R., McPherson, C. A., and Harry, G. J. (2016). Microglial M1/M2 polarization and metabolic states. *Br. J. Pharmacol.* 173, 649–665. doi: 10.1111/bph.13139

Pan, W. W., and Myers, M. G. Jr. (2018). Leptin and the maintenance of elevated body weight. *Nat. Rev. Neurosci.* 19, 95–105. doi: 10.1038/nrn.2017.168

Park, J., Min, J. S., Kim, B., Chae, U. B., Yun, J. W., Choi, M. S., et al. (2015). Mitochondrial ROS govern the LPS-induced pro-inflammatory response in microglia cells by regulating MAPK and NF-κB pathways. *Neurosci. Lett.* 584, 191–196. doi: 10.1016/j.neulet.2014.10.016

Pawate, S., Shen, Q., Fan, F., and Bhat, N. R. (2004). Redox regulation of glial inflammatory response to lipopolysaccharide and interferongamma. *J. Neurosci. Res.* 77, 540–551. doi: 10.1002/jnr.20180

Pfeuffer, M., Auinger, A., Bley, U., Kraus-Stojanowic, I., Laue, C., Winkler, P., et al. (2013). Effect of quercetin on traits of the metabolic syndrome, endothelial function and inflammation in men with different APOE isoforms. *Nutr. Metab. Cardiovasc. Dis.* 23, 403–409. doi: 10.1016/j.numecd.2011.08.010

Priller, J., Flügel, A., Wehner, T., Boentert, M., Haas, C. A., and Prinz, M. (2001). Targeting gene-modified hematopoietic cells to the central nervous system: use of green fluorescent protein uncovers microglial engraftment. *Nat. Med.* 7, 1356–1361. doi: 10.1038/nm1201-1356

Prinz, M., and Mildner, A. (2011). Microglia in the CNS: immigrants from another world. *Glia.* 59, 177–187. doi: 10.1002/glia.21104

Ramalho, A. F., Bombassaro, B., Dragano, N. R., Solon, C., Morari, J., and Fioravante, M. (2018). Dietary fats promote functional and structural changes in the median eminence blood/spinal fluid interface-the protective role for BDNF. *J. Neuroinflammation* 15:10. doi: 10.1186/s12974-017-1046-8

Rodríguez, E. M., Blázquez, J. L., and Guerra, M. (2010). The design of barriers in the hypothalamus allows the median eminence and the arcuate nucleus to enjoy private milieus: the former opens to the portal blood and the latter to the cerebrospinal fluid. *Peptides.* 31, 757–776. doi: 10.1016/j.peptides.2010.01.003

Saijo, K., and Glass, C. K. (2011). Microglial cell origin and phenotypes in health and disease. *Nat. Rev. Immunol.* 11, 775–787. doi: 10.1038/nri3086

Schaeffer, M., Langlet, F., Lafont, C., Molino, F., Hodson, D. J., Roux, T., et al. (2013). Rapid sensing of circulating ghrelin by hypothalamic appetite-modifying neurons. *Proc. Natl. Acad. Sci. U.S.A.* 110, 1512–1517. doi: 10.1073/pnas.1212137110

Schwartz, M. W., Woods, S. C., Porte, D. Jr., Seeley, R. J., and Baskin, D. G. (2000). Central nervous system control of food intake. *Nature* 404, 661–671. doi: 10.1038/35007534

Shanely, R. A., Knab, A. M., Nieman, D. C., Jin, F., McAnulty, S. R., and Landram, M. J. (2010). Quercetin supplementation does not alter antioxidant status in humans. *Free Radic. Res.* 44, 224–231. doi: 10.3109/10715760903407293

Spencer, S. J., D'Angelo, H., Soch, A., Watkins, L. R., Maier, S. F., and Barrientos, R. M. (2017). High-fat diet and aging interact to produce neuroinflammation and impair hippocampal- and amygdalar-dependent memory. *Neurobiol. Aging* 58, 88–101. doi: 10.1016/j.neurobiolaging.2017.06.014

Sumi, N., Nishioku, T., Takata, F., Matsumoto, J., Watanabe, T., and Shuto, H. (2010). Lipopolysaccharide-activated microglia induce dysfunction of the blood-brain barrier in rat microvascular endothelial cells co-cultured with microglia. *Cell Mol. Neurobiol.* 30, 247–253. doi: 10.1007/s10571-009-9446-7

Tang, Y., and Le, W. (2016). Differential roles of M1 and M2 microglia in neurodegenerative diseases. *Mol. Neurobiol.* 53, 1181–1194. doi: 10.1007/s12035-014-9070-5

Thaler, J. P., Yi, C. X., Schur, E. A., Guyenet, S. J., Hwang, B. H., Dietrich, M. O., et al. (2012). Obesity is associated with hypothalamic injury in rodents and humans. *J. Clin. Invest.* 122, 153–162. doi: 10.1172/JCI59660

Timper, K., and Brüning, J. C. (2017). Hypothalamic circuits regulating appetite and energy homeostasis: pathways to obesity. *Dis. Model Mech.* 10, 679–689. doi: 10.1242/dmm.026609

Valdearcos, M., Douglass, J. D., Robblee, M. M., Dorfman, M. D., Stifler, D. R., and Bennett, M. L. (2017). Microglial inflammatory signaling orchestrates the hypothalamic immune response to dietary excess and mediates obesity susceptibility. *Cell Metab.* 26, 185–197. doi: 10.1016/j.cmet.2017.05.015

Valdearcos, M., Robblee, M. M., and Benjamin, D. I. (2014). Microglia dictate the impact of saturated fat consumption on hypothalamic inflammation and neuronal function. *Cell Rep.* 9, 2124–2138. doi: 10.1016/j.celrep.2014.11.018

van de Sande-Lee, S., Pereira, F. R., Cintra, D. E., Fernandes, P. T., Cardoso, A. R., Garlipp, C. R., et al. (2011). Partial reversibility of hypothalamic dysfunction and changes in brain activity after body mass reduction in obese subjects. *Diabetes* 60, 1699–1704. doi: 10.2337/db10-1614

Velloso, L. A., and Schwartz, M. W. (2011). Altered hypothalamic function in diet-induced obesity. *Int. J. Obes.* 35, 1455–1465. doi: 10.1038/ijo.2011.56

Waise, T. M. Z., Toshinai, K., Naznin, F., NamKoong, C., Md Moin, A. S., Sakoda, H., et al. (2015). One-day high-fat diet induces inflammation in the nodose ganglion and hypothalamus of mice. *Biochem. Biophys. Res. Commun.* 464, 1157–1162. doi: 10.1016/j.bbrc.2015.07.097

Wang, Z., Liu, D., Wang, F., Liu, S., Zhao, S., Ling, E. A., et al. (2012). Saturated fatty acids activate microglia via Toll-like receptor 4/NF-kappaB signalling. *Br. J. Nutr.* 107, 229–241. doi: 10.1017/S0007114511002868

Wirenfeldt, M., Dissing-Olesen, L., Babcock, A. A., Nielsen, M., Meldgaard, M., and Zimmer, J. (2007). Population control of resident and immigrant microglia by mitosis and apoptosis. *Am. J. Pathol.* 171, 617–631. doi: 10.2353/ajpath.2007.061044

Xu, H., Xiao, T., Chen, C. H., Li, W., Meyer, C. A., and Wu, Q. (2015). Sequence determinants of improved CRISPR sgRNA design. *Genome Res.* 25, 1147–1157. doi: 10.1101/gr.191452.115

Yang, J., Kim, C., Tu, T., Kim, M., Goto, T., Kawada, T., et al. (2017a). Quercetin protects Obesity-Induced hypothalamic inflammation by reducing microglia-mediated inflammatory responses via HO-1 induction. *Nutrients* 9:650. doi: 10.3390/nu9070650

Yang, X., Xu, S., Qian, Y., and Xiao, Q. (2017b). Resveratrol regulates microglia M1/M2 polarization via PGC-1α in conditions of neuroinflammatory injury. *Brain Behav. Immun.* 64, 162–172. doi: 10.1016/j.bbi.2017.03.003

Zhang, X., Zhang, G., Zhang, H., Karin, M., Bai, H., and Cai, D. (2008). Hypothalamic IKKβ/NF-κB and ER stress link overnutrition to energy imbalance and obesity. *Cell* 135, 61–73. doi: 10.1016/j.cell.2008.07.043

Zhong, L., Zhang, Z. L., Li, X., Liao, C., Mou, P., Wang, T., et al. (2017). TREM2/DAP12 complex regulates inflammatory responses in microglia via the JNK signaling pathway. *Front. Aging Neurosci.* 9:204. doi: 10.3389/fnagi.2017.00204

Zhou, D., Huang, C., Lin, Z., Zhan, S., Kong, L., Fang, C., et al. (2014). Macrophage polarization and function with emphasis on the evolving roles of coordinated regulation of cellular signaling pathways. *Cell. Signal.* 26, 192–197. doi: 10.1016/j.cellsig.2013.11.004

Zhuang, P., Shou, Q., Lu, Y., Wang, G., Qiu, J., Wang, J., et al. (2017). Arachidonic acid sex-dependently affects obesity through linking gut microbiota-driven inflammation to hypothalamus-adipose-liver axis. *Biochim. Biophys. Acta Mol. Basis Dis.* 1863, 2715–2726. doi: 10.1016/j.bbadis.2017.07.003

9

Glucose Homeostasis is not Affected in a Murine Model of Parkinson's Disease Induced by 6-OHDA

*Felipe Azevedo Gomes[1], Rafael Appel Flores[2], Maciel Alencar Bruxel[2], Flávia Natividade da Silva[3], Eduardo Luiz Gasnhar Moreira[2,3], Daniel Breseghello Zoccal[4], Rui Daniel Prediger[1] and Alex Rafacho[1,2,3]**

[1] Postgraduate Program in Pharmacology, Federal University of Santa Catarina, Florianópolis, Brazil, [2] Multicenter Postgraduate Program in Physiological Sciences, Federal University of Santa Catarina, Florianópolis, Brazil, [3] Department of Physiological Sciences, Center of Biological Sciences, Federal University of Santa Catarina, Florianópolis, Brazil, [4] Department of Physiology and Pathology, School of Dentistry, São Paulo State University, Araraquara, Brazil

***Correspondence:**
Alex Rafacho
alex.rafacho@ufsc.br

There is a mutual relationship between metabolic and neurodegenerative diseases. However, the causal relationship in this crosstalk is unclear and whether Parkinson's disease (PD) causes a posterior impact on metabolism remains unknown. Considering that, this study aimed to evaluate the appearance of possible changes in metabolic homeostasis due to 6-hydroxydopamine (6-OHDA) administration, a neurotoxin that damage dopaminergic neurons leading to motor impairments that resemble the ones observed in PD. For this, male Wistar rats received bilateral 6-OHDA administration in the dorsolateral striatum, and the motor and metabolic outcomes were assessed at 7, 21, or 35 days post-surgical procedure. Dexamethasone, a diabetogenic glucocorticoid (GC), was intraperitoneally administered in the last 6 days to challenge the metabolism and reveal possible metabolic vulnerabilities caused by 6-OHDA. Controls received only vehicles. The 6-OHDA-treated rats displayed a significant decrease in locomotor activity, exploratory behavior, and motor coordination 7 and 35 days after neurotoxin administration. These motor impairments paralleled with no significant alteration in body mass, food intake, glucose tolerance, insulin sensitivity, and biochemical parameters (plasma insulin, triacylglycerol, and total cholesterol levels) until the end of the experimental protocol on days 35–38 post-6-OHDA administration. Moreover, hepatic glycogen and fat content, as well as the endocrine pancreas mass, were not altered in rats treated with 6-OHDA at the day of euthanasia (38th day after neurotoxin administration). None of the diabetogenic effects caused by dexamethasone were exacerbated in rats previously treated with 6-OHDA. Thus, we conclude that bilateral 6-OHDA administration in the striatum causes motor deficits in rats with no impact on glucose and lipid homeostasis and does not exacerbate the adverse effects caused by excess GC. These observations indicate that neurodegeneration of dopaminergic circuits in the 6-OHDA rats does not affect the metabolic outcomes.

Keywords: glucocorticoid, glycemia, lipids, liver, pancreatic islets, Parkinson's disease

INTRODUCTION

The first description of Parkinson's disease (PD) was made by James Parkinson in the early nineteenth century (Pearce, 1989). It is considered the second most prevalent neurodegenerative disease in the world, affecting approximately 1% of the world population over 60 years (Schapira, 2009). The disease is characterized by a slow and progressive loss of dopaminergic neurons from the substantia nigra resulting in a gradual loss of motor functions (Stern et al., 2012). At the diagnosis period, approximately 40% of the dopaminergic neurons are intact and the presence of dopamine in the striatum is restricted to approximately 20–30% of the normal condition (Riederer and Wuketich, 1976). The primary etiology of the disease is not yet well known. However, epidemiological studies associate the etiology with several risk factors such as neuronal aging, genetic and environmental factors, viruses and inadequate eating habits (Marttila et al., 1977; Gorell et al., 1997; Mattson, 2003; Steenland et al., 2006; Goldman, 2010).

A classic animal model of PD is obtained through the neurotoxin 6-hydroxydopamine (6-OHDA), a substance that does not cross the blood-brain barrier and therefore requires its administration to be performed directly on the substantia nigra *pars compacta* (SNpc) or on the striatum (Jackson-Lewis et al., 2012). As demonstrated for the first time by Ungerstedt (1968), an intranigral injection of 6-OHDA in rats rapidly eliminates about 60% of tyrosine hydroxylase (TH)-positive neurons in this brain area, with the subsequent loss of TH-positive terminals in the striatum (Blandini et al., 2008). However, when administered at the striatum, the neurotoxin promotes a slower and progressive degeneration and subsequent loss of neurons in the SNpc, which also occurs in PD context (Sauer and Oertel, 1994; Przedborski et al., 1995; Lee et al., 1996).

Several studies have suggested an association between metabolic-related diseases (i.e., diabetes *mellitus*) and neurodegenerative diseases. Some authors have suggested that diabetes *mellitus* type 2 (T2DM) is one of the risk factors for the development of neurodegenerative diseases such as PD (Hu et al., 2007; Klimek et al., 2015; Pagano et al., 2018). In addition, a higher prevalence of T2DM was reported in patients with PD (Pressley et al., 2003). Although there are some associations between metabolic outcomes and PD, or vice versa, an observational study reports that the prevalence of T2DM in patients with PD is similar to the prevalence of individuals without PD (Becker et al., 2008). Scigliano et al. (2006) reported a lower prevalence of DM2 in patients diagnosed with PD; whereas no differences were found in the risk of developing PD between eutrophic patients and diabetic patients (Simon et al., 2007). However, it is known that PD can damage several brain areas and may affect regions involved in metabolic control such as the hypothalamus (Dayan et al., 2018).

The pathophysiological process of PD is complex since it may involve environmental, genetic and inflammatory risk factors that are not yet well understood. In addition, remains unknown whether the brain damage observed in PD can negatively affect peripheral metabolic aspects such as glycemia, lipidemia, glucose tolerance, and peripheral insulin sensitivity. Thus, there is no definition of which the causal factor is; whether the metabolic dysfunctions favor the development of PD or, if the contrary is true, or if both conditions can occur. Thus, due to the high prevalence of metabolic diseases and PD in elderly populations and the lack of knowledge about the relationship between PD and metabolic outcomes, we aimed to investigate the possible impact of murine model of motor dysfunctions caused by 6-OHDA on glycemic and lipid homeostasis. We also challenged these rats with dexamethasone, a diabetogenic drug, to verify how much these 6-OHDA-treated rats are vulnerable or not to glucocorticoid (GC) adverse effects. Our hypothesis is that rats with motor deficits caused by 6-OHDA administration will exhibit deterioration of glucose tolerance and insulin sensitivity and that these changes will be exacerbated when GCs were administered. Overall, we demonstrated that motor impairments caused by 6-OHDA treatment did not parallel with peripheral metabolic parameters either predispose rats to the diabetogenic GC effects.

MATERIALS AND METHODS

Ethics Statement

The experimental protocol was approved by the Federal University of Santa Catarina Committee for Ethics in Animal Experimentation (Approval ID: 4468101116) in accordance with the Brazilian National Council for Animal Experimentation Control (CONCEA).

Animals

Thirty-six adults male Wistar rats (starting weight 280–350 g) were housed in a temperature and humidity-controlled environment and kept on a 12-h light–dark cycle (lights on 06:00 – 18:00 h). All rats had *ad libitum* access to food (commercial standard chow for rats, Nuvilab CR-1; Nuvital, Brazil) and filtered tap water. The animals were supplied by the Federal University of Santa Catarina's Animal Breeding Center.

Experimental Design and Groups

Animals were acclimatized for a period of 8 weeks before being randomly assigned in two groups, followed by a new distribution in four experimental groups, as will be described in detail. Animals were submitted to a baseline rotarod assessment protocol and those who were successful in this test were included in the study and underwent stereotaxic surgery. On the first day, only 12% responded adequately to the rotarod test (**Figure 1A**). The rate of successful increased in the second test day and, on day 3, approximately 91% successfully achieve the inclusion criteria on the rotarod test. Approximately 8% did not adapt to the test and therefore did not follow to the surgical procedure. As shown in **Figure 1B**, rats were submitted to the open field test on the 7th and 35th days after the surgery and to a second test, rotarod test, on the 7th, 21st, and 35th postoperative days. The intraperitoneal (i.p.) glucose tolerance test (ipGTT) was performed on the 8th, 22nd, and 36th days of the experimental protocol, while the i.p. insulin tolerance test (ipITT) was applied on the

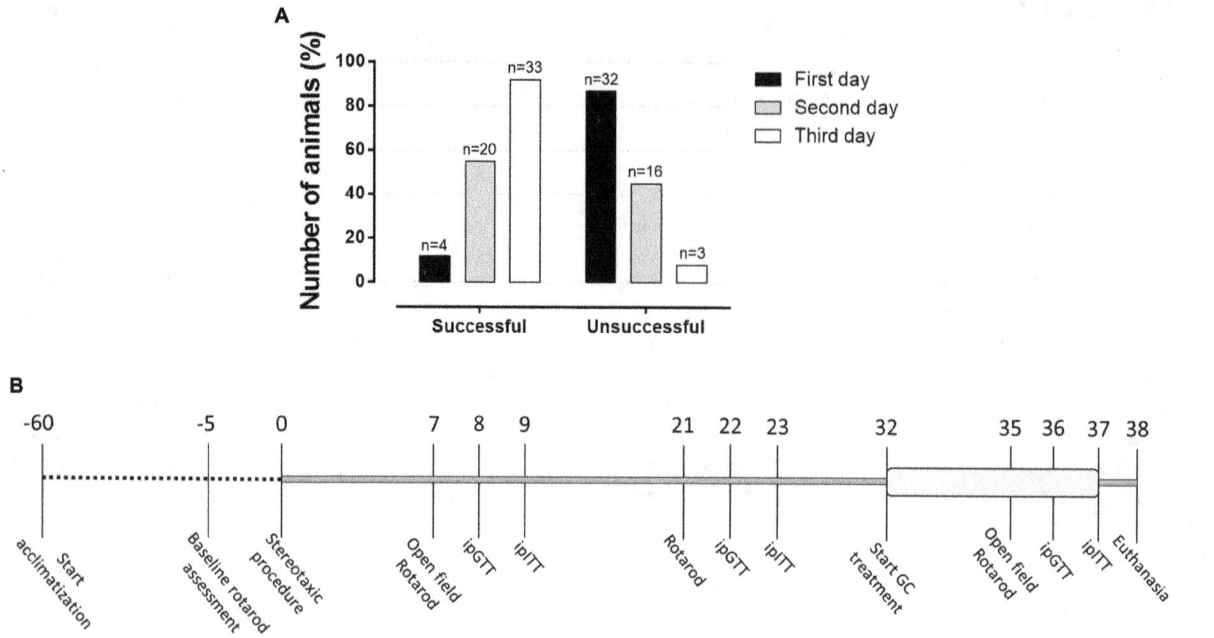

FIGURE 1 | Percentage of animals responsive to the rotarod basal motor protocol and experimental design. **(A)** This test was applied before to initiate the surgeries to identify those rats able to follow in the study. Around 12% of the animals responded to the rotarod test in the first attempt, which achieves approximately 91% of success on the third attempt day. **(B)** The number above line means days along experimental protocol with the respective experimental approaches applied in the study.

9th, 23rd, and 37th postoperative days. The treatment with dexamethasone started on the 32nd day, which lasted until the 37th day of the experimental protocol (6 days). On day 38, the animals were euthanized, and plasma and organs were collected for further biochemical analysis as described in the next sections.

Groups were defined as follow: initially, rats were randomly allocated in two experimental groups: (1) Control group (Control) ($n = 17$): rats treated only with vehicle via the intra-striatal administration (described in the next section), and (2) 6-hydroxydopamine group (6-OHDA) ($n = 16$): rats treated with 6-hydroxydopamine via the intra-striatal administration (described in the next section). Then, half of the animal from the Control and 6-OHDA groups were treated with dexamethasone composing the following groups, respectively: (3) Dexamethasone group (Dexa) ($n = 9$): received i.p. injection of dexamethasone (as described in other section), and (4) 6-hydroxydopamine+dexamethasone group (6-OHDA + Dexa) ($n = 8$): treated as 6-OHDA and Dexa groups. This experimental protocol was performed in two different sets of animals with half of the number of animals on each occasion.

Surgical Procedure

Before any surgical procedure, rats were anesthetized with ketamine/xylazine [75/10 mg/kg body mass (b.m.), i.p.]. 6-OHDA (20 μg in 3 μL and an infusion rate of 1 μL/min) (Sigma-Aldrich, St. Louis, MO, United States) was injected bilaterally into the dorsolateral striatum (DLS) at the coordinates: AP: +0.2 mm, ML: ±3.5 mm and DV: −4.8 mm to bregma (Paxinos and Watson, 1997), using a Hamilton 10 μL syringe with a 26-gauge needle connected to a 30-gauge cannula, whereas control rats received vehicle (saline solution). Then, the cannula was left untouchable for an additional minute to prevent backflow. This experimental procedure has been used in rats to generate motor impairments that resemble PD motor impairments (Rampersaud et al., 2012; Hegazy et al., 2017).

Dexamethasone Treatment

We used dexamethasone to generate an *in vivo* metabolic challenging considering the diabetogenic properties of this GC as previously demonstrated by several studies (Giozzet et al., 2008; Angelini et al., 2010; Rafacho et al., 2014). Dexamethasone disodium phosphate (Decadron®, Aché, Campinas, SP, Brazil) was daily injected, through i.p. vial, between 07:30 and 08:30 h, at a dose of 1 mg/kg, b.m., for the last 6 consecutive days.

Motor Tests

Open Field

This test was performed under a red-light (12 lux) condition and with controlled sound, temperature, and humidity. Animals were placed in an arena (100 × 100 cm) during 5 min for free exploration. The arena had smooth sidewalls, measuring 40 cm height, formed by odorless white painted metal and the base was made of concrete coated with black contact paper. The square base had 5 × 5 quadrants, each square with 400 cm^2 (20 × 20 cm). All experiments were recorded (Logitech C270, Lausanne, Switzerland), and the following parameters were analyzed: (1) number of squares crossed by the animal, which represents the locomotor activity; (2) number of rearing behavior, which represents the exploratory activity; (3) number of quadrants crossed peripherally or centrally, which allows identifying anxiety-related behaviors.

Rotarod

This test was applied to evaluate the motor coordination and balance of the animals. The equipment was prepared at three speeds: 12, 20, and 24 revolutions per minute (rpm). The change of speed occurred manually and involved shutdown of the equipment for each speed change. Thus, there was a brief interruption of the test between the rotational changes. All animals were exposed individually to the three different speed levels, consecutively. The baseline assessment protocol consisted of three trials in a constant 12 rpm speed. In the end, rats that remained in the rotarod for 1 min were included in the study and were underwent stereotaxic surgery (**Figure 1A**). This baseline assessment was initiated 5 days before stereotaxic surgery and was extended for three consecutive days (**Figure 1B**). On the 7th, 21st, and 35th postoperative days, animals were positioned in the rotarod apparatus, aiming to remain up to 2 min in each speed. The residence time (latency to fall) of each rat at each stage was measured with a conventional digital chronometer as an indicator of balance and motor coordination.

Measurements of *in vivo* Metabolic Parameters

Verification of body mass was performed every 3 days from the beginning of the experimental protocol to the day of euthanasia in a digital electronic balance (TECNAL; Piracicaba, SP, Brazil). Food intake was monitored as described for body mass. The determination of food intake was performed by weighing the remaining chow discounted from the total of that deposited 24 h before and the mass difference represents the daily amount ingested per cage. The average amount of food ingested per animal was obtained by the following formula [(total chow (g) ingested in the cage/number of rats per cage)/individual rat mass (g)] × 100. The results were expressed as grams (g) of food ingested per 100 g of body mass. During the dexamethasone treatment both body mass and food intake were daily measured, but for aesthetic reasons, only the initial and final measures of food intake were used in the line graph.

I.p. Glucose Tolerance Test (ipGTT)

The i.p. glucose tolerance test (ipGTT) was performed on 8th, 22nd, and 36th days of the experimental protocol in fasted (08 h) rats, with the experiments occurring around 16:00. The rats had the tip of the tail cut (no more than 1 mm) for blood collection. The first drop was discarded, and the second drop was used for the determination of blood glucose (time 0) using a glucometer (Accu-Chek Performa; Roche Diagnostics, GmbH, Mannheim, Germany). Immediately after, a 50% glucose solution pre-warmed at 36°C (2 g/kg, b.m.) was administered by i.p. injection and blood samples were collected from the tail tip at 30, 60, and 120 min for blood glucose measurements as described before (Giozzet et al., 2008; Motta et al., 2015). Area-under-glucose-curve (AUC) was obtained after normalization by the initial value.

I.p. Insulin Tolerance Test (ipITT)

The i.p. insulin tolerance test (ipITT) was performed on 9th, 23rd, and 37th days of the experimental protocol in fed rats, with the experiments occurring around 16:00. Blood collection at min 0 occurred as for ipGTT. Then, the animals received an i.p. injection of recombinant human insulin pre-warmed at 36°C (Biohulin® 1 IU/kg b.m.). Blood samples were posteriorly collected from the tail tip at 10, 20, and 40 min for blood glucose measurements (Giozzet et al., 2008; Protzek et al., 2016). AUC was obtained from normalized blood glucose values (expressed as % from min 0).

Euthanasia and Biochemical Analysis

On the 38th day, 24 h after the last dexamethasone administration, animals received a halothane super dosage (1 mL) (Tanohalo®, Cristália, Curitiba, PR, Brazil). Blood samples were collected through heart puncture with EDTA-NaF containing syringes (Glistab - Labtest; Lagoa Santa, MG, Brazil) and centrifuged at 400 *g* for 10 min at 21°C (Eppendorf 5810R). The plasma was separated and stored at −80°C until the posterior determination of insulin, total cholesterol, and triacylglycerol, according to manufacturer instructions and previously published data (dos Santos et al., 2014; Motta et al., 2015). Animals were then continuously perfused through the left ventricle with 20 mL of 0.9% NaCl containing 0.1% heparin followed by infusion of 200 mL of 4% paraformaldehyde (pH 7.4, Sigma-Aldrich). Organs of interest were carefully removed and weighed.

Liver Glycogen and Hepatic Triacylglycerol Content

Hepatic glycogen content was determined by a phenol-based assay according to a previous publication (Giozzet et al., 2008). Determination of hepatic triacylglycerol content was performed according to a previous publication (Gonçalves-Neto et al., 2014). The same hepatic lobe was used for collection of the fragments for all animals.

Hepatic Morphology

After perfusion, liver fragments (from the same lobe in all animals) were collected and fixed in 10% buffered formalin, pH 7.4, for 24 h, dehydrated and embedded in paraffin. Representative tissue sections (5 μm) were obtained on a rotating microtome (Leica) and placed on glass slides. Afterward, the slides were submitted to the staining procedure of Hematoxylin and Eosin for further morphological evaluation to verify the presence of lipids and glycogen according to Gonçalves-Neto et al. (2014).

The Relative Mass of the Endocrine Pancreas

After perfusion, pancreas fragments (splenic region) were collected and fixed in 4% paraformaldehyde for 24 h, dehydrated

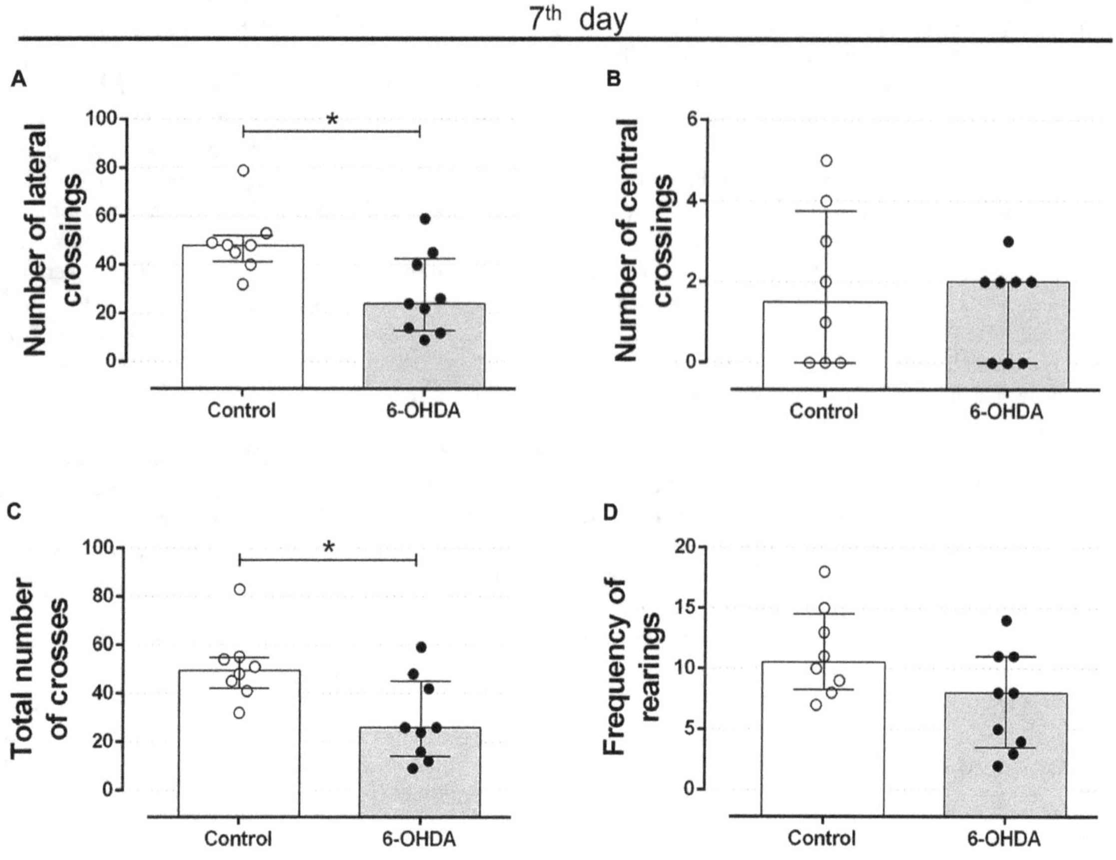

FIGURE 2 | Effect of 6-OHDA on the 7th day of the experimental protocol, in motor parameters evaluated in the open field test. **(A)** number of lateral crossings; **(B)** number of central crossings; **(C)** the total number of crosses (central + lateral); **(D)** average frequency of rearings. Data are median and interquartile range as they are asymmetrically distributed (nonparametric). *Indicates a significant difference compared to the respective control group using unpaired Mann–Whitney. $n = 8–9$, $p < 0.05$.

and embedded in paraffin. Representative tissue sections (5 μm) were obtained on a rotating microtome (Leica) and placed on glass slides. Afterward, the slides were submitted to the staining procedure of hematoxylin and eosin and later scanned by the AxioScan automatic slide scanner (ZEISS, Oberkochen, Germany) for quantification of the relative endocrine pancreatic mass and density of pancreatic islets. To obtain the relative mass data, the total area of the pancreas and pancreatic islets were calculated using the ZEN software (ZEISS). The sum of the areas corresponding to the pancreatic islets was divided by the total pancreas area and multiplied by 100 to obtain the percentage of endocrine pancreas area. To obtain the density of pancreatic islets the following relation was used: islet density = (total number of islets in section × 1000) divided by the total area of the pancreas analyzed. The result was expressed by the number of islets per 1000 μm^2 of pancreas area (Protzek et al., 2014).

Statistical Analysis

All analyses were performed using GraphPad Prism Version 6.01 software (GraphPad Inc., La Jolla, CA, United States). The results were expressed as the mean ± SD or mean ± SEM for parametric data or median and interquartile ranges for non-parametric data. The symmetry of the data was tested by Kolmogorov–Smirnov, Shapiro–Wilk, and D'Agostino and Pearson omnibus normality tests. It was considered symmetric if approved by at least one of three tests. Analysis of variance (two-way ANOVA) followed by Tukey's *post hoc* test was used for multiple comparisons of parametric data or Kruskal–Wallis followed by Dunn's *post hoc* when the variables presented an asymmetric distribution, while the categorical data were evaluated by the Person Chi-square test. Significance was set at $p < 0.05$.

RESULTS

Characterization of the 6-OHDA Model

Central Administration of 6-OHDA Caused Reduction in Locomotor Activity in the Open Field Test

Rats treated with 6-OHDA exhibited motor impairment on the 7th day after stereotaxic surgery. The number of lateral and

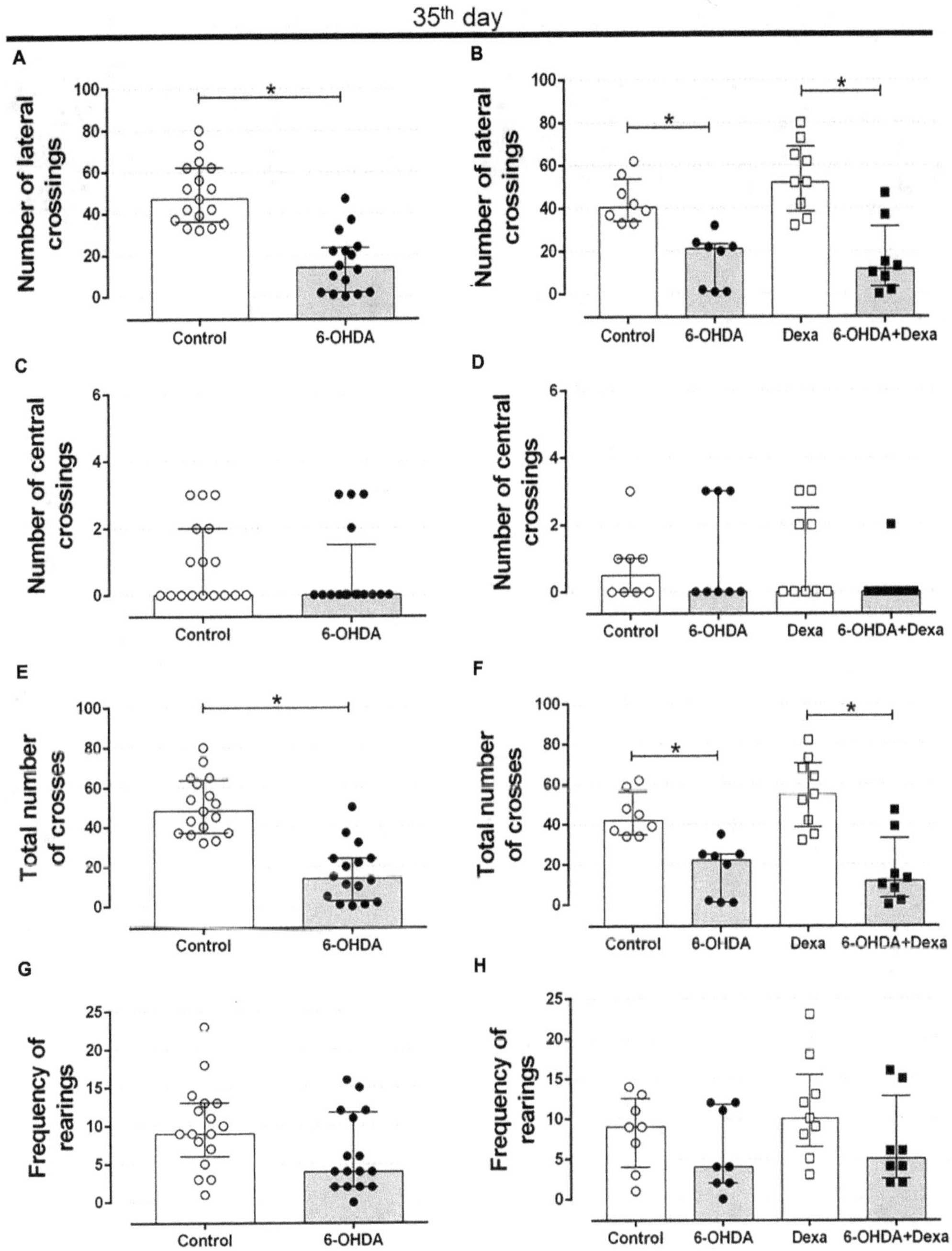

FIGURE 3 | Effect of 6-OHDA on the 35th day of the experimental protocol, in motor parameters evaluated in the open field test. **(A)** number of lateral crosses without distinction of dexamethasone treatment; **(B)** number of lateral crossings; **(C)** number of central crosses without distinction of dexamethasone treatment; **(D)** number of central crossings; **(E)** total number of crosses (central + lateral) without distinction of dexamethasone treatment; **(F)** total number of crosses (central + lateral); **(G)** frequency of rearings without distinction of dexamethasone treatment; **(H)** frequency of rearings. Data are median and interquartile range as they are asymmetrically distributed (nonparametric). *Indicates a significant difference compared to the respective control groups using unpaired Mann-Whitney in **(A,C,E,G)**, and Kruskal-Wallis with Dunn's *post hoc* test in **(B,D,F,H)**. $n = 16–17$ in **(A,C,E,G)**, and 8–9 in **(B,D,F,H)**, $p < 0.05$.

total crosses significantly reduced around 43% in the 6-OHDA group of rats, compared with the Control group (**Figures 2A,C**, respectively). No significant alterations were observed in the number of central crosses and in the frequency of rearing behavior (**Figures 2B,D**, respectively).

Motor impairment addressed on the open field test persisted until the end of experimental protocol (35 days after stereotaxic surgery and on the 3rd day of GC treatment) in rats treated with 6-OHDA, as observed by the significant reduction in the number of lateral crosses (62%) and in the number of total crosses (67%)

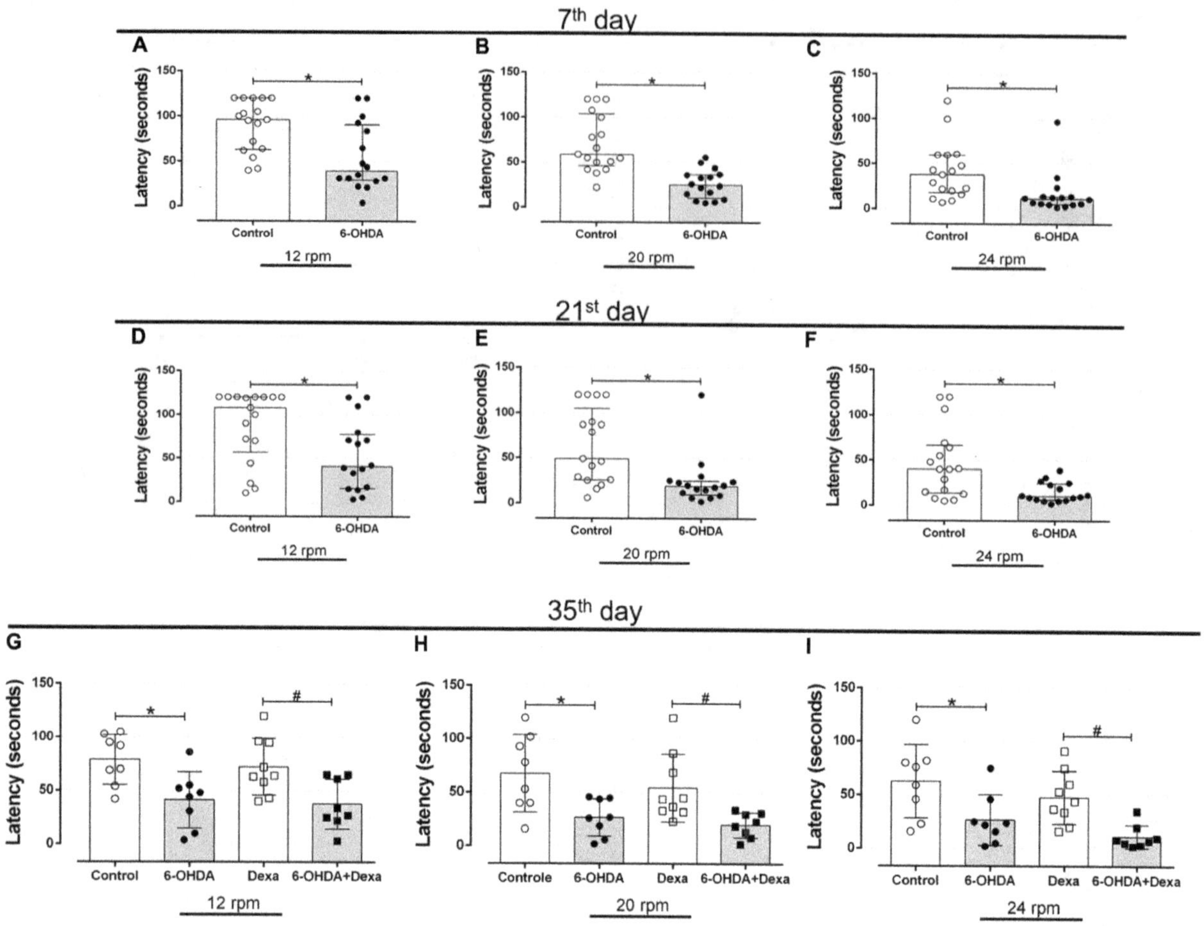

FIGURE 4 | Effect of 6-OHDA injection, on the 7th, 21st, 35th and day of the experimental protocol, in motor parameter evaluated in the rotarod test d. **(A–C)** Latency to fall in seconds at speeds of 12, 20, and 24 revolutions per minute (rpm) at the 7th, **(D–F)** 21st, and **(G–I)** 35th day. Data are median and interquartile range as they are asymmetrically distributed (non-parametric) in **(A–F)**, and mean ± SD in **(G–I)**. * and # Indicates a significant difference compared to the Control and Dexa groups, respectively, using unpaired Mann–Whitney in **(A–F)**, and ordinary two-way ANOVA with Tukey's *post hoc* test in **(G–I)**. $n = 16–17$ in **(A–F)**, and 8–9 in **(G–I)**, $p < 0.05$.

when compared with the Control group values (**Figures 3A,E**). This motor impairment was not attenuated or exacerbated by the GC treatment reinforcing the 6-OHDA effect (**Figures 3B,F**). There were no significant differences in the number of central crosses as well as in the number of rearing behavior in both 6-OHDA and 6-OHDA + Dexa groups compared to their respective Control groups (**Figures 3C,D,G,H**). Again, treatment with dexamethasone (Dexa and 6-OHDA + Dexa groups) exerted no impact on these parameters.

Central Administration of 6-OHDA Caused Reduction in Motor Coordination and Balance Impairments

Rotarod is considered a gold-standard method to evaluate motor coordination in rodents. Bilateral administration of 6-OHDA into the dorsolateral striatum resulted in impairment of the motor coordination of the animals. At the rate of 12 rpm (**Figure 4A**), the 6-OHDA group had a significant 39% reduction in the latency to rotarod fall on the 7th postoperative day, when compared to the Control group. In addition, the 6-OHDA group also showed a significant reduction of 63 and 60% at the speed of 20 and 24 rpm (**Figures 4B,C**, respectively).

The latency to fall from the rotarod equipment was very similar at day 21. The reduction in the latency to rotarod fall in the 6-OHDA group was of 40, 62, and 68% at the 12, 20, and 24 rpm speeds, respectively, demonstrating the significant persistence of motor impairment in relation to the Control group (**Figures 4D–F**).

The same pattern of latency to fall was observed on the 35th day of the experimental protocol (3rd day of GC treatment). The 6-OHDA group remained with a significant reduction of 46% in the rotarod permanence at 12 rpm (**Figure 4G**), 59% at 20 rpm (**Figure 4H**), and 54% at 24 rpm (**Figure 4I**), compared with the Control group. Treatment with dexamethasone did not influence the latency time to fall from rotarod, as observed in **Figures 4G–I**. Altogether, these findings confirm that bilateral administration of 6-OHDA in male rats is enough to cause motor dysfunctions.

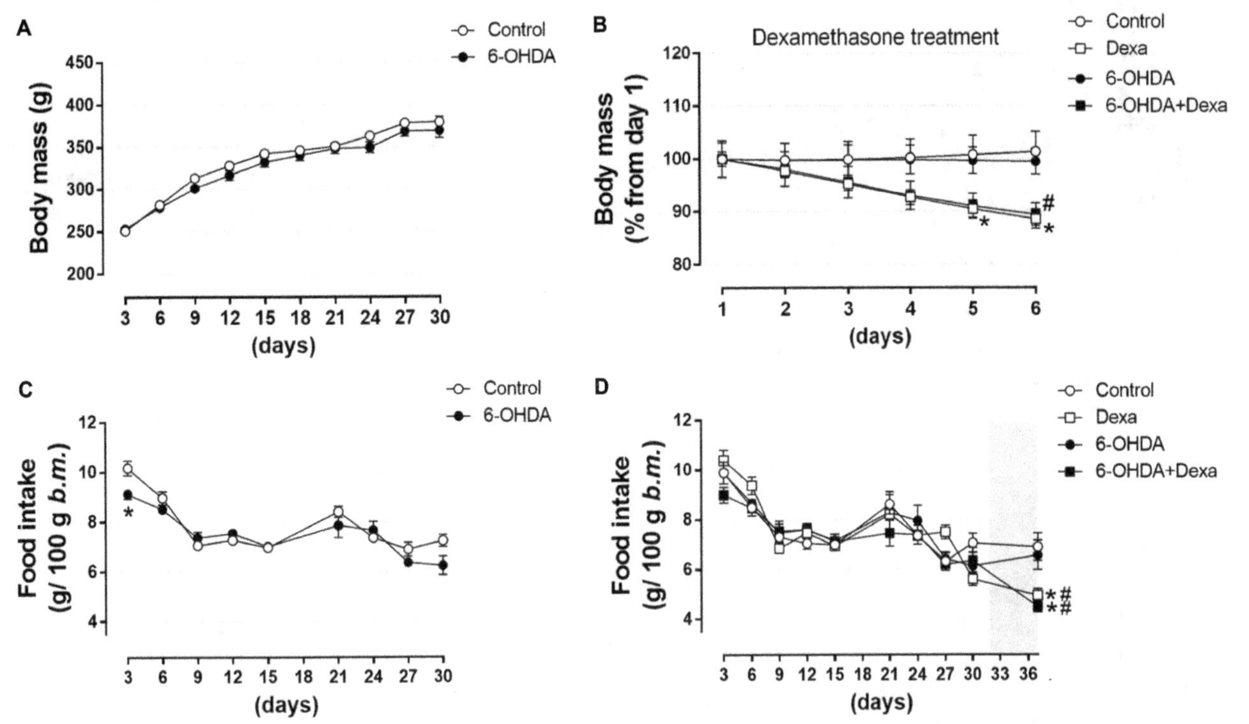

FIGURE 5 | Body mass and food intake over 36 days. **(A)** Body mass of Control and 6-OHDA groups in the first 30 days. **(B)** Normalized body mass (from the 1st day of treatment) of the Control, Dexa, 6-OHDA and 6-OHDA + Dexa groups during the 6 days of dexamethasone treatment. **(C)** Food intake of Control and 6-OHDA groups during the first 30 days. **(D)** Food intake of Control, Dexa, 6-OHDA, and 6-OHDA + Dexa groups during the whole experimental protocol. Data are mean ± SEM (SEM were applied only for aesthetic reasons). * and # Indicates a significant difference compared to the Control and 6-OHDA groups, respectively, using unpaired Student's t-test in **(A,C)**, and ordinary two-way ANOVA with repeated measures in **(B,D)**. n = 16–17 in **(A,C)**, and 8–9 in **(B,D)**, $p < 0.05$. The light gray color in **(D)** means the period of dexamethasone treatment (six consecutive days).

Central Administration of 6-OHDA Did Not Impact on Body Mass Gain and Food Intake

To verify whether motor dysfunctions resulted from treatment with 6-OHDA was associated to any alteration on murinometric parameters, and whether the treatment with dexamethasone was able to reveal any metabolic vulnerability in those animals, several parameters typical of metabolic studies were addressed. There were no differences in body mass between the Control and 6-OHDA groups during the first 30 days, before the beginning of dexamethasone treatment (**Figure 5A**). In the 32nd day, the metabolic challenge was initiated by treatment with dexamethasone. From this moment this parameter was analyzed in the four experimental groups. Both the Dexa and 6-OHDA + Dexa groups presented a significant reduction of ~11% in body mass at the end of the dexamethasone treatment (Δ 44 g and 39 g, respectively) (**Figure 5B**). Food intake was similar between Control and 6-OHDA groups when analyzed during the first 30 days of the experimental protocol, except for a transient reduction in the consumption of the 6-OHDA group in the first measure of the experimental protocol, when compared to the Control group (**Figure 5C**). In the 32nd day the metabolic challenge with dexamethasone started, and from this moment on, the parameter was analyzed in the four experimental groups. Both the Dexa and 6-OHDA + Dexa exhibited a significant reduction in food intake of 25 and 32%, respectively, at the end of dexamethasone treatment when compared to their respective controls (**Figure 5D**).

Central Administration of 6-OHDA Did Not Alter Glucose Tolerance and Insulin Sensitivity

To verify whether motor impairment caused by 6-OHDA may be associated with glucose homeostasis disturbances, we proceeded with analyzes of metabolic parameters to identify possible alterations associated with the neuromotor outcome. Considering glucose intolerance may anticipate the elevation in blood glucose, we assessed the glucose tolerance on the 8th, 22nd, and 36th days, and the insulin sensitivity on the 9th, 23rd, and 37th days of the experimental protocol. Rats treated with 6-OHDA exhibited a mild increase of blood glucose levels 30 min after an i.p. glucose *bolus* than the Control group (**Figure 6A**). The blood glucose values were 332 ± 17 mg/dL for the Control group and 388 ± 20 mg/dL for 6-OHDA group at min 30. However, this isolated alteration did not influence the area-under-curve (AUC) values, which revealed no changes in the overall glucose tolerance between the groups (**Figure 6C**). To verify whether motor impairment might be associated with an early change in insulin sensitivity, we performed ipITT on the 9th day of the experimental protocol. The insulin sensitivity remained unaltered in the 6-OHDA group compared

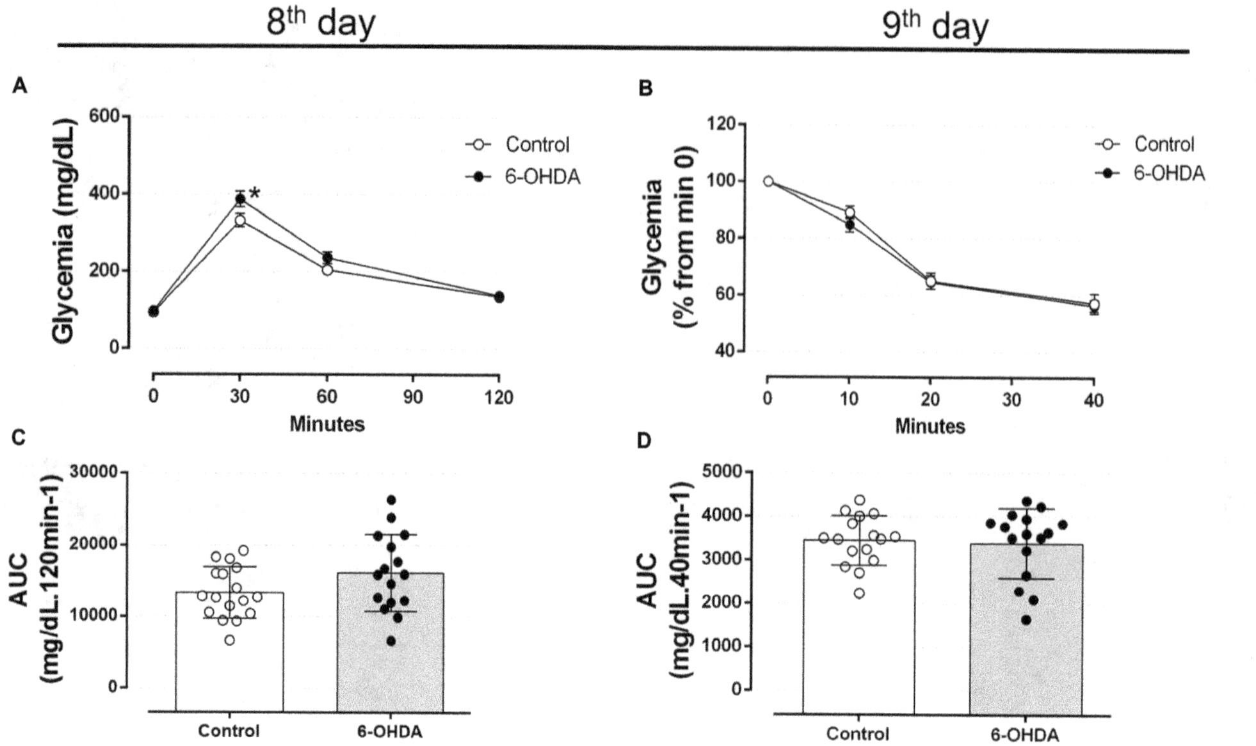

FIGURE 6 | Blood glucose values during the intraperitoneal glucose and insulin tolerance test on the 8th and 9th day of the experimental protocol. **(A)** Blood glucose values during the ipGTT on the 8th day. **(B)** Blood glucose values (normalized from min 0) during the ipITT on the 9th day. **(C)** Area-under-curve during ipGTT and **(D)** during ipITT. Data are mean ± SEM in **(A,B)**, and mean ± SD in **(C,D)** (SEM were applied only for aesthetic reasons). *Indicates a significant difference compared to the Control using ordinary two-way ANOVA with repeated measures. Unpaired Student's *t*-test was applied in **(C,D)**. $n = 16–17$, $p < 0.05$.

with the Control group (**Figures 6B,D**). The absolute fed blood glucose values on baseline of ipITT were 118 ± 7 and 121 ± 8 mg/dL for the Control and 6-OHDA groups, respectively ($n = 16–17$, NS).

The GTT values obtained in the 22nd postoperative day revealed no differences between the 6-OHDA and Control groups at 30, 60, and 120 min after intraperitoneal glucose load (**Figures 7A,C**). In addition, insulin sensitivity remained unaltered in the 23rd postoperative day in the 6-OHDA group when compared with the Control group (**Figures 7B,D**). The absolute fed blood glucose values on baseline of ipITT were 114 ± 5 and 112 ± 7 mg/dL for the Control and 6-OHDA groups, respectively ($n = 16–17$, NS).

On the 36th day of the experimental protocol (5th day of dexamethasone treatment), treatment with GC resulted in glucose intolerance in the Dexa and 6-OHDA + Dexa groups when compared with the respective Control and 6-OHDA groups, as observed at 30, 60, and 120 min (**Figure 8A**) and in the AUC values (**Figure 8C**). Again, motor dysfunction caused by 6-OHDA did parallel with normal glucose tolerance even after 36 days postoperative and was associated with no exacerbation in the glucose intolerance caused by GC treatment. Glucose intolerance caused by dexamethasone treatment occurred parallelly to a significant decrease in the insulin sensitivity as observed by the ipITT data obtained on the 37th day (**Figures 8B,D**). 6-OHDA administration did not affect insulin sensitivity *per se* or exacerbated the action of GC treatment. The absolute fed blood glucose values on baseline of ipITT were 116 ± 5, 119 ± 7, 155 ± 39, and 180 ± 34 mg/dL for the Control, 6-OHDA, Dexa and 6-OHDA + Dexa groups, respectively ($n = 8–9$, $p < 0.05$ for dexamethasone-treated rats when compared with their respective 6-OHDA groups; only dexamethasone effect).

Central Administration of 6-OHDA Did Not Affect Plasma Insulin, Triacylglycerol, and Total Cholesterol Levels

To verify whether motor impairment caused by bilateral 6-OHDA administration could be associated with alteration in peripheral glucose and lipid metabolism, we evaluated the insulinemia and some circulating lipid levels. As observed in **Figures 9A,B**, rats receiving dexamethasone (Dexa and 6-OHDA + Dexa groups) exhibited an increase in plasma insulin levels compared with their respective control groups due to GC effect. Motor dysfunction induced by 6-OHDA was not associated with changes in insulinemia compared to the Control group (**Figure 9A**) and did not exacerbate the elevation in insulinemia caused by GC. In a very similar fashion, groups treated with dexamethasone showed an increase in plasma triacylglycerol levels, compared to

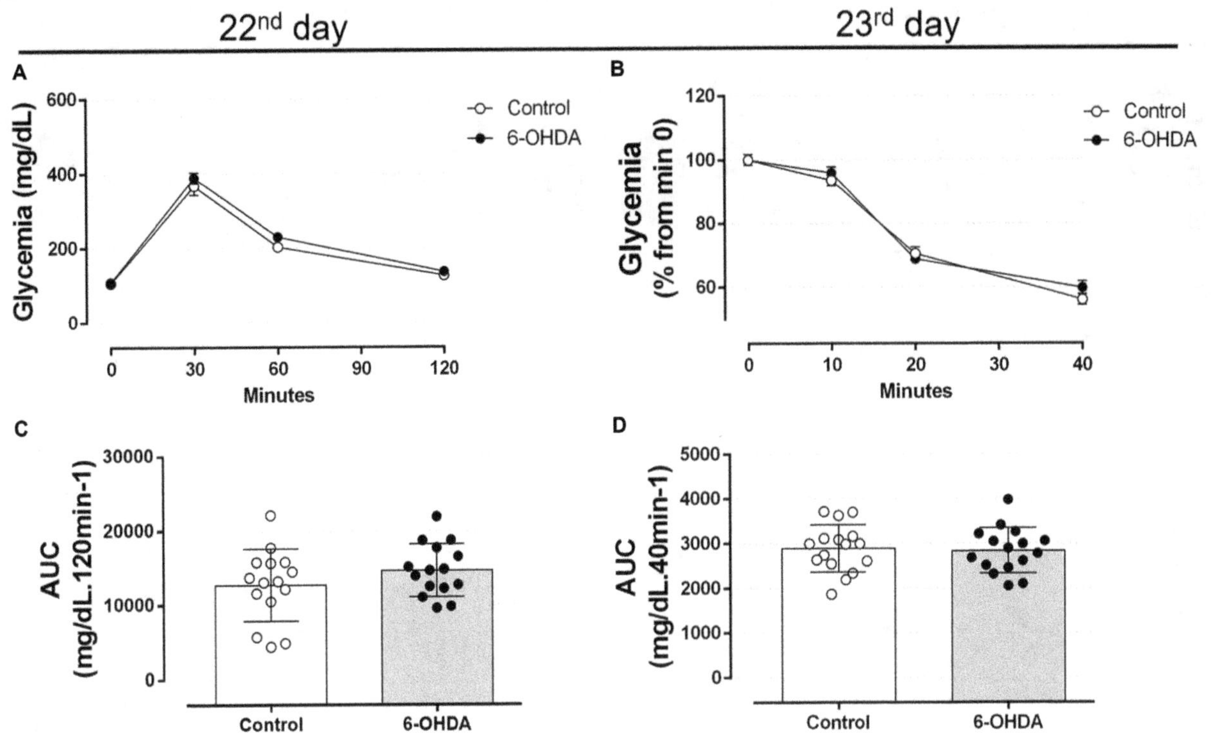

FIGURE 7 | Blood glucose values during the intraperitoneal glucose and insulin tolerance test on the 22nd and 23rd day of the experimental protocol. **(A)** Blood glucose values during the ipGTT on the 22nd day. **(B)** Blood glucose values (normalized from min 0) during the ipITT on the 23rd day. **(C)** Area-under-curve during ipGTT and **(D)** during ipITT. Data are mean ± SEM in **(A,B)**, and mean ± SD in **(C,D)** (SEM were applied only for aesthetic reasons). Ordinary two-way ANOVA with repeated measures was applied in **(A,B)**, whereas unpaired Student's t-test was applied in **(C,D)**. n = 16–17, $p < 0.05$.

their respective control groups (Control and 6-OHDA groups) (**Figure 9B**). No influence of 6-OHDA treatment *per se* was observed on this parameter. In addition, the four experimental groups evaluated did not show differences in plasma cholesterol levels (118, 108, 110, and 105 mg/dL for Control, Dexa, 6-OHDA and 6-OHDA + Dexa groups, respectively).

Central Administration of 6-OHDA Did Not Alter Hepatic Lipid and Glycogen Contents

The accumulation of ectopic lipids is a common outcome in the contexts of metabolic diseases. Thus, to verify whether treatment with 6-OHDA influenced these parameters, we collected hepatic fragments to perform biochemical and histological analyses. As illustrated in **Figures 10A,B**, central administration of 6-OHDA did not influence the content of triacylglycerol and glycogen in the liver, respectively. GC-treated groups (Dexa and 6-OHDA + Dexa groups) showed higher hepatic triacylglycerol and glycogen contents when compared with the Control and 6-OHDA groups.

The morphological analysis of the liver sections revealed a significant phenotype of glycogen deposition and microvesicle lipids distribution in both the dexamethasone-treated groups (**Table 1** and **Figures 10D,F**). Administration of 6-OHDA did not impact on lipid and glycogen content (**Table 1** and **Figure 10E**). As expected, none of the liver sections from the Control group exhibited signs of glycogen and triacylglycerol contents (**Table 1** and **Figure 10C**).

Central Administration of 6-OHDA Did Not Alter Adiposity and Metabolic Organ Masses

After perfusion and euthanasia of the animals, the relative mass of omental, epididymal, and retroperitoneal fat depots and metabolic organs were quantified. Neither 6-OHDA nor GC administration altered the visceral adiposity as observed in **Table 2**. Liver and spleen masses remained unaltered too. It was only observed a reduction in the adrenal gland mass in the 6-OHDA + Dexa group compared to the 6-OHDA group.

Central Administration of 6-OHDA Did Not Impact on Endocrine Pancreas Mass

Increase in the endocrine pancreas mass is an adaptive compensatory response to a reduction in peripheral insulin sensitivity. Thus, we evaluated whether motor dysfunction could be associated with the impairment of such expected adaptation in GC-treated rats. No differences were observed in the relative mass of the pancreas between the four groups (**Figure 11A**). The increase in the relative pancreatic islet mass caused by GC treatment was not affected by 6-OHDA treatment (**Figures 11B,D–G**). The increase of the relative mass was accompanied by a no significant increase of islet density

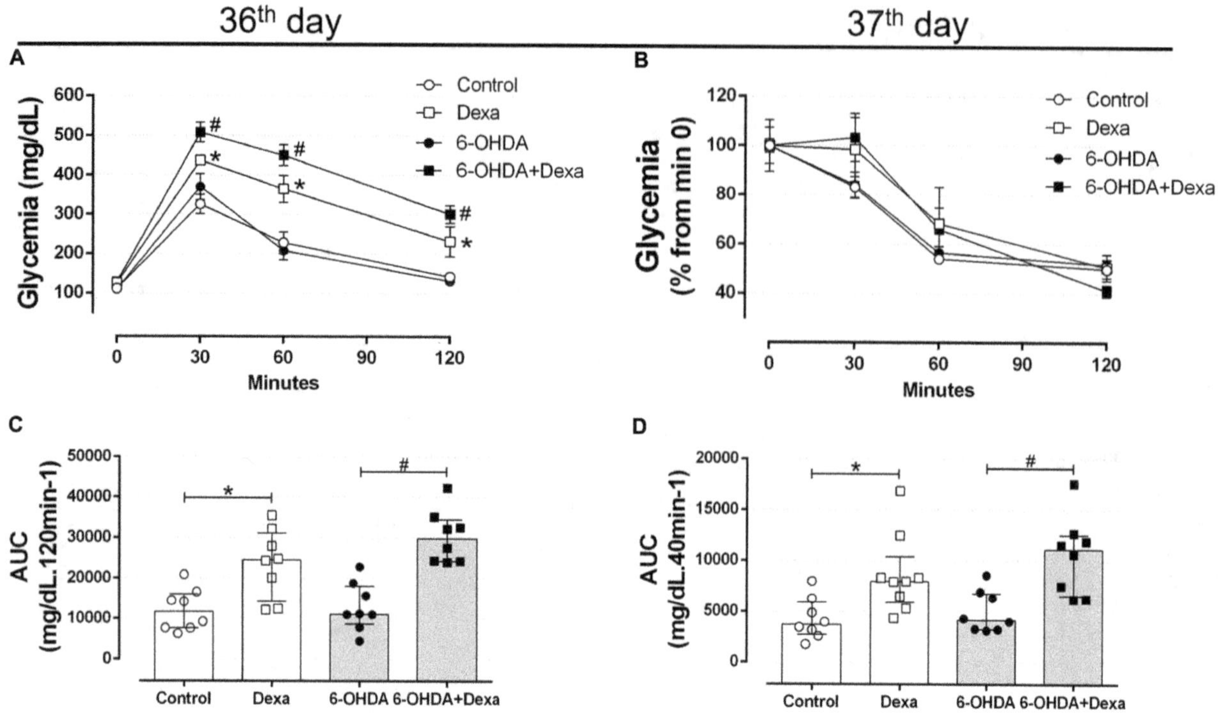

FIGURE 8 | Blood glucose values during the intraperitoneal glucose and insulin tolerance test on the 36th and 37th day of the experimental protocol. **(A)** Blood glucose values during the ipGTT on the 36th day. **(B)** Blood glucose values (normalized from min 0) during the ipITT on the 37th day. **(C)** Area-under-curve during ipGTT and **(D)** during ipITT. Data are mean ± SEM in **(A,B)** (SEM were applied only for aesthetic reasons), and median and interquartile range as they are asymmetrically distributed (nonparametric) in **(C,D)**. * and # Indicates a significant difference compared to the Control and 6-OHDA groups, respectively, using ordinary two-way ANOVA with repeated measures in **(A,B)**, or Kruskal–Wallis with Dunn's *post hoc* test in **(C,D)**. $n = 8–9$, $p < 0.05$.

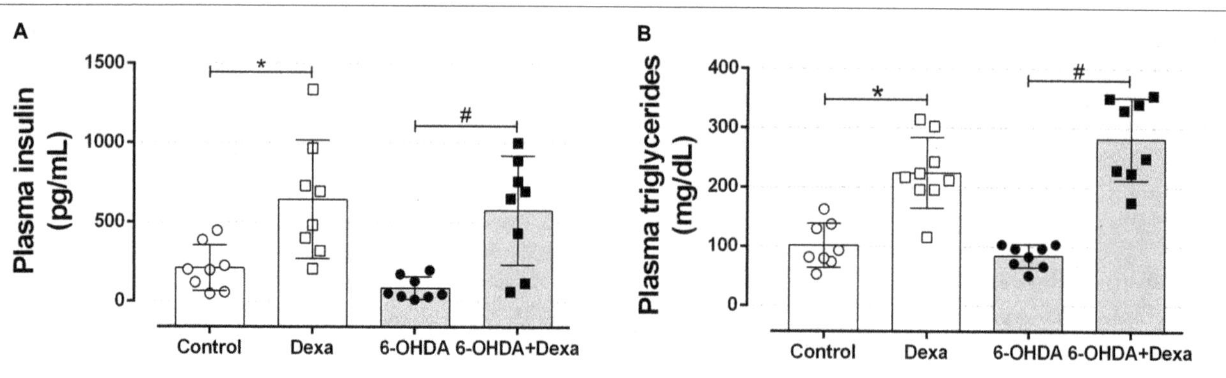

FIGURE 9 | Circulating parameters. **(A)** Plasma insulin and **(B)** triacylglycerol concentration at the day of euthanasia on the 38th day of the experimental protocol. Data are median and interquartile range as they are asymmetrically distributed (nonparametric). * and # Indicates a significant difference compared to the respective Control and 6-OHDA groups using Kruskal–Wallis with Dunn's *post hoc* test. $n = 8–9$, $p < 0.05$.

(number of islets per 1000 μm^2 of pancreas section) in the four experimental groups (**Figure 11C**).

DISCUSSION

In the present study, we investigated the impact of bilateral administration of 6-OHDA on the striatum of rats on metabolic parameters to verify whether a persistent motor dysfunction could affect the glucose and lipid homeostasis in a later period. Overall, we observed that central administration of 6-OHDA reproduced the motor dysfunction (i.e., impairment of locomotion and motor coordination) as evidenced in the open field and rotarod tests, which was persistent for the entire period of the experiment. This motor dysfunction was not associated with alteration of glucose tolerance and insulin sensitivity or circulating lipids levels and did not exacerbate the classical adverse effects of excessive GCs.

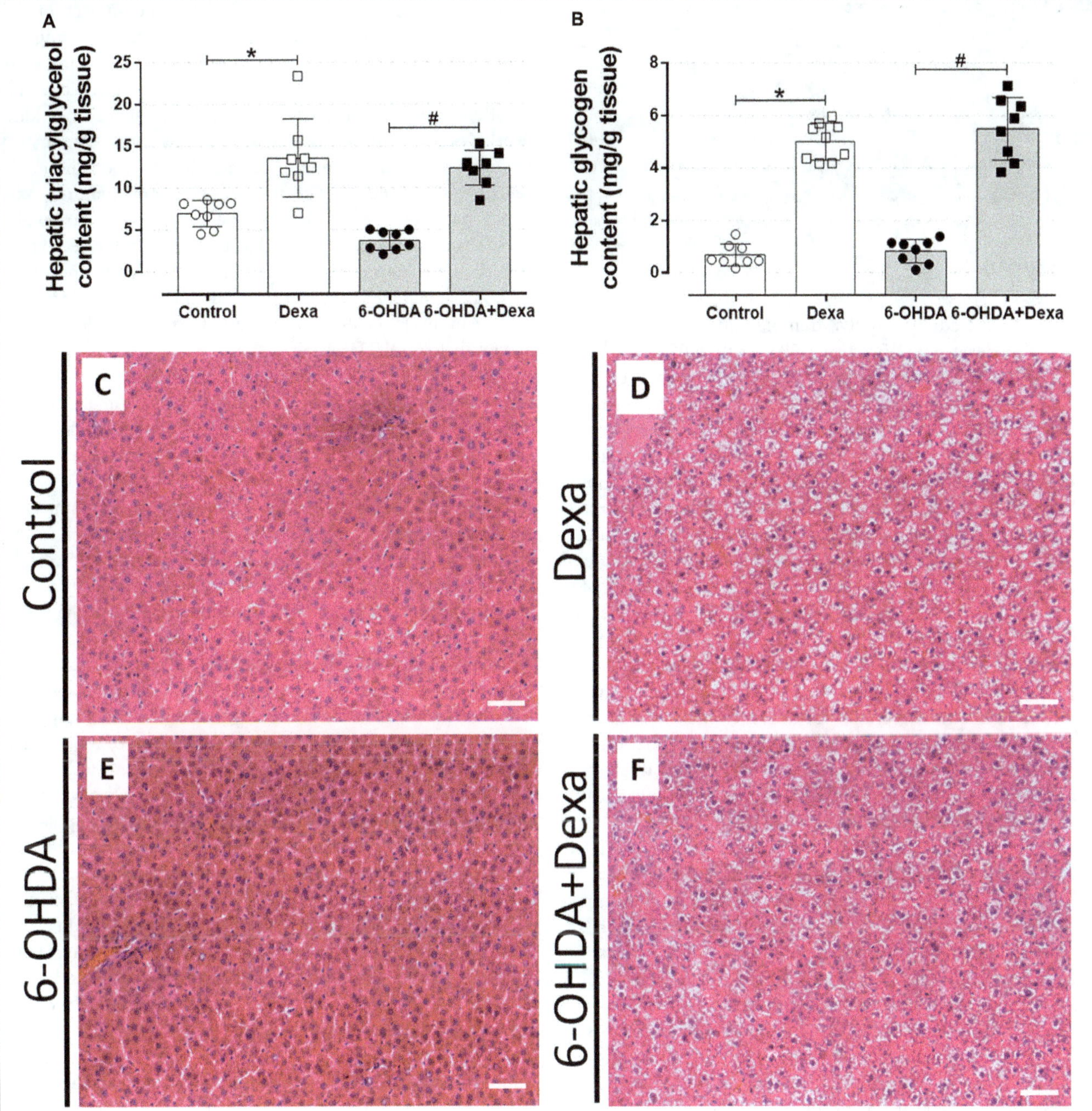

FIGURE 10 | Liver parameters. **(A)** Hepatic triacylglycerol and **(B)** glycogen content at the day of euthanasia on the 38th day of the experimental protocol. Data are mean ± SD. * and # indicate a significant difference compared to the respective Control and 6-OHDA groups using ordinary two-way ANOVA with Tukey's *post hoc* test. $n = 8–9$, $p < 0.05$. **(C–F)** Representative liver sections from all groups in 200x magnitude stained with Hematoxylin and Eosin. $n = 8–9$. Scale bar in **(C–F)** represents 25 μm.

To achieve a persistent motor dysfunction, we selected the PD rat model of bilateral 6-OHDA administration (Sauer and Oertel, 1994; Przedborski et al., 1995; Lee et al., 1996). With this approach occurs a neuronal lesion that gradually evolves from the nigrostriatal pathway, 1 day after the stereotaxic procedure, to the nigral cells, 1 week after injection, reaching the maximum degeneration between 2 and 3 weeks (Sauer and Oertel, 1994; Przedborski et al., 1995; Blandini et al., 2007). In addition, the dose of 20 μg administered in the striatum promotes a loss of dopaminergic cells varying between 20 and 85% in the SNpc region and 60–90% in the striatum region up to 2 weeks after the surgical procedure (Przedborski et al., 1995; Lee et al., 1996; Kirik et al., 1998; Blandini et al., 2007).

In human PD there is an extensive loss of dopaminergic neurons from the SNpc, resulting in a decline in dopamine concentrations of the striatum, which results in several motor

TABLE 1 | An indication of the presence of lipid and/or glycogen deposition.

	Lipids	Glycogen
Control	0/8	0/8
Dexa	8/9*	8/9*
6-OHDA	1/8	1/8
6-OHDA+Dexa	8/8#	8/8#

*Numbers indicate the presence of phenotype per total number of sections analyzed. Each section represents a different rat. * and # indicates a significant difference compared to the respective Control and 6-OHDA groups, respectively using Pearson Chi-square test, $p < 0.05$, n = 8–9.*

deficiencies including rigidity, tremor, and loss of postural reflexes (Riederer and Wuketich, 1976; Beal, 2005). In *in vivo* studies with rodents, dopaminergic loss resulting from the action of the 6-OHDA toxin and confirmation of motor impairments can be detected through analyses of motor behaviors. In our study, infusion of 6-OHDA into the dorsolateral striatum of rats resulted in motor impairment such as decreased locomotor activity at 7 and 35 days after 6-OHDA administration (**Figures 2, 3**). These results are supported by numerous previous studies. Bilateral administration of 20 μg of 6-OHDA in the dorsolateral striatum of rats promotes significant deficits in locomotor activity addressed in the open field test, 21 days after 6-OHDA administration (Matheus et al., 2016). Similarly, motor impairments were observed with unilateral administration of 10 μg of 6-OHDA in the striatum, which included a decrease in locomotion and exploratory behavior of male Wistar rats, observed 3 weeks after treatment with the 6-OHDA neurotoxin (Hegazy et al., 2017). Locomotor and exploratory deficits can also be achieved with bilateral 6-OHDA administration of 15 μg in the striatum of rats (Rampersaud et al., 2012).

In the present study, the 6-OHDA-treated rats also exhibited impaired motor coordination (**Figure 4**). This motor dysfunction is supported by several studies. For instance, the motor coordination was impaired after 1 week of unilateral 6-OHDA administration of 28 μg or bilateral 6-OHDA administration of 20 μg in rats (Monville et al., 2006; Kumar et al., 2012). These findings support our results demonstrating the validity of our experimental animal model. It is important to emphasize that 6-OHDA-lesioned rats displayed motor dysfunctions for the entire experimental protocol duration in the present study, corroborating findings from previous studies (Rampersaud et al., 2012; Matheus et al., 2016).

Although we were not searching for the impact of GC treatment on central outcomes, there is evidence suggesting that 7 days of treatment with dexamethasone (1 mg/kg b.m.) in 6-OHDA-treated mice may partially inhibit microglial activation by attenuating the production of proinflammatory cytokines (Kurkowska-Jastrzebska et al., 2004). This anti-inflammatory action of GCs could attenuate the degeneration of dopaminergic neurons in *in vivo* models of PD improving some motor deficits. In our study, no apparent attenuation that could be attributable to GCs were observed in the behavioral tests performed on the 35th day of the experimental protocol (4th day of exposure to GC). This apparent discrepancy can be explained, at least in part, because in this latter study with mouse the GC was administered previously to 6-OHDA lesion.

Murinometric data revealed no impact of 6-OHDA administration on body mass and on food intake in the present study (**Figure 5**). The nigrostriatal dopaminergic system plays an essential role in the regulation of appetite and body weight (Ungerstedt, 1971; Fibiger et al., 1973; Lénárd, 1977). In addition, there is evidence in mouse showing that hypothalamic arcuate nucleus (ARC) possesses TH-positive neurons and that these neurons play an orexigenic role in energy homeostasis (Zhang and van den Pol, 2016). Evidence obtained in animal models suggests that dopaminergic lesions greater than 95% induce adipsia and hypophagia (Ungerstedt, 1971; Sakai and Gash, 1994). However, in the present study, the animals were submitted to a lesion in the striatum that is expected to produce a slower progression of motor symptoms, which may have prevented any relevant influence on the control of food intake. Studies have shown that patients with PD tend to lose weight with disease progression, presenting a lower body weight when compared to the corresponding age-control population. Explanations for weight loss of PD patients include difficulty in chewing and swallowing, increased time required to eat, decreased olfactory and palatability, depression, and increased energy requirements intake due to muscular rigidity and involuntary movements (Beyer et al., 1995; Lorefält et al., 2006). Whether neurodegeneration in dopaminergic neurons outside striatum (i.e., hypothalamic ARC) in PD are also affected, and how much this can influence the metabolism from PD patients, is a question that merit investigation. Dayan et al. (2018) demonstrated that PD patients with symptoms of autonomic impairments exhibit disrupted thalamic-striatal-hypothalamic functional connectivity, suggesting the possible involvement

TABLE 2 | Organ masses (g/100 g body mass) on the day of euthanasia.

	Control	Dexa	6-OHDA	6-OHDA + Dexa
Omental fat	0.17[0.12;0.23]	0.17[0.16;0.24]	0.15[0.11;0.19]	0.16[0.09;0.24]
Epididymal fat	1.67[1.51;1.76]	1.85[1.48;1.87]	1.42[1.35;1.57]	1.68[1.18;2.25]
Retroperitoneal fat	1.58[1.43;2.12]	1.32[1.16;1.70]	1.38[1.12;1.53]	1.51[1.11;1.88]
Liver	4.15[3.83; 4.49]	4.92[4.24;5.05]	4.19[3.25;4.35]	4.46[4.11;4.93]
Spleen	0.18[0.16;0.19]	0.15[0.13;0.17]	0.18[0.17;0.19]	0.14[0.13;0.17]
Adrenals	0.02[0.01;0.02]	0.01[0.01;0.01]	0.02[0.01;0.02]	0.01[0.01;0.01]#

Results are expressed as a median ± interquartile range. The (#) indicates a significant difference compared to the 6-OHDA group using Kruskal–Wallis with Dunn's post hoc test. (n = 8, $p < 0.05$; see main text for a detailed description).

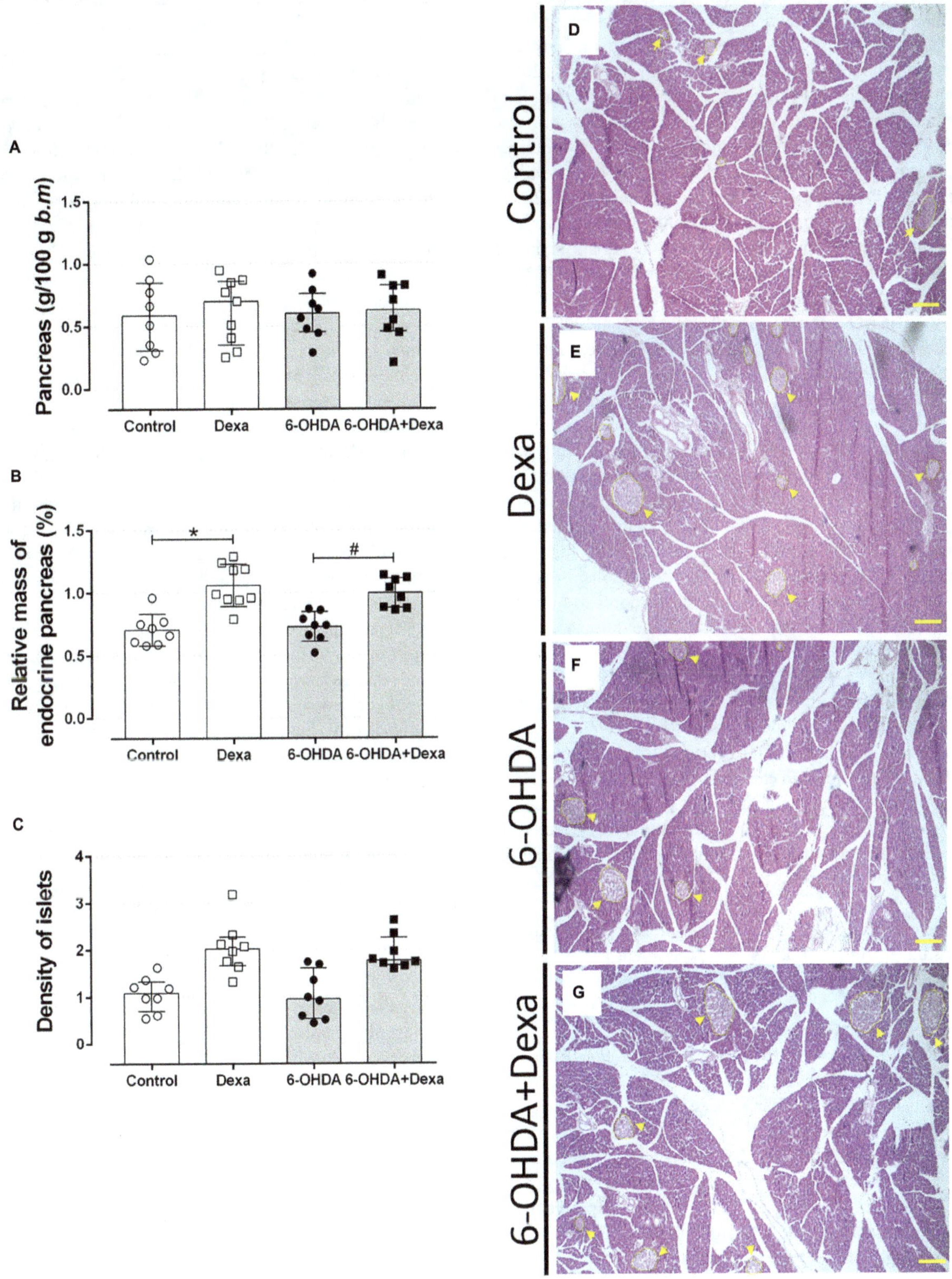

FIGURE 11 | Mass of endocrine pancreas. **(A)** The relative pancreas mass, **(B)** relative pancreatic islet mass, and **(C)** the islet density (islet number per 1000 μm^2 pancreas section) at the day of euthanasia on the 38th day of the experimental protocol. Data are mean ± SD. * and # Indicate a significant difference compared to the respective Control and 6-OHDA groups using ordinary two-way ANOVA with Tukey's *post hoc* test. n = 8–9, $p < 0.05$. **(D–G)** representative pancreas sections from all groups in 40x magnitude stained with Hematoxylin and Eosin. n = 8–9. Scale bar in **(D–G)** represents 200 μm. Yellow arrowheads are pointing to pancreatic islets.

of neural circuits that regulate autonomic function. Reduction in both body mass and food intake is a well-known adverse effect of high GC doses, as previously demonstrated in rats (Giozzet et al., 2008; dos Santos et al., 2014; Protzek et al., 2014). Numerous mechanisms by which GCs act on body mass and appetite includes: (i) suppression of osteoblastogenesis, as well as apoptosis of osteoblasts, decreasing bone density (Manolagas and Weinstein, 1999); (ii) increase of lipolysis in adipose tissue and catabolic effect on muscle tissue (Franco-Colin et al., 2000); (iii) decrease of expression of the orexigenic peptides NPY and AgRP (Liu et al., 2011); (iv) increase of circulating anorexigenic hormones insulin and leptin (Caldefie-Chézet et al., 2001; Giozzet et al., 2008; dos Santos et al., 2014; Protzek et al., 2014); and (v) by a negative water balance (Thunhorst et al., 2007).

Glucose tolerance and insulin sensitivity remained unaltered during the entire experimental protocol, despite the presence of consistent motor dysfunction caused by 6-OHDA administration (**Figures 6–8**). Some studies suggested the possible association between PD and impairment in insulin signaling. A study with rats submitted to the unilateral 6-OHDA administration of 12 μg in SNpc demonstrated an increase in serine phosphorylation of the insulin receptor substrate 2 that parallels with a depletion of dopamine (White, 2002; Morris et al., 2008). However, functional parameters reflecting the balance of glucose metabolism were not investigated by the authors. The presence of motor dysfunction caused by 6-OHDA did not exacerbate the known adverse effects of GC on glucose tolerance and insulin sensitivity in our study (**Figures 6–8**). The negative action of GC on glucose tolerance and in peripheral insulin sensitivity has been described in several clinical and preclinical studies (for a detailed review, refers to Pasieka and Rafacho, 2016). GCs treatment may alter glucose homeostasis through elevation of hepatic glucose output, reduction of skeletal muscle glucose uptake and an increase of adipose tissue lipolysis (Pasieka and Rafacho, 2016). Decreased insulin sensitivity is commonly accompanied by an increase in plasma insulin concentrations and an increase in the relative mass of pancreatic islets (Kahn et al., 1993), events observed in our GC-treated rats (**Figures 9, 11**). Although we did not evaluate the *in vivo* insulin secretion under ipGTT experiment, the suggestive insulin hypersecretion observed by our hyperinsulinemic rats was not enough to prevent glucose intolerance and this is supported by previous studies (Giozzet et al., 2008; Angelini et al., 2010; Protzek et al., 2014; dos Santos et al., 2014), an effect that was not exacerbated in 6-OHDA-treated rats.

The impairment in glucose homeostasis may be followed by an imbalance in lipid homeostasis. Consistent with the diabetogenic effects of GCs, dexamethasone-treated rats had increased levels of circulating triacylglycerides, with a parallel increase in hepatic fat content (**Figures 9B**, **10A** respectively). There is evidence demonstrating that GCs may increase circulating and hepatic triacylglycerol levels by inhibiting lipoprotein lipase in adipose tissue (Franco-Colin et al., 2000) and upregulating hepatic lipogenic enzymes (Motta et al., 2018). The presence of motor dysfunctions seemed to be innocuous on these lipidic measures. The relative masses of metabolic organs, except for the hypotrophy of adrenal gland mass in Dexa + 6-OHDA group, were unaltered and the perfusion process may have masked the visualization of these changes since these parenchymas retained fixative solution used for the perfusion procedure.

One of the limitations of our study resides in the fact that we did not appreciate the TH distribution or quantification by immunohistochemistry or western blot experiments, respectively. However, there is evidence for a sustained lesion in the striatum and in the SNpc up to 8 weeks after unilateral (Perlbarg et al., 2018) or bilateral (Oliveira et al., 2017; Fernandes-Junior et al., 2018) administration of 6-OHDA in rats. No motor function parameters were evaluated in these aforementioned studies demonstrating that not all studies include both analyses (motor analysis and TH immunostaining) to confirm the effectiveness of 6-OHDA administration.

The relationship between neurodegeneration and metabolic outcomes are complex and is difficult to predict which comes first. This crosstalk is influenced by numerous factors, which turn difficult to precisely define the causal factor(s). For instance, there is evidence linking the severity of neurodegeneration caused by 6-OHDA with a previous metabolic status (i.e., diet-induced obesity) in rats (Morris et al., 2010). Similarly, there is also evidence linking the inflammation of hypothalamus triggered by Aβ oligomers infusion with posterior disruption of metabolic homeostasis (Clarke et al., 2015), suggesting a relationship between central and peripheral components. With our current experimental design, we defined the independent factor (treatment with 6-OHDA) and then considered all metabolic outcomes as dependent variables, and by doing this we tried to isolate as much as possible the causal factor.

Recent evidence demonstrated the relationship between metabolic disorders and consequent negative prognostic for PD. For instance, coexistence of T2DM with PD lead to a faster motor progression and cognitive decline (Pagano et al., 2018) as well as reduction in the baseline dopamine transport availability in the caudate and ventral striatum, cortical thinning in the inferomedial temporal lobe that is also associated with reduced cognitive performances (Chung et al., 2018) when compared to patient with only PD. In addition, the content of the tau and α-synuclein in the cerebrospinal fluid is higher in patients with both PD and T2DM in relation to patients only with PD, and these markers are already upregulated in T2DM patients compared with healthy controls (Pagano et al., 2018), indicating a relationship between PD-pathology markers and T2DM. This mutual relationship is reinforced when considering the benefits of some antidiabetic drugs (i.e., agonists of glucagon-like peptide-1 receptor and inhibitors of dipeptidyl peptidase-4) exerts on the neurodegenerative process in patients with PD (Ashraghi et al., 2016).

A recent study conducted by Ter Horst et al. (2018) revealed that bilateral deep brain stimulation targeting the border of the nucleus accumbens (NAc) core and ventral anterior limb of the internal capsule ameliorates some metabolic aspects of patients with diabetes (i.e., improves the peripheral insulin sensitivity). This study also demonstrated that pharmacological dopamine deletion decreases insulin sensitivity, whereas optogenetic activation of NAc dopaminergic-receptor-1 neurons improves glucose tolerance in mice, suggesting that striatal dopamine signaling plays a role in glucose metabolism.

CONCLUSION

Our findings let us conclude that bilateral 6-OHDA administration in the dorsolateral striatum causes sustained motor impairments with no impact on glucose and lipid homeostasis and does not exacerbate the adverse effects caused by excess GC in glucose and lipid metabolism. These observations suggest that on this two-way road between PD and peripheral metabolism, it is probable that dopaminergic circuit dysfunction has a minor impact on metabolic outcomes.

AUTHOR CONTRIBUTIONS

AR, EM, FG, and RP contributed to the experimental design. FG, FdS, MB, and RF conducted the experiments. AR and FG contributed with analytic tools and data analysis, performed the data collection, and wrote up the manuscript. AR, DZ, and RP supplied reagents and materials. AR, EM, and FG contributed to the discussion of the experimental findings. All authors read and approved the manuscript's final format.

ACKNOWLEDGMENTS

The authors would like to thank the technical assistance of the Chronic Diseases Research Laboratory (LIDoC) and Multiuser Laboratory of Studies in Biology (LAMEB) staff for the technical assistance.

REFERENCES

Angelini, N., Rafacho, A., Boschero, A. C., and Bosqueiro, J. R. (2010). Involvement of the cholinergic pathway in glucocorticoid-induced hyperinsulinemia in rats. *Diabetes Res. Clin. Pract.* 87, 184–191. doi: 10.1016/j.diabres.2009.11.008

Ashraghi, M. R., Pagano, G., Polychronis, S., Niccolini, F., and Politis, M. (2016). Parkinson's disease, diabetes and cognitive impairment. *Recent. Pat. Endocr. Metab. Immune Drug Discov.* 10, 11–21. doi: 10.2174/1872214810999160628105549

Beal, M. F. (2005). Mitochondria take center stage in aging and neurodegeneration. *Ann. Neurol.* 58, 495–505. doi: 10.1002/ana.20624

Becker, C., Brobert, G. P., Johansson, S., Jick, S. S., and Meier, C. R. (2008). Diabetes in patients with idiopathic Parkinson's disease. *Diabetes Care* 31, 1808–1812. doi: 10.2337/dc08-0479

Beyer, P. L., Palarino, M. Y., Michalek, D., Busenbark, K., and Koller, W. C. (1995). Weight change and body composition in patients with Parkinson's disease. *J. Am. Diet. Assoc.* 95, 979–983. doi: 10.1016/S0002-8223(95)00269-3

Blandini, F., Armentero, M. T., and Martignoni, E. (2008). The 6-hydroxydopamine model: news from the past. *Parkinsonism Relat. Disord.* 14(Suppl. 2), 124–129. doi: 10.1016/j.parkreldis.2008.04.015

Blandini, F., Levandis, G., Bazzini, E., Nappi, G., and Armentero, M. T. (2007). Time-course of nigrostriatal damage, basal ganglia metabolic changes and behavioural alterations following intrastriatal injection of 6-hydroxydopamine in the rat: new clues from an old model. *Eur. J. Neurosci.* 25, 397–405. doi: 10.1111/j.1460-9568.2006.05285.x

Caldefie-Chézet, F., Moinard, C., Minet-Quinard, R., Gachon, F., Cynober, L., and Vasson, M. (2001). Dexamethasone treatment induces long-lasting hyperleptinemia and anorexia in old rats. *Metabolism* 50, 1054–1058. doi: 10.1053/meta.2001.2580

Chung, S. J., Jeon, S., Yoo, H. S., Kim, G., Oh, J. S., Kim, J. S., et al. (2018). Detrimental effect of type 2 diabetes mellitus in a large case series of Parkinson's disease. *Parkinsonism Relat. Disord.* doi: 10.1016/j.parkreldis.2018.08.023 [Epub ahead of print].

Clarke, J. R., Lyra, E., Silva, N. M., Figueiredo, C. P., Frozza, R. L., Ledo, J. H., et al. (2015). Alzheimer-associated Ab oligomers impact the central nervous system to induce peripheral metabolic deregulation. *EMBO Mol. Med.* 7, 190–210. doi: 10.15252/emmm.201404183

Dayan, E., Sklerov, M., and Browner, N. (2018). Disrupted hypothalamic functional connectivity in patients with PD and autonomic dysfunction. *Neurology* 90, 2051–2058. doi: 10.1212/WNL.0000000000005641

dos Santos, C., Ferreira, F. B., Gonçalves-Neto, L. M., Taboga, S. R., Boschero, A. C., and Rafacho, A. (2014). Age- and gender-related changes in glucose homeostasis in glucocorticoid-treated rats. *Can. J. Physiol. Pharmacol.* 92, 867–878. doi: 10.1139/cjpp-2014-0259

Fernandes-Junior, S. A., Carvalho, K. S., Moreira, T. S., and Takakura, A. C. (2018). Correlation between neuroanatomical and functional respiratory changes observed in an experimental model of Parkinson's disease. *Exp. Physiol.* 103, 1377–1389. doi: 10.1113/EP086987

Fibiger, H. C., Zis, A. P., and Mcgeer, E. G. (1973). Feeding and drinking deficits after 6-hydroxydopamine administration in the rat: similarities to the lateral hypothalamic syndrome. *Brain Res.* 55, 135–148. doi: 10.1016/0006-8993(73)90493-9

Franco-Colin, M., Tellez-Lopez, A. M., Quevedo-Corona, L., and Racotta, R. (2000). Effects of long-term high-sucrose and dexamethasone on fat depots, liver fat, and lipid fuel fluxes through the retroperitoneal adipose tissue and splanchnic area in rats. *Metabolism* 49, 1289–1294. doi: 10.1053/meta.2000.9522

Giozzet, V. A. G., Rafacho, A., Boschero, A. C., Carneiro, E. M., and Bosqueiro, J. R. (2008). Dexamethasone treatment in vivo counteracts the functional pancreatic islet alterations caused by malnourishment in rats. *Metabolism* 57, 617–624. doi: 10.1016/j.metabol.2007.12.004

Goldman, S. M. (2010). Trichloroethylene and Parkinson's disease: dissolving the puzzle. *Expert Rev. Neurother.* 10, 835–837. doi: 10.1586/ern.10.61

Gonçalves-Neto, L. M., Ferreira, F. B., Souza, L., dos Santos, C., Boschero, A. C., Facundo, V. A., et al. (2014). Disruption of glucose tolerance caused by glucocorticoid excess in rats is partially prevented, but not attenuated, by arjunolic acid. *Indian J. Exp. Biol.* 52, 972–982.

Gorell, J. M., Johnson, C. C., Rybicki, B. A., Peterson, E. L., Kortsha, G. X., Brown, G. G., et al. (1997). Occupational exposures to metals as risk factors for Parkinson's disease. *Neurology* 48, 650–658. doi: 10.1212/WNL.48.3.650

Hegazy, M. A., Maklad, H. M., Samy, D. M., Abdelmonsif, D. A., El Sabaa, B. M., and Elnozahy, F. Y. (2017). Cerium oxide nanoparticles could ameliorate behavioral andneurochemical impairments in 6-hydroxydopamine induced Parkinson's disease in rats. *Neurochem. Int.* 108, 361–371. doi: 10.1016/j.neuint.2017.05.011

Hu, G., Jousilahti, P., Bidel, S., Antikainen, R., and Tuomilehto, J. (2007). Type 2 diabetes and the risk of Parkinson's disease. *Diabetes Care* 30, 842–847. doi: 10.2337/dc06-2011

Jackson-Lewis, V., Blesa, J., and Przedborski, S. (2012). Animal models of Parkinson's disease. *Parkinsonism Relat. Disord.* 18, 183–185. doi: 10.1016/S1353-8020(11)70057-8

Kahn, S. E., Prigeon, R. L., McCulloch, D. K., Boyko, E. J., Bergman, R. N., Schwartz, M. W., et al. (1993). Quantification of the relationship between insulin sensitivity and beta-cell function in human subjects. Evidence for a hyperbolic function. *Diabetes* 42, 1663–1672. doi: 10.2337/diab.42.11.1663

Kirik, D., Rosenblad, C., and Bjorklund, A. (1998). Characterization of behavioral and neurodegenerative changes following partial lesions of the nigrostriatal dopamine system induced by intrastriatal 6-hydroxydopamine in the rat. *Exp. Neurol.* 152, 259–277. doi: 10.1006/exnr.1998.6848

Klimek, P., Kautzky-Willer, A., Chmiel, A., Schiller-Frühwirth, I., and Thurner, S. (2015). Quantification of diabetes comorbidity risks across life using nation-wide big claims data. *PLoS Comput. Biol.* 11:1004125. doi: 10.1371/journal.pcbi.1004125

Kumar, A., Sharma, N., Gupta, A., Kalonia, H., and Mishra, J. (2012). Neuroprotective potential of atorvastatin and simvastatin (HMG-CoA reductase inhibitors) against 6-hydroxydopamine (6-OHDA) induced Parkinson-like symptoms. *Brain Res.* 1471, 13–22. doi: 10.1016/j.brainres.2012.06.050

Kurkowska-Jastrzebska, I., Litwin, T., Joniec, I., Ciesielska, A., Przybyłkowski, A., Członkowski, A., et al. (2004). Dexamethasone protects against dopaminergic neurons damage in a mouse model of Parkinson's disease. *Int. Immunopharmacol.* 4, 1307–1318. doi: 10.1016/j.intimp.2004.05.006

Lee, C. S., Sauer, H., and Bjorklund, A. (1996). Dopaminergic neuronal degeneration and motor impairments following axon terminal lesion by instrastriatal 6-hydroxydopamine in the rat. *Neuroscience* 72, 641–653. doi: 10.1016/j.brainres.2009.03.026

Lénárd, L. (1977). Sex-dependent body weight loss after bilateral 6-hydroxydopamine injection into the globus pallidus. *Brain Res.* 128, 559–568. doi: 10.1016/0006-8993(77)90183-4

Liu, X. Y., Shi, J. H., Du, W. H., Fan, Y. P., Hu, X. L., Zhang, C. C., et al. (2011). Glucocorticoids decrease body weight and food intake and inhibit appetite regulatory peptide expression in the hypothalamus of rat. *Exp. Ther. Med.* 2, 977–984. doi: 10.3892/etm.2011.292

Lorefält, B., Ganowiak, W., Wissing, U., Granérus, A. K., and Unosson, M. (2006). Food habits and intake of nutrients in elderly patients with Parkinson's disease. *Gerontology* 52, 160–168. doi: 10.1159/000091825

Manolagas, S. C., and Weinstein, R. S. (1999). New developments in the pathogenesis and treatment of steroid-induced osteoporosis. *J. Bone Miner. Res.* 14, 1061–1066. doi: 10.1359/jbmr.1999.14.7.1061

Marttila, R. J., Arstila, P., Nikoskelainen, J., Halonen, P. E., and Rinne, U. K. (1977). Viral antibodies in the sera from patients with Parkinson disease. *Eur. Neurol.* 15, 25–33. doi: 10.1159/000114785

Matheus, F. C., Rial, D., Real, J. I., Lemos, C., Ben, J., Guaita, G. O., et al. (2016). Decreased synaptic plasticity in the medial prefrontal cortex underlies short-term memory deficits in 6-OHDA-lesioned rats. *Behav. Brain Res.* 301, 43–54. doi: 10.1016/j.bbr.2015.12.011

Mattson, M. P. (2003). Will caloric restriction and folate protect against AD and PD? *Neurology* 60, 690–695. doi: 10.1212/01.WNL.0000042785.02850.11

Monville, C., Torres, E. M., and Dunnett, S. B. (2006). Comparison of incremental and accelerating protocols of the rotarod test for the assessment of motor deficits in the 6-OHDA model. *J. Neurosci. Methods* 158, 219–223. doi: 10.1016/j.jneumeth.2006.06.001

Morris, J. K., Bomhoff, G. L., Stanford, J. A., and Geiger, P. C. (2010). Neurodegeneration in an animal model of Parkinson's disease is exacerbated by a high-fat diet. *Am. J. Physiol. Regul. Integr. Comp. Physiol.* 299, 1082–1090. doi: 10.1152/ajpregu.00449.2010

Morris, J. K., Zhang, H., Gupte, A. A., Bomhoff, G. L., Stanford, J. A., and Geiger, P. C. (2008). Measures of striatal insulin resistance in a 6-hydroxydopamine model of Parkinson's disease. *Brain Res.* 1240, 185–195. doi: 10.1016/j.brainres.2008.08.089

Motta, K., Barbosa, A. M., Bobinski, F., Boschero, A. C., and Rafacho, A. (2015). JNK and IKKβ phosphorylation is reduced by glucocorticoids in adipose tissue from insulin-resistant rats. *J. Steroid Biochem. Mol. Biol.* 145, 1–12. doi: 10.1016/j.jsbmb.2014.09.024

Motta, K., Gomes, P. R. L., Sulis, P. M., Bordin, S., and Rafacho, A. (2018). Dexamethasone Administration During Late Gestation Has No Major Impact on Lipid Metabolism, but Reduces Newborn Survival Rate in Wistar Rats. *Front. Physiol.* 9:783. doi: 10.3389/fphys.2018.00783

Oliveira, L. M., Tuppy, M., Moreira, T. S., and Takakura, A. C. (2017). Role of the locus coeruleus catecholaminergic neurons in the chemosensory control of breathing in a Parkinson's disease model. *Exp. Neurol.* 293, 172–180. doi: 10.1016/j.expneurol.2017.04.006

Pagano, G., Polychronis, S., Wilson, H., Giordano, B., Ferrara, N., Niccolini, F., et al. (2018). Diabetes mellitus and Parkinson disease. *Neurology* 90, e1654–e1662. doi: 10.1212/WNL.0000000000005475

Pasieka, A. M., and Rafacho, A. (2016). Impact of glucocorticoid excess on glucose tolerance: clinical and preclinical evidence. *Metabolites* 6, 1–24. doi: 10.3390/metabo6030024

Paxinos, G., and Watson, C. (1997). *The Rat Brain in Stereotaxic Coordinates*, 3rd Edn. Amsterdam. Elsevier.

Pearce, J. M. (1989). Aspects of the history of Parkinson's disease. *J. Neurol. Neurosurg. Psychiatry* 52(Suppl.), 6–10. doi: 10.1136/jnnp.52.Suppl.6

Perlbarg, V., Lambert, J., Butler, B., Felfli, M., Valabrègue, R., Privat, A. L., et al. (2018). Alterations of the nigrostriatal pathway in a 6-OHDA rat model of Parkinson's disease evaluated with multimodal MRI. *PLoS One* 13:0202597. doi: 10.1371/journal.pone.0202597

Pressley, J. C., Louis, E. D., Tang, M. X., Cote, L., Cohen, P. D., Glied, S., et al. (2003). The impact of comorbid disease and injuries on resource use and expenditures in parkinsonism. *Neurology* 60, 87–93. doi: 10.1212/WNL.60.1.87

Protzek, A. O., Costa-Júnior, J. M., Rezende, L. F., Santos, G. J., Araújo, T. G., Vettorazzi, J. F., et al. (2014). Augmented β-cell function and mass in glucocorticoid-treated rodents are associated with increased islet Ir-β /AKT/mTOR and decreased AMPK/ACC and AS160 signaling. *Int. J. Endocrinol.* 2014:983453. doi: 10.1155/2014/983453

Protzek, A. O., Rezende, L. F., Costa-Júnior, J. M., Ferreira, S. M., Cappelli, A. P., de Paula, F. M., et al. (2016). Hyperinsulinemia caused by dexamethasone treatment is associated with reduced insulin clearance and lower hepatic activity of insulin-degrading enzyme. *J. Steroid Biochem. Mol. Biol.* 155, 1–8. doi: 10.1016/j.jsbmb.2015.09.020

Przedborski, S., Levivier, M., Jiang, H., Ferreira, M., Jackson-Lewis, V., Donaldson, D., et al. (1995). Dose-dependent lesions of the dopaminergic nigrostriatal pathway induced by intrastriatal injection of 6-hydroxydopamine. *Neuroscience* 67, 631–647. doi: 10.1016/0306-4522(95)00066-R

Rafacho, A., Gonçalves-Neto, L. M., Santos-Silva, J. C., Alonso-Magdalena, P., Merino, B., Taboga, R., et al. (2014). Pancreatic alpha-cell dysfunction contributes to the disruption of glucose homeostasis and compensatory insulin hypersecretion in glucocorticoid-treated rats. *PLoS One* 9:93531. doi: 10.1371/journal.pone.0093531

Rampersaud, N., Harkavyi, A., Giordano, G., Lever, R., Whitton, J., and Whitton, P. S. (2012). Exendin-4 reverses biochemical and behavioral deficits in a pre-motor 5 rodent model of Parkinson's disease with combined noradrenergic and serotonergic 6 lesions. *Neuropeptides* 46, 183–193. doi: 10.1016/j.npep.2012.07.004

Riederer, P., and Wuketich, S. (1976). Time course of nigrostriatal degeneration in parkinson's disease. A detailed study of influential factors in human brain amine analysis. *J. Neural Transm.* 38, 277–301. doi: 10.1007/BF01249445

Sakai, K., and Gash, D. M. (1994). Effect of bilateral 6-OHDA lesions of the substantia nigra on locomotor activity in the rat. *Brain Res.* 633, 144–150. doi: 10.1016/0006-8993(94)91533-4

Sauer, H., and Oertel, W. H. (1994). Progressive degeneration of nigrostriatal dopamine neurons following intrastriatal terminal lesions with 6-hydroxydopamine: a combined retrograde tracing and immunocytochemical study in the rat. *Neuroscience* 59, 401–415. doi: 10.1016/0306-4522(94)90605-X

Schapira, A. H. (2009). Neurobiology and treatment of Parkinson's disease. *Trends Pharmacol. Sci.* 30, 41–47. doi: 10.1016/j.tips.2008.10.005

Scigliano, G., Musicco, M., Soliverim, P., Piccolom, I., Ronchettim, G., and Girottim, F. (2006). Reduced risk factors for vascular disorders in Parkinson disease patients: a casecontrol study. *Stroke* 37, 1184–1188. doi: 10.1161/01.STR.0000217384.03237.9c

Simon, K. C., Chen, H., Schwarzschild, M., and Ascherio, A. (2007). Hypertension, hypercholesterolemia, diabetes, and the risk of Parkinson disease. *Neurology* 69, 1688–1695. doi: 10.1212/01.wnl.0000271883.45010.8a

Steenland, K., Hein, M. J., Cassinelli, R. T., Prince, M. M., Nilsen, N. B., Whelan, E. A., et al. (2006). Polychlorinated biphenyls and neurodegenerative disease mortality in an occupational cohort. *Epidemiology* 17, 8–13. doi: 10.1097/01.ede.0000190707.51536.2b

Stern, M. B., Lang, A., and Poewe, W. (2012). Toward a redefinition of Parkinson's disease. *Mov. Disord.* 27, 54–60. doi: 10.1002/mds.24051

Ter Horst, K. W., Lammers, N. M., Trinko, R., Opland, D. M., Figee, M., Ackermans, M. T., et al. (2018). Striatal dopamine regulates systemic glucose metabolism in humans and mice. *Sci. Transl. Med.* 10:eaar3752. doi: 10.1126/scitranslmed.aar3752

Thunhorst, R. L., Beltz, T. G., and Johnson, A. K. (2007). Glucocorticoids increase salt appetite by promoting water and sodium excretion. *Am. J. Physiol. Regul. Integr. Comp. Physiol.* 293, 1444–1451. doi: 10.1152/ajpregu.00294.2007

Ungerstedt, U. (1968). 6-hydroxy-dopamine induced degeneration of central monoamine neurons. *Eur. J Pharmacol.* 5, 107–110. doi: 10.1016/0014-2999(68)90164-7

Ungerstedt, U. (1971). Adipsia and aphagia after 6-hydroxydopamine induced degeneration of the nigrostriatal dopamind system. *Acta Physiol. Stand. Suppl.* 367, 95–122. doi: 10.1111/j.1365-201X.1971.tb11001.x

White, M. F. (2002). IRS proteins and the common path to diabetes. *Am. J. Physiol.* 283, 413–422. doi: 10.1152/ajpendo.00514.2001

Zhang, X., and van den Pol, A. N. (2016). Hypothalamic arcuate nucleus tyrosine hydroxylase neurons play orexigenic role in energy homeostasis. *Nat. Neurosci.* 19, 1341–1347. doi: 10.1038/nn.4372

10

Deep Brain Stimulation for Obesity: A Review and Future Directions

Douglas A. Formolo[1,2], *Joana M. Gaspar*[3,4], *Hiago M. Melo*[1,2], *Tuany Eichwald*[3,4], *Ramiro Javier Zepeda*[5], *Alexandra Latini*[3,4], *Michael S. Okun*[6] *and Roger Walz*[1,2,6,7,8]*

[1] *Center for Applied Neuroscience, University Hospital, Federal University of Santa Catarina, Florianópolis, Brazil,* [2] *Graduate Program in Neuroscience, Federal University of Santa Catarina, Florianópolis, Brazil,* [3] *Laboratory of Bioenergetics and Oxidative Stress, Department of Biochemistry, Federal University of Santa Catarina, Florianópolis, Brazil,* [4] *Graduate Program in Biochemistry, Department of Biochemistry, Federal University of Santa Catarina, Florianópolis, Brazil,* [5] *Department of Neuroscience, Faculty of Medicine, Chile University and Health Science Institute, O'Higgins University, Santiago, Chile,* [6] *Fixel Institute for Neurological Diseases, Department of Neurology, University of Florida, Gainesville, FL, United States,* [7] *Graduate Program in Medical Sciences, Federal University of Santa Catarina, Florianópolis, Brazil,* [8] *Department of Internal Medicine, University Hospital, Federal University of Santa Catarina, Florianópolis, Brazil*

Correspondence:
Roger Walz
rogerwalz@hotmail.com

The global prevalence of obesity has been steadily increasing. Although pharmacotherapy and bariatric surgeries can be useful adjuvants in the treatment of morbid obesity, they may lose long-term effectiveness. Obesity result largely from unbalanced energy homeostasis. Palatable and densely caloric foods may affect the brain overlapped circuits involved with homeostatic hypothalamus and hedonic feeding. Deep brain stimulation (DBS) consists of delivering electrical impulses to specific brain targets to modulate a disturbed neuronal network. In selected patients, DBS has been shown to be safe and effective for movement disorders. We review all the cases reports and series of patients treated with DBS for obesity using a PubMed search and will address the following obesity-related issues: (i) the hypothalamic regulation of homeostatic feeding; (ii) the reward mesolimbic circuit and hedonic feeding; (iii) basic concepts of DBS as well as the rationale for obesity treatment; (iv) perspectives and challenges in obesity DBS. The small number of cases provides preliminary evidence for the safety and the tolerability of a potential DBS approach. The ventromedial (n = 2) and lateral (n = 8) hypothalamic nuclei targets have shown mixed and disappointing outcomes. Although nucleus accumbens (n = 7) targets were more encouraging for the outcomes of body weight reduction and behavioral control for eating, there was one suicide reported after 27 months of follow-up. The authors did not attribute the suicide to DBS therapy. The identification of optimal brain targets, appropriate programming strategies and the development of novel technologies will be important as next steps to move DBS closer to a clinical application. The identification of electrical control signals may provide an opportunity for closed-loop adaptive DBS systems to address obesity. Metabolic and hormonal sensors such as glycemic levels, leptin, and ghrelin levels are candidate control signals for DBS. Focused excitation or alternatively inhibition of regions of the hypothalamus may provide better outcomes compared to non-selective DBS. Utilization of the NA delta oscillation or other physiological markers from one or multiple regions in obesity-related brain network is a promising approach. Experienced multidisciplinary team will be critical to improve the risk-benefit ratio for this approach.

Keywords: obesity, deep brain stimulation, hypothalamus, nucleus accumbens, metabolic disorders, neuroinflammation

INTRODUCTION

According to the World Health Organization (WHO), obesity is defined as an abnormal and excessive fat accumulation. The increase in fat mass is a major health problem and is a risk factor for the development of several metabolic complications. Obesity decreases the quality of life and decreases life expectancy. The incidence of obesity has continued to rise rapidly during the last several decades. Similarly, the prevalence of obesity has been rising in most countries worldwide, and its prevalence has doubled in more than seventy countries over the last four decades. It was estimated that in 2015 there were a total of 603.7 million obese adults (body mass index [BMI] > 30 kg/m^2) and 107.7 million obese children (defined as a BMI at or above the 95th percentile). Approximately 1.9 billion adults are by definition overweight (BMI > 25 kg/m^2) (Gonzalez-Muniesa et al., 2017). The rising prevalence of obesity has been associated with a higher incidence of chronic metabolic disorders including type 2 diabetes. Both diseases share similar features including early cognitive dysfunction and a substantial socio-economic impact (Gaspar et al., 2016; Remor et al., 2018).

The etiology of obesity results from a complex interaction of several factors, including socioeconomic status, genetics, epigenetics, cultural features, and lifestyle. The obesity problem is even more complex with a link to compulsive eating behaviors and to depression (Val-Laillet et al., 2015; Ivezaj et al., 2016). Although no cause-and-effect relationship has been conclusively established, a systematic review revealed that obesity and depression had a significant and bidirectional association. The association with anxiety was modest but potentially important (Rajan and Menon, 2017). Despite its multifactorial etiology, a general consensus has emerged that the majority of obesity cases result from the combination of an increase in food intake along with a decrease in energy expenditure which together results in excessive fat accumulation. In most cases, obesity is a preventable disease and is largely dependent on lifestyle. Living a healthy lifestyle has recently become more of a challenge with elevated levels of stress, reduction of physical activity and the availability of palatable foods that are high in sugar, fat, and calories. The increased availability of an energy-dense diet, high in saturated fat and sugar, has been strongly associated with weight gain and increased adiposity, precipitating a strong change in energy balance not only resulting from a simple increase in energy intake (McClelland et al., 2013).

The palatable and densely caloric foods affect brain circuits involved with the control of energy metabolism in the hypothalamus and those involved with reward and humor perception within the limbic system. In predisposed, individuals this combination may result in overeating patterns and manifest as a "food addiction" or "food abuse." This phenomenon can increase the difficulty in achieving a long-term successful reduction of caloric intake by non-pharmacological and pharmacological approaches. This phenomenon has also increased the challenges of bariatric surgery for individuals with morbid obesity (Stice et al., 2013). Additionally, genetic factors might contribute to vulnerability to weight gain that, in combination with the environment precipitants result in brain network changes. This may reinforce the desire for food intake even if this desire is incongruent with the aspiration to reduce weight (Horstmann, 2017). Neuromodulation for the regulation of homeostatic and hedonic feeding has been suggested as a potential approach.

We review all the cases reports and series of patients treated with DBS for obesity using a PubMed search and will address the following obesity-related issues: (i) the hypothalamic regulation of homeostatic feeding; (ii) the reward mesolimbic circuit and hedonic feeding; (iii) basic concepts of DBS as well as the rationale for obesity treatment; (iv) perspectives and challenges in obesity DBS.

HYPOTHALAMUS, HOMEOSTATIC FEEDING, AND OBESITY

Homeostatic feeding is necessary for basic metabolic processes and survival (Rossi and Stuber, 2018). Energy homeostasis which is defined as a balance between food intake and energy expenditure is regulated primarily by the hypothalamus. The hypothalamus regulates food intake and energy expenditure but also regulates peripheral glucose and lipid homeostasis as well as metabolism (Morton et al., 2014; Timper and Bruning, 2017).

The discovery of the hypothalamus as a key center for energy homeostasis had its genesis with the studies of Hetherington and Ranson (1940) which revealed that adiposity increased in rats with hypothalamic lesions. Additionally, the discovery of leptin in 1996, by Zhang et al. (1994) opened new pathways for the molecular understanding of the role of the hypothalamus in the regulation of food intake and energy expenditure.

The **Figure 1** shows the interconnected hypothalamic nuclei, including the arcuate nucleus (ARC), the paraventricular nucleus (PVN), the ventromedial nucleus (VMN), the dorsomedial nucleus, and the lateral hypothalamic area (LHA) in both the healthy and the obesity state. Due to its privileged anatomical location, ARC is the principal region to receive and to sense afferent signals (nutrients and hormones) from the gut and the brainstem, as well as the region that processes efferent signals capable of modulating both food intake and energy expenditure. Two well-defined neuronal populations within the ARC have been described and each has been characterized by the expression of specific neuropeptides. These neuronal populations have potent effects on energy homeostasis namely, proopiomelanocortin (POMC) and agouti-related protein/neuropeptide Y (AgRP/NPY) (Morton et al., 2014; Sohn, 2015; Timper and Bruning, 2017). However, more recently it was identified that there was a third neuronal population which expressed tyrosine hydroxylase and had orexigenic characteristics (Zhang and van den Pol, 2016). All of these neuronal populations express high levels of hormone receptors (e.g., insulin, leptin, ghrelin, GLP-1, among others) and these receptors seem to facilitate a response to metabolic signals and to reflect the energy state of the organism as well as to control energy homeostasis (**Figure 1A**).

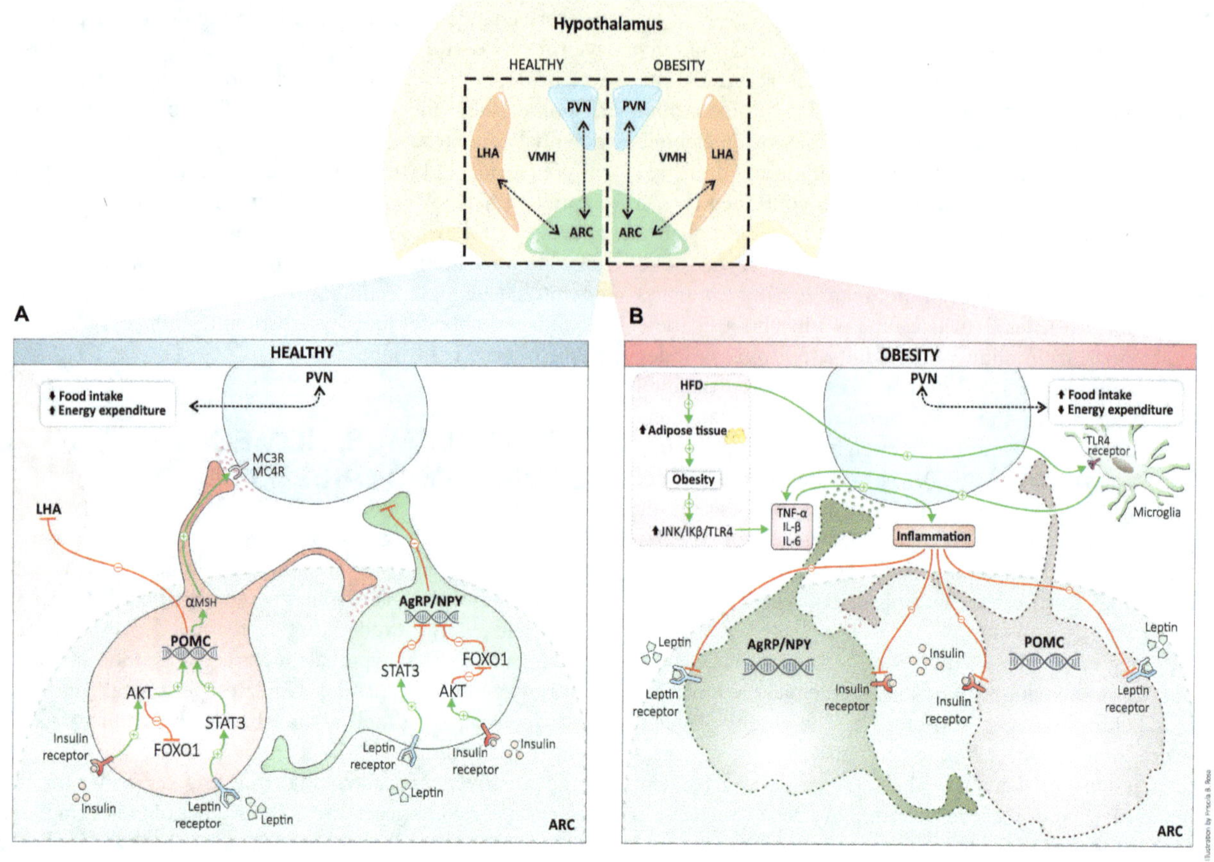

FIGURE 1 | Hypothalamic regulation of energy homeostasis in healthy (blue) and obesity (pink). The neuronal populations in the arcuate nucleus of the hypothalamus, POMC, and AgRP, senses and integrates peripheral adipostatic hormones (insulin and leptin), that circulate in levels proportionate to nutritional status and adipose tissue stores. Under the physiological postprandial state, insulin and leptin bind to respective receptors, both in POMC and AgRP neurons regulating the transcription of neuropeptides. Leptin and insulin signaling pathway stimulates POMC peptide transcription (activation of POMC neurons) and inhibits the transcription of AgRP neuropeptide (leading to AgRP neuronal inhibition). POMC neuronal activation involves the processing of POMC with the formation of α-MSH that is an agonist of MC4R in PVN neurons. PVN activation culminates in satiety (decreased food intake) and stimulation of energy expenditure **(A)**. High-fat diet consumption and obesity induces a whole-body chronic inflammatory state. Proinflammatory cytokines produced during inflammation are responsible for hypothalamic insulin and leptin resistance, and consequently, the neuronal control of energy homeostasis is disrupted inducing an increase in food intake and a decrease in energy homeostasis **(B)**. AgRP, agouti-related protein; Akt, protein kinase B; ARC, arcuate nucleus; FOXO1, forkhead box protein O1; IL-1β, interleukin-1β; IL-6, interleukin-6; JNK, c-Jun N-terminal kinases; LHA, lateral hypothalamus; MC4R, melanocortin 4 receptor; NPY, neuropeptide Y; POMC, proopiomelanocortin; α-MSH, alpha-melanocyte-stimulating hormone; PVN, paraventricular nucleus; STAT3, Signal transducer and activator of transcription 3; TLR4, toll-like receptor 4; TNF-α, tumor necrosis factor-α; VMH, ventromedial hypothalamus.

The anorexigenic neurons, the POMC, are activated by adiposity signals, such as leptin, insulin, and some nutrients. The binding of leptin to its receptor induces the phosphorylation of the transcription factor STAT3 and this reaction upregulates POMC expression (Hakansson and Meister, 1998; Lee et al., 2018). Neuronal insulin signaling induces phosphorylation of forkhead box protein O1 (FOXO1), which is also a transcription factor that increases the expression of POMC (Belgardt et al., 2008). POMC is a neuropeptide that is post-translationally processed in several active peptides, including α and β melanocyte-stimulating hormone (MSH) and β-endorphins (Liotta et al., 1980; Wardlaw, 2011). After activation, neuronal projections of POMC neurons activate second-order neurons in the PVN, acting on the melanocortin receptors (MC3R/MC4R) leading to a decrease in food intake and to an activation of energy expenditure. The activation of POMC neurons has been shown to decrease body weight (Cheung et al., 1997; Wardlaw, 2011; Mountjoy, 2015). By contrast, the second population of AgRP/NPY neurons, inhibited by leptin and activated by fasting and ghrelin, has been shown to have a potent orexigenic effect, increasing food intake and decreasing energy expenditure (Wu et al., 2014). Ghrelin is primarily produced by stomach cells under fasting conditions. Ghrelin modulates feeding behavior and metabolism through the ghrelin receptor. The ghrelin receptor is abundantly expressed in the hypothalamus, mainly in AgRP/NPY neurons. AgRPq/NPY neurons are depolarized and activated by ghrelin. Concomitantly, ghrelin hyperpolarizes and inhibits POMC neurons (Kamegai et al., 2000; Al Massadi et al., 2017). In the fed state, AgRP expression is suppressed by leptin. Under fasting conditions (no leptin release) there is an increase in AgRP and consequent increases in food behavior and adiposity. Activation of these neuronal populations leads to a release of AgRP, which is an antagonist of the MC4 receptor, and it inhibits PVN neurons. This process blocks the satiety feeling and stimulates feeding behavior through activation of lateral hypothalamic neurons (LHA) (**Figure 1A**) (Hahn et al., 1998; Luquet et al., 2005; Sohn, 2015).

Obesity is considered by many experts to be a low-grade chronic inflammatory condition. For several years, it was believed that the link between peripheral insulin resistance and obesity was a consequence of several variable factors including feeding patterns, consumption of high-fat diets, sedentary lifestyle and also that obesity occurred from stress. All of these factors are involved in the induction of systemic inflammation which can result in changes in metabolic and endocrine signaling (Hotamisligil, 2017). The expansion of white adipose tissue which occurs during the development of obesity produces proinflammatory cytokines (TNF-α, IL-1β, and IL-6) through the activation of intracellular serine kinases, such as JNK and IkB kinase. These kinases participate in the induction of insulin resistance (see review, Hotamisligil, 2017). Inflammation is also a hallmark in the brain of rodents under peripheral metabolic dysregulation (Remor et al., 2018), and in the hypothalamus of diet-induced obesity models (De Souza et al., 2005; Wang et al., 2012) (**Figure 1B**). Besides neuroinflammation, hypothalamic dysregulation induced by high-fat diets can result in an increase in markers of oxidative stress, endoplasmic reticulum stress, autophagy defects and changes in the rate of apoptosis and neuronal regeneration (Cavadas et al., 2016).

Unlike inflammation in peripheral tissues, which develops as a consequence of obesity, hypothalamic inflammatory signaling, microglia activation, and gliosis is observed during the first week of high fat diet consumption. They can also be observed prior to weight gain and in ARC (Thaler et al., 2012). A growing body of studies has demonstrated that saturated fatty acids are the trigger for early hypothalamic inflammation and are mediated mainly by microglial cells and astrocytes (Kleinridders et al., 2009; Gupta et al., 2012; Valdearcos et al., 2014, 2017; Mendes et al., 2018). Toll-like receptor 4 (TLR4) can be activated by saturated fatty acids, inducing the activity of NF-κB which transactivates gene expression of various proinflammatory cytokines and oxidative stress (Zhang et al., 2008; Kleinridders et al., 2009; Milanski et al., 2009). NF-κB also activates the expression of the suppressor of cytokine signaling 3 (SOCS3) which promotes negative feedback in the insulin and leptin intracellular signaling pathways, potentially linking hypothalamic inflammation with central leptin and insulin resistance (Valdearcos et al., 2015). Blocking the inflammatory process in the hypothalamus can prevent diet induced obesity and insulin/leptin resistance (Kleinridders et al., 2009; Valdearcos et al., 2014, 2017; Mendes et al., 2018) (**Figure 1B**).

Neuroinflammatory damage to ARC neurons might disrupt integrated circuitry, including the communication with the downstream effector nucleus (such as PVN and LHN), and may generate a pathologic activation pattern that disturbs energy homeostasis. Targeting hypothalamic structures with DBS could thus possibly lead to weight loss and reduction in binge eating behavior if the appropriate circuits can be selectively activated or inactivated (Whiting et al., 2013).

REWARD CIRCUITS, HEDONIC FEEDING, AND OBESITY

The reward circuit structures have been implicated in motivation and desire, associative learning, and in emotions with a pleasure component related to reward. 'Liking' mechanisms include hedonic circuits that connect forebrain limbic structures such as NA and ventral pallidum (where opioid/endocannabinoid/orexin signals can amplify sensory pleasure). 'Wanting' mechanisms include larger opioid networks in NA, striatum, and amygdala that extend beyond the hedonic hotspots, as well as mesolimbic dopamine systems, and corticolimbic glutamate signals that interact with those systems (Berridge et al., 2010). Hedonic feeding is driven by sensory perception or pleasure involving reward structures and these also show a close anatomic and functional relationship with the hypothalamus and the homeostatic feeding (Rossi and Stuber, 2018). Hyperpalatable foods may be potentially "addictive" and have been compared to drugs of abuse. The cues that predict drug and food reward activate similar regions that have been implicated in reward and reward learning. The circuits involved include the mesolimbic dopamine system, which projects from the ventral tegmental area (VTA) to the NA (Stice et al., 2008). Functional MRI has shown that blood oxygen dependent signal (BOLD) in the NA is selectively increased during the perception of pleasant, emotionally arousing pictures and during mental imagery of pleasant, emotional scenes (Sabatinelli et al., 2007; Costa et al., 2010). In comparison to lean individuals, obese individuals experience greater activation in the gustatory cortex and somatosensory regions in response to anticipation and consumption of food (consummatory and anticipatory food reward) and experience a weaker activation in the striatum during food intake (Stice et al., 2008). The findings of reward responsivity in obese people can be inherited (genetic predisposition) or can result from repeated food intake or from both scenarios (Berridge et al., 2010).

On the other hand, the incidental finding of increased weight gain after discontinuation of pharmacological dopaminergic in rats suggested that hypofunctioning of dopamine circuits related to overstimulation by high palatable function could contribute to obesity (Reinholz et al., 2008). The Taq1A minor (A1) allele of the gene codifying dopamine receptors 2 and 3 (DRD2/3 gene) is associated with lower DRD2/3 density and has been found to exist in higher frequencies in obese subjects (Dang et al., 2016). In rodents, reduced DA transmission has been well documented in the striatum of obese rats (Johnson and Kenny, 2010; Rada et al., 2010). The results were in agreement with the earlier report showing lower striatal levels of D2 receptors of obese subjects in comparison to controls in 2001 (Wang et al., 2001). However, a large sample of adult subjects (n = 130, age between 18 and 81 years), Dang et al. (2016) show no association between o relation between DRD2/3 and BMI (range from underweight to extreme obesity) after controlling for age distribution. Besides that, a randomized pilot study with a dopamine agonist (cabergoline) treatment for 16 weeks did not affect significantly the weight loss, but improve the glucose tolerance (Gibson et al., 2012). Also, genetic studies in humans have suggested that striatal D2Rs for obesity etiology have been considered somewhat controversial. Experts have questioned the reward deficiency theory of "food addiction" (Benton and Young, 2016). Recently Labouesse et al. (2018) outlined a causal relationship between striatal D2Rs and obesity in mice. These authors showed that high striatal D2R during development increased the risk for obesity in the mouse and that obesogenic diets were necessary to reveal the full effects of the D2R on obesity in the mouse. This data suggested that diet was an important cofactor along with the genetic predisposition.

Although the genetic and neuroimaging studies in humans and the experimental findings in rodents suggest a complex role for the reward-related dopaminergic system in obesity, the results support the use of this circuit as a target for "stimulation" or "inhibition" by DBS.

DEEP BRAIN STIMULATION

Based partially on the notion that high-frequency stimulation could suppress extrapyramidal tremor during functional ablative neurosurgery (Hassler et al., 1960; Alberts et al., 1965, 1966), Benabid et al. (1987) moved the field toward chronic stimulation with high-frequency continuous stimulation (130 Hz) of the thalamic nucleus ventralis intermedius for essential tremor and for parkinsonian tremor. He showed that DBS could be applied bilaterally without pseudobulbar and cognitive side-effects, an important observation as this was the major shortcoming of bilateral lesion therapy. Collectively, these observations consolidated the concept that high-frequency DBS could provide a "functional" lesion or alternatively modulation of a relevant brain network (Grill et al., 2004). We do not completely understand the mechanism of action of DBS, however, there seem to be important associated neurophysiological, neurochemical, neurovascular, neurogenic, neurochemical (e.g., glial cells), and neuro-oscillatory changes. The application of DBS should always be focused to selectively influence a specific and even multiple brain targets to modulate a relevant neural network. It should only be applied to alleviate human suffering (Benabid et al., 1987; Miocinovic et al., 2013; Williams and Okun, 2013; Okun, 2014).

The target size and the anatomical relationship to adjacent structures should be carefully considered during surgical planning. Presently, most DBS leads contain four platinum/iridium cone shape electrodes around the lead with a 1.27 mm diameter and 1.5 mm length. The spacing between each electrode can be 1.5 mm or 0.5 mm providing, respectively, a total of 10.5 mm or 7.5 mm length distance between the deepest and the most superficial electrode borders. There are newer models with eight contacts and segmented leads with variable spacing. The DBS leads are inserted by stereotactic surgery into the targeted brain structure, and an extension wire is subcutaneously tunneled to connect the implanted pulse generator (IPG) to the DBS lead (Oluigbo et al., 2012; Okun, 2014; Klooster et al., 2016). The IPG delivers adjustable pulses through the quadripolar electrodes and can be programmed to many settings based on voltage (or current in newer devices) amplitude, pulse width, and frequency (Hassler et al., 1960; Alberts et al., 1966; Benabid et al., 1991; Kuncel and Grill, 2004; Kringelbach et al., 2007; Brocker and Grill, 2013; Udupa and Chen, 2015). The DBS can be switched ON or OFF on demand (Oluigbo et al., 2012) in some paradigms. When the monopolar configuration is utilized a large sphere of current is generated and when bipolar is used the current is more restricted and elliptical. Newer devices may provide multiple independent current sources as well as segmented leads which can be used to steer or shape the current.

Deep brain stimulation has steadily become a safer procedure especially when an experienced multidisciplinary approach is applied. Severe adverse events are usually less than 5% in well-selected cases (Shukla et al., 2015). DBS is FDA approved in the United States for the treatment of advanced Parkinson's disease (Odekerken et al., 2013), dystonia (Meoni et al., 2017), and essential tremor (Barbe et al., 2018) and also has a humanitarian device exemption for dystonia and obsessive-compulsive disorder. DBS has been utilized in several refractory neuropsychiatric disorders including Tourette syndrome, depression (Schlaepfer et al., 2013), post-traumatic stress disorder (Koek et al., 2014), epilepsy (Salanova, 2018), obsessive-compulsive disorder (Goodman et al., 2010), pain (Farrell et al., 2018), Alzheimer's disease (Leoutsakos et al., 2018); drug addiction (Wang et al., 2018) and appetite disorders (Whiting et al., 2018).

Several observations have described a "feeling of happiness" accompanied by smile that progressed to natural laughter with DBS applied to the internal capsule/NA region for obsessive-compulsive disorder (Okun et al., 2004, 2007; Springer et al., 2006; Haq et al., 2011). Mood elevation during stimulation-induced smiles and laughter could be transient and was found to habituate with chronic NA stimulation (Springer et al., 2006; Haq et al., 2011). Rarely DBS induced mood elevation or "manic-like" symptoms in PD which were rapidly reversed with IPG reprogramming. Also, non-mood-related symptoms may also occur. Responses such as taste, smell, and smile were strongly associated with the most ventral lead positions. Similarly, physiological responses – for example, autonomic changes, increased breathing rate, sweating, nausea, cold sensation, heat sensation, fear, panic and panic episodes were significantly associated with ventral stimulation (Okun et al., 2007). Some authors showed that resistant depression treated with medial forebrain bundle DBS may improve over weeks to months (Schlaepfer et al., 2013; Fenoy et al., 2016). Perhaps most compelling was a paper by Halpern et al. (2011) which showed a delta oscillation in NA that was associated with feeding behavior in the mouse. These investigators also explored the use of neuromodulation applied to the NA in the animal and in one human case (an OCD case) as a method to modulate this "feeding" oscillation.

Taken together, clinical observations have shown that modulation can affect different limbic symptoms and this response can be exhibit variable latency. Neuromodulation for obesity treatment will need to consider the overlapping circuits involved with hedonic and homeostatic feeding. Selectivity of a DBS treatment to specific cells using optogenetics may also be a viable approach (Creed et al., 2015; Lüscher et al., 2015; Mastro et al., 2017).

HYPOTHALAMIC DBS AS APPLIED TO OBESITY

The hypothalamic nuclei have become targets for DBS therapy in obesity because of the known association with vegetative functions, social behavior, food behavior and control of metabolism. Human hypothalamus is a 0.7 cm^3 volume and it is functionally heterogeneous and complex. It is located below the thalamus and it forms the lateral walls and floor of the third ventricle (Saper, 2004). The four hypothalamic nuclei directly involved with appetite control and food behavior are the VMH, LHA, DMH, PVN, and ARC (Lemaire et al., 2013; Barbosa et al., 2017). These are the nuclei of interest for neuromodulation.

Classical ablative studies have established VMN as the "satiety center," and LHA as the "feeding center." This dichotomy has, however, been replaced by a more complex hypothalamic neural network coupled to hormonal, metabolic and energy regulation signals (Lacan et al., 2008) as shown in **Figure 1**. In both rodent models and in humans obesity has been associated with hypothalamic gliosis and neuronal injury and this has been raised by some experts as a concern for future neuromodulation therapy (Thaler et al., 2012). Variations in the pattern of gliosis and also of neuronal injury distribution may impact local and distal neuroplasticity and may have implications for clinical outcome. The two nuclei require different stimulation frequencies to produce their therapeutic effects (Hamani et al., 2008; Wilent et al., 2010). Moreover, as previously described, systemic metabolic signals under fasting or non-fasting conditions (such as leptin and ghrelin) have antagonistic effects over ARC neurons (namely the POMC and AgRP) and result in the selective activation of PVN or LHA, which either favors weight loss or stimulates food behavior (Morton et al., 2014; Timper and Bruning, 2017).

As shown in **Figure 1**, in healthy conditions the PVN activation culminates in satiety (decreased food intake) and stimulation of energy expenditure. This nucleus is modulated by the anorexigenic POMC and orexigenic AgRP/NPY neurons from ARC nucleus. It has been suggested that to be effective for obesity, the PVN should be activated by a device directly implanted into the nucleus itself or in the ARC nucleus that projects to the PVN. A DBS neuromodulation approach of the ARC to treat obesity would preferably activate selectively the anorexigenic POMC and/or inactivate the orexigenic AgRP/NPY neurons. Because obesity is associated with complex changes in the neurophysiology of the POMC and AgRP/NPY neurons (see **Figure 1**), the result of ARC neuromodulation by DBS on the PVN in obese patients is tricky and an optogenetic manipulation may be a preferred approach. Also, because the PVN and ARC nuclei are relatively small, their selective modulation by DBS remains a barrier.

The DMH has been implicated in day-time feeding, in emotional responses to stress and when lesioned in male and female patients has been shown to be associated with persistent impotence and loss of libido (Meyers, 1962; Barbosa et al., 2017). Implications for DMH as a target for DBS in obesity remain to be explored.

The series and case reports about the VMH, LHA, and NA as DBS targets for obesity are discussed below and also summarized in **Table 1**.

Ventral Medial Hypothalamus DBS

Hamani et al. (2008) performed the first DBS trial to treat human obesity. The trial was inspired by the positive results obtained from preclinical (Halpern et al., 2011; Prinz and Stengel, 2018) and clinical studies, and it revealed that inhibition of the hypothalamus resulted in decreased food intake and weight loss (De Salles et al., 2018). Hamani et al. (2008) implanted DBS leads bilaterally in the ventral hypothalamus of one 50-year-old man with a life-long history of obesity (190.5 kg; BMI, 55.1 kg/m^2). The first stimulation parameter settings (130 Hz, 60 μs, and 2.8 V) did not reveal a significant effect (e.g., weight loss) during the first 6 months following surgery. Interesting, after a slight adjustment (50 Hz, 210 μs, and 3–4 V) the patient had a consequent weight loss (12 kg) without significant dietary changes and a reduction in food craving (Hamani et al., 2008). Because the patient reported difficulties in sleeping, the stimulation was turned off at night. The patient then began to eat at night and had increased weight (Wilent et al., 2010; Whiting et al., 2013). Wilent et al. (2010) used the same target as Hamani et al. (2008), however, in their case the stimulation (135 Hz, 60 μs, and 1–7 V) was associated with an unexpected panic event, and resulted in the interruption of the treatment.

An open-label clinical trial of hypothalamic DBS for morbid obesity is currently in progress and six patients will be included (De Salles et al., 2018). The subjects are required to have a BMI greater than 40 kg/m^2 or to have undergone bariatric surgery with therapeutic failure, as defined by BMI $\geq$ 35 kg/m^2 (must be 5 years after the procedure). Subjects must have no obesity comorbidities such as diabetes or cardiopulmonary abnormalities. The trial aims to assess the safety, identify possible side effects, and to optimize stimulation parameters in a paradigm of continuous VMH-DBS. Additionally, the study aims to determine if continuous VMH-DBS will lead to weight loss associated with changes in body composition, basal metabolism or food intake control (De Salles et al., 2018).

Lateral Hypothalamic Area (LHA) DBS

Weight gain has been observed in patients with PD treated with the subthalamic nucleus (STN) DBS and globus pallidus internus (GPi) DBS (Novakova et al., 2007). The weight gain could be an influence of spreading electrical currents into hypothalamic pathways though this remains speculative. There are also other factors including impulse control and dyskinesia reduction which could confound the finding. Nevertheless, it is interesting that STN and GPi DBS for Parkinson's disease have both been associated with weight gain.

TABLE 1 | Series and cases reports of patients treated with DBS for obesity.

References	Target	Stimulations parameters	*N*	Efficacy assessments	Follow-up (months)	Main results	Side effects
Hamani et al., 2008	Ventromedial hypothalamus (bilateral)	50 Hz, 210 μs and 3–4 V	1 (♂)	Body weight Neuropsychological assessment Binge eating	5 months	↓ Body weight ↑ Memory	Warming sensation (>4 V), flashes of light
Wilent et al., 2010	Ventral medial hypothalamus (bilateral)	135 Hz, 60 μs and 1–7 V	1 (♀)	–	–	–	Panic attack (increase in heart rate and blood pressure and anxiety feelings)
Whiting et al., 2013	Lateral hypothalamic (bilateral)	185 Hz, 90 μs and 1–7 V	3 (2♀; 1♂)	Body weight Psychological testing Binge Eating Scale Body shape Quality of life	35 months	↓ Body weight (2/3) ↓ Binge eating behaviors (1/3) No changes in Psychological Scores and life quality (3/3) ↑ Body image	Nausea, anxiety or "hot of flushed" sensations during programming changes
Talakoub et al., 2017	Lateral hypothalamic (bilateral)	8 Hz, 90 μs, and 3 V	1 (♂) a Prader–Willi	Local field potentials (LFPs) from the DBS contacts during acute evaluation during hunger and satiety.		Exposure to food-related cues during hunger induced an increase in beta/low-gamma activity. Satiety was marked by alpha rhythms (8 Hz). Alpha frequency DBS delivered prior to and during food intake resulted in sensation of fullness without effects on crave for food. Body weight was not reported.	None
Franco et al., 2018	Lateral hypothalamic (bilateral)	Off (2 months) 40 Hz (1 month) 15 days washout 130 Hz (1 month)	4 (2♀; 2♂) all were Prader–Willi	Calorimetry, bioimpedanciometry, neuropsychological assessments, hormonal levels, blood workup, and sleep studies	6 months	No major effects on anthropometric and calorimetric variables, hormonal levels, blood workup, sleep and neuropsychological evaluation	Two had stimulation-induced manic symptoms, one improves with discontinuation of DBS and one required topiramate increase. One removes the system because infection and one successfully treated with antibiotics
Mantione et al., 2010	Nucleus accumbens (bilateral)	185 Hz, 90 μs and 3.5 V	1 (♀)	Psychological assessment (anxiety and depression) Body weight	24 months	↓Obsessive–compulsive symptoms ↓Body weight ↓ Anxiety ↓ Depression	None reported
Harat et al., 2016	Nucleus accumbens (bilateral)	130 Hz, 208 μs and 2–3, 75 mA	1 (♀)	Body weight, body mass index, and neuropsychological assessment	14 months	↓ Weight ↓ BMI Without neuropsychological impairment	None
Tronnier et al., 2018	Nucleus accumbens (bilateral)	130 Hz, 90 μs and 3–4 V	1 (♀)	Body weight, Binge Eating Scale, Weight Efficacy Life-Style, Depression Scales, SF36 mood, simples mood	14 months	↓ Body weight ↓ Resist desire to eat and binge eating behaviors ↓ Depressed symptoms ↑ Mood and quality of life	Difficulties to falling sleep
Rezai et al., 2018	Nucleus accumbens (bilateral)	Not reported (high-frequency)	3 (♀)	Body weight, body mass index	36 months	One patient finished the follow-up period with ↓ weight and ↓ BMI Two patients did not complete the trial	One patient withdrew from the study with 13 months; one patient completed suicide after 27 months in the study, non-attributed to DBS (see the main text)

A right-side LHA hypothalamotomy lesion in two patients and bilateral in one (staged over 3 months) resulted in a transient decrease in caloric intake. This finding was compared to two patients with transient stimulation but no lesion(s) (Quaade et al., 1974).

In 2013, the first DBS treatment with electrodes implanted in the LHA was performed in three patients, (two females). All patients were previously treated with gastric bypass between 2001 and 2003 (Whiting et al., 2013). During the intraoperative microelectrode recording isolated but not discernible firing patterns were recorded. Microstimulation within the LHA produced sensations of nausea and thermal responses while more ventromedial microstimulation (presumably within the VMH) resulted in an anxiety or panic response. DBS was initiated 2 months after surgery. No significant weight loss trends were observed when DBS was programmed utilizing standard settings similar to the high-frequency parameters used for movement disorder surgery. Weight loss trends were observed when monopolar DBS stimulation was applied via specific contacts found to be associated with an increase in the resting metabolic rate as measured in a respiratory chamber. After 35 months of follow-up, two patients lost weight and one had a decrease in binge eating behaviors. There were no significant neuropsychological changes across patients and no significant side effects were reported.

Hyperphagia in Prader–Willi syndrome (PWS) is an important cause of genetic obesity. Recently, Talakoub et al. (2017) recorded the local field potentials (LFPs) from the DBS contacts implanted in the LHA of a 19-year-old Prader–Willi male patient undergoing DBS for obesity. During hunger exposure to food-related cues, there was an induced increase in beta/low-gamma activity. During satiety, the recordings were marked by alpha rhythms. An alpha frequency DBS was delivered prior to and during food intake. The patient reported a sensation of fullness but had a persistent food craving. The long-term effects have yet to be reported (Talakoub et al., 2017).

Franco et al. (2018) described four patients (two males) with Prader–Willi syndrome, treated with lateral hypothalamus DBS. The cohorts age ranged from 18 to 28 and their mean (SD) baseline BMI was 39.6 (11.1). Two patients had previous bariatric surgery. All patients had psychiatric comorbidities, including skin picking, nail biting, aggressive behavior, hypersexuality, episodes of hypomania, psychosis, and impulsiveness. These behaviors were reported as adequately controlled with medications. After DBS implantation, the treatment included the following phases: titration (1–2 months), stimulation off (2 months), low-frequency DBS (40 Hz; 1 month), washout (15 days), high-frequency DBS (130 Hz; 1 month), and long-term follow-up (6 months). Six months after receiving DBS at the "best" settings, the patients had a mean 9.6% increase in weight, a 5.8% increase in BMI, an 8.4% increase in abdominal circumference, a 4.2% increase in neck circumference, a 5.3% increase in the percentage of body fat, and a 0% change in calorimetry (as compared to baseline). The hormonal levels and results of a blood workup, sleep studies, and neuropsychological evaluations were unchanged by DBS therapy. Two patients developed manic symptoms during the titration phase, one improved with DBS programming and one required an increase in topiramate. One patient was receiving preoperative testosterone injections for hypogonadism, which infrequently resulted in priapism. One episode of priapism during the titration phase required drainage. One patient developed an infection over the connector site thought to be associated with skin picking 7 months following treatment. The family requested explantation since the device was ineffective for obesity. Another patient developed a superficial infection over IPG 1 month after the implant and this issue was successfully addressed with antibiotics.

NUCLEUS ACCUMBENS DBS

The first clinical report on NA DBS was published by Mantione et al. (2010) who treated refractory obsessive-compulsive disorder with associated nicotine dependence and also obesity (Mantione et al., 2010). In this study, a 47-year-old female patient weighed 107 kg with a height of 170 cm, corresponding to a BMI of 37 was implanted with a monopolar DBS (185 Hz, 90 μs, and 3.5 V). The clinical team utilized the two deepest contacts (0 and 1) for initial programming (accumbens region) and adjusted it using the more dorsal 1 and 2 contacts 3 weeks later, when she gradually started to improve her obsessive-compulsive symptoms. Within 5 months the Yale-Brown Obsessive-Compulsive Scale scores decreased from 38 to 2 and she reported reducing the time spent on obsessions and compulsions from 20 h a day to less than 1 h a day. The HAM-A (subclinical anxiety) and the HAM-D (subclinical depression) gradually decreased from 17 to 2 and 11 to 3, respectively. Seven months after surgery she realized she was no longer dependent on her compulsions, but that she was still dependent on her cigarettes. She stopped smoking and stated she did not crave cigarettes and did not experience withdrawal symptoms. The 2-year follow-up evaluation showed her weight was 71 kg, she was not smoking and she had no desire to start smoking. She scored 1 on the Yale-Brown Obsessive-Compulsive Scale, 3 on the HAM-A, and 3 on the HAM-D.

More recently in 2016, Harat et al. (2016) described a 19-year-old woman with obesity associated with a hypothalamic region that was damaged by a craniopharyngioma (neurosurgery was in 2004). She was approved for bariatric surgery but preferred DBS surgery. She was treated with bilateral NA DBS (130 Hz, 208 μs, and 2–3.75 mA). After 14 months her weight was reduced from 151.4 kg to 138 kg and her BMI from 53 to 48. No neuropsychological or other side effects were observed as a result of the surgery (Harat et al., 2016).

Tronnier et al. (2018) reported that bilateral NA DBS (130 Hz, 90 μs, and 4 V) decreased body weight, BMI and binge behavior without significant psychological impairment in a woman who was followed for 14-months. She had depression resistant to electroconvulsive therapy (ECT). Her peak weight in November 2013 was 183.6 kg which at a height of 167 cm translated to a BMI of 66. In March 2015, she underwent gastric bypass surgery after a course of behavioral therapy for her obesity and it was reported to have limited success. Because the temporary improvement of depression was less than 2 weeks and further antidepressant medication was not successful, the decision was made for treatment with NA DBS in November 2015. Morbid obesity of the patient was considered a secondary target of the DBS procedure. After DBS surgery, her weight loss accelerated to 2.85 kg/month. At the time of writing of this report (12/2016) her body weight has continuously decreased to 106 kg, corresponding to a BMI of 38. Her depressive symptoms have also been reported to be significantly reduced. Interestingly, the weight loss was accompanied with heightened feelings of "self-efficacy of ingestive behavior" that was not felt following bariatric surgery. This case raised the issue as to whether obesity associated with depression could be addressed with NA DBS.

Rezai et al. (2018) described their experience with NA DBS for obesity in three female patients followed by their multidisciplinary team. The inclusion criteria were age between 22 and 60 years, "extreme obesity" defined as BMI > 40, and patients had to fail Rou-en-Y gastric bypass surgery. Although all patients lost weight with DBS, only one participant successfully completed the 3-year trial, losing 100 pounds with a 30% BMI reduction (55.7–39.3). After 13 months in the study, one subject requested explantation. One patient died as a result of a completed suicide after 27 months into the study. All patients had significant psychiatric illness and during the trial reported major psychosocial stressors including family violence, divorce, job loss, family illness, and pet death. The study team concluded that DBS itself was not responsible for the suicide, patient withdrawal or explantation. Regarding the association between obesity and suicide, a recent systematic review and meta-analysis of 15 prospective studies showed an inverse association between obesity with suicide mortality and attempted suicide (Amiri and Behnezhad, 2018). The mechanisms related to an association between DBS and suicide are not understood but the recent Veterans Affairs study with a long term follow-up did not show an association with STN and GPi DBS and suicide (Weintraub et al., 2013). One confounding factor has been the early reports of suicide led most major groups to implement more careful pre-operative screening and post-operative monitoring.

Rezai et al. (2018) has suggested the following strategies to reduce suicide risk (i) Requirement of close psychiatric monitoring by clinicians trained in bariatric psychiatry and mandatory psychological therapy during the study period; (ii) Requirement of subject commitment to compliance with the study requirements and close involvement with a social support system and a study partner (a family member or close friend committed to the trial with the subject) from the subject's environment; (iii) Upfront consideration should be given to the long-term follow-up of the DBS system after the trial conclusion and should be discussed with the subjects and family support system in advance of implantation.

Finally, because of its assumed role in reward-related behavior, the ventral anterior limb of the internal capsule (vALIC) could be a potential target for obesity DBS. However, Linssen et al. (2017) reported no significant change in body weight on a group level after vALIC DBS (mean follow-up was 3.8 years, range 10 months to 8.7 years) for either obsessive-compulsive disorder (n = 30) or major depressive disorder (n = 16). The average baseline BMI in their sample of 46 patients was 28.0 (SD 7.3), with 26 (57%) being overweight (BMI 25–30, n = 11), obese (BMI 30–40, n = 12), or morbidly obese (BMI ≥ 40, n = 3).

CONCLUSION AND FINAL REMARKS

Prevention of obesity is a worldwide issue. It will required broad changes in the worldwide pattern of food ingestion and physical activity. The cost-effectiveness of innovations must be taken into account in epidemiological terms. However, in selected cases of morbid obesity, DBS, similar to gastric surgery, may in the future be refined into a therapeutic modality. Hypothalamic DBS for obesity has been shown to be reasonably safe in well-selected patients. The effectiveness has, however, not been shown to be robust or reproducible. Based on both biological plausibility and on observational studies, the NA has emerged as an alternative obesity DBS target.

Future studies should also focus on better understanding the patient characteristics most likely to benefit from obesity DBS (Tronnier et al., 2018). Specific DBS targets may be optimal for specific clinical phenotypes. The therapy could thus become more personalized (Famm et al., 2013).

The identification of electrical control signals may provide an opportunity for closed-loop adaptive DBS systems to address obesity (Carron et al., 2013; Kuhn and Volkmann, 2017). Metabolic and hormonal sensors such as glycemic levels (Christiansen et al., 2018), leptin and ghrelin levels are candidate control signals for DBS.

Newer approaches for obesity DBS should be explored. Focused excitation or alternatively inhibition of regions of the hypothalamus may provide better outcomes compared to non-selective DBS. Utilization of the delta oscillation (Halpern et al., 2011) or other physiological markers from one or multiple regions in the obesity network is a promising approach.

Finally, it will be important to implement expert multidisciplinary screening teams as well as post-operative monitoring to lessen the occurrence of neuropsychiatric adverse events.

AUTHOR CONTRIBUTIONS

DF, JG, HM, TE, RZ, AL, and RW wrote the manuscript. TE, JG, and DF elaborated the tables and figures. AL, JG, MO, and RW participated in the conception of the idea and revised the manuscript.

FUNDING

AL and RW are Research Fellows from CNPq (Brazilian Council for Scientific and Technologic Development, Brazil). AL and RW were supported by PRONEX Program of FAPESC/CNPq (NENASC Project). DF, HM, and TE are supported by scholarships from CAPES. JG was supported by CNPq (401842/2018-5). RZ is supported by Fondecyt n 11140757. MO serves as a consultant for the National Parkinson Foundation, and has received research grants from NIH, NPF, the Michael J. Fox

Foundation, the Parkinson Alliance, Smallwood Foundation, the Bachmann-Strauss Foundation, the Tourette Syndrome Association, and the UF Foundation. MO's DBS research is supported by: R01 NR014852 and R01NS096008. MO has previously received honoraria, but in the past >60 months has received no support from industry. MO has received royalties for publications with Demos, Manson, Amazon, Smashwords, Books4Patients, and Cambridge (movement disorders books). MO is an associate editor for New England Journal of Medicine Journal Watch Neurology. MO has participated in CME and educational activities on movement disorders (in the last 36) months sponsored by PeerView, Prime, QuantiaMD, WebMD, Medicus, MedNet, Henry Stewart, and by Vanderbilt University. The institution and not MO receives grants from Medtronic, Abbvie, Allergan, and ANS/St. Jude, and the PI has no financial interest in these grants. MO has participated as a site PI and/or co-PI for several NIH, foundation, and industry sponsored trials over the years but has not received honoraria.

REFERENCES

Al Massadi, O., Lopez, M., Tschop, M., Dieguez, C., and Nogueiras, R. (2017). Current understanding of the hypothalamic ghrelin pathways inducing appetite and adiposity. *Trends Neurosci.* 40, 167–180. doi: 10.1016/j.tins.2016.12.003

Alberts, W. W., Feinstein, B., Levin, G., and Wright, E. W. Jr. (1966). Electrical stimulation of therapeutic targets in waking dyskinetic patients. *Electroencephalogr. Clin. Neurophysiol.* 20, 559–566. doi: 10.1016/0013-4694(66)90020-4

Alberts, W. W., Feinstein, B., Levin, G., Wright, E. W. Jr., Darland, M. G., and Scott, E. L. (1965). Stereotaxic surgery for parkinsonism. Clinical results and stimulation thresholds. *J. Neurosurg.* 23, 174–183. doi: 10.3171/jns.1965.23.2.0174

Amiri, S., and Behnezhad, S. (2018). Body mass index and risk of suicide: a systematic review and meta-analysis. *J. Affect. Disord.* 238, 615–625. doi: 10.1016/j.jad.2018.05.028

Barbe, M. T., Reker, P., Hamacher, S., Franklin, J., Kraus, D., Dembek, T. A., et al. (2018). DBS of the PSA and the VIM in essential tremor: a randomized, double-blind, crossover trial. *Neurology* 91, e543–e550. doi: 10.1212/WNL.0000000000005956

Barbosa, D. A. N., De Oliveira-Souza, R., Monte Santo, F., De Oliveira Faria, A. C., Gorgulho, A. A., and De Salles, A. A. F. (2017). The hypothalamus at the crossroads of psychopathology and neurosurgery. *Neurosurg. Focus* 43:E15. doi: 10.3171/2017.6.FOCUS17256

Belgardt, B. F., Husch, A., Rother, E., Ernst, M. B., Wunderlich, F. T., Hampel, B., et al. (2008). PDK1 deficiency in POMC-expressing cells reveals FOXO1-dependent and -independent pathways in control of energy homeostasis and stress response. *Cell Metab.* 7, 291–301. doi: 10.1016/j.cmet.2008.01.006

Benabid, A. L., Pollak, P., Gervason, C., Hoffmann, D., Gao, D. M., Hommel, M., et al. (1991). Long-term suppression of tremor by chronic stimulation of the ventral intermediate thalamic nucleus. *Lancet* 337, 403–406. doi: 10.1016/0140 6736(91)91175-T

Benabid, A. L., Pollak, P., Louveau, A., Henry, S., and De Rougemont, J. (1987). Combined (thalamotomy and stimulation) stereotactic surgery of the VIM thalamic nucleus for bilateral Parkinson disease. *Appl. Neurophysiol.* 50, 344–346. doi: 10.1159/000100803

Benton, D., and Young, H. A. (2016). A meta-analysis of the relationship between brain dopamine receptors and obesity: a matter of changes in behavior rather than food addiction? *Int. J. Obes.* 40(Suppl. 1), S12–S21. doi: 10.1038/ijo.2016.9

Berridge, K. C., Ho, C. Y., Richard, J. M., and Difeliceantonio, A. G. (2010). The tempted brain eats: pleasure and desire circuits in obesity and eating disorders. *Brain Res.* 1350, 43–64. doi: 10.1016/j.brainres.2010.04.003

Brocker, D. T., and Grill, W. M. (2013). Principles of electrical stimulation of neural tissue. *Handb. Clin. Neurol.* 116, 3–18. doi: 10.1016/B978-0-444-53497-2.00001-2

Carron, R., Chaillet, A., Filipchuk, A., Pasillas-Lepine, W., and Hammond, C. (2013). Closing the loop of deep brain stimulation. *Front. Syst. Neurosci.* 7:112. doi: 10.3389/fnsys.2013.00112

Cavadas, C., Aveleira, C. A., Souza, G. F., and Velloso, L. A. (2016). The pathophysiology of defective proteostasis in the hypothalamus - from obesity to ageing. *Nat. Rev. Endocrinol.* 12, 723–733. doi: 10.1038/nrendo.2016.107

Cheung, C. C., Clifton, D. K., and Steiner, R. A. (1997). Proopiomelanocortin neurons are direct targets for leptin in the hypothalamus. *Endocrinology* 138, 4489–4492. doi: 10.1210/endo.138.10.5570

Christiansen, M. P., Klaff, L. J., Brazg, R., Chang, A. R., Levy, C. J., Lam, D., et al. (2018). A prospective multicenter evaluation of the accuracy of a novel implanted continuous glucose sensor: PRECISE II. *Diabetes Technol. Ther.* 20, 197–206. doi: 10.1089/dia.2017.0142

Costa, V. D., Lang, P. J., Sabatinelli, D., Versace, F., and Bradley, M. M. (2010). Emotional imagery: assessing pleasure and arousal in the brain's reward circuitry. *Hum. Brain Mapp.* 31, 1446–1457. doi: 10.1002/hbm.20948

Creed, M., Pascoli, V. J., and Lüscher, C. (2015). Addiction therapy. Refining deep brain stimulation to emulate optogenetic treatment of synaptic pathology. *Science* 347, 659–664. doi: 10.1126/science.1260776

Dang, L. C., Samanez-Larkin, G. R., Castrellon, J. J., Perkins, S. F., Cowan, R. L., and Zald, D. H. (2016). Associations between dopamine D2 receptor availability and BMI depend on age. *Neuroimage* 138, 176–183. doi: 10.1016/j.neuroimage.2016.05.044

De Salles, A. A. F., Barbosa, D. A. N., Fernandes, F., Abucham, J., Nazato, D. M., Oliveira, J. D., et al. (2018). An open-label clinical trial of hypothalamic deep brain stimulation for human morbid obesity: BLESS study protocol. *Neurosurgery* 83, 800–809. doi: 10.1093/neuros/nyy024

De Souza, C. T., Araujo, E. P., Bordin, S., Ashimine, R., Zollner, R. L., Boschero, A. C., et al. (2005). Consumption of a fat-rich diet activates a proinflammatory response and induces insulin resistance in the hypothalamus. *Endocrinology* 146, 4192–4199. doi: 10.1210/en.2004-1520

Famm, K., Litt, B., Tracey, K. J., Boyden, E. S., and Slaoui, M. (2013). Drug discovery: a jump-start for electroceuticals. *Nature* 496, 159–161. doi: 10.1038/496159a

Farrell, S. M., Green, A., and Aziz, T. (2018). The current state of deep brain stimulation for chronic pain and its context in other forms of neuromodulation. *Brain Sci.* 8:E158. doi: 10.3390/brainsci8080158

Fenoy, A. J., Schulz, P., Selvaraj, S., Burrows, C., Spiker, D., Cao, B., et al. (2016). Deep brain stimulation of the medial forebrain bundle: distinctive responses in resistant depression. *J. Affect. Disord.* 203, 143–151. doi: 10.1016/j.jad.2016.05.064

Franco, R. R., Fonoff, E. T., Alvarenga, P. G., Alho, E. J. L., Lopes, A. C., Hoexter, M. Q., et al. (2018). Assessment of safety and outcome of lateral hypothalamic deep brain stimulation for obesity in a small series of patients with prader-willi syndrome. *JAMA Netw. Open* 1:e185275. doi: 10.1001/jamanetworkopen.2018.5275

Gaspar, J. M., Baptista, F. I., Macedo, M. P., and Ambrosio, A. F. (2016). Inside the diabetic brain: role of different players involved in cognitive decline. *ACS Chem. Neurosci.* 7, 131–142. doi: 10.1021/acschemneuro.5b00240

Gibson, C. D., Karmally, W., Mcmahon, D. J., Wardlaw, S. L., and Korner, J. (2012). Randomized pilot study of cabergoline, a dopamine receptor agonist: effects on body weight and glucose tolerance in obese adults. *Diabetes Obes. Metab.* 14, 335–340. doi: 10.1111/j.1463-1326.2011.01534.x

Gonzalez-Muniesa, P., Martinez-Gonzalez, M. A., Hu, F. B., Despres, J. P., Matsuzawa, Y., Loos, R. J. F., et al. (2017). Obesity. *Nat. Rev. Dis. Primers* 3:17034. doi: 10.1038/nrdp.2017.34

Goodman, W. K., Foote, K. D., Greenberg, B. D., Ricciuti, N., Bauer, R., Ward, H., et al. (2010). Deep brain stimulation for intractable obsessive compulsive disorder: pilot study using a blinded, staggered-onset design. *Biol. Psychiatry* 67, 535–542. doi: 10.1016/j.biopsych.2009.11.028

Grill, W. M., Snyder, A. N., and Miocinovic, S. (2004). Deep brain stimulation creates an informational lesion of the stimulated nucleus. *Neuroreport* 15, 1137–1140. doi: 10.1097/00001756-200405190-00011

Gupta, S., Knight, A. G., Gupta, S., Keller, J. N., and Bruce-Keller, A. J. (2012). Saturated long-chain fatty acids activate inflammatory signaling in astrocytes. *J. Neurochem.* 120, 1060–1071. doi: 10.1111/j.1471-4159.2012.07660.x

Hahn, T. M., Breininger, J. F., Baskin, D. G., and Schwartz, M. W. (1998). Coexpression of Agrp and NPY in fasting-activated hypothalamic neurons. *Nat. Neurosci.* 1, 271–272. doi: 10.1038/1082

Hakansson, M. L., and Meister, B. (1998). Transcription factor STAT3 in leptin target neurons of the rat hypothalamus. *Neuroendocrinology* 68, 420–427. doi: 10.1159/000054392

Halpern, C. H., Torres, N., Hurtig, H. I., Wolf, J. A., Stephen, J., Oh, M. Y., et al. (2011). Expanding applications of deep brain stimulation: a potential therapeutic role in obesity and addiction management. *Acta Neurochir.* 153, 2293–2306. doi: 10.1007/s00701-011-1166-3

Hamani, C., Mcandrews, M. P., Cohn, M., Oh, M., Zumsteg, D., Shapiro, C. M., et al. (2008). Memory enhancement induced by hypothalamic/fornix deep brain stimulation. *Ann. Neurol.* 63, 119–123. doi: 10.1002/ana.21295

Haq, I. U., Foote, K. D., Goodman, W. G., Wu, S. S., Sudhyadhom, A., Ricciuti, N., et al. (2011). Smile and laughter induction and intraoperative predictors of response to deep brain stimulation for obsessive-compulsive disorder. *Neuroimage* 54(Suppl. 1), S247–S255. doi: 10.1016/j.neuroimage.2010.03.009

Harat, M., Rudas, M., Zielinski, P., Birska, J., and Sokal, P. (2016). Nucleus accumbens stimulation in pathological obesity. *Neurol. Neurochir. Pol.* 50, 207–210. doi: 10.1016/j.pjnns.2016.01.014

Hassler, R., Riechert, T., Mundinger, F., Umbach, W., and Ganglberger, J. A. (1960). Physiological observations in stereotaxic operations in extrapyramidal motor disturbances. *Brain* 83, 337–350. doi: 10.1093/brain/83.2.337

Hetherington, A. W., and Ranson, S. W. (1940). Hypothalamic lesions and adiposity in the rat. *Anat. Rec. Banner* 78, 149–172. doi: 10.1002/ar.1090780203

Horstmann, A. (2017). It wasn't me; it was my brain - Obesity-associated characteristics of brain circuits governing decision-making. *Physiol. Behav.* 176, 125–133. doi: 10.1016/j.physbeh.2017.04.001

Hotamisligil, G. S. (2017). Inflammation, metaflammation and immunometabolic disorders. *Nature* 542, 177–185. doi: 10.1038/nature21363

Ivezaj, V., White, M. A., and Grilo, C. M. (2016). Examining binge-eating disorder and food addiction in adults with overweight and obesity. *Obesity* 24, 2064–2069. doi: 10.1002/oby.21607

Johnson, P. M., and Kenny, P. J. (2010). Dopamine D2 receptors in addiction-like reward dysfunction and compulsive eating in obese rats. *Nat. Neurosci.* 13, 635–641. doi: 10.1038/nn.2519

Kamegai, J., Tamura, H., Shimizu, T., Ishii, S., Sugihara, H., and Wakabayashi, I. (2000). Central effect of ghrelin, an endogenous growth hormone secretagogue, on hypothalamic peptide gene expression. *Endocrinology* 141, 4797–4800. doi: 10.1210/endo.141.12.7920

Kleinridders, A., Schenten, D., Konner, A. C., Belgardt, B. F., Mauer, J., Okamura, T., et al. (2009). MyD88 signaling in the CNS is required for development of fatty acid-induced leptin resistance and diet-induced obesity. *Cell Metab.* 10, 249–259. doi: 10.1016/j.cmet.2009.08.013

Klooster, D. C., De Louw, A. J., Aldenkamp, A. P., Besseling, R. M., Mestrom, R. M., Carrette, S., et al. (2016). Technical aspects of neurostimulation: focus on equipment, electric field modeling, and stimulation protocols. *Neurosci. Biobehav. Rev.* 65, 113–141. doi: 10.1016/j.neubiorev.2016.02.016

Koek, R. J., Langevin, J. P., Krahl, S. E., Kosoyan, H. J., Schwartz, H. N., Chen, J. W., et al. (2014). Deep brain stimulation of the basolateral amygdala for treatment-refractory combat post-traumatic stress disorder (PTSD): study protocol for a pilot randomized controlled trial with blinded, staggered onset of stimulation. *Trials* 15:356. doi: 10.1186/1745-6215-15-356

Kringelbach, M. L., Jenkinson, N., Owen, S. L., and Aziz, T. Z. (2007). Translational principles of deep brain stimulation. *Nat. Rev. Neurosci.* 8, 623–635. doi: 10.1038/nrn2196

Kuhn, A. A., and Volkmann, J. (2017). Innovations in deep brain stimulation methodology. *Mov. Disord.* 32, 11–19. doi: 10.1002/mds.26703

Kuncel, A. M., and Grill, W. M. (2004). Selection of stimulus parameters for deep brain stimulation. *Clin. Neurophysiol.* 115, 2431–2441. doi: 10.1016/j.clinph.2004.05.031

Labouesse, M. A., Sartori, A. M., Weinmann, O., Simpson, E. H., Kellendonk, C., and Weber-Stadlbauer, U. (2018). Striatal dopamine 2 receptor upregulation during development predisposes to diet-induced obesity by reducing energy output in mice. *Proc. Natl. Acad. Sci. U.S.A.* 115, 10493–10498. doi: 10.1073/pnas.1800171115

Lacan, G., De Salles, A. A., Gorgulho, A. A., Krahl, S. E., Frighetto, L., Behnke, E. J., et al. (2008). Modulation of food intake following deep brain stimulation of the ventromedial hypothalamus in the vervet monkey. Laboratory investigation. *J. Neurosurg.* 108, 336–342. doi: 10.3171/JNS/2008/108/2/0336

Lee, S., Lee, J., Kang, G. M., and Kim, M. S. (2018). Leptin directly regulate intrinsic neuronal excitability in hypothalamic POMC neurons but not in AgRP neurons in food restricted mice. *Neurosci. Lett.* 681, 105–109. doi: 10.1016/j.neulet.2018.05.041

Lemaire, J. J., Nezzar, H., Sakka, L., Boirie, Y., Fontaine, D., Coste, A., et al. (2013). Maps of the adult human hypothalamus. *Surg. Neurol. Int.* 4, S156–S163. doi: 10.4103/2152-7806.110667

Leoutsakos, J. S., Yan, H., Anderson, W. S., Asaad, W. F., Baltuch, G., Burke, A., et al. (2018). Deep brain stimulation targeting the fornix for mild alzheimer dementia (the ADvance Trial): a two year follow-up including results of delayed activation. *J. Alzheimers Dis.* 64, 597–606. doi: 10.3233/JAD-180121

Linssen, R. S. N., Oudijn, M. S., Mantione, M., Van Den Munckhof, P., Denys, D., and Schuurman, P. R. (2017). Body weight changes after deep brain stimulation for obsessive-compulsive disorder or depression. *Stereotact. Funct. Neurosurg.* 95, 348–351. doi: 10.1159/000480665

Liotta, A. S., Loudes, C., Mckelvy, J. F., and Krieger, D. T. (1980). Biosynthesis of precursor corticotropin/endorphin-, corticotropin-, alpha-melanotropin-, beta-lipotropin-, and beta-endorphin-like material by cultured neonatal rat hypothalamic neurons. *Proc. Natl. Acad. Sci. U.S.A.* 77, 1880–1884. doi: 10.1073/pnas.77.4.1880

Luquet, S., Perez, F. A., Hnasko, T. S., and Palmiter, R. D. (2005). NPY/AgRP neurons are essential for feeding in adult mice but can be ablated in neonates. *Science* 310, 683–685. doi: 10.1126/science.1115524

Lüscher, C., Pascoli, V., and Creed, M. (2015). Optogenetic dissection of neural circuitry: from synaptic causalities to blue prints for novel treatments of behavioral diseases. *Curr. Opin. Neurobiol.* 35, 95–100. doi: 10.1016/j.conb.2015.07.005

Mantione, M., Van De Brink, W., Schuurman, P. R., and Denys, D. (2010). Smoking cessation and weight loss after chronic deep brain stimulation of the nucleus accumbens: therapeutic and research implications: case report. *Neurosurgery* 66:E218; discussion E218. doi: 10.1227/01.NEU.0000360570.40339.64

Mastro, K. J., Zitelli, K. T., Willard, A. M., Leblanc, K. H., Kravitz, A. V., and Gittis, A. H. (2017). Cell-specific pallidal intervention induces long-lasting motor recovery in dopamine-depleted mice. *Nat. Neurosci.* 20, 815–823. doi: 10.1038/nn.4559

McClelland, J., Bozhilova, N., Campbell, I., and Schmidt, U. (2013). A systematic review of the effects of neuromodulation on eating and body weight: evidence from human and animal studies. *Eur. Eat. Disord. Rev.* 21, 436–455. doi: 10.1002/erv.2256

Mendes, N. F., Gaspar, J. M., Lima-Júnior, J. C., Donato, J. Jr., Velloso, L. A., and Araújo, E. P. (2018). TGF-beta1 down-regulation in the mediobasal hypothalamus attenuates hypothalamic inflammation and protects against diet-induced obesity. *Metabolism* 85, 171–182. doi: 10.1016/j.metabol.2018.04.005

Meoni, S., Fraix, V., Castrioto, A., Benabid, A. L., Seigneuret, E., Vercueil, L., et al. (2017). Pallidal deep brain stimulation for dystonia: a long term study. *J. Neurol. Neurosurg. Psychiatry* 88, 960–967. doi: 10.1136/jnnp-2016-315504

Meyers, R. (1962). Three cases of myoclonus alleviated by bilateral ansotomy, with a note on postoperative alibido and impotence. *J. Neurosurg.* 19, 71–81. doi: 10.3171/jns.1962.19.1.0071

Milanski, M., Degasperi, G., Coope, A., Morari, J., Denis, R., Cintra, D. E., et al. (2009). Saturated fatty acids produce an inflammatory response predominantly through the activation of TLR4 signaling in hypothalamus: implications for the pathogenesis of obesity. *J. Neurosci.* 29, 359–370. doi: 10.1523/JNEUROSCI.2760-08.2009

Miocinovic, S., Somayajula, S., Chitnis, S., and Vitek, J. L. (2013). History, applications, and mechanisms of deep brain stimulation. *JAMA Neurol.* 70, 163–171. doi: 10.1001/2013.jamaneurol.45

Morton, G. J., Meek, T. H., and Schwartz, M. W. (2014). Neurobiology of food intake in health and disease. *Nat. Rev. Neurosci.* 15, 367–378. doi: 10.1038/nrn3745

Mountjoy, K. G. (2015). Pro-opiomelanocortin (POMC) neurones, POMC-derived peptides, melanocortin receptors and obesity: how understanding of this system has changed over the last decade. *J. Neuroendocrinol.* 27, 406–418. doi: 10.1111/jne.12285

Novakova, L., Ruzicka, E., Jech, R., Serranova, T., Dusek, P., and Urgosik, D. (2007). Increase in body weight is a non-motor side effect of deep brain stimulation of the subthalamic nucleus in Parkinson's disease. *Neuro Endocrinol. Lett.* 28, 21–25.

Odekerken, V. J., Van Laar, T., Staal, M. J., Mosch, A., Hoffmann, C. F., Nijssen, P. C., et al. (2013). Subthalamic nucleus versus globus pallidus bilateral deep brain stimulation for advanced Parkinson's disease (NSTAPS study): a randomised controlled trial. *Lancet Neurol.* 12, 37–44. doi: 10.1016/S1474-4422(12)70264-8

Okun, M. S. (2014). Deep-brain stimulation–entering the era of human neural-network modulation. *N. Engl. J. Med.* 371, 1369–1373. doi: 10.1056/NEJMp1408779

Okun, M. S., Bowers, D., Springer, U., Shapira, N. A., Malone, D., Rezai, A. R., et al. (2004). What's in a "smile?" Intra-operative observations of contralateral smiles induced by deep brain stimulation. *Neurocase* 10, 271–279. doi: 10.1080/13554790490507632

Okun, M. S., Mann, G., Foote, K. D., Shapira, N. A., Bowers, D., Springer, U., et al. (2007). Deep brain stimulation in the internal capsule and nucleus accumbens region: responses observed during active and sham programming. *J. Neurol. Neurosurg. Psychiatry* 78, 310–314. doi: 10.1136/jnnp.2006.095315

Oluigbo, C. O., Salma, A., and Rezai, A. R. (2012). Deep brain stimulation for neurological disorders. *IEEE Rev. Biomed. Eng.* 5, 88–99. doi: 10.1109/RBME.2012.2197745

Prinz, P., and Stengel, A. (2018). Deep brain stimulation-possible treatment strategy for pathologically altered body weight? *Brain Sci.* 8:E19. doi: 10.3390/brainsci8010019

Quaade, F., Vaernet, K., and Larsson, S. (1974). Stereotaxic stimulation and electrocoagulation of the lateral hypothalamus in obese humans. *Acta Neurochir.* 30, 111–117. doi: 10.1007/BF01405759

Rada, P., Bocarsly, M. E., Barson, J. R., Hoebel, B. G., and Leibowitz, S. F. (2010). Reduced accumbens dopamine in Sprague-Dawley rats prone to overeating a fat-rich diet. *Physiol. Behav.* 101, 394–400. doi: 10.1016/j.physbeh.2010.07.005

Rajan, T. M., and Menon, V. (2017). Psychiatric disorders and obesity: a review of association studies. *J. Postgrad. Med.* 63, 182–190. doi: 10.4103/jpgm.JPGM_712_16

Reinholz, J., Skopp, O., Breitenstein, C., Bohr, I., Winterhoff, H., and Knecht, S. (2008). Compensatory weight gain due to dopaminergic hypofunction: new evidence and own incidental observations. *Nutr. Metab.* 5:35. doi: 10.1186/1743-7075-5-35

Remor, A. P., Da Silva, R. A., De Matos, F. J., Glaser, V., De Paula Martins, R., Ghisoni, K., et al. (2018). Chronic metabolic derangement-induced cognitive deficits and neurotoxicity are associated with REST inactivation. *Mol. Neurobiol.* 56, 1539–1557. doi: 10.1007/s12035-018-1175-9

Rezai, A. R., Krishna, V., Bogner, J., Kramer, D., Needleman, B., Emerson, A. M., et al. (2018). Letter: feasibility of nucleus accumbens deep brain stimulation for morbid, treatment-refractory obesity. *Neurosurgery* 82, E136–E137. doi: 10.1093/neuros/nyx630

Rossi, M. A., and Stuber, G. D. (2018). Overlapping brain circuits for homeostatic and hedonic feeding. *Cell Metab.* 27, 42–56. doi: 10.1016/j.cmet.2017.09.021

Sabatinelli, D., Bradley, M. M., Lang, P. J., Costa, V. D., and Versace, F. (2007). Pleasure rather than salience activates human nucleus accumbens and medial prefrontal cortex. *J. Neurophysiol.* 98, 1374–1379. doi: 10.1152/jn.00230.2007

Salanova, V. (2018). Deep brain stimulation for epilepsy. *Epilepsy Behav.* 88S, 21–24. doi: 10.1016/j.yebeh.2018.06.041

Saper, C. B. (2004). "Hypothalamus," in *The Human Nervous System*, 2nd Edn, eds G. Paxinos and J. Mai (Philadelphia, PA: Elsevier).

Schlaepfer, T. E., Bewernick, B. H., Kayser, S., Madler, B., and Coenen, V. A. (2013). Rapid effects of deep brain stimulation for treatment-resistant major depression. *Biol. Psychiatry* 73, 1204–1212. doi: 10.1016/j.biopsych.2013.01.034

Shukla, A. W., Bona, A. R., and Walz, R. (2015). "Troubleshooting in DBS," in *Deep Brain Stimulation*, ed. R. Mehanna (New York, NY: Nova Science Publishers), 213–261.

Sohn, J. W. (2015). Network of hypothalamic neurons that control appetite. *BMB Rep.* 48, 229–233. doi: 10.5483/BMBRep.2015.48.4.272

Springer, U. S., Bowers, D., Goodman, W. K., Shapira, N. A., Foote, K. D., and Okun, M. S. (2006). Long-term habituation of the smile response with deep brain stimulation. *Neurocase* 12, 191–196. doi: 10.1080/13554790600646995

Stice, E., Figlewicz, D. P., Gosnell, B. A., Levine, A. S., and Pratt, W. E. (2013). The contribution of brain reward circuits to the obesity epidemic. *Neurosci. Biobehav. Rev.* 37, 2047–2058. doi: 10.1016/j.neubiorev.2012.12.001

Stice, E., Spoor, S., Bohon, C., Veldhuizen, M. G., and Small, D. M. (2008). Relation of reward from food intake and anticipated food intake to obesity: a functional magnetic resonance imaging study. *J. Abnorm. Psychol.* 117, 924–935. doi: 10.1037/a0013600

Talakoub, O., Paiva, R. R., Milosevic, M., Hoexter, M. Q., Franco, R., Alho, E., et al. (2017). Lateral hypothalamic activity indicates hunger and satiety states in humans. *Ann. Clin. Transl. Neurol.* 4, 897–901. doi: 10.1002/acn3.466

Thaler, J. P., Yi, C. X., Schur, E. A., Guyenet, S. J., Hwang, B. H., Dietrich, M. O., et al. (2012). Obesity is associated with hypothalamic injury in rodents and humans. *J. Clin. Invest.* 122, 153–162. doi: 10.1172/JCI59660

Timper, K., and Bruning, J. C. (2017). Hypothalamic circuits regulating appetite and energy homeostasis: pathways to obesity. *Dis. Model. Mech.* 10, 679–689. doi: 10.1242/dmm.026609

Tronnier, V. M., Rasche, D., Thorns, V., Alvarez-Fischer, D., Munte, T. F., and Zurowski, B. (2018). Massive weight loss following deep brain stimulation of the nucleus accumbens in a depressed woman. *Neurocase* 24, 49–53. doi: 10.1080/13554794.2018.1431678

Udupa, K., and Chen, R. (2015). The mechanisms of action of deep brain stimulation and ideas for the future development. *Prog. Neurobiol.* 133, 27–49. doi: 10.1016/j.pneurobio.2015.08.001

Valdearcos, M., Douglass, J. D., Robblee, M. M., Dorfman, M. D., Stifler, D. R., Bennett, M. L., et al. (2017). Microglial inflammatory signaling orchestrates the hypothalamic immune response to dietary excess and mediates obesity susceptibility. *Cell Metab.* 26, 185–197.e3. doi: 10.1016/j.cmet.2017.05.015

Valdearcos, M., Robblee, M. M., Benjamin, D. I., Nomura, D. K., Xu, A. W., and Koliwad, S. K. (2014). Microglia dictate the impact of saturated fat consumption on hypothalamic inflammation and neuronal function. *Cell Rep.* 9, 2124–2138. doi: 10.1016/j.celrep.2014.11.018

Valdearcos, M., Xu, A. W., and Koliwad, S. K. (2015). Hypothalamic inflammation in the control of metabolic function. *Annu. Rev. Physiol.* 77, 131–160. doi: 10.1146/annurev-physiol-021014-071656

Val-Laillet, D., Aarts, E., Weber, B., Ferrari, M., Quaresima, V., Stoeckel, L. E., et al. (2015). Neuroimaging and neuromodulation approaches to study eating behavior and prevent and treat eating disorders and obesity. *Neuroimage Clin.* 8, 1–31. doi: 10.1016/j.nicl.2015.03.016

Wang, G. J., Volkow, N. D., Logan, J., Pappas, N. R., Wong, C. T., Zhu, W., et al. (2001). Brain dopamine and obesity. *Lancet* 357, 354–357. doi: 10.1016/S0140-6736(00)03643-6

Wang, T. R., Moosa, S., Dallapiazza, R. F., Elias, W. J., and Lynch, W. J. (2018). Deep brain stimulation for the treatment of drug addiction. *Neurosurg. Focus* 45:E11. doi: 10.3171/2018.5.FOCUS18163

Wang, X., Ge, A., Cheng, M., Guo, F., Zhao, M., Zhou, X., et al. (2012). Increased hypothalamic inflammation associated with the susceptibility to obesity in rats exposed to high-fat diet. *Exp. Diabetes Res.* 2012:847246. doi: 10.1155/2012/847246

Wardlaw, S. L. (2011). Hypothalamic proopiomelanocortin processing and the regulation of energy balance. *Eur. J. Pharmacol.* 660, 213–219. doi: 10.1016/j.ejphar.2010.10.107

Weintraub, D., Duda, J. E., Carlson, K., Luo, P., Sagher, O., Stern, M., et al. (2013). Suicide ideation and behaviours after STN and GPi DBS surgery for Parkinson's disease: results from a randomised, controlled trial. *J. Neurol. Neurosurg. Psychiatry* 84, 1113–1118. doi: 10.1136/jnnp-2012-304396

Whiting, A. C., Oh, M. Y., and Whiting, D. M. (2018). Deep brain stimulation for appetite disorders: a review. *Neurosurg. Focus* 45:E9. doi: 10.3171/2018.4.FOCUS18141

Whiting, D. M., Tomycz, N. D., Bailes, J., De Jonge, L., Lecoultre, V., Wilent, B., et al. (2013). Lateral hypothalamic area deep brain stimulation for refractory obesity: a pilot study with preliminary data on safety, body weight, and energy metabolism. *J. Neurosurg.* 119, 56–63. doi: 10.3171/2013.2.JNS12903

Wilent, W. B., Oh, M. Y., Buetefisch, C. M., Bailes, J. E., Cantella, D., Angle, C., et al. (2010). Induction of panic attack by stimulation of the ventromedial hypothalamus. *J. Neurosurg.* 112, 1295–1298. doi: 10.3171/2009.9.JNS09577

Williams, N. R., and Okun, M. S. (2013). Deep brain stimulation (DBS) at the interface of neurology and psychiatry. *J. Clin. Invest.* 123, 4546–4556. doi: 10.1172/JCI68341

Wu, Q., Lemus, M. B., Stark, R., Bayliss, J. A., Reichenbach, A., Lockie, S. H., et al. (2014). The temporal pattern of cfos activation in hypothalamic, cortical, and brainstem nuclei in response to fasting and refeeding in male mice. *Endocrinology* 155, 840–853. doi: 10.1210/en.2013-1831

Zhang, X., and van den Pol, A. N. (2016). Hypothalamic arcuate nucleus tyrosine hydroxylase neurons play orexigenic role in energy homeostasis. *Nat. Neurosci.* 19, 1341–1347. doi: 10.1038/nn.4372

Zhang, X., Zhang, G., Zhang, H., Karin, M., Bai, H., and Cai, D. (2008). Hypothalamic IKKbeta/NF-kappaB and ER stress link overnutrition to energy imbalance and obesity. *Cell* 135, 61–73. doi: 10.1016/j.cell.2008.07.043

Zhang, Y., Proenca, R., Maffei, M., Barone, M., Leopold, L., and Friedman, J. M. (1994). Positional cloning of the mouse obese gene and its human homologue. *Nature* 372, 425–432. doi: 10.1038/372425a0

11

Hypoxia Inducible Factor as a Central Regulator of Metabolism – Implications for the Development of Obesity

Joana M. Gaspar[1,2] *and Lício A. Velloso*[3,4*]

[1] *Post-Graduation in Biochemistry, Department of Biochemistry, Federal University of Santa Catarina, Florianópolis, Brazil,* [2] *Laboratório de Bioenergética e Estresse Oxidativo, Departamento de Bioquímica, Centro de Ciências Biológicas, Universidade Federal de Santa Catarina, Florianópolis, Brazil,* [3] *Laboratory of Cell Signaling, Obesity and Comorbidities Research Center, University of Campinas, Campinas, Brazil,* [4] *National Institute of Science and Technology on Neuroimmunomodulation, Rio de Janeiro, Brazil*

Correspondence:
Lício A. Velloso
lavelloso.unicamp@gmail.com

The hypothalamus plays a major role in the regulation of food intake and energy expenditure. In the last decade, it was demonstrated that consumption of high-fat diets triggers the activation of an inflammatory process in the hypothalamus, inducing neurofunctional alterations and contributing to the development of obesity. Hypoxia-inducible factors (HIFs) are key molecules that regulate cellular responses to inflammation and hypoxia, being essential for the normal cell function and survival. Currently, evidence points to a role of HIF pathway in metabolic regulation that could also be involved in the progression of obesity and metabolic diseases. The challenge is to understand how HIF modulation impacts body mass gain and metabolic disorders such as insulin resistance. Distinct animal models with tissue-specific knocking-out or overexpression of hypoxia signaling pathway genes revealed a cell-specificity in the activation of HIF pathways, and some of them have opposite phenotypes among the various HIFs gain- and loss-of-function mouse models. In this review, we discuss the major findings that provide support for a role of HIF pathway involvement in the regulation of metabolism, especially in glucose and energy homeostasis.

Keywords: HIF complex, obesity, metabolic disorders, inflammation, hypothalamus, energy homeostasis

INTRODUCTION

Obesity has reached epidemic proportions around the world. It is characterized by excessive and abnormal fat mass accumulation, associated with chronic low-grade systemic inflammation, which predispose to metabolic diseases. In 2015, in the adult population, a total of 603.7 million were obese and approximately 1.9 billion were overweight. In addition, childhood obesity has increased considerably raising concern issues on the future of public health in the world (Collaborators et al., 2017; Gregg and Shaw, 2017).

Obesity has a multifactorial and complex etiology, involving the combination of genetic and epigenetic factors, life style, and socioeconomic status, which result in increased food intake, decreased energy expenditure, and also changes in nutrient utilization and metabolism, ultimately leading to a positive energy balance. The aberrant expansion of white adipose tissue, through hyperplasia as well as hypertrophy, promotes insufficient intra-adipose blood perfusion resulting in hypoxia. These niches of hypoxia are partially responsible for white adipose tissue inflammation and insulin resistance (Jiang et al., 2011; Lee et al., 2011, 2014; Krishnan et al., 2012; Michailidou et al., 2015). Hypoxia-inducible factor-α (HIF-α) is a fundamental transcription factor involved in the oxygen homeostasis that induces inflammation and insulin resistance in obesity. In addition, the abnormal regulation of HIF complex is involved in the development of obesity, fatty liver disease, and type 2 diabetes (Virtue and Vidal-Puig, 2011; Girgis et al., 2012). Moreover, recent data show that HIF has important functions in the hypothalamus, the region of the brain that controls energy balance and metabolism (Lando et al., 2002; Bento and Pereira, 2011; Zhang et al., 2011; Ban et al., 2014).

Currently, the approaches used to treat obesity include behavioral counseling for reducing caloric intake and increasing physical activity, the use of some pharmacological compounds that reduce hunger and caloric harvesting from the gut and bariatric surgery. However, these interventions have not proven effective in providing long term weight loss, highlighting the importance of development of new strategies to tackle obesity (Gonzalez-Muniesa et al., 2017; Narayanaswami and Dwoskin, 2017; Srivastava and Apovian, 2018). Several animal studies manipulating HIF pathways highlight the involvement of this transcriptional factor in the pathogenesis of obesity placing it as a potential target for the treatment of obesity and diabetes. The current challenge is to understand how HIF modulation might impact body weight gain and metabolic disorders such as insulin resistance. Here, we review data that have contributed to expand the current understanding of how HIF regulates whole body metabolism and how it is affected by nutritional and immune signals that are involved in the pathophysiology of obesity and metabolic disorders.

HYPOTHALAMIC REGULATION OF ENERGY EXPENDITURE

The regulation of energy homeostasis is a highly integrated and regulated process aimed at maintaining the stability of body energy stores over time. Neurons located in the hypothalamus are the most important components of the complex system that regulates energy flux in the body. Hypothalamic neurons respond to peripheral signals controlling food intake and energy expenditure on a homeostatic way, and also integrate with limbic and cortical areas to coordinate the hedonic responses to food (Timper and Bruning, 2017; Rossi and Stuber, 2018).

The hypothalamus, located at the base of the forebrain and around the walls of third ventricle, is at a privileged location to receive afferent signals from the periphery through the bloodstream, and also from the brainstem. These signals inform hypothalamic neurons about the magnitude of the energy stores in body. In turn, the neurons respond providing signals that regulate hunger and energy expenditure, as well as systemic glucose and lipid metabolism (Williams and Schwartz, 2011; Kim et al., 2018). The hypothalamus is composed by several nuclei arrayed in a three-dimensional organization, each with distinct neuronal connections and functions, including the arcuate nucleus (ARC), paraventricular nucleus (PVN), ventromedial nucleus (VMN), dorsomedial nucleus (DMN), and lateral hypothalamic area (LHA; Baroncini et al., 2012; Kim et al., 2018).

The role of the hypothalamus in feeding and metabolism was first demonstrated in the 1940s, when severe hypophagia was observed after large lesions centered on the lateral hypothalamus (Hetherington and Ranson, 1940). Conversely, lesions on the VMH and ARC induced hyperphagia and obesity (Marshall and Mayer, 1956; Olney, 1969). Such studies led to the definition of the central role played by the hypothalamic nuclei controlling satiety and hunger (Timper and Bruning, 2017; Kim et al., 2018).

The strategic location of ARC in proximity to the median eminence places its neurons in close contact with a special type of blood/spinal fluid interface that is less restrictive than the classical blood/brain barrier (Haddad-Tovolli et al., 2017). Due to this anatomical particularity, ARC neurons are exposed to systemic oscillations of hormone and nutrient levels providing rapid and dynamic information required for optimal regulation of whole body energy homeostasis. Within the ARC, there are three main neuronal subpopulations: a subpopulation of anorexigenic neurons that co-express cocaine and amphetamine-related transcript (CART) and proopiomelanocortin (POMC; Vrang et al., 1999; Yaswen et al., 1999); and two subpopulations of orexigenic neurons, one co-expressing neuropeptide Y (NPY) and agouti-related protein (AgRP; Hahn et al., 1998; Luquet et al., 2005), and another expressing tyrosine hydroxylase (TH; Zhang and van den Pol, 2015, 2016). ARC neurons communicate with other hypothalamic areas (PVN, DMN, and LHA) involved in appetite regulation.

Hormonal Regulation

The identification of leptin in 1994 (Zhang et al., 1994) is a hallmark that provided advance in the characterization of hypothalamic pathways/mechanisms involved in the regulation of energy homeostasis. Leptin is secreted by adipose tissue and circulates at concentrations proportional to fat mass providing key signals for the regulation of food intake (**Figure 1**). Leptin binds to the long form of the leptin receptor, Ob-Rb, both in POMC and AgRP neurons in the hypothalamus. POMC neurons are activated by leptin, while AgRP neurons are inhibited (Cheung et al., 1997; Williams and Schwartz, 2011; Lee et al., 2018). Insulin is also an important regulator of food intake and energy expenditure. Insulin receptors are distributed all over the brain, particularly in hypothalamic neurons and upon ligand-induced stimulation it activates POMC neurons and inhibit food intake (Woods et al., 1979; Belgardt et al., 2008; **Figure 1**).

Activation of POMC neurons induces the release of α-melanocyte-stimulating hormone (α-MSH) that is an endogenous agonist of the melanocortin 3 and 4 receptors (MC3-R and MC4-R), mostly localized in the PVN (Cowley et al., 2001; Mountjoy, 2015). Conversely, AgRP is an endogenous antagonist of MC4-R in the PVN. The inhibition of AgRP neurons by leptin blocks the activation of PVN neurons, which results in the inhibition of synaptic activation, increasing food intake and consequently decreasing energy expenditure (Ollmann et al., 1997; Mizuno and Mobbs, 1999; Lee et al., 2018).

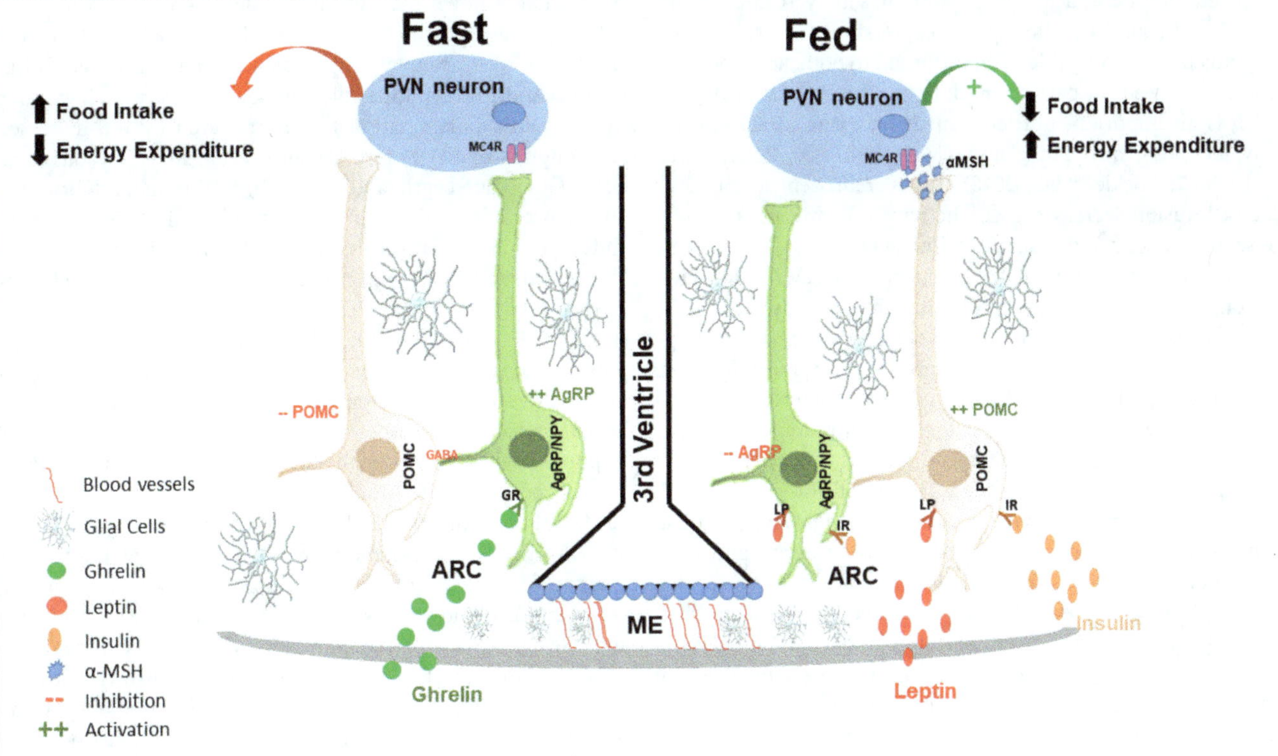

FIGURE 1 | Hypothalamic regulation of energy homeostasis: the hypothalamus senses and integrates peripheral adipostatic hormones that circulate in levels proportionate to nutritional status and adipose tissue stores. Under fasting conditions ghrelin, secreted by the stomach, binds to its receptor in AgRP neurons in the ARC, leading to its activation. AgRP neuronal activation increased the release of AgRP that is an antagonist of MC4R in the PVN neurons; at the same time, AgRP neurons also release of GABA neurotransmitter that inhibited POMC neurons, and consequently increasing appetite and decreased energy expenditures. In the fed state, insulin and leptin act directly on their receptors, both in POMC and AgRP neurons in the ARC of the hypothalamus to control energy homeostasis; insulin and leptin induce inhibition of AgRP and activation of POMC neurons. POMC neuronal activation involves the processing of POMC with formation of α-MSH that is an agonist of MC4R and consequently activating PVN neurons. PVN activation culminates in satiety (decreased food intake) and stimulation of energy expenditure. AgRP, agouti related protein; MC4R, melanocortin 4 receptor; GABA, gamma-aminobutyric acid; POMC, proopiomelanocortin; α-MSH, alpha-melanocyte-stimulating hormone; PVN, paraventricular nucleus.

Ghrelin is yet another hormone that is involved in hypothalamic neuronal regulation. It is primarily produced by the stomach in fasting condition and has the property of inducing food intake, through the activation of ghrelin receptors expressed predominantly in AgRP neurons (Al Massadi et al., 2017). Thus, AgRP/NPY neurons are activated by fasting and ghrelin (Kamegai et al., 2000; Nakazato et al., 2001; Tang-Christensen et al., 2004; Betley et al., 2015), leading to a greater release of AgRP; therefore, stimulating appetite. Furthermore, AgRP neuronal activation also leads to the release of gamma-aminobutyric acid (GABA) and NPY that inhibit POMC neurons (Cowley et al., 2001; Atasoy et al., 2012) providing further increase in food intake.

Nutrient Sensing

There are extensive data indicating that in addition to hormonal factors, hypothalamic neurons can also sense nutrients (glucose, lipids, and some amino acids, such as leucine) to modulate food intake and energy expenditure (Loftus et al., 2000) and also to regulate systemic glucose and lipid levels (Obici et al., 2002b; Chari et al., 2010; Thorens, 2012).

The first demonstration that hypothalamus can sense nutritional status came from studies of Miselis and Epstein (1975), showing that the induction of glucoprivation in hypothalamus increases feeding behavior. Thereafter, two hypothalamic neuronal subpopulations were defined as glucose-excited (GE), found mostly in the lateral ARC, and glucose-inhibited (GI) neurons, found in the medial ARC (Wang et al., 2004; Thorens, 2012). Later on, studies demonstrated that GE are predominantly POMC neurons (Parton et al., 2007), whereas GI are predominantly AgRP (Chalmers et al., 2014). Hypothalamic increase of glucose concentration results in a decrease in AgRP mRNA levels and to an activation of POMC neurons, which leads to decreased food intake, decreased hepatic glucose production and increased insulin secretion (Thorens, 2012).

Energy depletion is sensed by mechanisms that activate catabolic pathways to mobilize cellular components for the provision of energy, such as autophagy and 5′ AMP-activated protein kinase (AMPK). AMPK is a central enzyme for the regulation of whole body metabolism, its activation increases fatty acid oxidation, glucose uptake, and stimulates glycolysis and mitochondrial biogenesis (Ha et al., 2015). In POMC and AgRP neuronal populations, the activation of AMPK acts as a nutrient sensor and as a regulator of satiety (Claret et al., 2007; Kola, 2008), by altering the expression of orexigenic or anorexigenic neuropeptides. Alterations in hypothalamic glucose concentration act in part by modulating the activity of AMPK which is an important nutrient sensor in several tissues in the body, including the hypothalamus (Minokoshi et al., 2004; Claret et al., 2007; Lockie et al., 2018). Intracerebroventricular (icv) glucose infusion decreases AMPK activity in POMC neurons and consequently reduces food intake (Zhang et al., 2011). However, low glucose concentration induces activation of AMPK (in AgRP neurons) leading to increased food intake and body mass gain, this effect is inhibited by insulin and leptin. Briefly, AMPK is inhibited by high glucose concentrations or by refeeding that decrease the expression of AgRP and NPY (Claret et al., 2007; Chalmers et al., 2014). High glucose concentration can induce depolarization in POMC neurons leading to its activation (Parton et al., 2007). Thus, the combined actions of glucose in AgRP and POMC neurons provide anorexigenic signals through a pathway distinct but yet integrated with the pathway controlled by hormones.

Autophagy is an evolutionary conserved mechanism that provides an alternative form of energy to the starved cell. Some evidence suggests that autophagy is closely involved in the hypothalamic regulation of food intake (Kaushik et al., 2011, 2012; Singh and Cuervo, 2011; Portovedo et al., 2015; Oh et al., 2016). Long-term fasting was shown increase autophagy in AgRP neurons resulting in increased expression of the neuropeptide AgRP and thus, increasing food intake (Kaushik et al., 2011). In POMC neurons, the impairment of autophagy induces an increase in food consumption and body weight gain (Malhotra et al., 2015). Recently, it was demonstrated that autophagy that occurs in hypothalamic neuronal populations is induced/regulated by the activation of AMPK. Under low-glucose availability AMPK-induced autophagy regulates appetite by regulating neuropeptide expression NPY and POMC (Oh et al., 2016).

Fatty acids and the amino acid leucine also regulate food intake via hypothalamus. Enzymes and intermediates of fatty acid metabolism function as energy sensors for hypothalamic response to fats. The icv administration of long-chain fatty acids can trigger a hypothalamic response to inhibit food intake and regulate glucose homeostasis (decrease in plasma insulin and glucose levels and also reduction of hepatic glucose production; Obici et al., 2002a). The mechanism behind regulation of food intake is likely mediated by the decreased expression of orexigenic hypothalamic NPY and AgRP levels (Obici et al., 2002a; Morgan et al., 2004; Chari et al., 2010). A summarized view of the physiological hypothalamic control of food intake and energy expenditure is shown in **Figure 1**.

OBESITY-ASSOCIATED HYPOTHALAMIC DYSFUNCTION

In non-pathological conditions, hypothalamic neurons are programed to respond to hormones, nutrients, and neural signals maintaining whole body energy homeostasis. However, several studies have shown that during the development of obesity, a defective regulation of this system plays a major role in the emergence of a positive energy balance. The main mechanism behind abnormal hypothalamic function in obesity is a low-grade hypothalamic inflammation that is triggered by the increased consumption of dietary fats (De Souza et al., 2005; Cavadas et al., 2016; Guillemot-Legris and Muccioli, 2017; Jais and Bruning, 2017). Activation of Toll-like receptor-4 (TLR4), induction of endoplasmic reticulum stress, and activation of isozyme protein kinase C-theta (PKC-theta) have all been identified as important mediators of the dietary fats induced inflammation (Benoit et al., 2009; Milanski et al., 2009). The consumption of large portions of predominantly saturated dietary fats promotes a rapid (as early as one day) increase in the expression of proinflammatory cytokines in the hypothalamus. Most of this response is dependent on the activation of resident microglia (Thaler et al., 2012; Morari et al., 2014; Valdearcos et al., 2014, 2017). If the consumption of dietary fats is interrupted after short time, the inflammation will disappear without major damage. However, if the consumption of dietary fats persists, peripheral myeloid cells will be recruited to the hypothalamus and the chronicity of inflammation will provoke damage to neurons (Moraes et al., 2009; Souza et al., 2016; Valdearcos et al., 2017). Studies have shown that in diet-induced obesity, the hypothalamic neurons are afflicted by abnormal mitochondrial turnover, abnormal function of the ubiquitin/proteasome system, and abnormal regulation of autophagy (Horvath et al., 2010; Ignacio-Souza et al., 2014; Portovedo et al., 2015; Carraro et al., 2017). Initially, neurons become resistant to the actions of leptin and insulin; however, as inflammation persists, neuronal apoptosis will appear. POMC neurons are more sensitive to the damage inflicted by inflammation and after some time, an imbalance in the orexigenic and anorexigenic hypothalamic neuronal subpopulations can act to boost body mass gain (Souza et al., 2016). Taken together all of these studies suggest that hypothalamic neuroinflammation could be a cause rather than a consequence of diet-induced obesity and metabolic dysfunction. Defining the details involved in the regulation and response to hypothalamic inflammation may help identifying potential targets to prevent and treat obesity.

HIF CANONICAL PATHWAY AND CELLULAR FUNCTIONS

Hypoxia-inducible factors (HIFs) are basic helix-loop-helix transcription factors that act as master regulators of hypoxia activated gene expression, allowing the adaptation to hypoxia (Semenza et al., 1991; Wang et al., 1995). HIF is a heterodimer complex composed by two subunits, α-subunit (oxygen sensitive) and a β-subunit [constitutively expressed, and also called aryl hydrocarbon receptor nuclear translocator (ARNT)]. In mammalian cells, there are three major α subunits isoforms, 1α, 2α (also known as endothelial PAS domain-containing protein 1, EPAS1), and 3α. HIF-1α subunit is ubiquitously expressed and 2α is selectively expressed in tissue-restricted manner (e.g., in vascular endothelial cells and myeloid-derived cells). Both

HIF1α and HIF2α function mainly as transcriptional activators, regulating several biological processes, such as angiogenesis, glucose, fatty acid, cholesterol, and mitochondrial metabolism and inflammation (Greer et al., 2012; Semenza, 2014). HIF3α has very weak transcriptional capacity, compared to other HIFs isoforms. A splicing isoform generated from HIF3α, inhibitory PAS (Per/Arnt/Sim) domain protein (IPAS), can function as a dominant negative regulator of HIF1α. This splicing isoform of HIF3 α can function as a negative feedback loop regulation of adaptive responses to hypoxia/ischemia (Makino et al., 2002).

Under normoxia, the hydroxylation of a proline and asparagine residues suppresses HIF transcriptional activity. Specifically, under normal oxygen conditions, α-subunits are hydroxylated in two conserved proline residues (405 and 531) within the O_2-dependent degradation domain, by prolyl-hydroxylases domain proteins (PHDs; Epstein et al., 2001). The hydroxylation of α-subunit function as a target for von Hippel-Lindau tumor suppressor protein (pVHL), and is subsequently ubiquitylated by the Elongin BC/Cul2/pVHL ubiquitin–ligase complex, a marker for 26S proteasome degradation (Maxwell et al., 1999; Ivan et al., 2001; Jaakkola et al., 2001; Greer et al., 2012). HIF-α subunit is also hydroxylated in an asparagine residue (803) that blocks the association with coactivators. This hydroxylation is mediated by an asparaginyl hydroxylase factor inhibiting HIF-1 (FIH-1; Lando et al., 2002). Together, the oxygen-dependent enzymes, prolyl and asparaginyl hydroxylases, are critical regulatory components of the hypoxic response pathway, regulating both stability and transcriptional activity of HIF complex (Greer et al., 2012; **Figure 2**).

The canonical pathway of HIF activation defines that under low O_2 concentration, α-subunits are no longer hydroxylated by PHDs and neither degraded by the proteasome. Instead, this promotes stabilization of α-subunit that translocates to the nucleus and dimerizes with ARNT/HIF-1β subunit recruiting coactivators such as Creb Binding Protein (CBP)/p300. This transcriptional complex binds to hypoxia-response elements (HREs), within the promoter of target genes, and transactivates gene expression that regulates the adaptive response to hypoxia (Semenza et al., 1991; Greer et al., 2012; Semenza, 2014; **Figure 2**).

In addition to hypoxia, HIF stabilization and transcription activity can be regulated by several other factors, such as reactive oxygen species (ROS), nitric oxide (NO), metabolic intermediates of the tricarboxylic acid (TCA) cycle (such as succinate and fumarate), proinflammatory mediators [tumor necrosis factor-α (TNF-α), interleukine-1β (IL-1β)] and also hormonal factors. The regulation of HIF can occur by increasing its stabilization, by inhibiting both enzymes PHD and FIH, and also by the recruitment and posttranslational modification of cofactors that potentiate the transcriptional complex (Lando et al., 2002).

Hypoxia-inducible factor regulates several genes that promote the adaptation to hypoxia [for example, vascular endothelial growth factor (VEGF), erythropoietin, and glucose transporter-1 (GLUT1)] and also genes that promote a metabolic switch to glycolysis through the transcriptional regulation of key metabolic enzymes [for example, pyruvate dehydrogenase kinase 1 (PDK1), lactate dehydrogenase A (LDHA), and glycogen phosphorylase L (PYGL)]. The transcriptional regulation of these metabolic enzymes by HIF-1 activation under oxygen deprivation stimulates glucose intake, glycolysis, and lactate production to provide ATP. In liver, hypoxia-activated HIF-1 leads to an increase hepatic glucose production by transactivation of phosphoenolpyruvate carboxykinase (PEPCK), a rate-limiting enzyme in gluconeogenesis, gene in liver (Choi et al., 2005).

In obesity, the expansion of adipose tissue (hypertrophy and hyperplasia) creates hypoxia niches that are involved in the inflammatory process and insulin resistance that culminates in hyperglycemia (Halberg et al., 2009; Fujisaka et al., 2013). HIF-1α mRNA and protein are enhanced in adipose tissue in a model of diet-induced obesity, by a mechanism that involves adipogenesis, insulin, and hypoxia (He et al., 2011). Both in obese patients and in animal models of obesity, there is an association between reduced oxygen pressure in adipose depots and macrophage and T cell infiltration (Ye et al., 2007; Pasarica et al., 2009; Fujisaka et al., 2013), highlighting the role of HIF pathway in the development of inflammation.

In the last decade, it has been suggested a broad range of functions including embryonic development, immunity and metabolism (Frede et al., 2006; Semenza, 2014; Corcoran and O'Neill, 2016). When changes in metabolism occur, multiple signals (O_2, CO_2, ROS, immunometabolism, and ATP) emanate from the mitochondria. These signals regulate HIF response, which in turn promote major changes in immune cell function and subsequently affects distinct cellular and organic functions (Peyssonnaux et al., 2007; Jantsch et al., 2008; Corcoran and O'Neill, 2016). Therefore, HIF is a key cellular metabolic sensor all over the body.

Immune Regulation of HIF

Despite the fact that HIF regulation has primarily been thought oxygen concentration, several studies have showed that HIF-1α can have an oxygen-independent regulation, such as in response to hyperglycemia, oxidative stress, and inflammatory proteins (Cramer et al., 2003; Catrina, 2014; Corcoran and O'Neill, 2016). Hypoxia is an important factor in the pathophysiology of a number of human diseases (e.g., obesity, insulin resistance, diabetes, Alzheimer disease, and aging) that are characterized by the presence of inflammatory processes (Eltzschig and Carmeliet, 2011; Iyalomhe et al., 2017). Hypoxia can also lead to the production of oxygen radicals, which, as well, have important implications in these diseases. Nevertheless, HIF-1α can also act as a neuroprotective factor following some neuronal insults, activating survival genes, and promoting the adaptation to oxidative stress and inflammation.

Proinflammatory cytokines (TNF-α and IL-1β) can upregulate HIF-1α, by a mechanism that inhibits PHD enzymes with stabilization of HIF activity; conversely, HIF-1 transcriptional activity can downregulate receptors for inflammatory cytokines, attenuating the neuroinflammation (Dehne and Brune, 2009; Xing and Lu, 2016; Iyalomhe et al., 2017).

The molecular mechanism of HIF activation induced by neuroinflammation involves the activation of TLRs and subsequent activation of the mitogen-activated protein kinase (MAPK) pathway and nuclear factor kappa-light-chain-enhancer of activated B cells (NF-kb), which transactivate HIF-1α under

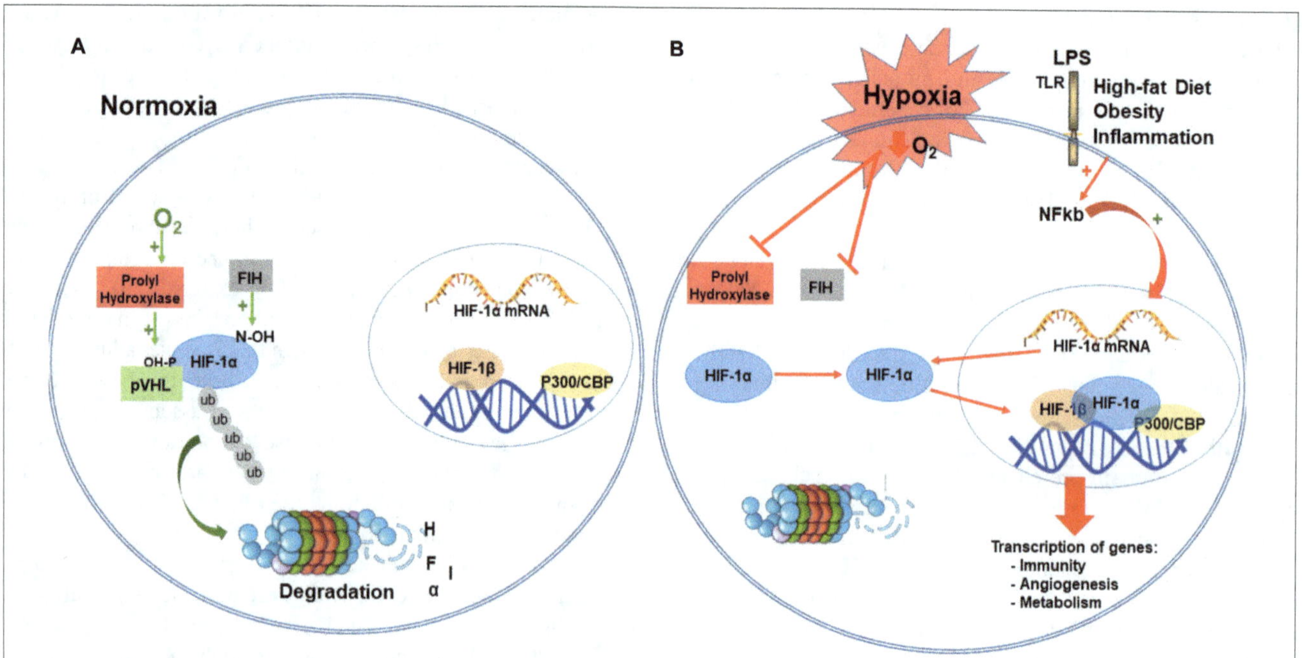

FIGURE 2 | Hypoxia-inducible factor-1 regulation. Under normoxia, HIF-1α is hydroxylated on proline residues 402 and 564 by prolyl hydroxylases (PHD). This hydroxylation is a target for von Hippel-Lindau protein (VHL) binding, a E3 ligase that targets HIF-1α for ubiquitination and proteasomal degradation. Factor inhibiting HIF-1 (FIH-1) hydroxylated an asparagine residue (803) that blocks the binding of the coactivator p300/CBP **(A)**. Under hypoxia, PDH and FIH are inhibited and HIF-1α is stabilized to dimerize with HIF-1β, and binds to target genes at the DNA, recruits p300, and activates transcription of several genes involved in immunity, angiogenesis, metabolism, survival, and proliferation. Immune and inflammatory stimuli can also regulate the HIF pathway, primarily via activation of Toll-like receptors (TRL) and NF-kB activation. NF-Kb is translocated to the nucleus where it regulates the expression of HIF- α mRNA **(B)**. CBP/p300, Creb Binding Protein/p300; LPS, lipopolysaccharide; PHD, prolyl hydroxylases; VHL, von Hippel-Lindau protein; FIH-1, factor inhibiting HIF-1; P-OH, hydroxylation in proline residues; N-OH, hydroxylation in asparaginyl residues; TLR-4, Toll-like receptors; ub, ubiquitin; NF-kB, nuclear factor kappa-light-chain-enhancer of activated B cells.

normal oxygen tension (Frede et al., 2006; Spirig et al., 2010). Neuroinflammation induced upregulation of HIF-1α suggests the involvement of neuronal survival pathway during inflammatory neurological insults, particularly in the early stages of the process.

In hypothalamus, HIF-1α is increased after short-term high-fat diet consumption, before the onset of body weight gain (Gaspar et al., 2018). The inhibition of HIF signaling in ARC of mice fed a HFD induces hypothalamic inflammation, with increased expression of TLR4, TNFα, and IL-1β, and is associated with an increase in body mass gain and glucose intolerance (Gaspar et al., 2018). Taken together, these results and the fact that consumption of saturated fats is involved in the biogenesis of obesity (Thaler et al., 2012; Valdearcos et al., 2014), it is possible that HIF-1α stabilization is a regulator and a protective factor against saturated fatty acids induced-neuroinflammation, regulating energy expenditure and metabolism.

CENTRAL REGULATION OF METABOLISM BY HIF

The hypothalamus has a critical role in the regulation of energy homeostasis and whole-body metabolism. Changes in hypothalamic nutrient and hormonal sensors play important roles in the genesis of obesity and metabolic disorders. Studies performed at high altitude, in conditions of hypobaric hypoxia, have demonstrated a progressive loss of body mass, caused by the decrease in food intake and thus inducing an energy deficit possibly due to hypobaric hypoxia (Westerterp-Plantenga et al., 1999; Westerterp and Kayser, 2006). In these studies, Wasterterp and colleagues exposed eight men for 31 days to simulated stay in high altitudes with palatable food provided *ad libitum*. They observed a decrease in body mass in 5 ± 2 kg with a 40% reduction in energy intake as a result of a decrease in appetite. Changes in appetite can occur by central mechanisms of energy homeostasis regulation, but also by an increase in leptin secretion (Tschop et al., 1998). Weight loss due to hypobaric hypoxia was also observed in obese patients; in high altitude, obese subjects presented increased leptin levels and higher metabolic rate (Lippl et al., 2010). Populations that live at high altitude had a lower prevalence of impaired fasting glucose and type 2 diabetes compared with low altitude living populations (Santos et al., 2001).

The combination of these studies and the fact that hypothalamus, mainly the ARC, express high levels of both HIF-1α and HIF-2α (Zhang et al., 2011; Gaspar et al., 2018), raised the question of how central HIF activity regulates food intake and whole-body metabolism. HIF-1α is expressed in POMC neurons, in astrocytes and microglial cells within the ARC (Gaspar et al., 2018).

Mice with a neuronal-specific loss for the FIH-1α presented reduced body weight, decreased fat accumulation, elevated metabolic rate, hyperventilation, enhanced insulin sensitivity, and improved glucose and lipid metabolism; in addition, they are resistant to body weight gain and hepatic steatosis induced by high-fat feeding (Zhang et al., 2010). However, this study does not demonstrate which brain region was responsible for this metabolic regulation, since FIH was deleted in whole-body neuronal cells. FIH neuronal deletion, and consequently increased activity of HIF-1a induces an increased in food intake besides the beneficial effects of whole body weight. FIH is an enzyme that is negative regulator of other proteins such SOCS (Ferguson et al., 2007), that suppress leptin signaling. FIH can also regulate several other proteins such as Notch receptors, p105 and IkBa (Cockman et al., 2006; Coleman et al., 2007), which make a difficult task to for the determination of direct FIH action as a regulator of food intake trough HIF signaling. Since many of these metabolic processes are controlled by neuronal regulatory circuits located in the hypothalamus, at least in part the neuronal HIF-1α activity regulates systemic metabolism through the modulation of afferent neural connections.

Another study showed that HIF is present in the hypothalamus and is upregulated by the local availability of glucose and its metabolites (Zhang et al., 2011). In this study, the authors demonstrate that under glucose availability in HIF can function as a glucose sensor that specifically binds to the promoter of pomc gene, upregulation the POMC expression. HIF loss-of-function specifically in POMC neurons caused increase in food intake, decrease in basal metabolism, and consequently increasing fat mass and weight gain to promote obesity development (Zhang et al., 2011).

Furthermore, endothelial HIF in hypothalamus also has a main role for central regulation of metabolism. The knockdown of endothelium HIF-1α, resulted in impairment of glucose uptake in the ARC and decreased POMC neuronal activity; following caloric deprivation, mice presented increased caloric intake as compared to control (Varela et al., 2017). Taken together, both studies suggested that hypothalamic HIF regulates glucose uptake in the ARC and consequently controls neuronal POMC adaptation to the changing metabolic environment, important for regulation of energy homeostasis mechanisms (**Figure 3A**).

Recently, we demonstrated using bioinformatics analysis, that hypothalamic HIF-1 transcripts are directly correlated with hypothalamic transcripts for proteins involved in inflammation, apoptosis and autophagy; in addition, hypothalamic HIF-1 expression is directly correlated with the phenotype of increased energy expenditure (Gaspar et al., 2018). High-fat diet induced increases in protein expression of hypothalamic HIF-1α; ARC

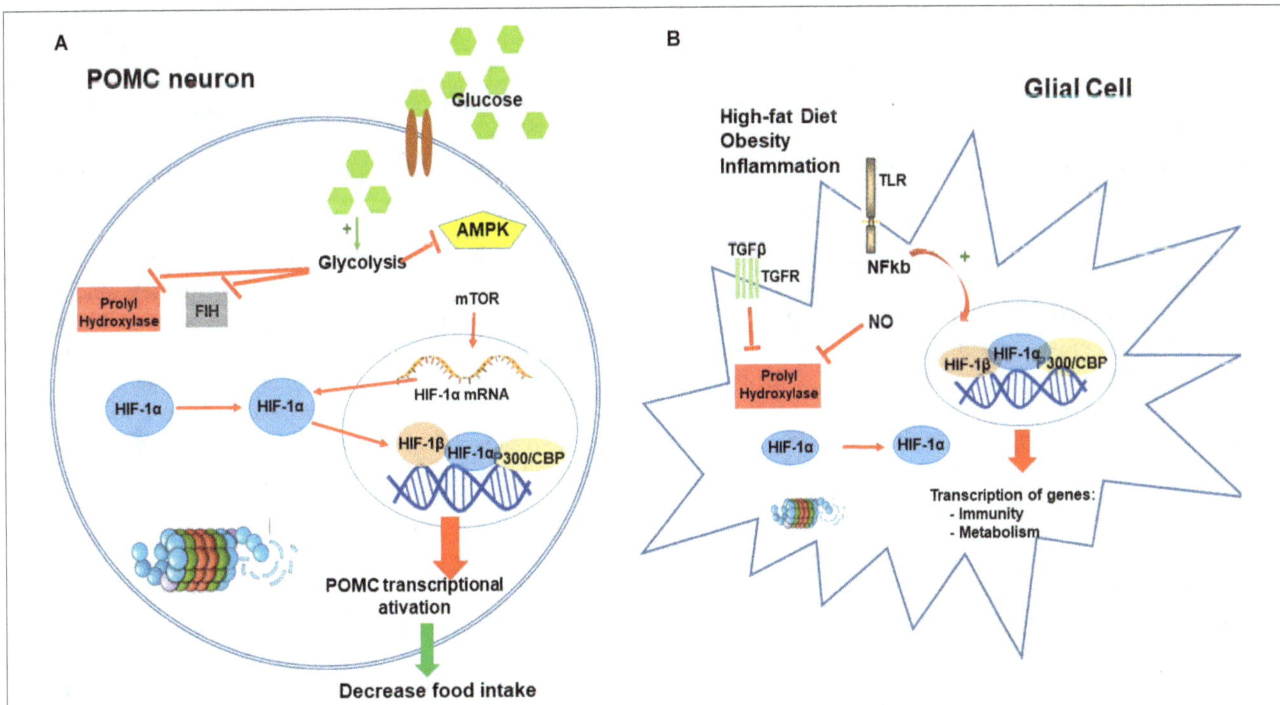

FIGURE 3 | Hypoxia-inducible factor-1 regulation of food intake. HIF in POMC neurons can function as a glucose sensor. After a meal, the increase in neuronal concentration activates neuronal glycolysis producing pyruvate, lactate, and intermediaries from the tricarboxylic acid (TCA) cycle. These metabolites inhibit PHD and FIH enzymes leading to the HIF stabilization. Conversely, these metabolites also block AMPK activation that regulates and increase the expression of HIF-α mRNA. Increase in HIF induces its translocation to the nucleus to bind POMC promoter and consequently stimulating the transactivation of POMC **(A)**. Obesity and consumption of high-fat diet induces an inflammatory condition in the hypothalamus, mostly driven by microglia and glial cells. Our main hypothesis is that inflammation in hypothalamic glial cells (increased TGF-β, TLR4 signaling, and increased NO production) leads to a stabilization of HIF that consequently transactivates several genes involved in the regulation of metabolism and inflammatory process as a compensatory mechanism for the nutritional excess **(B)**. CBP/p300, Creb Binding Protein/p300; PHD, prolyl hydroxylases; FIH-1, factor inhibiting HIF-1; AMPK, 5′ AMP-activated protein kinase; POMC, proopiomelanocortin.

inhibition of HIF-1 resulted in further increase in body mass, decreased basal metabolic rate, increased hypothalamic inflammation, and glucose intolerance (Gaspar et al., 2018; **Figure 3B**).

Orexins are hypothalamic neuropeptides involved in the regulatory network of food intake. One of the orexin-responsive genes is HIF-1α; upon orexin stimulus, HIF-1α gene expression is increased, resulting in increased glucose uptake and glycolytic activity. This provides evidence to support the important role of HIF-1 as a transcription factor in the hormone-mediated regulation of hunger (Sikder and Kodadek, 2007).

Also in the liver HIF proteins have important roles in the regulation of glucose and lipid metabolism. Diet-induced obesity induces an upregulation of hepatic HIF-1α (Ochiai et al., 2011), as a compensatory mechanism for metabolic regulation. Mice with liver-specific deletion of HIF-1α exhibited more severe impairment of glucose tolerance and peripheral insulin-resistance than control littermates; these changes were accompanied by a significant reduction of hepatic glucose uptake (Ochiai et al., 2011). Mice with liver specific deletion of HIF-1β, had increased hepatic gluconeogenesis, increased lipogenic gene expression, and impaired glucose tolerance, similar to what happened in type 2 diabetes (Wang et al., 2009).

Despite the importance hypothalamic and hepatic HIF-1α as regulator of energy, glucose, and lipid homeostasis, the increased expression/stability of HIF-1α during the expansion of white adipose tissue is implicated in the inflammatory process and insulin resistance (Ye et al., 2007; Pasarica et al., 2009; Fujisaka et al., 2013; Sun et al., 2013). Both in obese patients and in animal models of obesity, there is an association between reduced oxygen pressure in adipose depots and macrophage and T cell infiltration (Ye et al., 2007; Pasarica et al., 2009; Fujisaka et al., 2013; Lee et al., 2014; Taylor et al., 2014), highlighting the role of HIF pathway in the development of inflammation. However, obese mice deficient in adipocyte-specific HIF2 displayed dysregulation in thermogenesis under cold exposure, as a result of reduced levels of UCP1 and brown adipose tissue impairment (Garcia-Martin et al., 2015). In fact, in brown adipose tissue, HIF complex (isoform 2) is one of the factors that contribute to the upregulation of thermogenesis as an adaptation to obesity (protective effect) through UCP-1 expression (Vucetic et al., 2011; Garcia-Martin et al., 2015).

Thus, HIF-1 can control BAT activity through both direct and indirect mechanisms. In addition, the induction of HIF activity in neuronal cells (neuron-specific FIH null mice) is involved in the regulation of respiration, energy balance, and lipid metabolism (Zhang et al., 2010). Thus, HIF has emerged as an important component of the hypothalamic neuronal machinery involved in the control of body mass and metabolism (Zhang et al., 2011).

In conclusion, HIF has important functions in the regulation of whole body energy homeostasis (both in regulation of food intake, but also in thermogenesis) and also in the hepatic glucose and lipid metabolism. These functions are both directly in the peripheral organs, but also through central nervous system regulation (Zhang et al., 2010, 2011; Gaspar et al., 2016). Considering the positive metabolic results observed in patients under high altitude (hypobaric hypoxia), it is suggested that whole body activation of HIF signaling can have more beneficial than pathological effects against metabolic complications. However, caution should be taken since chronic systemic HIF1α inactivation (genetic or pharmacological manipulation) attenuates WAT expansion and obesity (Sun et al., 2013; Soro-Arnaiz et al., 2016) despite of the HIF1a-dependent beneficial metabolic effects in the hypothalamus. Specifically, in the hypothalamic, HIF-1α is an important nutrient sensor and regulator of energy metabolism; it is also implicated in the regulation of hypothalamic neuroinflammation during the development of obesity. Hypothalamic inhibition of HIF-1α aggravates obesity-associated metabolic phenotype; this highlights the hypothalamic HIF-1α as a potential target for therapeutic intervention against obesity.

CONCLUDING REMARKS

Both human and experimental data support an important role for hypothalamic HIF-1 in the regulation body weight, glucose homeostasis, and liver metabolism. Modulation of specific and selective central/ hypothalamic HIF in obesity can function as a protective mechanism to reduce the negative impact of hypothalamic dysfunction thus, placing tissue specific HIF-1 activation as a potential therapeutic target for the pharmacological management of obesity and type 2 diabetes. Along the role of HIF-1α in the white adipose tissue development, it might be possible that HIF1α actions favoring obesity in WAT overrides that HIF1α-dependent repression of food intake. Nevertheless, further biological, pharmacological, and clinical studies are needed to provide an extended understanding of the mechanisms and molecular players involved in the different cellular responses of HIF in the central mechanisms of energy homeostasis and also during the course of development of obesity and diabetes.

AUTHOR CONTRIBUTIONS

Both authors contributed to the writing, editing, and discussion of the manuscript.

REFERENCES

Al Massadi, O., Lopez, M., Tschop, M., Dieguez, C., and Nogueiras, R. (2017). Current understanding of the hypothalamic ghrelin pathways inducing appetite and adiposity. *Trends Neurosci.* 40, 167–180. doi: 10.1016/j.tins.2016.12.003

Atasoy, D., Betley, J. N., Su, H. H., and Sternson, S. M. (2012). Deconstruction of a neural circuit for hunger. *Nature* 488, 172–177. doi: 10.1038/nature11270

Ban, J. J., Ruthenborg, R. J., Cho, K. W., and Kim, J. W. (2014). Regulation of obesity and insulin resistance by hypoxia-inducible factors. *Hypoxia* 2, 171–183. doi: 10.2147/HP.S68771

Baroncini, M., Jissendi, P., Balland, E., Besson, P., Pruvo, J. P., Francke, J. P., et al. (2012). MRI atlas of the human hypothalamus. *Neuroimage* 59, 168–180. doi: 10.1016/j.neuroimage.2011.07.013

Belgardt, B. F., Husch, A., Rother, E., Ernst, M. B., Wunderlich, F. T., Hampel, B., et al. (2008). PDK1 deficiency in POMC-expressing cells reveals FOXO1-dependent and -independent pathways in control of energy homeostasis and stress response. *Cell Metab.* 7, 291–301. doi: 10.1016/j.cmet.2008.01.006

Benoit, S. C., Kemp, C. J., Elias, C. F., Abplanalp, W., Herman, J. P., Migrenne, S., et al. (2009). Palmitic acid mediates hypothalamic insulin resistance by altering PKC-theta subcellular localization in rodents. *J. Clin. Invest.* 119, 2577–2589. doi: 10.1172/JCI36714

Bento, C. F., and Pereira, P. (2011). Regulation of hypoxia-inducible factor 1 and the loss of the cellular response to hypoxia in diabetes. *Diabetologia* 54, 1946–1956. doi: 10.1007/s00125-011-2191-8

Betley, J. N., Xu, S., Cao, Z. F. H., Gong, R., Magnus, C. J., Yu, Y., et al. (2015). Neurons for hunger and thirst transmit a negative-valence teaching signal. *Nature* 521, 180–185. doi: 10.1038/nature14416

Carraro, R. S., Souza, G. F., Solon, C., Razolli, D. S., Chausse, B., Barbizan, R., et al. (2017). Hypothalamic mitochondrial abnormalities occur downstream of inflammation in diet-induced obesity. *Mol. Cell. Endocrinol.* 460, 238–245. doi: 10.1016/j.mce.2017.07.029

Catrina, S. B. (2014). Impaired hypoxia-inducible factor (HIF) regulation by hyperglycemia. *J. Mol. Med.* 92, 1025–1034. doi: 10.1007/s00109-014-1166-x

Cavadas, C., Aveleira, C. A., Souza, G. F., and Velloso, L. A. (2016). The pathophysiology of defective proteostasis in the hypothalamus - from obesity to ageing. *Nat. Rev. Endocrinol.* 12, 723–733. doi: 10.1038/nrendo.2016.107

Chalmers, J. A., Jang, J. J., and Belsham, D. D. (2014). Glucose sensing mechanisms in hypothalamic cell models: glucose inhibition of AgRP synthesis and secretion. *Mol. Cell. Endocrinol.* 382, 262–270. doi: 10.1016/j.mce.2013.10.013

Chari, M., Lam, C. K. L., Lam, T. K. T., and le Coutre, J. (2010). Hypothalamic fatty acid sensing in the normal and disease states," in *Fat Detection: Taste, Texture, and Post Ingestive Effect*, ed. J. P. Montmayeur (Boca Raton, FL: CRC Press).

Cheung, C. C., Clifton, D. K., and Steiner, R. A. (1997). Proopiomelanocortin neurons are direct targets for leptin in the hypothalamus. *Endocrinology* 138, 4489–4492. doi: 10.1210/endo.138.10.5570

Choi, J. H., Park, M. J., Kim, K. W., Choi, Y. H., Park, S. H., An, W. G., et al. (2005). Molecular mechanism of hypoxia-mediated hepatic gluconeogenesis by transcriptional regulation. *FEBS Lett.* 579, 2795–2801. doi: 10.1016/j.febslet.2005.03.097

Claret, M., Smith, M. A., Batterham, R. L., Selman, C., Choudhury, A. I., Fryer, L. G., et al. (2007). AMPK is essential for energy homeostasis regulation and glucose sensing by POMC and AgRP neurons. *J. Clin. Invest.* 117, 2325–2336. doi: 10.1172/JCI31516

Cockman, M. E., Lancaster, D. E., Stolze, I. P., Hewitson, K. S., McDonough, M. A., Coleman, M. L., et al. (2006). Posttranslational hydroxylation of ankyrin repeats in IkappaB proteins by the hypoxia-inducible factor (HIF) asparaginyl hydroxylase, factor inhibiting HIF (FIH). *Proc. Natl. Acad. Sci. U.S.A.* 103, 14767–14772. doi: 10.1073/pnas.0606877103

Coleman, M. L., McDonough, M. A., Hewitson, K. S., Coles, C., Mecinovic, J., Edelmann, M., et al. (2007). Asparaginyl hydroxylation of the Notch ankyrin repeat domain by factor inhibiting hypoxia-inducible factor. *J. Biol. Chem.* 282, 24027–24038. doi: 10.1074/jbc.M704102200

Collaborators, G. B. D. O., Afshin, A., Forouzanfar, M. H., Reitsma, M. B., Sur, P., Estep, K., et al. (2017). Health effects of overweight and obesity in 195 countries over 25 years. *N. Engl. J. Med.* 377, 13–27. doi: 10.1056/NEJMoa1614362

Corcoran, S. E., and O'Neill, L. A. (2016). HIF1alpha and metabolic reprogramming in inflammation. *J. Clin. Invest.* 126, 3699–3707. doi: 10.1172/JCI84431

Cowley, M. A., Smart, J. L., Rubinstein, M., Cerdan, M. G., Diano, S., Horvath, T. L., et al. (2001). Leptin activates anorexigenic POMC neurons through a neural network in the arcuate nucleus. *Nature* 411, 480–484. doi: 10.1038/35078085

Cramer, T., Yamanishi, Y., Clausen, B. E., Forster, I., Pawlinski, R., Mackman, N., et al. (2003). HIF-1alpha is essential for myeloid cell-mediated inflammation. *Cell* 112, 645–657. doi: 10.1016/S0092-8674(03)00154-5

De Souza, C. T., Araujo, E. P., Bordin, S., Ashimine, R., Zollner, R. L., Boschero, A. C., et al. (2005). Consumption of a fat-rich diet activates a proinflammatory response and induces insulin resistance in the hypothalamus. *Endocrinology* 146, 4192–4199. doi: 10.1210/en.2004-1520

Dehne, N., and Brune, B. (2009). HIF-1 in the inflammatory microenvironment. *Exp. Cell Res.* 315, 1791–1797. doi: 10.1016/j.yexcr.2009.03.019

Eltzschig, H. K., and Carmeliet, P. (2011). Hypoxia and inflammation. *N. Engl. J. Med.* 364, 656–665. doi: 10.1056/NEJMra0910283

Epstein, A. C., Gleadle, J. M., McNeill, L. A., Hewitson, K. S., O'Rourke, J., Mole, D. R., et al. (2001). *C. elegans* EGL-9 and mammalian homologs define a family of dioxygenases that regulate HIF by prolyl hydroxylation. *Cell* 107, 43–54. doi: 10.1016/S0092-8674(01)00507-4

Ferguson, J. E. III, Wu, Y., Smith, K., Charles, P., Powers, K., Wang, H., et al. (2007). ASB4 is a hydroxylation substrate of FIH and promotes vascular differentiation via an oxygen-dependent mechanism. *Mol. Cell. Biol.* 27, 6407–6419. doi: 10.1128/MCB.00511-07

Frede, S., Stockmann, C., Freitag, P., and Fandrey, J. (2006). Bacterial lipopolysaccharide induces HIF-1 activation in human monocytes via p44/42 MAPK and NF-kappaB. *Biochem. J.* 396, 517–527. doi: 10.1042/BJ20051839

Fujisaka, S., Usui, I., Ikutani, M., Aminuddin, A., Takikawa, A., Tsuneyama, K., et al. (2013). Adipose tissue hypoxia induces inflammatory M1 polarity of macrophages in an HIF-1alpha-dependent and HIF-1alpha-independent manner in obese mice. *Diabetologia* 56, 1403–1412. doi: 10.1007/s00125-013-2885-1

Garcia-Martin, R., Alexaki, V. I., Qin, N., Rubin, de Celis, M. F., Economopoulou, M., et al. (2015). Adipocyte-specific hypoxia-inducible factor 2alpha deficiency exacerbates obesity-induced brown adipose tissue dysfunction and metabolic dysregulation. *Mol. Cell. Biol.* 36, 376–393. doi: 10.1128/MCB.00430-15

Gaspar, J. M., Baptista, F. I., Macedo, M. P., and Ambrosio, A. F. (2016). inside the diabetic brain: role of different players involved in cognitive decline. *ACS Chem. Neurosci.* 7, 131–142. doi: 10.1021/acschemneuro.5b00240

Gaspar, J. M., Mendes, N. F., Correa-da-Silva, F., Lima-Junior, J. C., Gaspar, R. C., Ropelle, E. R., et al. (2018). Downregulation of HIF complex in the hypothalamus exacerbates diet-induced obesity. *Brain Behav. Immun.* 73, 550–561. doi: 10.1016/j.bbi.2018.06.020

Girgis, C. M., Cheng, K., Scott, C. H., and Gunton, J. E. (2012). Novel links between HIFs, type 2 diabetes, and metabolic syndrome. *Trends Endocrinol. Metab.* 23, 372–380. doi: 10.1016/j.tem.2012.05.003

Gonzalez-Muniesa, P., Martinez-Gonzalez, M. A., Hu, F. B., Despres, J. P., Matsuzawa, Y., Loos, R. J. F., et al. (2017). Obesity. *Nat Rev Dis Primers* 3:17034. doi: 10.1038/nrdp.2017.34

Greer, S. N., Metcalf, J. L., Wang, Y., and Ohh, M. (2012). The updated biology of hypoxia-inducible factor. *EMBO J.* 31, 2448–2460. doi: 10.1038/emboj.2012.125

Gregg, E. W., and Shaw, J. E. (2017). Global health effects of overweight and obesity. *N. Engl. J. Med.* 377, 80–81. doi: 10.1056/NEJMe1706095

Guillemot-Legris, O., and Muccioli, G. G. (2017). Obesity-Induced Neuroinflammation: Beyond the Hypothalamus. *Trends Neurosci.* 40, 237–253. doi: 10.1016/j.tins.2017.02.005

Ha, J., Guan, K. L., and Kim, J. (2015). AMPK and autophagy in glucose/glycogen metabolism. *Mol. Aspects Med.* 46, 46–62. doi: 10.1016/j.mam.2015.08.002

Haddad-Tovolli, R., Dragano, N. R. V., Ramalho, A. F. S., and Velloso, L. A. (2017). Development and function of the blood-brain barrier in the context of metabolic control. *Front. Neurosci.* 11:224. doi: 10.3389/fnins.2017.00224

Hahn, T. M., Breininger, J. F., Baskin, D. G., and Schwartz, M. W. (1998). Coexpression of Agrp and NPY in fasting-activated hypothalamic neurons. *Nat. Neurosci.* 1, 271–272. doi: 10.1038/1082

Halberg, N., Khan, T., Trujillo, M. E., Wernstedt-Asterholm, I., Attie, A. D., Sherwani, S., et al. (2009). Hypoxia-inducible factor 1alpha induces fibrosis and insulin resistance in white adipose tissue. *Mol. Cell. Biol.* 29, 4467–4483. doi: 10.1128/mcb.00192-09

He, Q., Gao, Z., Yin, J., Zhang, J., Yun, Z., and Ye, J. (2011). Regulation of HIF-1{alpha} activity in adipose tissue by obesity-associated factors: adipogenesis, insulin, and hypoxia. *Am. J. Physiol. Endocrinol. Metab.* 300, E877–E885. doi: 10.1152/ajpendo.00626.2010

Hetherington, A. W., and Ranson, S. W. (1940). Hypothalamic lesions and adiposity in the rat. *Anat. Rec.* 78, 149–172. doi: 10.1002/ar.1090780203

Horvath, T. L., Sarman, B., Garcia-Caceres, C., Enriori, P. J., Sotonyi, P., Shanabrough, M., et al. (2010). Synaptic input organization of the melanocortin system predicts diet-induced hypothalamic reactive gliosis and obesity. *Proc. Natl. Acad. Sci. U.S.A.* 107, 14875–14880. doi: 10.1073/pnas.100428 2107

Ignacio-Souza, L. M., Bombassaro, B., Pascoal, L. B., Portovedo, M. A., Razolli, D. S., Coope, A., et al. (2014). Defective regulation of the ubiquitin/proteasome system in the hypothalamus of obese male mice. *Endocrinology* 155, 2831–2844. doi: 10.1210/en.2014-1090

Ivan, M., Kondo, K., Yang, H., Kim, W., Valiando, J., Ohh, M., et al. (2001). HIFalpha targeted for VHL-mediated destruction by proline hydroxylation: implications for O2 sensing. *Science* 292, 464–468. doi: 10.1126/science.1059817

Iyalomhe, O., Swierczek, S., Enwerem, N., Chen, Y., Adedeji, M. O., Allard, J., et al. (2017). The role of hypoxia-inducible factor 1 in mild cognitive impairment. *Cell Mol. Neurobiol.* 37, 969–977. doi: 10.1007/s10571-016-0440-6

Jaakkola, P., Mole, D. R., Tian, Y. M., Wilson, M. I., Gielbert, J., Gaskell, S. J., et al. (2001). Targeting of HIF-alpha to the von Hippel-Lindau ubiquitylation complex by O2-regulated prolyl hydroxylation. *Science* 292, 468–472. doi: 10.1126/science.1059796

Jais, A., and Bruning, J. C. (2017). Hypothalamic inflammation in obesity and metabolic disease. *J. Clin. Invest.* 127, 24–32. doi: 10.1172/JCI88878

Jantsch, J., Chakravortty, D., Turza, N., Prechtel, A. T., Buchholz, B., Gerlach, R. G., et al. (2008). Hypoxia and hypoxia-inducible factor-1 alpha modulate lipopolysaccharide-induced dendritic cell activation and function. *J. Immunol.* 180, 4697–4705. doi: 10.4049/jimmunol.180.7.4697

Jiang, C., Qu, A., Matsubara, T., Chanturiya, T., Jou, W., Gavrilova, O., et al. (2011). Disruption of hypoxia-inducible factor 1 in adipocytes improves insulin sensitivity and decreases adiposity in high-fat diet-fed mice. *Diabetes Metab. Res. Rev.* 60, 2484–2495. doi: 10.2337/db11-0174

Kamegai, J., Tamura, H., Shimizu, T., Ishii, S., Sugihara, H., and Wakabayashi, I. (2000). Central effect of ghrelin, an endogenous growth hormone secretagogue, on hypothalamic peptide gene expression. *Endocrinology* 141, 4797–4800. doi: 10.1210/endo.141.12.7920

Kaushik, S., Arias, E., Kwon, H., Lopez, N. M., Athonvarangkul, D., Sahu, S., et al. (2012). Loss of autophagy in hypothalamic POMC neurons impairs lipolysis. *EMBO Rep.* 13, 258–265. doi: 10.1038/embor.2011.260

Kaushik, S., Rodriguez-Navarro, J. A., Arias, E., Kiffin, R., Sahu, S., Schwartz, G. J., et al. (2011). Autophagy in hypothalamic AgRP neurons regulates food intake and energy balance. *Cell Metab.* 14, 173–183. doi: 10.1016/j.cmet.2011.06.008

Kim, K. S., Seeley, R. J., and Sandoval, D. A. (2018). Signalling from the periphery to the brain that regulates energy homeostasis. *Nat. Rev. Neurosci.* 19, 185–196. doi: 10.1038/nrn.2018.8

Kola, B. (2008). Role of AMP-activated protein kinase in the control of appetite. *J. Neuroendocrinol.* 20, 942–951. doi: 10.1111/j.1365-2826.2008.01745.x

Krishnan, J., Danzer, C., Simka, T., Ukropec, J., Walter, K. M., Kumpf, S., et al. (2012). Dietary obesity-associated Hif1alpha activation in adipocytes restricts fatty acid oxidation and energy expenditure via suppression of the Sirt2-NAD + system. *Genes Dev.* 26, 259–270. doi: 10.1101/gad.180406.111

Lando, D., Peet, D. J., Gorman, J. J., Whelan, D. A., Whitelaw, M. L., and Bruick, R. K. (2002). FIH-1 is an asparaginyl hydroxylase enzyme that regulates the transcriptional activity of hypoxia-inducible factor. *Genes Dev.* 16, 1466–1471. doi: 10.1101/gad.991402

Lee, K. Y., Gesta, S., Boucher, J., Wang, X. L., and Kahn, C. R. (2011). The differential role of Hif1beta/Arnt and the hypoxic response in adipose function, fibrosis, and inflammation. *Cell Metab.* 14, 491–503. doi: 10.1016/j.cmet.2011.08.006

Lee, S., Lee, J., Kang, G. M., and Kim, M. S. (2018). Leptin directly regulate intrinsic neuronal excitability in hypothalamic POMC neurons but not in AgRP neurons in food restricted mice. *Neurosci. Lett.* 681, 105–109. doi: 10.1016/j.neulet.2018.05.041

Lee, Y. S., Kim, J. W., Osborne, O., Oh, D. Y., Sasik, R., Schenk, S., et al. (2014). Increased adipocyte O2 consumption triggers HIF-1alpha, causing inflammation and insulin resistance in obesity. *Cell* 157, 1339–1352. doi: 10.1016/j.cell.2014.05.012

Lippl, F. J., Neubauer, S., Schipfer, S., Lichter, N., Tufman, A., Otto, B., et al. (2010). Hypobaric hypoxia causes body weight reduction in obese subjects. *Obesity* 18, 675–681. doi: 10.1038/oby.2009.509

Lockie, S. H., Stark, R., Mequinion, M., Ch'ng, S., Kong, D., Spanswick, D. C., et al. (2018). Glucose availability predicts the feeding response to ghrelin in male mice, an effect dependent on AMPK in AgRP neurons. *Endocrinology* 159, 3605–3614. doi: 10.1210/en.2018-00536

Loftus, T. M., Jaworsky, D. E., Frehywot, G. L., Townsend, C. A., Ronnett, G. V., Lane, M. D., et al. (2000). Reduced food intake and body weight in mice treated with fatty acid synthase inhibitors. *Science* 288, 2379–2381. doi: 10.1126/science.288.5475.2379

Luquet, S., Perez, F. A., Hnasko, T. S., and Palmiter, R. D. (2005). NPY/AgRP neurons are essential for feeding in adult mice but can be ablated in neonates. *Science* 310, 683–685. doi: 10.1126/science.1115524

Makino, Y., Kanopka, A., Wilson, W. J., Tanaka, H., and Poellinger, L. (2002). Inhibitory PAS domain protein (IPAS) is a hypoxia-inducible splicing variant of the hypoxia-inducible factor-3alpha locus. *J. Biol. Chem.* 277, 32405–32408. doi: 10.1074/jbc.C200328200

Malhotra, R., Warne, J. P., Salas, E., Xu, A. W., and Debnath, J. (2015). Loss of Atg12, but not Atg5, in pro-opiomelanocortin neurons exacerbates diet-induced obesity. *Autophagy* 11, 145–154. doi: 10.1080/15548627.2014.998917

Marshall, N. B., and Mayer, J. (1956). Specificity of gold thioglucose for ventromedial hypothalamic lesions and hyperphagia. *Nature* 178, 1399–1400. doi: 10.1038/1781399a0

Maxwell, P. H., Wiesener, M. S., Chang, G. W., Clifford, S. C., Vaux, E. C., Cockman, M. E., et al. (1999). The tumour suppressor protein VHL targets hypoxia-inducible factors for oxygen-dependent proteolysis. *Nature* 399, 271–275. doi: 10.1038/20459

Michailidou, Z., Morton, N. M., Moreno Navarrete, J. M., West, C. C., Stewart, K. J., Fernandez-Real, J. M., et al. (2015). Adipocyte pseudohypoxia suppresses lipolysis and facilitates benign adipose tissue expansion. *Diabetes Metab. Res. Rev.* 64, 733–745. doi: 10.2337/db14-0233

Milanski, M., Degasperi, G., Coope, A., Morari, J., Denis, R., Cintra, D. E., et al. (2009). Saturated fatty acids produce an inflammatory response predominantly through the activation of TLR4 signaling in hypothalamus: implications for the pathogenesis of obesity. *J. Neurosci.* 29, 359–370. doi: 10.1523/JNEUROSCI.2760-08.2009

Minokoshi, Y., Alquier, T., Furukawa, N., Kim, Y. B., Lee, A., Xue, B., et al. (2004). AMP-kinase regulates food intake by responding to hormonal and nutrient signals in the hypothalamus. *Nature* 428, 569–574. doi: 10.1038/nature02440

Miselis, R. R., and Epstein, A. N. (1975). Feeding induced by intracerebroventricular 2-deoxy-D-glucose in the rat. *Am. J. Physiol.* 229, 1438–1447. doi: 10.1152/ajplegacy.1975.229.5.1438

Mizuno, T. M., and Mobbs, C. V. (1999). Hypothalamic agouti-related protein messenger ribonucleic acid is inhibited by leptin and stimulated by fasting. *Endocrinology* 140, 814–817. doi: 10.1210/endo.140.2.6491

Moraes, J. C., Coope, A., Morari, J., Cintra, D. E., Roman, E. A., Pauli, J. R., et al. (2009). High-fat diet induces apoptosis of hypothalamic neurons. *PLoS One* 4:e5045. doi: 10.1371/journal.pone.0005045

Morari, J., Anhe, G. F., Nascimento, L. F., de Moura, R. F., Razolli, D., Solon, C., et al. (2014). Fractalkine (CX3CL1) is involved in the early activation of hypothalamic inflammation in experimental obesity. *Diabetes Metab. Res. Rev.* 63, 3770–3784. doi: 10.2337/db13-1495

Morgan, K., Obici, S., and Rossetti, L. (2004). Hypothalamic responses to long-chain fatty acids are nutritionally regulated. *J. Biol. Chem.* 279, 31139–31148. doi: 10.1074/jbc.M400458200

Mountjoy, K. G. (2015). Pro-Opiomelanocortin (POMC) neurones, POMC-derived peptides, melanocortin receptors and obesity: how understanding of this system has changed over the last decade. *J. Neuroendocrinol.* 27, 406–418. doi: 10.1111/jne.12285

Nakazato, M., Murakami, N., Date, Y., Kojima, M., Matsuo, H., Kangawa, K., et al. (2001). A role for ghrelin in the central regulation of feeding. *Nature* 409, 194–198. doi: 10.1038/35051587

Narayanaswami, V., and Dwoskin, L. P. (2017). Obesity: current and potential pharmacotherapeutics and targets. *Pharmacol. Ther.* 170, 116–147. doi: 10.1016/j.pharmthera.2016.10.015

Obici, S., Feng, Z., Morgan, K., Stein, D., Karkanias, G., and Rossetti, L. (2002a). Central administration of oleic acid inhibits glucose production and food intake. *Diabetes Metab. Res. Rev.* 51, 271–275.

Obici, S., Zhang, B. B., Karkanias, G., and Rossetti, L. (2002b). Hypothalamic insulin signaling is required for inhibition of glucose production. *Nat. Med.* 8, 1376–1382. doi: 10.1038/nm798

Ochiai, D., Goda, N., Hishiki, T., Kanai, M., Senoo-Matsuda, N., Soga, T., et al. (2011). Disruption of HIF-1alpha in hepatocytes impairs glucose metabolism in diet-induced obesity mice. *Biochem. Biophys. Res. Commun.* 415, 445–449. doi: 10.1016/j.bbrc.2011.10.089

Oh, T. S., Cho, H., Cho, J. H., Yu, S. W., and Kim, E. K. (2016). Hypothalamic AMPK-induced autophagy increases food intake by regulating NPY and POMC expression. *Autophagy* 12, 2009–2025. doi: 10.1080/15548627.2016.1215382

Ollmann, M. M., Wilson, B. D., Yang, Y. K., Kerns, J. A., Chen, Y., Gantz, I., et al. (1997). Antagonism of central melanocortin receptors in vitro and in vivo by agouti-related protein. *Science* 278, 135–138. doi: 10.1126/science.278.5335.135

Olney, J. W. (1969). Brain lesions, obesity, and other disturbances in mice treated with monosodium glutamate. *Science* 164, 719–721. doi: 10.1126/science.164.3880.719

Parton, L. E., Ye, C. P., Coppari, R., Enriori, P. J., Choi, B., Zhang, C. Y., et al. (2007). Glucose sensing by POMC neurons regulates glucose homeostasis and is impaired in obesity. *Nature* 449, 228–232. doi: 10.1038/nature06098

Pasarica, M., Sereda, O. R., Redman, L. M., Albarado, D. C., Hymel, D. T., Roan, L. E., et al. (2009). Reduced adipose tissue oxygenation in human obesity: evidence for rarefaction, macrophage chemotaxis, and inflammation without an angiogenic response. *Diabetes Metab. Res. Rev.* 58, 718–725. doi: 10.2337/db08-1098

Peyssonnaux, C., Cejudo-Martin, P., Doedens, A., Zinkernagel, A. S., Johnson, R. S., and Nizet, V. (2007). Cutting edge: essential role of hypoxia inducible factor-1alpha in development of lipopolysaccharide-induced sepsis. *J. Immunol.* 178, 7516–7519. doi: 10.4049/jimmunol.178.12.7516

Portovedo, M., Ignacio-Souza, L. M., Bombassaro, B., Coope, A., Reginato, A., Razolli, D. S., et al. (2015). Saturated fatty acids modulate autophagy's proteins in the hypothalamus. *PLoS One* 10:e0119850. doi: 10.1371/journal.pone.0119850

Rossi, M. A., and Stuber, G. D. (2018). Overlapping brain circuits for homeostatic and hedonic feeding. *Cell Metab.* 27, 42–56. doi: 10.1016/j.cmet.2017.09.021

Santos, J. L., Perez-Bravo, F., Carrasco, E., Calvillan, M., and Albala, C. (2001). Low prevalence of type 2 diabetes despite a high average body mass index in the Aymara natives from Chile. *Nutrition* 17, 305–309. doi: 10.1016/S0899-9007(00)00551-7

Semenza, G. L. (2014). Oxygen sensing, hypoxia-inducible factors, and disease pathophysiology. *Annu. Rev. Pathol.* 9, 47–71. doi: 10.1146/annurev-pathol-012513-104720

Semenza, G. L., Nejfelt, M. K., Chi, S. M., and Antonarakis, S. E. (1991). Hypoxia-inducible nuclear factors bind to an enhancer element located 3' to the human erythropoietin gene. *Proc. Natl. Acad. Sci. U.S.A.* 88, 5680–5684. doi: 10.1073/pnas.88.13.5680

Sikder, D., and Kodadek, T. (2007). The neurohormone orexin stimulates hypoxia-inducible factor-1 activity. *Genes Dev.* 21, 2995–3005. doi: 10.1101/gad.1584307

Singh, R., and Cuervo, A. M. (2011). Autophagy in the cellular energetic balance. *Cell Metab.* 13, 495–504. doi: 10.1016/j.cmet.2011.04.004

Soro-Arnaiz, I., Li, Q. O. Y., Torres-Capelli, M., Melendez-Rodriguez, F., Veiga, S., Veys, K., et al. (2016). Role of mitochondrial complex iv in age-dependent obesity. *Cell Rep.* 16, 2991–3002. doi: 10.1016/j.celrep.2016.08.041

Souza, G. F., Solon, C., Nascimento, L. F., De-Lima-Junior, J. C., Nogueira, G., Moura, R., et al. (2016). Defective regulation of POMC precedes hypothalamic inflammation in diet-induced obesity. *Sci. Rep.* 6:29290. doi: 10.1038/srep29290

Spirig, R., Djafarzadeh, S., Regueira, T., Shaw, S. G., von Garnier, C., Takala, J., et al. (2010). Effects of TLR agonists on the hypoxia-regulated transcription factor HIF-1alpha and dendritic cell maturation under normoxic conditions. *PLoS One* 5:e0010983. doi: 10.1371/journal.pone.0010983

Srivastava, G., and Apovian, C. (2018). Future Pharmacotherapy for obesity: new anti-obesity drugs on the horizon. *Curr. Obes. Rep.* 7, 147–161. doi: 10.1007/s13679-018-0300-4

Sun, K., Halberg, N., Khan, M., Magalang, U. J., and Scherer, P. E. (2013). Selective inhibition of hypoxia-inducible factor 1alpha ameliorates adipose tissue dysfunction. *Mol. Cell. Biol.* 33, 904–917. doi: 10.1128/MCB.00951-12

Tang-Christensen, M., Vrang, N., Ortmann, S., Bidlingmaier, M., Horvath, T. L., and Tschop, M. (2004). Central administration of ghrelin and agouti-related protein (83-132) increases food intake and decreases spontaneous locomotor activity in rats. *Endocrinology* 145, 4645–4652. doi: 10.1210/en.2004-0529

Taylor, C. T., Kent, B. D., Crinion, S. J., McNicholas, W. T., and Ryan, S. (2014). Human adipocytes are highly sensitive to intermittent hypoxia induced NF-kappaB activity and subsequent inflammatory gene expression. *Biochem. Biophys. Res. Commun.* 447, 660–665. doi: 10.1016/j.bbrc.2014.04.062

Thaler, J. P., Yi, C. X., Schur, E. A., Guyenet, S. J., Hwang, B. H., Dietrich, M. O., et al. (2012). Obesity is associated with hypothalamic injury in rodents and humans. *J. Clin. Invest.* 122, 153–162. doi: 10.1172/jci59660

Thorens, B. (2012). Sensing of glucose in the brain. *Handb. Exp. Pharmacol.* 209, 277–294. doi: 10.1007/978-3-642-24716-3_12

Timper, K., and Bruning, J. C. (2017). Hypothalamic circuits regulating appetite and energy homeostasis: pathways to obesity. *Dis. Model Mech.* 10, 679–689. doi: 10.1242/dmm.026609

Tschop, M., Strasburger, C. J., Hartmann, G., Biollaz, J., and Bartsch, P. (1998). Raised leptin concentrations at high altitude associated with loss of appetite. *Lancet* 352, 1119–1120. doi: 10.1016/S0140-6736(05)79760-9

Valdearcos, M., Douglass, J. D., Robblee, M. M., Dorfman, M. D., Stifler, D. R., Bennett, M. L., et al. (2017). Microglial inflammatory signaling orchestrates the hypothalamic immune response to dietary excess and mediates obesity susceptibility. *Cell Metab.* 26, 185–197.e3. doi: 10.1016/j.cmet.2017.05.015

Valdearcos, M., Robblee, M. M., Benjamin, D. I., Nomura, D. K., Xu, A. W., and Koliwad, S. K. (2014). Microglia dictate the impact of saturated fat consumption on hypothalamic inflammation and neuronal function. *Cell Rep.* 9, 2124–2138. doi: 10.1016/j.celrep.2014.11.018

Varela, L., Suyama, S., Huang, Y., Shanabrough, M., Tschop, M. H., Gao, X. B., et al. (2017). Endothelial HIF-1alpha enables hypothalamic glucose uptake to drive POMC Neurons. *Diabetes Metab. Res. Rev.* 66, 1511–1520. doi: 10.2337/db16-1106

Virtue, S., and Vidal-Puig, A. (2011). Nothing Iffy about HIF in the Hypothalamus. *PLoS Biol.* 9:e1001116. doi: 10.1371/journal.pbio.1001116

Vrang, N., Larsen, P. J., Clausen, J. T., and Kristensen, P. (1999). Neurochemical characterization of hypothalamic cocaine- amphetamine-regulated transcript neurons. *J. Neurosci.* 19:RC5.

Vucetic, M., Otasevic, V., Korac, A., Stancic, A., Jankovic, A., Markelic, M., et al. (2011). Interscapular brown adipose tissue metabolic reprogramming during cold acclimation: Interplay of HIF-1alpha and AMPKalpha. *Biochim. Biophys. Acta* 1810, 1252–1261. doi: 10.1016/j.bbagen.2011.09.007

Wang, G. L., Jiang, B. H., Rue, E. A., and Semenza, G. L. (1995). Hypoxia-inducible factor 1 is a basic-helix-loop-helix-PAS heterodimer regulated by cellular O2 tension. *Proc. Natl. Acad. Sci. U.S.A.* 92, 5510–5514. doi: 10.1073/pnas.92.12.5510

Wang, R., Liu, X., Hentges, S. T., Dunn-Meynell, A. A., Levin, B. E., Wang, W., et al. (2004). The regulation of glucose-excited neurons in the hypothalamic arcuate nucleus by glucose and feeding-relevant peptides. *Diabetes Metab. Res. Rev.* 53, 1959–1965. doi: 10.2337/diabetes.53.8.1959

Wang, X. L., Suzuki, R., Lee, K., Tran, T., Gunton, J. E., Saha, A. K., et al. (2009). Ablation of ARNT/HIF1beta in liver alters gluconeogenesis, lipogenic gene expression, and serum ketones. *Cell Metab.* 9, 428–439. doi: 10.1016/j.cmet.2009.04.001

Westerterp, K. R., and Kayser, B. (2006). Body mass regulation at altitude. *Eur. J. Gastroenterol. Hepatol.* 18, 1–3. doi: 10.1097/00042737-200601000-00001

Westerterp-Plantenga, M. S., Westerterp, K. R., Rubbens, M., Verwegen, C. R., Richelet, J. P., and Gardette, B. (1999). Appetite at "high altitude" [Operation Everest III (Comex-'97)]: a simulated ascent of Mount Everest. *J. Appl. Physiol.* (1985) 87, 391–399. doi: 10.1152/jappl.1999.87.1.391

Williams, D. L., and Schwartz, M. W. (2011). Neuroanatomy of body weight control: lessons learned from leptin. *J. Clin. Invest.* 121, 2152–2155. doi: 10.1172/JCI58027

Woods, S. C., Lotter, E. C., McKay, L. D., and Porte, D. Jr. (1979). Chronic intracerebroventricular infusion of insulin reduces food intake and body weight of baboons. *Nature* 282, 503–505. doi: 10.1038/282503a0

Xing, J., and Lu, J. (2016). HIF-1alpha activation attenuates IL-6 and TNF-alpha pathways in hippocampus of rats following transient global Ischemia. *Cell Physiol. Biochem.* 39, 511–520. doi: 10.1159/000445643

Yaswen, L., Diehl, N., Brennan, M. B., and Hochgeschwender, U. (1999). Obesity in the mouse model of pro-opiomelanocortin deficiency responds to peripheral melanocortin. *Nat. Med.* 5, 1066–1070. doi: 10.1038/12506

Ye, J., Gao, Z., Yin, J., and He, Q. (2007). Hypoxia is a potential risk factor for chronic inflammation and adiponectin reduction in adipose tissue of ob/ob and dietary obese mice. *Am. J. Physiol. Endocrinol. Metab.* 293, E1118–E1128. doi: 10.1152/ajpendo.00435.2007

Zhang, H., Zhang, G., Gonzalez, F. J., Park, S. M., and Cai, D. (2011). Hypoxia-inducible factor directs POMC gene to mediate hypothalamic glucose sensing and energy balance regulation. *PLoS Biol.* 9:e1001112. doi: 10.1371/journal.pbio.1001112

Zhang, N., Fu, Z., Linke, S., Chicher, J., Gorman, J. J., Visk, D., et al. (2010). The asparaginyl hydroxylase factor inhibiting HIF-1alpha is an essential regulator of metabolism. *Cell Metab.* 11, 364–378. doi: 10.1016/j.cmet.2010.03.001

Zhang, X., and van den Pol, A. N. (2015). Dopamine/tyrosine hydroxylase neurons of the hypothalamic arcuate nucleus release GABA, communicate with dopaminergic and other arcuate neurons, and respond to dynorphin, Met-Enkephalin, and Oxytocin. *J. Neurosci.* 35, 14966–14982. doi: 10.1523/JNEUROSCI.0293-15.2015

Zhang, X., and van den Pol, A. N. (2016). Hypothalamic arcuate nucleus tyrosine hydroxylase neurons play orexigenic role in energy homeostasis. *Nat. Neurosci.* 19, 1341–1347. doi: 10.1038/nn.4372

Zhang, Y., Proenca, R., Maffei, M., Barone, M., Leopold, L., and Friedman, J. M. (1994). Positional cloning of the mouse obese gene and its human homologue. *Nature* 372, 425–432. doi: 10.1038/372425a0

12

Neurochemical Modifications in the Hippocampus, Cortex and Hypothalamus of Mice Exposed to Long-Term High-Fat Diet

Blanca Lizarbe[1,2], Ana Francisca Soares[1], Sara Larsson[3,4] and João M. N. Duarte[3,4]*

[1] Laboratory for Functional and Metabolic Imaging, École Polytechnique Fédérale de Lausanne, Lausanne, Switzerland, [2] Instituto de Investigaciones Biomédicas "Alberto Sols", Consejo Superior de Investigaciones Científicas – Universidad Autónoma de Madrid, Madrid, Spain, [3] Department of Experimental Medical Science, Faculty of Medicine, Lund University, Lund, Sweden, [4] Wallenberg Centre for Molecular Medicine, Faculty of Medicine, Lund University, Lund, Sweden

***Correspondence:**
João M. N. Duarte
joao.duarte@med.lu.se

Metabolic syndrome and diabetes impact brain function and metabolism. While it is well established that rodents exposed to diets rich in saturated fat develop brain dysfunction, contrasting results abound in the literature, likely as result of exposure to different high-fat diet (HFD) compositions and for varied periods of time. In the present study, we investigated alterations of hippocampal-dependent spatial memory by measuring Y-maze spontaneous alternation, metabolic profiles of the hippocampus, cortex and hypothalamus by ^{1}H magnetic resonance spectroscopy (MRS), and levels of proteins specific to synaptic and glial compartments in mice exposed for 6 months to different amounts of fat (10, 45, or 60% of total energy intake). Increasing the dietary amount of fat from 10 to 45% or 60% resulted in obesity accompanied by increased leptin, fasting blood glucose and insulin, and reduced glucose tolerance. In comparison to controls (10%-fat), only mice fed the 60%-fat diet showed increased fed glycemia, as well as plasma corticosterone that has a major impact on brain function. HFD-induced metabolic profile modifications measured by ^{1}H MRS were observed across the three brain areas in mice exposed to 60%- but not 45%-fat diet, while both HFD groups displayed impaired hippocampal-dependent memory. HFD also affected systems involved in neuro- or gliotransmission in the hippocampus. Namely, relative to controls, 60%-fat-fed mice showed reduced SNAP-25, PSD-95 and syntaxin-4 immunoreactivity, while 45%-fat-fed mice showed reduced gephyrin and syntaxin-4 immunoreactivity. For both HFD levels, reductions of the vesicular glutamate transporter vGlut1 and levels of the vesicular GABA transporter were observed in the hippocampus and hypothalamus, relative to controls. Immunoreactivity against GFAP and/or Iba-1 in the hypothalamus was higher in mice exposed to HFD than controls, suggesting occurrence of gliosis. We conclude that different levels of dietary fat result in distinct neurochemical alterations in the brain.

Keywords: glucose, insulin, diabetes, brain metabolism, synaptic dysfunction, gliosis

INTRODUCTION

The ever-increasing life expectancy has led to a dramatic increase in the prevalence of age-associated disorders namely metabolic syndrome and type 2 diabetes (T2D), and neurodegenerative disorders, such as Alzheimer's disease (AD). Notably, there is a growing body of epidemiological evidence suggesting that both metabolic syndrome and T2D increase the risk of developing age-related cognitive decline, mild cognitive impairment, vascular dementia, and AD (Frisardi et al., 2010; Duarte, 2015).

In addition to the many components of metabolic syndrome that may affect brain function, brain insulin resistance is a proposed mechanistic link between T2D and AD. Indeed, post-mortem analyses of brains from dementia patients revealed that insulin receptors are downregulated, and pointed toward a major role of neuronal insulin resistance in the etiology of AD (Steculorum et al., 2014; Duarte, 2015). Insulin receptors are widely distributed in the brain (Havrankova et al., 1978; Hill et al., 1986). Insulin and insulin-like growth factor 1 (IGF-1), which have converging signaling pathways in the brain, regulate the neuronal control of energy and glucose homeostasis by acting on hypothalamic nuclei (Steculorum et al., 2014), and also regulate cognitive processes through its actions on neurotransmission, synaptic plasticity, and neurogenesis within cortical and hippocampal circuits (Fernandez and Torres-Alemán, 2012).

A number of components of the metabolic syndrome such as hyperglycemia, microvascular complications, insulin resistance, dyslipidemia and hypertension occur in diabetes, and are risk factors for cognitive dysfunction (Duarte, 2015; Moheet et al., 2015). Although this combination of factors with potential impact on the central nervous system makes the mechanisms of diabetes-induced brain dysfunction difficult to study, research on different rodent models of diabetes have found that diabetic conditions lead to synaptic deterioration that results in defective neurotransmission and synaptic plasticity (Duarte et al., 2009, 2012a; Calvo-Ochoa et al., 2014), as well as neuroinflammation and astrogliosis (Saravia et al., 2002; Baydas et al., 2003; Duarte et al., 2009, 2012a; Calvo-Ochoa et al., 2014).

Changes in the cellular integrity of neurons and astrocytes are likely reflected on brain metabolic regulation, as well as metabolic profiles. Indeed, studies employing MRS, which allow to quantify brain metabolite profiles in a non-invasive manner, have generally identified reduced levels of the putative neuronal marker *N*-acetylaspartate, as well as increased in *myo*-inositol content (a proposed marker of astrocyte density) in brains of subjects with both AD and diabetes, relative to healthy individuals (reviewed in Duarte, 2016). Accordingly, altered metabolite profiles have been also reported in the brain of diabetes and HFD-induced obesity models (van der Graaf et al., 2004; Duarte et al., 2009; Wang et al., 2012; Lizarbe et al., 2018; Ribeiro et al., 2018).

In the present study, we tested the hypothesis that the severity of the metabolic syndrome is related to the degree of neurochemical alterations, as well as brain function deficits. For that, mice were fed diets containing different amounts of fat during 6 months, which lead to different degrees of glucose intolerance and insulin resistance (Soares et al., 2018). We then evaluated spatial memory performance, metabolic profiles of the hippocampus, cortex and hypothalamus, and levels of proteins specific to synaptic and glial compartments.

Abbreviations: Aβ, amyloid β; AD, Alzheimer's disease; ANOVA, analysis of variance; CRLB, Cramér-Rao lower bound; GABA, γ-aminobutyrate; HFD, high-fat diet; IGF-1, insulin-like growth factor 1; LSD, least significant difference; MOPS, 3-(*N*-morpholino)propanesulfonic acid; MRS, magnetic resonance spectroscopy; NAAG, *N*-acetylaspartylglutamate; TBS, Tris-buffered saline; T2D, type 2 diabetes; VOI, volume of interest.

MATERIALS AND METHODS

Animals

Animal experiments were performed with the approval by the local ethics committee (Service de la Consommation et des Affaires Vétérinaires, Epalinges, Switzerland). Sample size estimation was based on previous MRS experiments (Gapp et al., 2017; Lizarbe et al., 2018). Eleven-week-old male C57BL/6J mice were purchased from Charles River (L'Arbresle, France), and housed in groups of 3–4 on a 12-h light-dark cycle with lights on at 07:00, room temperature at 21–23°C, and humidity at 55–60%. Mice were randomly split in three groups (n = 11/group), and dietary interventions started after 1 week of acclimatization to the facility, i.e., at 3 months of age. During 6 months, mice were fed standardized diets containing 10%, 45%, or 60% of kilocalories from lard-based fat (D12450B, D12451, D12492, Research Diets, New Brunswick, NJ, United States), as previously detailed (Soares et al., 2018). Food and tap water were provided *ad libitum*. After this 6-month housing period, the following procedures were carried out sequentially with 2 days of interval: behavior experiments, one MRS scan session, glucose tolerance tests, tissue collection.

Behavioral Tasks

Exploratory behavior and locomotor activity of mice was evaluated over a 5-min period in the dark, using a squared open field arena measuring 30 cm × 30 cm and 25 cm high, divided in four squares of 15 cm × 15 cm. The number of crossings in these squares and the number of rearing movements with forepaws were quantified as horizontal and vertical activity, respectively. Rearing with the forepaws pressed against the walls was not considered.

Spontaneous alternation was observed in a Y-maze (Duarte et al., 2012a), with each arm of 30 cm long, 5 cm wide, and 25 cm height, converging to an equal angle. Mice were placed at the bottom of one arm in the Y-maze and were allowed to explore freely all three arms for a single 8-min session in the dark. The recorded spontaneous alternation behavior was used to access hippocampal-dependent spatial memory. If the mouse remembers the arm it has just explored, it will then enter the other arm of the maze instead. Complete spontaneous alternation was defined as successive entries into the three arms and expressed as fraction of the possible alternations in the respective test. In additionally to the open field test, the number of entries in the arms of the maze also allowed to access locomotor activity.

Magnetic Resonance Spectroscopy (MRS)

All experiments were carried out in a 14.1 T magnet with a horizontal bore of 26 cm (Magnex Scientific, Abingdon, United Kingdom), equipped with a 12-cm internal diameter gradient coil insert (400mT/m, 200μs), and interfaced to a DirectDrive console (Agilent Technologies, Palo Alto, CA, United States). Radio frequency transmission and reception were achieved with a home-built quadrature surface coil composed of two geometrically decoupled single-turn loops of 12 mm inner diameter resonating at 600 MHz. Spontaneously breathing mice were anesthetized with 1–1.5% isoflurane (Animalcare Ltd., York, United Kingdom) in a 1:1 O_2:air mixture, and fixed in a home-built mouse holder with a bite bar and two ear inserts. Body temperature was maintained at 37°C by warm water circulation. Respiration and temperature were continuously monitored using a MR-compatible system (Small Animal Instruments, Inc., Stony Brook, NY, United States). Volumes of interest (VOI) were placed in the dorsal hippocampus (1.2 mm × 2.0 mm × 2.1 mm), cortex (0.8 mm × 4.0 mm × 1.6 mm) or hypothalamus (1.8 mm × 2.7 mm × 1.8 mm) according to anatomical landmarks in T_2-weighted fast-spin-echo images. Field homogeneity in the VOI was achieved with FAST(EST)MAP (Gruetter and Tkác, 2000). Spectra were acquired using SPECIAL with echo time of 2.8 ms and repetition time of 4 s (Mlynárik et al., 2006). We accumulated 210, 320, and 400 scans for the cortex, hippocampus, and hypothalamus, respectively. The order of scanning the regions was random.

The concentrations of brain metabolites were determined with LCModel (Stephen Provencher Inc., Oakville, ON, Canada), including a Mac spectrum in the database and using the unsuppressed water signal measured from the same VOI as internal reference (Gapp et al., 2017). The following metabolites were included in the analysis: alanine, ascorbate, aspartate, creatine, γ-aminobutyrate (GABA), glutamine, glutamate, glutathione, glycine, glycerophosphorylcholine, glucose, lactate, *myo*-inositol, *N*-acetylaspartate, *N*-acetylaspartylglutamate (NAAG), phosphorylethanolamine, phosphorylcholine, phosphocreatine, *scyllo*-inositol, taurine. The Cramér-Rao lower bound (CRLB) was provided by LCModel as a measure of the reliability of the quantification for each metabolite. In most measured spectra, *scyllo*-inositol was below the detection limit, and was excluded from subsequent data analyses. Alanine in the hypothalamus was also below the detection limit. Remaining metabolites had CRLB below 30%. Given the substantial overlap between phosphorylcholine and glycerophosphorylcholine signals, total choline levels are reported.

Three mice (one on 45% fat diet, two on 60% fat diet) were excluded from the study because of abnormally high glutamine concentration in all brain regions investigated, which suggests the occurrence of congenital portosystemic shunting (Cudalbu et al., 2013).

Glucose Tolerance Test

After a 6-h fast starting at 07:00, a blood sample was collected to determine glucose and insulin levels. Then mice were given an oral load of glucose (1.5 g/kg), and blood glucose was measured after 15, 30, 60, 90, and 120 min from the tail tip with the Breeze glucometer (Bayer, Zürich, Switzerland).

Tissue Collection

Mice were briefly anesthetized with isoflurane (2% in air). Glycemia under isoflurane anesthesia was measured using the Ascensia Contour glucometer (Bayer). A blood sample was collected from the descending aorta, and then mice were decapitated. The brain was rapidly removed, and brain regions were dissected in ice-cold phosphate-buffered saline (PBS; in mmol/L: 137 NaCl, 2.7 KCl, 1.5 KH_2PO_4, 8.1 Na_2HPO_4, pH 7.4). Brain and plasma samples were stored at −80°C until further processing.

Western Blot

Tissue samples were homogenized with a needle sonicator in lysis buffer [in mmol/L: 150 NaCl, 1 ethylenediaminetetraacetic acid (EDTA), 50 tris(hydroxymethyl)aminomethane (Tris)-HCl, 1% (v/v) Triton X-100, 0.5% (w/v) sodium deoxycholate, 0.5% (w/v) sodium dodecylsulfate (SDS), pH 8.0] containing protease inhibitors (Roche, Switzerland). The homogenate was then maintained in constant agitation for 2 h at 4°C. After centrifugation at 3,000 × *g* for 10 min at 4°C to remove major debris, the supernatant was saved. Total protein content was determined with the bicinchoninic acid assay (kit from Pierce, Thermo Fisher Scientific, Göteborg, Sweden).

Samples were then diluted in NuPAGE-LDS sample buffer [in mmol/L: 141 Tris-base, 106 Tris-HCl, 50 dithiothreitol, 0.51 EDTA, 0.22 Coomassie Brilliant Blue G-250, 0.175 phenol red, 2% (w/v) lithium dodecylsulfate, 10% glycerol, pH 8.5] and heated for 2 min at 95°C, 2–20 μg of protein were loaded in precast NuPAGE Novex 4–12% polyacrylamide gradient gels (Invitrogen, Thermo Fisher Scientific), along with molecular weight standards (Precision Plus Protein standards from Bio-Rad, Sundbyberg, Sweden), and electrophoresis was carried out at 125 V in a 3-(*N*-morpholino)propanesulfonic acid (MOPS) running buffer (in mmol/L: 50 MOPS, 50 Tris Base, 1 EDTA, 0.1% SDS, pH 7.7).

Proteins were transferred onto 0.45 μm polyvinylidene difluoride membranes (GE Life Sciences, Sweden) in a buffer composed of 192 mmol/L glycine, 25 mmol/L Tris and 20% (v/v) methanol (pH 9.2). The membranes were subsequently blocked for 90 min in 5% (w/v) low-fat milk (VWR, Stockholm, Sweden) solution prepared in Tris-buffered saline (TBS) (in mmol/L: 20 Tris, 137 NaCl, pH 7.46) with 0.1% (v/v) tween-20 (TBS-T), and were then incubated with primary antibodies (**Table 1**) over night at 4°C. After three 15-min washes in TBS-T containing 1% (w/v) milk, membranes were incubated with the respective secondary antibodies conjugated with horseradish peroxidase (**Table 1**)

TABLE 1 | Antibodies employed in the present study.

Antigen	Host	Dilution	Supplier	Molecular weight (kDa)*
Primary antibodies:				
Gephyrin	R	1:500	Abcam (#ab181382)	90–95
GFAP	R	1:2,000	Abcam (#ab68428)	49–51
Iba-1	G	1:500	Sigma-Aldrich (#SAB2500041)	15–20
PSD-95	R	1:2,000	Abcam (#ab76115)	90–95
SNAP-25	R	1:5,000	Abcam (#ab109105)	25–26
Synaptophysin	R	1:10,000	Abcam (#ab32127)	34–36
Syntaxin-1	R	1:1,000	Sigma-Aldrich (#S1172)	34–39
Syntaxin-4	R	1:1,000	Abcam (#ab184545)	31–39
vGAT	R	1:1,000	Abcam (#ab42939)	53–55
vGluT1	R	1:2,000	Abcam (#ab180188)	61–62
vGluT2	R	1:1,000	Abcam (#ab216463)	63–65
HRP-conjugated secondary antibodies:				
Rabbit IgG	D	1 : 10 000	Abcam (#ab6802)	
Goat IgG	D	1 : 10 000	GeneTex (#GTX232040-01)	

*HRP, horseradish peroxidase; D, donkey; G, goat; R, rabbit. *Molecular weight range observed in the present study.*

for 1 h at room temperature. After the second antibody, the membranes were washed three more times in TBS-T and developed in the ChemiDoc (Bio-Rad) using the SuperSignal West Pico PLUS Chemiluminescent substrate (Thermo Scientific).

Biochemical Analyses

Plasma corticosterone and leptin were assayed with ELISA kits from Abcam (Cambridge, United Kingdom). Plasma insulin concentration was determined using the mouse insulin ELISA kit from Mercodia (Uppsala, Sweden).

Statistical Analysis

All results were analyzed using analysis of variance (ANOVA), followed by independent comparisons with the Fisher's least significant difference (LSD) test. For the analyses of metabolite concentrations, the three brain regions were analyzed together as repeated measures, and *post hoc* analyses were only performed in case of significant effects of fat or fat-region interaction at $P < 0.05$. Results are presented as mean ± SEM unless otherwise stated.

RESULTS

Chronic exposure to HFD resulted in development of obesity, mild hyperglycemia, glucose intolerance, and hyperinsulinemia (**Figure 1**). Weight gain was proportional to the dietary fat content ($F = 64.2$, $P < 0.001$, **Figure 1A**). Fed glycemia was modified by HFD ($F = 9.1$, $P = 0.001$, **Figure 1B**), being significantly increased in 60%-fat fed mice compared to controls (+56 ± 14%, $P < 0.001$) and to 45%-fat fed mice (+45 ± 13%, $P = 0.002$). Mice under 10%- and 45%-fat diets showed similar fed glycemia. After fasting for 6 h, mice showed a glycemia that was proportional to the amount of fat in the diet ($F = 23.1$; $P < 0.001$, **Figure 1C**), while insulinemia was similarly increased in both HFD groups compared to controls ($F = 9.2$, $P < 0.001$, **Figure 1D**). The diet also had an effect on the fasting glycemia to plasma insulin ratio ($F = 3.6$, $P = 0.041$) that is commonly taken as an indicator of insulin sensitivity. In particular, compared to controls (10%-fat fed mice), the ratio of glucose to insulin was reduced by 94 ± 42% ($P = 0.034$) and 95 ± 42% ($P = 0.033$) in mice from the 45%-fat or 60%-fat groups, respectively. An oral glucose tolerance test after this fasting period revealed an impairment of blood glucose clearance that was also proportional to the amount of fat present in the diet ($F = 14.6$, $P < 0.001$, **Figure 1E**). This is especially clear when looking at the glycemia at 2 h post the glucose administration ($F = 13.5$, $P < 0.001$, **Figure 1F**), with 60%-fat fed mice displaying increased glycemia compared to both 45%-fat fed mice (+32 ± 14%, $P = 0.033$) and controls (+109 ± 21%, $P < 0.001$). HFD also affected the circulating concentrations of corticosterone ($F = 4.2$, $P = 0.025$, **Figure 1G**) and leptin ($F = 19.0$, $P < 0.001$, **Figure 1H**). In *post hoc* tests, corticosterone was only significantly different between mice under diets with 10% and 60% fat (+32 ± 11%, $P = 0.007$), while leptin was similarly increased in both HFD groups compared to controls.

Spatial Memory

Exposure to HFD resulted in impaired spatial memory performance, measured as spontaneous alternation in the Y-maze ($F = 3.8$, $P = 0.030$, **Figure 2A**). In particular, there was a reduction of the Y-maze spontaneous alternation in mice consuming both the 45%-fat diet (−11 ± 5%, $P = 0.028$) and 60%-fat diet (−10 ± 4%, $P = 0.025$), relative to controls. Diet also had an effect on the number of entries in the maze arms ($F = 8.2$, $P = 0.001$), but not resulting in major impairment of exploratory behavior, which was also assessed in the open-field test (**Figure 2B**). Nevertheless, mice exposed to both 45%-fat and 60%-fat diets showed a reduction in locomotor activity, that is reduced number of crossing events between quadrants of the arena ($F = 5.5$, $P = 0.008$), and reduced vertical explorations of the arena's space, that is rearing events ($F = 3.8$, $P = 0.030$). Nevertheless, the observed reduction activity did not impair the analysis of spontaneous alteration behavior as it is normalized for the number of possible complete alternations, and there were sufficient arm entries in the Y-maze (**Figure 2A**).

Metabolic Profiles

Proton spectra were acquired with an average SNR of 18 ± 3 (standard deviation across all brain areas). Typical spectra are shown in **Figure 3**. Linewidths at half-height were 11.2 ± 3.0 Hz, 16.2 ± 4.0 Hz and 13.6 ± 2.2 Hz (mean with standard deviation) in the hippocampus, cortex and hypothalamus, respectively.

The amount of fat in the diet significantly impacted the levels of creatine ($F = 13.7$, $P < 0.001$, **Figure 4A**), which also varied across analyzed brain areas (region effect $F = 55.1$, $P < 0.001$; interaction $F = 0.9$, $P = 0.506$). Although phosphocreatine levels were not impacted by HFD exposure (**Figure 4B**), the content

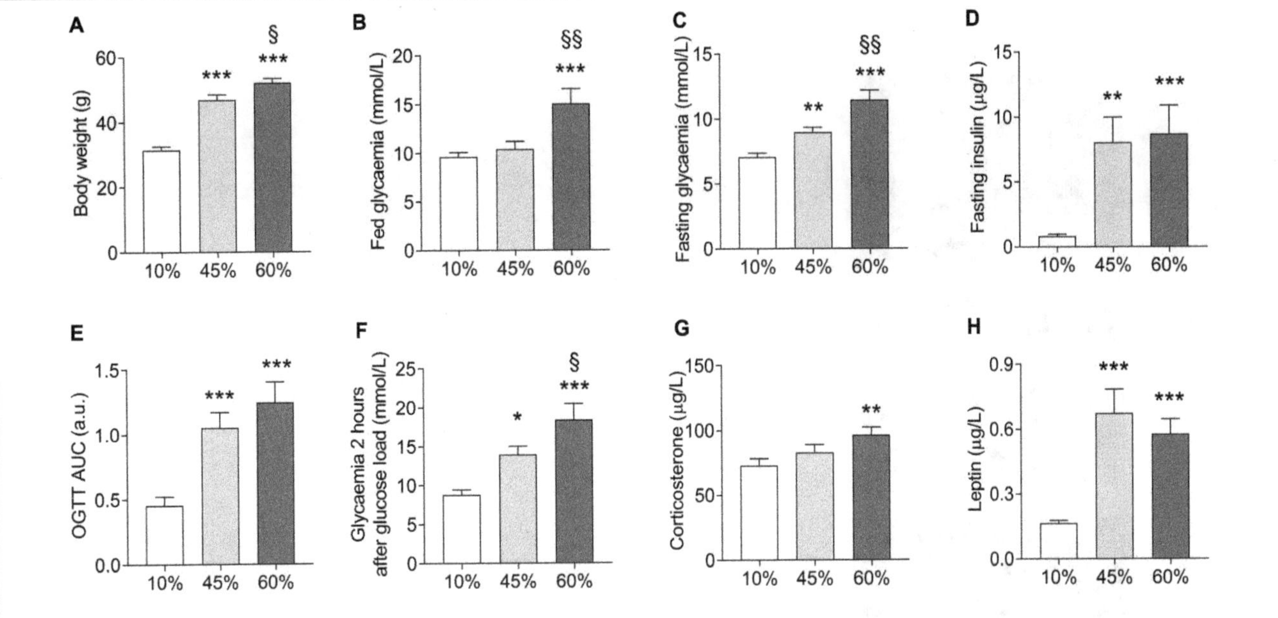

FIGURE 1 | HFD-induced changes on body weight **(A)**, fed glycemia **(B)**, glycemia **(C)**, and plasma insulin **(D)** after a 6-h fasting, area under the curve (AUC) of an oral glucose tolerance test (OGTT) with 1.5 g/kg of glucose **(E)** and glycemia measured 2 h after the glucose load **(F)**, and plasma corticosterone **(G)** and leptin **(H)** concentrations. Data are mean ± SEM. Symbols indicate significant differences in LSD tests after significant ANOVA, comparing HFD fed mice (45% fat or 60%-fat) and controls (10%-fat; $^{*}P < 0.05$, $^{**}P < 0.01$; $^{***}P < 0.001$), or the diets containing 45% and 60% fat (§ $P < 0.05$, §§ $P < 0.01$).

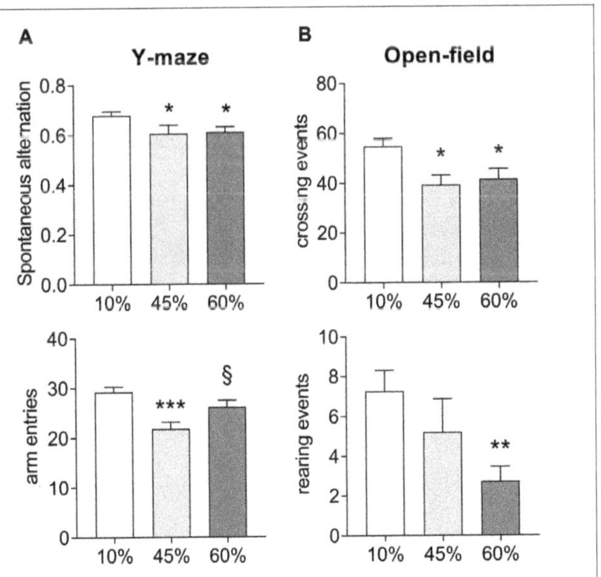

FIGURE 2 | Impact of HFD exposure on the performance in the Y-maze **(A)** and the open-field arena **(B)**. Data are mean ± SEM. Symbols indicate significant differences in LSD tests after significant ANOVA, comparing HDF fed mice (45% fat or 60%-fat) and controls (10%-fat; $^{*}P < 0.05$, $^{**}P < 0.01$; $^{***}P < 0.001$), or the diets containing 45% and 60% fat (§ $P < 0.05$).

of fat was associated to reductions of the phosphocreatine-to-creatine ratio ($F = 13.1$, $P = 0.009$, **Figure 4C**), which suggests impaired energy metabolism. This effect was particularly prominent in the cortex (−31%, $P = 0.003$) and hypothalamus (−20%, $P = 0.050$), and not significant in the hippocampus (−13%, $P = 0.303$) of the 60%-fat group compared to controls.

High-fat diet caused a general increase of glutamine levels ($F = 7.9$, $P = 0.050$, **Figure 4D**), and there was also an effect of brain region on glutamine levels (region $F = 33.3$, $P < 0.0001$; interaction $F = 0.9$, $P = 0.717$), and *post hoc* analyses revealed a significant increase the hippocampus of mice fed 60%-fat diet relative to controls (+21 ± 10%, $P = 0.036$), as well as relative to mice fed 45%-fat diet (+27 ± 10%, $P = 0.011$). Interestingly glutamate levels were not significantly affected by the diet (**Figure 4E**). Brain concentrations the neuro-transmitting amino acids GABA (**Figure 4F**), glycine (**Figure 4G**), and aspartate (**Figure 4H**) also remained unaltered by HFD exposure.

The levels of the neuronal marker *N*-acetylaspartate showed a significant diet-region interaction (interaction $F = 6.7$, $P = 0.006$; region $F = 44.2$, $P < 0.001$; fat $F = 4.5$, $P = 0.066$, **Figure 4I**). *Post hoc* analyses identified an increase of *N*-acetylaspartate concentration in the hippocampus of mice exposed to 60%-fat diet compared to controls (+11 ± 4%, $P = 0.007$), and compared to 45%-fat fed mice (+18 ± 4%, $P < 0.001$).

N-Acetylaspartylglutamate levels were modified by fat content in the diet ($F = 12.8$, $P = 0.015$, **Figure 4J**) and varied across brain areas ($F = 20.4$, $P < 0.001$), without interaction ($F = 0.5$, $P = 0.918$). However, no significant changes were detected in *post hoc* analyses between controls and mice in either HFD group. However, significant differences were observed between 45%-fat and 60%-fat groups in the cortex (+36 ± 22%, $P = 0.005$) and hippocampus (+46 ± 20%, $P = 0.046$).

We found a diet-region interaction effect on the concentration of glutathione (interaction $F = 9.8$, $P = 0.047$; region $F = 10.9$, $P = 0.006$; diet $F = 2.7$, $P = 0.247$, **Figure 4K**). *Post hoc* analyses showed a significant increase of hippocampal glutathione levels

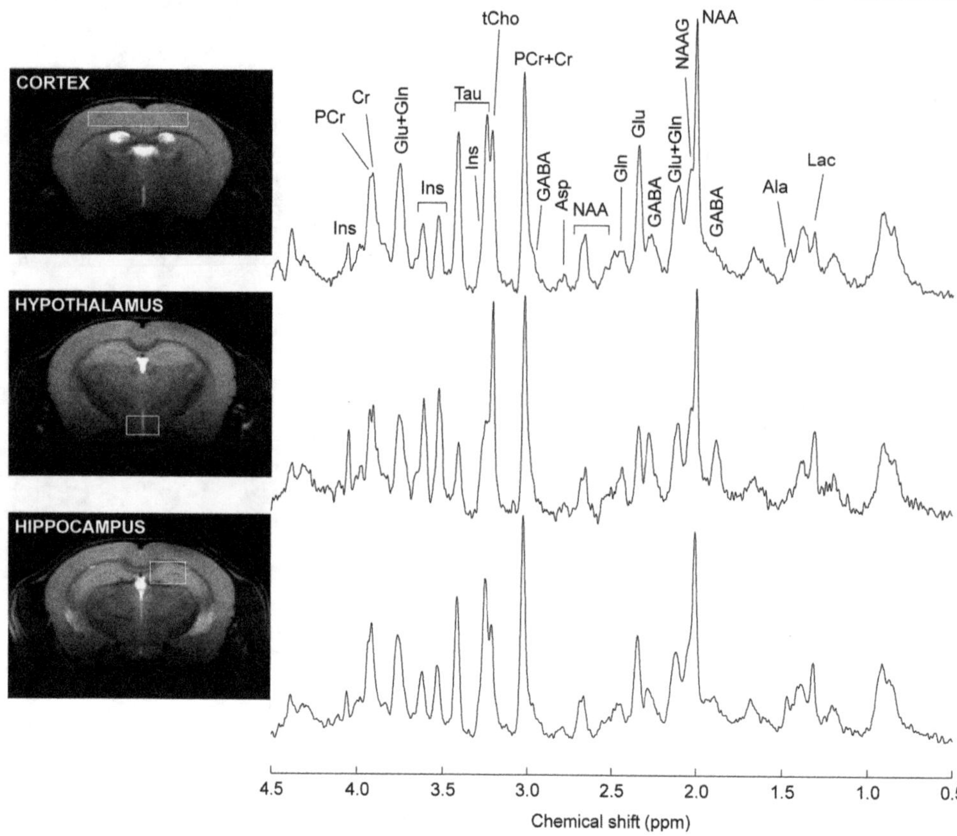

FIGURE 3 | Typical spectra recorded from the mouse hippocampus, cortex and hypothalamus. Spectra were acquired with SPECIAL at 14.1 T. For signal enhancement of the displayed spectra, a Gaussian apodization (gf = 0.08, gfs = 0.02) was applied prior Fourier transformation. Lac, lactate; Ala, alanine; GABA, γ-aminobutyrate; NAA, *N*-acetylaspartate; NAAG, *N*-acetylaspartylglutamate; Glu, glutamate; Gln, glutamine; Asp, aspartate, Cr, creatine; PCr, phosphocreatine; tCho, total choline-containing compounds; Tau, taurine; Ins, *myo*-inositol.

in the 60%-fat group compared to controls (+35 ± 13%, $P = 0.011$). The concentrations of the antioxidant Asc were not significantly modified by HFD exposure (**Figure 4L**).

There was a significant diet-region interaction effect on the concentration of *myo*-inositol (interaction $F = 4.9$, $P = 0.029$; region $F = 45.4$, $P < 0.001$; diet $F = 5.2$, $P = 0.071$, **Figure 4M**). *Post hoc* analyses indicated that the increase of *myo*-inositol was exclusive to the hypothalamus (+18 ± 5%, $P < 0.001$ for mice exposed to 60%-fat diet vs. controls; and +18 ± 5%, $P < 0.001$ vs. 45%-fat).

High-fat diet caused an increase of taurine levels ($F = 1.3$, $P = 0.047$, **Figure 4N**), which also varied across the three brain regions ($F = 85.9$, $P < 0.001$) without diet-region interaction ($F = 0.2$, $P = 0.788$). *Post hoc* analyses showed a significant difference of hippocampal taurine content between the mice exposed 60%-fat diet and controls (+12 ± 0.5%, $P = 0.022$).

The concentration of total choline-containing compounds was affected by HFD exposure ($F = 6.8$, $P = 0.001$, **Figure 4O**) and varied across brain regions ($F = 68.1$, $P < 0.001$) without interaction between the two factors ($F = 1.8$, $P = 0.149$). The content of total choline was significantly higher in mice exposed to 60%-fat diet in the hippocampus (+17 ± 6%, $P = 0.007$ vs. controls; +14 ± 6%, $P = 0.018$ vs. 45%-fat) and hypothalamus (+16 ± 4%, $P < 0.001$ vs. controls; +15 ± 4%, $P < 0.001$ vs. 45%-fat), but not in the cortex.

A significant diet-region interaction effect was observed on phosphorylethanolamine levels (interaction $F = 8.7$, $P = 0.022$; region $F = 19.8$, $P < 0.0001$; fat $F = 3.2$, $P = 0.252$, **Figure 4P**). *Post hoc* analyses identified a 40 ± 16% reduction of phosphorylethanolamine concentration in the cortex of mice exposed to 45%-fat diet compared to controls ($P = 0.017$). Such reduction in mice exposed to the 60%-fat diet did not reach statistical significance (−24 ± 17%, $P = 0.148$). The concentration of phosphorylethanolamine in the hypothalamus was different between the two HFD groups ($P = 0.009$).

Brain glucose levels were increased with the amount of fat in the diet ($F = 12.6$, $P = 0.037$, **Figure 4Q**) with no region ($F = 0.8$, $P = 0.513$) or interaction ($F = 4.4$, $P = 0.146$) effects. Compared to control mice, mice exposed to 60%-fat diet displayed a glucose concentration increase of 84 ± 25% in the hippocampus ($P < 0.001$) and of 41 ± 20% in the cortex ($P = 0.049$), but negligible in the hypothalamus (+16 ± 21%, $P = 0.442$).

We observed a significant diet-region interaction effect on the levels of lactate (interaction $F = 11.9$, $P = 0.005$, region $F = 10.1$, $P = 0.002$, fat $F = 6.9$, $P = 0.080$,

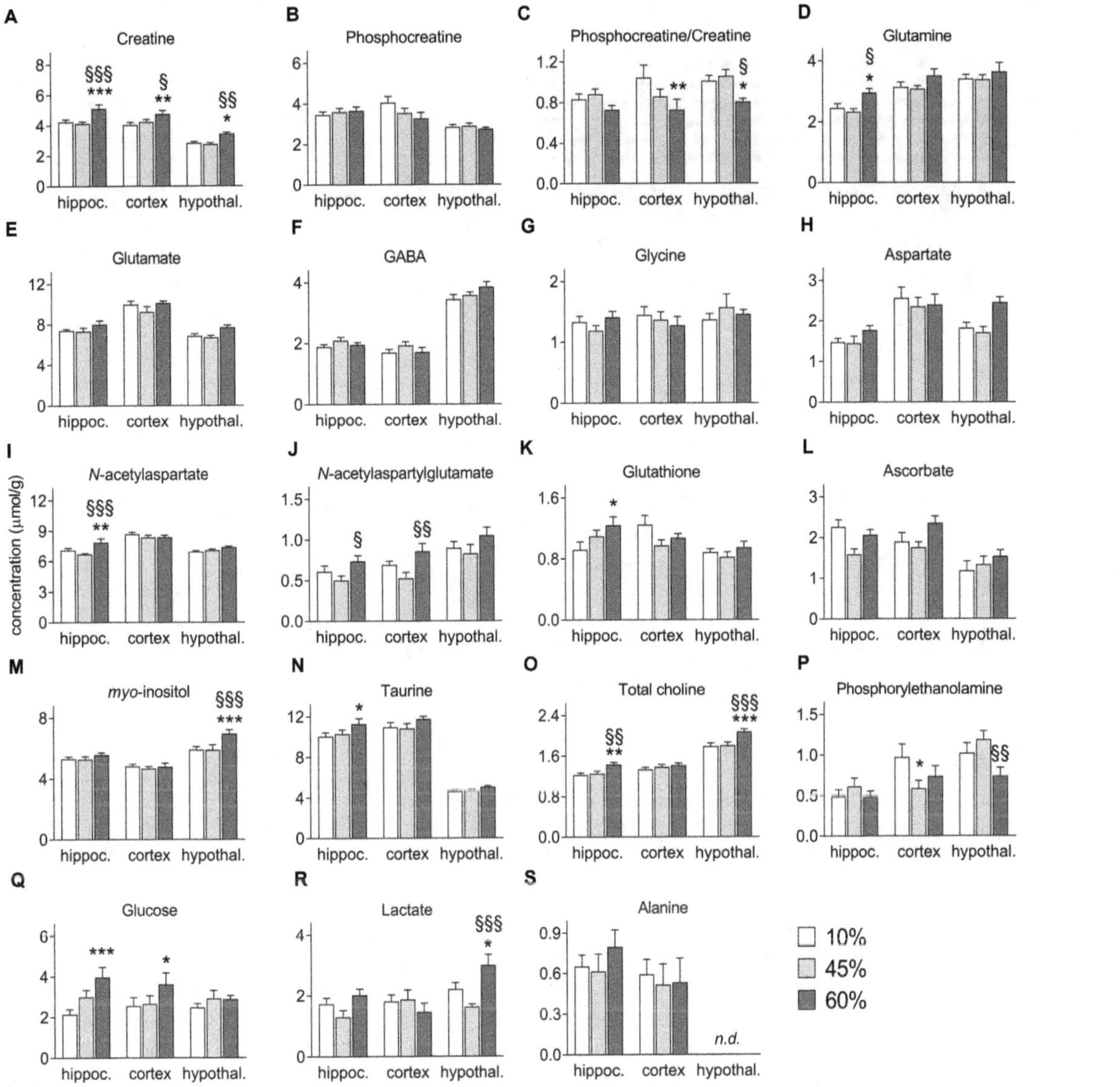

FIGURE 4 | Concentrations of metabolites in the hippocampus (hippoc.), cortex and hypothalamus (hypothal.) of mice fed diets containing 10%, 45%, and 60% fat. Panels **(A–S)** show alterations of each metabolite as presented in the text. Data are mean ± SEM (μmol/g). Symbols indicate significant differences in LSD tests after significant ANOVA, comparing HFD fed mice (45% fat or 60%-fat) and controls (10%-fat; *$P < 0.05$, **$P < 0.01$; ***$P < 0.001$), or the diets containing 45% and 60% fat (§ $P < 0.05$, §§ $P < 0.01$, §§§ $P < 0.001$).

Figure 4R). *Post hoc* analyses identified an increase of lactate concentration in the hypothalamus of mice exposed to 60%-fat diet compared to controls (+36 ± 16%, $P = 0.025$), and compared to 45%-fat fed mice (+84 ± 21%, $P < 0.001$). Levels of alanine were not significantly modified by HFD exposure (**Figure 4S**).

Synaptic Degeneration

In order to infer on synaptic degeneration, we measured the density of proteins located in synapses (**Figure 5**). Levels of synaptophysin were not significantly impacted by HFD exposure in any of the brain regions investigated (hippocampus $F = 2.4$, $P = 0.112$; cortex $F = 1.5$, $P = 0.250$; hypothalamus $F = 0.4$, $P = 0.661$), although one may notice a tendency for reduced synaptophysin content in the hippocampus of HFD mice relative to controls ($P = 0.054$ and $P = 0.090$ for 45% and 60%-fat versus controls, respectively). Also levels of syntaxin-1 were similar across experimental groups in the hippocampus ($F = 0.9$, $P = 0.414$), cortex ($F = 1.8$, $P = 0.240$) and hypothalamus ($F = 0.3$, $P = 0.764$). The synaptosomal-associated protein SNAP-25 was modified in the hippocampus of HFD-exposed mice ($F = 6.8$, $P = 0.029$), but not in the cortex or hypothalamus. In particular, SNAP-25 in the hippocampus on mice the fed 60%-fat diet was reduced by 25 ± 8% ($P = 0.021$) when compared to controls and by 26 ± 8% ($P = 0.017$) when compared to 45%-fat fed mice. Levels of syntaxin-4, which is another protein

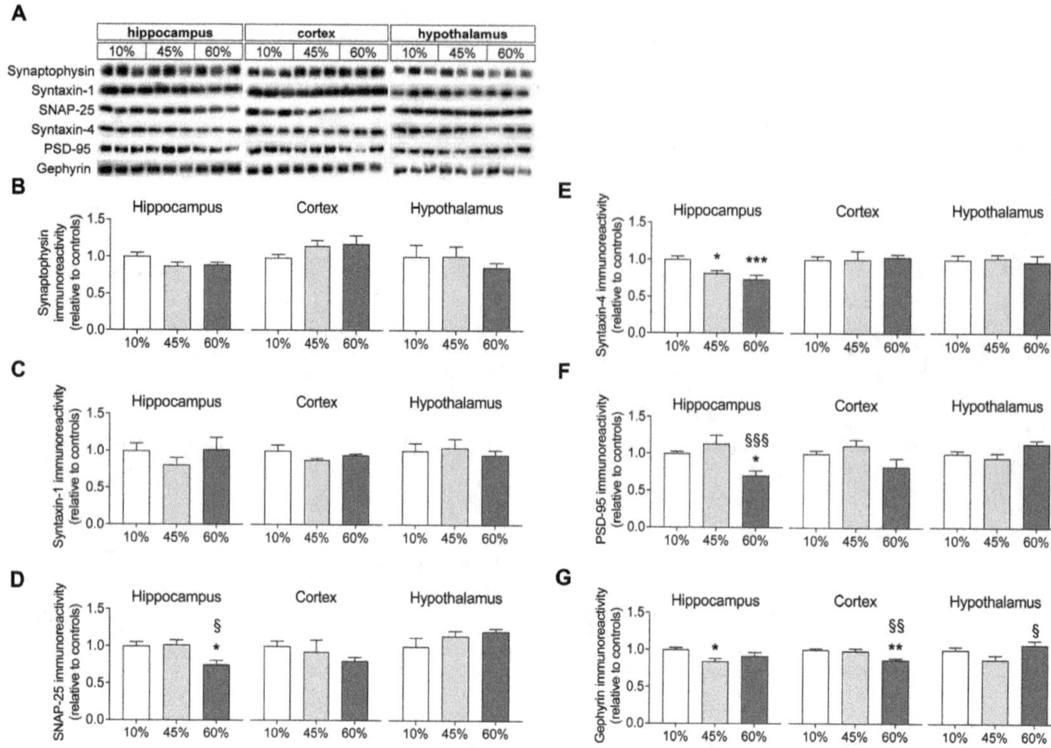

FIGURE 5 | HFD-induced changes on levels of synaptic proteins. **(A)** Shows typical Western blot of synaptophysin **(B)**, syntaxin-1 **(C)**, SNAP-25 **(D)**, syntaxin-4 **(E)**, PSD-95 **(F)**, and gephyrin **(G)**. Samples from three mice of each group were loaded in SDS-PAGE gels (2 μg of protein of syntaxin-1 and synaptophysin, 5 μg of protein for the remaining proteins). Measured immunoreactivity was normalized to the average of the three controls (10%-fat group, white bar) to allow pooling data from different gels. Data are mean ± SEM of $n = 6$. Symbols indicate significant differences in LSD tests after significant ANOVA, comparing HFD fed mice (45% fat or 60%-fat) and controls (10%-fat; $^{*}P < 0.05$, $^{**}P < 0.01$; $^{***}P < 0.001$), or the diets containing 45% and 60% fat (§ $P < 0.05$, §§ $P < 0.01$).

of the exocytosis machinery of nerve terminals but mainly occurring in processes of astrocytes (Tao-Cheng et al., 2015), were reduced in the hippocampus ($F = 9.2$, $P = 0.002$) but not cortex ($F = 0.1$, $P = 0.932$) or hypothalamus ($F = 0.1$, $P = 0.887$). In particular, when compared to controls, syntaxin-4 in the hippocampus was reduced by 19 ± 5% ($P = 0.011$) and 27 ± 7% ($P < 0.001$) in mice fed 45%-fat and 60%-fat diets, respectively.

Proteins from the post-synaptic region of synapses were also modified by HFD feeding. Diet impacted the postsynaptic density protein PSD-95 levels in the hippocampus ($F = 8.1$, $P = 0.002$) but not cortex ($F = 2.9$, $P = 0.076$) or hypothalamus ($F = 3.3$, $P = 0.067$). PSD-95 levels were reduced in the hippocampus of mice fed the 60%-fat diet by 30 ± 7% ($P = 0.012$) when compared to controls, and by 38 ± 13% ($P < 0.001$) when compared to mice fed the 45%-fat diet. Levels of gephyrin, another protein from the post-synaptic zone, varied with the amount of fat in the diet in the hippocampus ($F = 3.8$, $P = 0.044$), cortex ($F = 8.8$, $P = 0.003$) and hypothalamus ($F = 3.9$, $F = 0.035$). Compared to controls, the 45%-fat diet caused a significant reduction of gephyrin levels in the hippocampus (−16 ± 5%, $P = 0.014$). In the cortex, 60%-fat diet mice showed reduced gephyrin relative to the other groups (−13 ± 3%, $P = 0.002$ vs. controls; −12 ± 4%, $P = 0.004$ vs. 45%-fat diet). In the hypothalamus there was a reduction of −18 ± 8% in gephyrin levels in mice fed 45%-fat diet versus 60%-fat diet ($P = 0.011$).

We further measured the relative levels of vesicular glutamate and GABA transporters (vGluT1/2 and vGAT; **Figure 6**). The amount of fat in the diet was associated with a reduction of vGluT1 levels in the mouse hippocampus ($F = 7.9$, $P = 0.005$) and hypothalamus ($F = 4.3$, $P = 0.033$) but not in the cortex ($F = 1.5$, $P = 0.297$). In the hippocampus, both 45%-fat and 60%-fat fed mice showed significantly reduced vGluT1 levels when compared to controls (−38 ± 9%, $P = 0.001$ for 45%-fat diet; −22 ± 7%, $P = 0.032$ for 60%-fat diet). The same was observed in the hypothalamus (−39 ± 14%, $P = 0.015$ for 45%-fat diet; −32 ± 16%, $P = 0.039$ for 60%-fat diet). HFD exposure impacted levels of vGluT2 in the mouse cortex ($F = 10.3$, $P = 0.001$) and hypothalamus ($F = 3.9$, $P = 0.043$) but not in the hippocampus ($F = 0.3$, $P = 0.748$). In the cortex, mice fed 60%-fat diet showed increased cortical vGluT2 relative to the other groups (+25 ± 6%, $P < 0.001$ vs. controls; +24 ± 7%, $P = 0.001$ vs. 45%-fat diet). In the hypothalamus, we observed a significant reduction of vGluT2 levels in mice fed 45%-fat diet (−28 ± 8%, $P = 0.014$ vs. controls). Levels of vGAT were affected by HFD exposure in the hippocampus ($F = 3.6$, $P = 0.044$) and hypothalamus ($F = 3.6$, $P = 0.049$). The hippocampus of mice exposed to both 45%-fat and 60%-fat diet showed less vGAT levels than controls (−25 ± 9%, $P = 0.024$

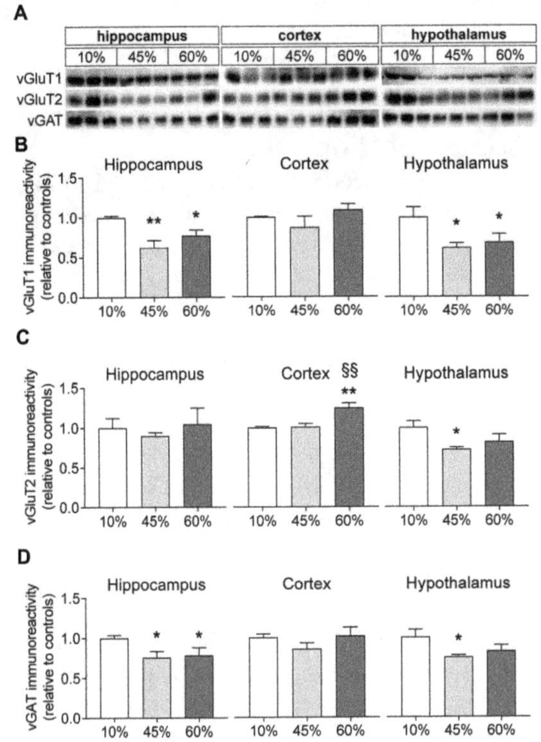

FIGURE 6 | HFD-induced changes on levels of vesicular glutamate and GABA transporters. **(A)** Shows representative Western blots of vGluT1 **(B)**, vGluT2 **(C)**, and vGAT **(D)**. Samples from three mice of each group were loaded in SDS-PAGE gels (20 μg of protein). Measured immunoreactivity was normalized to the average of the three controls (10%-fat group, white bar) to allow pooling data from different gels. Data are mean ± SEM of $n = 6$. Symbols indicate significant differences in LSD tests after significant ANOVA, comparing HFD fed mice (45% fat or 60%-fat) and controls (10%-fat; $^*P < 0.05$, $^{**}P < 0.01$), or the diets containing 45% and 60% fat ($^{\S\S}P < 0.01$).

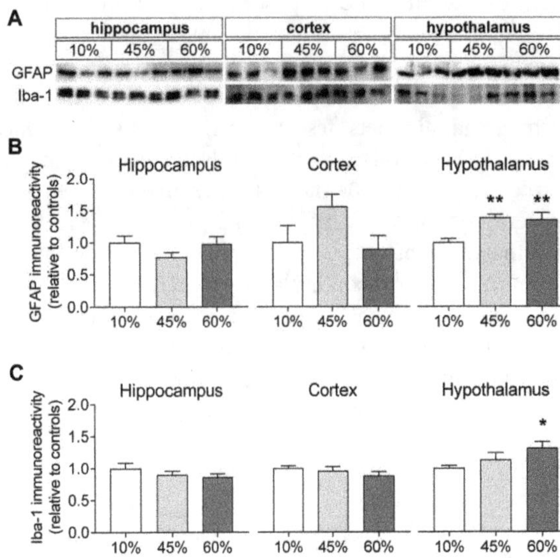

FIGURE 7 | HFD-induced changes on levels of glia-specific proteins. **(A)** Shows typical Western blot of GFAP **(B)** and Iba-1 **(C)**. Samples from three mice of each group were loaded in SDS-PAGE gels (20 μg of protein). Measured immunoreactivity was normalized to the average of the three controls (10%-fat group, white bar) to allow pooling data from different gels. Data are mean ± SEM of $n = 6$. Symbols indicate significant differences in LSD tests after significant ANOVA, comparing HFD fed mice (45% fat or 60%-fat) and controls (10%-fat; $^*P < 0.05$, $^{**}P < 0.01$). No significant differences were observed between the two HFD groups.

for 45%-fat diet; −22 ± 10%, $P = 0.042$ for 60%-fat diet). In the hypothalamus, the reduction of vGAT was significant only in mice exposed to 45%-fat diet (−25 ± 10%, $P = 0.018$ vs. controls).

Gliosis Markers

To infer on the modification of glial compartments, we measured the levels of glia-specific proteins (**Figure 7**). The glial fibrillary acidic protein (GFAP) that is specific to astrocytes was modified by fat levels in the diet in the hypothalamus ($F = 7.8$, $P = 0.005$), but not in the hippocampus ($F = 1.6$, $P = 0.235$) and cortex ($F = 2.6$, $P = 0.155$). Relative to controls, the hypothalamus of mice exposed to 45%-fat diet displayed a 38 ± 7% increase of GFAP immunoreactivity ($P = 0.003$), and a similar increase was observed for mice on the 60%-fat diet (+35 ± 12%, $P = 0.005$). Also the ionized calcium-binding adapter molecule 1 (iba-1), a protein present in microglial cells, showed increased levels in the hypothalamus ($F = 3.5$, $P = 0.045$), but not in the hippocampus ($F = 1.1$, $P = 0.352$) and cortex ($F = 1.1$, $P = 0.360$). In particular, there was a 31 ± 10% increase of iba-1 immunoreactivity in the hypothalamus of mice exposed to 60%-fat diet compared to controls ($P = 0.014$).

DISCUSSION

The present results show that mice chronically exposed to a lard-based HFD develop glucose intolerance associated to reduced insulin sensitivity, impaired hippocampal-dependent spatial memory, and neurochemical alterations in the hippocampus, cortex and hypothalamus. While metabolic profiles of the hippocampus, cortex and hypothalamus were modified in mice fed 60%-fat but not 45%-fat diet, when compared to controls, memory dysfunction was observed in both HFD groups. Accordingly, levels of proteins required for adequate synaptic function were found modified in mice fed diets containing fat at either 45% or 60%, relative to controls. This indicates that synaptic dysfunction may occur in the brain upon diet-induced obesity in the absence of major changes of metabolite concentrations. Nevertheless, this does not exclude the presence of alterations in the rate of certain metabolic pathways.

Modifications of Energy Metabolism

A general reduction of the phosphocreatine-to-creatine ratio was prominent in 60%-fat fed mice, when compared to the other groups, which suggests a disruption of mechanisms regulating metabolism and maintaining the cellular energy status in the brain. HFD exposure resulted in changes of glucose concentration in the hippocampus and cortex that were parallel to the changes in fed glycemia. However, this was not observed in the hypothalamus, where glucose levels were similar in all diets tested. This suggests that glucose transport and metabolism is differently adapted to the mild hyperglycemia state of 60%-fat fed mice, likely related to the glucose-sensing ability of the hypothalamus. In line with this, the hypothalamus of mice exposed to 60%-fat, but not the hippocampus and cortex, displayed higher levels of lactate than the other experimental groups. The measurement of basal metabolite concentrations, however, does not provide insight into metabolic pathways, namely glycolysis and tricarboxylic acid cycle. By employing ^{13}C MRS with ^{13}C-labeled glucose we have previously demonstrated that energy metabolism is altered in the hypothalamus upon high-fat feeding (Lizarbe et al., 2018). Modifications of brain energy metabolism were reported in rats fed a fat-rich diet for 3 weeks, namely reduced glucose utilization and increased astrocytic metabolism (Melø et al., 2006). Recently, we also reported that a rat model of lean T2D, the Goto-Kakizaki rat, displays impaired neuronal oxidative metabolism and reduced glutamate-glutamine cycle rate, as well as exacerbated oxidative metabolism in astrocytes (Girault et al., 2018). The relative contributions of fatty acids and glucose as available brain energy substrates, and of neurodegeneration-associated metabolic changes to brain energy dysfunction deserve further investigation. Previous experiments suggest that HFD exposure increases the utilization of fat in detriment of glucose oxidation, at least in the hypothalamus (Lizarbe et al., 2018). This observation, together with the present findings of higher lactate and lower glucose concentrations, leads us to speculate that long-term HFD exposure results in increased glycolysis in for lactate production while other available substrates, such as fats, are metabolized in the tricarboxylic acid cycle.

Osmolarity Regulation

Changes of the phosphocreatine-to-creatine ratio were due to increases in the creatine concentration rather than decreases of phosphocreatine (see **Figures 4A–C**), which is in line with the relevance of creatine levels for osmolarity regulation. Osmolarity control in the brain is considered to occur via the concentrations of not only creatine but also taurine and *myo*-inositol, since hyper-osmolarity causes their accumulation (Gullans and Verbalis, 1993). Also *N*-acetylaspartate, which is present in large concentrations in neurons, has been proposed to act as a brain osmolyte (Taylor et al., 1994; Gotoh et al., 1997), and is effectively released to the interstitial space upon osmotic challenges (Sager et al., 1997; Bothwell et al., 2001). Accordingly, taurine and *N*-acetylaspartate in the hippocampus, and *myo*-inositol in the hypothalamus were also increased upon exposure to 60% but not 45% fat in the diet. It should be noted that these modifications in brain osmolytes follow the plasma glucose concentration in the fed state, as well as corticosterone levels, which were significantly higher in 60%-fat fed mice than the other groups. Indeed, in addition to chronic hyperglycemia, it cannot be excluded that glucocorticoid-mediated signaling plays a role in diabetes-induced impaired brain metabolism and function (discussed in Girault et al., 2018).

Metabolic Indications of Neurodegeneration

N-Acetylaspartate reductions are often associated to impaired mitochondrial integrity in neurons, as well as lipid and myelin biosynthesis (Duarte et al., 2012b). Metabolism of *N*-acetylaspartate is compartmentalized between neurons and oligodendrocytes and serves for myelination. *N*-acetylaspartate is mainly stored in neurons, being synthesized from mitochondrial acetyl-CoA and Asp (Baslow, 2003), and its de-acetylation occurs in oligodendrocytes (Kirmani et al., 2002), where it can replenish both acetyl-CoA and oxaloacetate (through aspartate) pools providing carbon skeletons for both energy production and local lipid synthesis, required in the myelination process. In line with this role of *N*-acetylaspartate, Canavan disease is characterized by accumulation of *N*-acetylaspartate due to impaired de-acetylation in oligodendrocytes, which is associated to defects in myelin synthesis and deposition (Chakraborty et al., 2001). Indeed, it was recently suggested that high-fat feeding has an impact on myelination, namely by promoting the loss of oligodendrocyte progenitor cells and mature oligodendrocytes (Yoon et al., 2016).

A significant increase of hippocampal glutathione levels was observed in the 60%-fat group relative to controls, while there was a tendency for reduced glutathione levels in the cortex. It should be noted that the levels of glutathione measured by MRS include both reduced and oxidized forms, which are not distinguishable. Although lower ratio of reduced-to-oxidized glutathione has been reported in short-term HFD feeding (e.g., Alzoubi et al., 2018), no change of brain levels of oxidized and reduced glutathione, or their ratio upon long-term HFD exposure (Li et al., 2013). It should be noted however that Li et al. (2013) reported a non-significant increase of 15–20% of hippocampal reduced glutathione in high- versus low-fat-fed mice, in line with the present observation. It is likely that a total glutathione increase in the hippocampus might reflect a compensatory mechanism to oxidative stress upon chronic HFD exposure. In fact, the brain of HFD-fed mice displays impaired redox homeostasis, including: (1) enhanced activity of enzymes that generate free radicals, such as xanthine oxidase or NADPH oxidase; (2) reduced activity of enzymes with antioxidant action, namely glutathione peroxidase and catalase; (3) increased concentration of free radicals; (4) and oxidative damage to lipids and proteins (e.g., Morrison et al., 2010; Li et al., 2013; Charradi et al., 2017; Liu et al., 2017; Alzoubi et al., 2018; Maciejczyk et al., 2018). Accordingly, the hippocampus of mice fed a 60%-fat diet for 4 months also shows impaired signaling mediated by the transcription factor NRF2 which protects against brain oxidative damage (Morrison et al., 2010). Namely, Morrison et al. (2010) reported HFD-induced reductions of NRF2 protein levels, NRF2-DNA binding activity, and levels of the NRF2 responsive proteins in the hippocampus.

Interestingly, impaired cellular redox regulation in the brain has been proposed to impact oligodendrocyte proliferation (consistent with increased levels of *N*-acetylaspartate, discussed above), which has implications on the maintenance of myelin sheets around axons, and thus brain connectivity (see Corcoba et al., 2016 and references there in).

The content of total choline was significantly higher in hippocampus and hypothalamus, but not cortex. The main contributors to the choline peaks in MRS are the water-soluble glycerophosphorylcholine and phosphorylcholine, which are involved in membrane lipid metabolism (Duarte et al., 2012b). Namely, it is precursor of phosphatidylcholine and, in turn, of sphingomyelin, which is necessary for adequate myelination of axons (Oshida et al., 2003), and is implicated in immune responses (Li et al., 2015). In contrast to phosphorylcholine, a HDF-induced reduction of phosphorylethanolamine concentration was observed in the cortex. It is interesting to note that besides these changes in the concentration of phosphorylethanolamine in the cortex, no other significant metabolic alterations were observed between mice fed the diet containing 45% of fat and those in the control group. Altogether, these results point to alterations on phospholipid metabolism with possible implications on plasma membrane permeability, maintenance of action potentials and conduction of electric impulses, and on events that involve membrane deformation, fusion and fission, such as transcellular signaling, vesicular release of neurotransmitters, gliotransmitters or neuromodulators, mitochondrial dynamics, and autophagy (Aureli et al., 2015; Krols et al., 2016; Lauwers et al., 2016; van Echten-Deckert and Alam, 2018). In addition, lipid metabolism is important for membrane reorganization of astrocytes and microglia in neuroinflammation, which have been proposed to be reflected on MRS-detected changes of choline-containing compounds (discussed in Duarte et al., 2012b). In our study, total choline increased with HFD in the hippocampus and hypothalamus, while increased levels of GFAP and Iba-1, which are signs of inflammation, were exclusively observed in the hypothalamus. These results support the notion that MRS markers do not distinguish neuroinflammation from neurodegeneration and other processes (Zahr et al., 2014; Pardon et al., 2016).

Taurine is an amino acid that, although it is present at 1 μmol/g in the human brain, it reaches relatively large concentrations in the rodent brain (above 5 μmol/g in rats and above 8 μmol/g in mice; Duarte, 2016), thus playing a major role as osmolyte (Duarte et al., 2009 and references therein). Taurine is released from both neurons and glial cells (Hada et al., 1998), and acts as an agonist at receptors of the GABAergic and glycinergic neurotransmission systems (Albrecht and Schousboe, 2005). In the present study, HFD exposure caused a reduction of proteins associated to inhibitory neurotransmission (gephyrin and vGAT), suggesting that increased taurine might be a compensatory mechanism for the loss of inhibitory tone. Moreover, taurine is transported into the mitochondrial matrix where it buffers pH to the optimal value for isocitrate dehydrogenase, which is one of the key enzymes of the tricarboxylic acid cycle regulating energy metabolism and oxidative phosphorylation, contributes to stabilize the pH gradient across the inner-membrane, and thus helps preserving mitochondrial function and preventing oxidative damage (Hansen et al., 2010). Therefore, this HFD-induced increase of taurine levels in the is likely a beneficial adaptation of the brain.

Microgliosis and Astrogliosis

Increased levels of *myo*-inositol have been suggested to represent astrogliosis in the neurodegeneration-associated inflammatory process (discussed in Duarte et al., 2012b). The HFD-associated increased *myo*-inositol of the present study was exclusive to the hypothalamus. Interestingly, the hypothalamus was also the sole brain region to show significantly HFD-associated increased levels of glial specific proteins, namely GFAP and Iba-1 that are present in astrocytes and microglia, respectively. This overexpression of GFAP and Iba-1 is thus indicative of HFD-associated hyper-reactivity of astrocytes (astrogliosis) and microglia (microgliosis), as we reported recently (Lizarbe et al., 2018). Brain disorders are accompanied by neuroinflammation with astrogliosis and microgliosis generally in response to damage of nearby neuronal processes, but gliosis might become deleterious for the neurons upon chronicity (López-Valdés and Martínez-Coria, 2016). A transient increase in levels of pro-inflammatory cytokines was observed in the hypothalamus within 1–3 days of HFD exposure (e.g., Thaler et al., 2012; Waise et al., 2015), which might constitute a protective or reparative inflammatory process. In contrast, the hypothalamic gliosis in chronic HFD exposure (present study) is likely neurotoxic and has been suggested to participate in the genesis of obesity-associated diabetes since it may cause alterations of food intake, energy expenditure, insulin secretion, hepatic glucose production and metabolism of glucose and fats (Rahman et al., 2018).

The hippocampus and cortex of HFD-exposed mice did not show signs of gliosis, when compared to controls (no significant increase in levels of *myo*-inositol, GFAP or Iba-1). Despite the general consensus that neuroinflammation and astrogliosis occur in insulin resistance and T2D (Saravia et al., 2002; Baydas et al., 2003; Duarte et al., 2009, 2012a; Calvo-Ochoa et al., 2014), conflicting results have been reported regarding astrogliosis in memory-related brain areas upon HFD exposure. This is likely due to the distinct study designs, diet compositions, fat origin, age and/or species. Recent studies do not find HFD-induced increased levels of GFAP in the rat hippocampus (Raider et al., 2016; Ribeiro et al., 2018). In contrast, Tarantini et al. found that mice exposed to a 60%-fat diet from 3 to 8 months of age show mild behavior deficits and neuroinflammation, which are exacerbated by exposure to a cellular stress induced by deletion of the transcription factor *nrf2* that regulates the expression of antioxidant proteins, thus protecting against oxidative damage (Tarantini et al., 2018). A particularly interesting study by Tsai et al. (2018) found that GFAP levels increase in the hippocampus of mice exposed to 60%-fat diet for 3 months, relative to controls, and that HFD consumption leads to a reduction of the length and ramification of astrocytic processes in the CA1 and CA3 regions but not the dentate gyrus of the hippocampus. This retraction of astrocytic processes is of importance for the metabolic support that astrocytes should provide to neurons and their synapses (Sonnay et al., 2017), and in fact Tsai et al. (2018) also reported that HFD reduced levels of the astrocytic glutamate carriers GLT-1 and GLAST in the hippocampus, without changes of glutamine synthase levels. Soontornniyomkij et al. (2016) also found that 5 months of HFD exposure does not change levels of glutamine synthetase in the hippocampus of 5-month-old mice, although HFD increases the density of this protein in aged mice. Altogether, these observations suggest impaired glutamate-glutamine cycle rate that, in turn, may result in glutamatergic dysfunction and consequent accumulation of glutamine in astrocytes. Consistent with impaired glutamate release, we observed reduced levels of vesicular glutamate transporters, mainly vGluT1. However, care should be taken when interpreting changes on levels of carriers and enzymes because they may not reflect changes of their activity in the brain *in vivo*.

Moreover, as mentioned above, observations from different diet-induced obesity studies should be compared with caution. For example, in contrast to the reduced levels of glutamate carriers caused by a 60% HFD (Tsai et al., 2018), hippocampal slices prepared from mice fed a 45%-fat diet for only 2 months displayed enhanced glutamate uptake, increased density of glutamate carriers and reduced levels of the glutamate degrading enzymes glutamine synthetase and GABA-decarboxylase, compared to slices from controls (Valladolid-Acebes et al., 2012). Based on our results, we believe that the exposure to diets containing fat at 45% or 60% elicits different degenerative processes rather than resulting from a simple dose-response phenotype.

Glutamine synthesis takes place in astrocytes (Sonnay et al., 2017). In our study, HFD caused indeed an increase of glutamine levels in the 60%-fat group (but not the 45%-fat) relative to controls, which was particularly significant in the hippocampus. In line with our observations, increased hippocampal glutamine-to-creatine ratio was recently reported in Wistar rats exposed to a 60%-diet from 8 to 12 months of age (Ribeiro et al., 2018). In young adult Fisher 344 rats under a 60%-fat diet for 5 months, Raider et al. (2016) also observed a tendency for higher hippocampal glutamine concentration, and a significantly increased glutamine-to-glutamate ratio, relative to controls. This study, however, reported lower levels of *myo*-inositol and creatine in high versus low fat-fed rats (Raider et al., 2016), contrasting to the findings of the present study (discussed above).

Dysfunction in Excitatory and Inhibitory Synapses

N-Acetylaspartylglutamate (NAAG) levels increased in the cortex and hippocampus with HFD exposure. Similar NAAG changes were observed in HFD-exposed rats (Raider et al., 2016). NAAG is synthetized from ATP-dependent condensation of *N*-acetylaspartate and glutamate in neurons, packed into synaptic vesicles of presynaptic terminals, including those of pyramidal neurons in the cortex and limbic system, is co-released with glutamate, and acts as an antagonist of the glycine site of the NMDA receptor (Duarte and Xin, 2018 and referenced therein). Importantly, NAAG also acts on the metabotropic type II glutamate receptor mGluR3 inhibiting the release of neurotransmitters, such as glutamate, GABA and glycine (Neale, 2011). In HFD-exposed mice, increased NAAG levels would thus reduce glutamatergic neurotransmission by both inhibiting the activity of NMDA receptors and augmenting the negative feedback of glutamate release through its agonist action on presynaptic mGluR3 receptors. High NAAG concentration might prevent glutamate excitotoxicity, which is important when astrocytes have impaired glutamate clearance (see above), but on the other hand sufficient glutamatergic activity is necessary for proper function, including memory performance.

Consistent with reduced rate of the glutamate-glutamine cycle and with synaptic dysfunction in general, we observed a reduction in the levels of some pre- and post-synaptic proteins and of vesicular glutamate and GABA transporters in mice exposed to diets containing either 45% or 60%, relative to controls. We measured the density of two presynaptic proteins that are target SNARE (Soluble *N*-ethylmaleimide-sensitive factor Attachment protein REceptor) proteins required for vesicle fusion, namely syntaxin-1 and SNAP-25 (Söllner et al., 1993), and the density of synaptophysin that is a major component of presynaptic vesicles (Valtorta et al., 2004). SNAP-25 was reduced in the hippocampus of mice fed 60%-fat diet, when compared to controls, and there was also a tendency for hippocampal synaptophysin levels to be reduced with increasing fat content in the diet. Similar results were found for the density of vGluT1 and vGAT in the hippocampus, which suggest a reduction of the number of excitatory and inhibitory synaptic vesicles that are available for neurotransmission. Deficits in gliotransmission cannot be excluded since vesicular transporters are present in both neurons and astrocytes (see Schubert et al., 2011 and references therein). Therefore, we further measured the levels of syntaxin-4. While syntaxin-1 is mostly located in neurons, namely in the plasma membrane of the presynaptic terminal, syntaxin-4 is particularly concentrated in glial cells, namely in peri-synaptic astrocytic processes (Schubert et al., 2011; Tao-Cheng et al., 2015). In fact, the level of syntaxin-4 was also found reduced in the hippocampus of mice from either HFD group, confirming also a dysfunction at the level of gliotransmission. We further measured the density of PSD-95 that is associated to excitatory postsynaptic densities (Hunt et al., 1996), and gephyrin that is present at the inhibitory postsynaptic density, where it interacts with glycine and γ-aminobutyric acid type A ($GABA_A$) receptors (Maric et al., 2011). In the hippocampus, HFD also led to a reduction of PSD-95 (60%-fat group only) and of gephyrin (only significant for 45%-fat), compared to controls. Reduced level PSD-95 in the hippocampus of 45%-fat fed mice (for 2 weeks) relative to controls was also reported previously (Arnold et al., 2014). This synaptic dysfunction might be an important contributor for the hippocampal-dependent spatial memory impairment that was measured through the reduced spontaneous alternation in the Y-maze. In the cortex, only the levels of gephyrin were reduced in 60% fat fed mice versus controls, suggesting reduced inhibitory tone by the GABAergic system. In the hypothalamus, only vesicular neurotransmitter transporters and not the remaining measured synaptic proteins were reduced by HFD exposure, suggesting reduced neurotransmission capacity in both orexigenic and anorexigenic neurons (Meister, 2007; Moraes et al., 2009).

CONCLUSION

In sum, increasing the dietary amount of lard-based fat from 10 to 45% or 60% of the total energy intake leads to obesity accompanied by increased fasting blood glucose and insulin (pointing toward reduced insulin sensitivity), reduced glucose tolerance and increased plasma leptin. However, compared to controls (10%-fat) increased fed glycemia and plasma corticosterone were only observed in the 60%-fat fed mice. Exposure to both 45%-fat and 60%-fat diets resulted in deterioration of systems involved in neuro- and gliotransmission in the hippocampus, and in impaired spatial memory performance. Metabolic alterations measured by ^{1}H MRS were generally observed in mice exposed to 60%-fat but not 45%-fat diet. Therefore, we conclude that different features of the metabolic syndrome result in distinct neurochemical alterations in the brain, all likely contributing for memory impairment. Moreover, chronically increased blood glucose and/or corticosterone appear to be main drivers for changes in brain metabolite levels.

AUTHOR CONTRIBUTIONS

JD designed the study and wrote the manuscript. All authors performed the experiments, analyzed the data, and revised the manuscript.

REFERENCES

Albrecht, J., and Schousboe, A. (2005). Taurine interaction with neurotransmitter receptors in the CNS: an update. *Neurochem. Res.* 30, 1615–1621. doi: 10.1007/s11064-005-8986-6

Alzoubi, K. H., Mayyas, F. A., Mahafzah, R., and Khabour, O. F. (2018). Melatonin prevents memory impairment induced by high-fat diet: role of oxidative stress. *Behav. Brain Res.* 336, 93–98. doi: 10.1016/j.bbr.2017.08.047

Arnold, S. E., Lucki, I., Brookshire, B. R., Carlson, G. C., Browne, C. A., Kazi, H., et al. (2014). High fat diet produces brain insulin resistance, synaptodendritic abnormalities and altered behavior in mice. *Neurobiol. Dis.* 67, 79–87. doi: 10.1016/j.nbd.2014.03.011

Aureli, M., Grassi, S., Prioni, S., Sonnino, S., and Prinetti, A. (2015). Lipid membrane domains in the brain. *Biochim. Biophys. Acta* 1851, 1006–1016. doi: 10.1016/j.bbalip.2015.02.001

Baslow, M. H. (2003). *N*-acetylaspartate in the vertebrate brain: metabolism and function. *Neurochem. Res.* 28, 941–953. doi: 10.1023/A:1023250721185

Baydas, G., Nedzvetskii, V. S., Tuzcu, M., Yasar, A., and Kirichenko, S. V. (2003). Increase of glial fibrillary acidic protein and S-100B in hippocampus and cortex of diabetic rats: effects of vitamin E. *Eur. J. Pharmacol.* 462, 67–71. doi: 10.1016/S0014-2999(03)01294-9

Bothwell, J. H., Rae, C., Dixon, R. M., Styles, P., and Bhakoo, K. K. (2001). Hypo-osmotic swelling-activated release of organic osmolytes in brain slices: implications for brain oedema *in vivo*. *J. Neurochem.* 77, 1632–1640. doi: 10.1046/j.1471-4159.2001.00403.x

Calvo-Ochoa, E., Hernández-Ortega, K., Ferrera, P., Morimoto, S., and Arias, C. (2014). Short-term high-fat-and-fructose feeding produces insulin signaling alterations accompanied by neurite and synaptic reduction and astroglial activation in the rat hippocampus. *J. Cereb. Blood Flow Metab.* 34, 1001–1008. doi: 10.1038/jcbfm.2014.48

Chakraborty, G., Mekala, P., Yahya, D., Wu, G., and Ledeen, R. W. (2001). Intraneuronal *N*-acetylaspartate supplies acetyl groups for myelin lipid synthesis: evidence for myelin-associated aspartoacylase. *J. Neurochem.* 78, 736–745. doi: 10.1046/j.1471-4159.2001.00456.x

Charradi, K., Mahmoudi, M., Bedhiafi, T., Kadri, S., Elkahoui, S., Limam, F., et al. (2017). Dietary supplementation of grape seed and skin flour mitigates brain oxidative damage induced by a high-fat diet in rat: gender dependency. *Biomed. Pharmacother.* 87, 519–526. doi: 10.1016/j.biopha.2017.01.015

Corcoba, A., Steullet, P., Duarte, J. M. N., van de Looij, Y., Monin, A., Cuenod, M., et al. (2016). Glutathione deficit affects the integrity and function of the fimbria/fornix and anterior commissure in mice: relevance for schizophrenia. *Int. J. Neuropsychopharmacol.* 19, 1–11. doi: 10.1093/ijnp/pyv110

Cudalbu, C., McLin, V. A., Lei, H., Duarte, J. M. N., Rougemont, A. L., Oldani, G., et al. (2013). The C57BL/6 mouse exhibits sporadic congenital portosystemic shunts. *PLoS One* 8:e69782. doi: 10.1371/journal.pone.0069782

Duarte, J. M. N. (2015). Metabolic alterations associated to brain dysfunction in diabetes. *Aging Dis.* 6, 304–321. doi: 10.14336/AD.2014.1104

Duarte, J. M. N. (2016). Metabolism in the diabetic brain: neurochemical profiling by 1H magnetic resonance spectroscopy. *J. Diabetes Metab. Disord.* 3:011. doi: 10.24966/DMD-201X/100011

Duarte, J. M. N., Agostinho, P. M., Carvalho, R. A., and Cunha, R. A. (2012a). Caffeine consumption prevents diabetes-induced memory impairment and synaptotoxicity in the hippocampus of NONcNZO10/LtJ mice. *PLoS One* 7:e21899. doi: 10.1371/journal.pone.0021899

Duarte, J. M. N., Carvalho, R. A., Cunha, R. A., and Gruetter, R. (2009). Caffeine consumption attenuates neurochemical modifications in the hippocampus of streptozotocin-induced diabetic rats. *J. Neurochem.* 111, 368–379. doi: 10.1111/j.1471-4159.2009.06349.x

Duarte, J. M. N., Lei, H., Mlynárik, V., and Gruetter, R. (2012b). The neurochemical profile quantified by in vivo 1H NMR spectroscopy. *Neuroimage* 61, 342–362. doi: 10.1016/j.neuroimage.2011.12.038

Duarte, J. M. N., and Xin, L. (2018). Magnetic resonance spectroscopy in schizophrenia: evidence for glutamatergic dysfunction and impaired energy metabolism. *Neurochem. Res.* doi: 10.1007/s11064-018-2521-z [Epub ahead of print]. doi: 10.1007/s11064-018-2521-z

Fernandez, A. M., and Torres-Alemán, I. (2012). The many faces of insulin-like peptide signalling in the brain. *Nat. Rev. Neurosci.* 13, 225–239. doi: 10.1038/nrn3209

Frisardi, V., Solfrizzi, V., Seripa, D., Capurso, C., Santamato, A., Sancarlo, D., et al. (2010). Metabolic-cognitive syndrome: a cross-talk between metabolic syndrome and Alzheimer's disease. *Ageing Res. Rev.* 9, 399–417. doi: 10.1016/j.arr.2010.04.007

Gapp, K., Corcoba, A., van Steenwyk, G., Mansuy, I. M., and Duarte, J. M. N. (2017). Brain metabolic alterations in mice subjected to postnatal traumatic stress and in their offspring. *J. Cereb. Blood Flow Metab.* 37, 2423–2432. doi: 10.1177/0271678X16667525

Girault, F.-M., Sonnay, S., Gruetter, R., and Duarte, J. M. N. (2018). Alterations of brain energy metabolism in type 2 diabetic Goto-Kakizaki rats measured in vivo by 13C magnetic resonance spectroscopy. *Neurotox. Res.* doi: 10.1007/s12640-017-9821-y [Epub ahead of print].

Gotoh, M., Davies, S. E., and Obrenovitch, T. P. (1997). Brain tissue acidosis: effects on the extracellular concentration of *N*-acetylaspartate. *J. Neurochem.* 69, 655–661. doi: 10.1046/j.1471-4159.1997.69020655.x

Gruetter, R., and Tkáč, I. (2000). Field mapping without reference scan using asymmetric echo-planar techniques. *Magn. Reson. Med.* 43, 319–323. doi: 10.1002/(SICI)1522-2594(200002)43:2<319::AID-MRM22>3.0.CO;2-1

Gullans, S. R., and Verbalis, J. G. (1993). Control of brain volume during hyperosmolar and hypoosmolar conditions. *Annu. Rev. Med.* 44, 289–301. doi: 10.1146/annurev.me.44.020193.001445

Hada, J., Kaku, T., Morimoto, K., Hayashi, Y., and Nagai, K. (1998). Activation of adenosine A2 receptors enhances high K^+-evoked taurine release from rat hippocampus: a microdialysis study. *Amino Acids* 15, 43–52. doi: 10.1007/BF01345279

Hansen, S. H., Andersen, M. L., Cornett, C., Gradinaru, R., and Grunnet, N. (2010). A role for taurine in mitochondrial function. *J. Biomed. Sci.* 17(Suppl. 1):S23. doi: 10.1186/1423-0127-17-S1-S23

Havrankova, J., Roth, J., and Brownstein, M. (1978). Insulin receptors are widely distributed in the central nervous system of the rat. *Nature* 272, 827–829. doi: 10.1038/272827a0

Hill, J. M., Lesniak, M. A., Pert, C. B., and Roth, J. (1986). Autoradiographic localization of insulin receptors in rat brain: prominence in olfactory and limbic areas. *Neuroscience* 17, 1127–1138. doi: 10.1016/0306-4522(86)90082-5

Hunt, C. A., Schenker, L. J., and Kennedy, M. B. (1996). PSD-95 is associated with the postsynaptic density and not with the presynaptic membrane at forebrain synapses. *J. Neurosci.* 16, 1380–1388. doi: 10.1523/JNEUROSCI.16-04-01380.1996

Kirmani, B. F., Jacobowitz, D. M., Kallarakal, A. T., and Namboodiri, M. A. (2002). Aspartoacylase is restricted primarily to myelin synthesizing cells in the CNS: therapeutic implications for Canavan disease. *Brain Res. Mol. Brain Res.* 107, 176–182. doi: 10.1016/S0169-328X(02)00490-4

Krols, M., van Isterdael, G., Asselbergh, B., Kremer, A., Lippens, S., Timmerman, V., et al. (2016). Mitochondria-associated membranes as hubs for neurodegeneration. *Acta Neuropathol.* 131, 505–523. doi: 10.1007/s00401-015-1528-7

Lauwers, E., Goodchild, R., and Verstreken, P. (2016). Membrane lipids in presynaptic function and disease. *Neuron* 90, 11–25. doi: 10.1016/j.neuron.2016.02.033

Li, L., Wang, Z., and Zuo, Z. (2013). Chronic intermittent fasting improves cognitive functions and brain structures in mice. *PLoS One* 8:e66069. doi: 10.1371/journal.pone.0066069

Li, M., Fan, P., and Wang, Y. (2015). Integrative approaches for lipid analysis. *Pharmacologia* 6, 213–234. doi: 10.5567/pharmacologia.2015.213.234

Liu, Y., Zhang, Q., Wang, L., Wang, H., Sun, T., Xia, H., et al. (2017). The α-lipoic acid improves high-fat diet-induced cerebral damage through inhibition of oxidative stress and inflammatory reaction. *Environ. Toxicol. Pharmacol.* 56, 219–224. doi: 10.1016/j.etap.2017.09.018

Lizarbe, B., Cherix, A., Duarte, J. M. N., Cardinaux, J. R., and Gruetter, R. (2018). High-fat diet consumption alters energy metabolism on the mouse hypothalamus. *Int. J. Obesity* doi: 10.1038/s41366-018-0224-9 [Epub ahead of print]. doi: 10.1038/s41366-018-0224-9

López-Valdés, H. E., and Martínez-Coria, H. (2016). The role of neuroinflammation in age-related dementias. *Rev. Invest. Clin.* 68, 40–48.

Maciejczyk, M., Żebrowska, E., Zalewska, A., and Chabowski, A. (2018). Redox balance, antioxidant defense, and oxidative damage in the hypothalamus and cerebral cortex of rats with high fat diet-induced insulin resistance. *Oxid. Med. Cell. Longev.* 2018:6940515. doi: 10.1155/2018/6940515

Maric, H. M., Mukherjee, J., Tretter, V., Moss, S. J., and Schindelin, H. (2011). Gephyrin-mediated γ-aminobutyric acid type A and glycine receptor clustering relies on a common binding site. *J. Biol. Chem.* 286, 42105–42114. doi: 10.1074/jbc.M111.303412

Meister, B. (2007). Neurotransmitters in key neurons of the hypothalamus that regulate feeding behavior and body weight. *Physiol. Behav.* 92, 263–271. doi: 10.1016/j.physbeh.2007.05.021

Melø, T. M., Nehlig, A., and Sonnewald, U. (2006). Neuronal-glial interactions in rats fed a ketogenic diet. *Neurochem. Int.* 48, 498–507. doi: 10.1016/j.neuint.2005.12.037

Mlynárik, V., Gambarota, G., Frenkel, H., and Gruetter, R. (2006). Localized short-echo-time proton MR spectroscopy with full signal-intensity acquisition. *Magn. Reson. Med.* 56, 965–970. doi: 10.1002/mrm.21043

Moheet, A., Mangia, S., and Seaquist, E. R. (2015). Impact of diabetes on cognitive function and brain structure. *Ann. N. Y. Acad. Sci.* 1353, 60–71. doi: 10.1111/nyas.12807

Moraes, J. C., Coope, A., Morari, J., Cintra, D. E., Roman, E. A., Pauli, J. R., et al. (2009). High-fat diet induces apoptosis of hypothalamic neurons. *PLoS One* 4:e5045. doi: 10.1371/journal.pone.0005045

Morrison, C. D., Pistell, P. J., Ingram, D. K., Johnson, W. D., Liu, Y., Fernandez-Kim, S. O., et al. (2010). High fat diet increases hippocampal oxidative stress and cognitive impairment in aged mice: implications for decreased Nrf2 signaling. *J. Neurochem.* 114, 1581–1589. doi: 10.1111/j.1471-4159.2010.06865.x

Neale, J. H. (2011). *N*-acetylaspartylglutamate is an agonist at mGluR3 *in vivo* and *in vitro*. *J. Neurochem.* 119, 891–895. doi: 10.1111/j.1471-4159.2011.07380.x

Oshida, K., Shimizu, T., Takase, M., Tamura, Y., Shimizu, T., and Yamashiro, Y. (2003). Effects of dietary sphingomyelin on central nervous system myelination in developing rats. *Pediatr. Res.* 53, 589–593. doi: 10.1203/01.PDR.0000054654.73826.AC

Pardon, M. C., Yanez Lopez, M., Yuchun, D., Marjańska, M., Prior, M., Brignell, C., et al. (2016). Magnetic Resonance Spectroscopy discriminates the response to microglial stimulation of wild type and Alzheimer's disease models. *Sci. Rep.* 6:19880. doi: 10.1038/srep19880

Rahman, M. H., Bhusal, A., Lee, W. H., Lee, I. K., and Suk, K. (2018). Hypothalamic inflammation and malfunctioning glia in the pathophysiology of obesity and diabetes: Translational significance. *Biochem. Pharmacol.* 153, 123–133. doi: 10.1016/j.bcp.2018.01.024

Raider, K., Ma, D., Harris, J. L., Fuentes, I., Rogers, R. S., Wheatley, J. L., et al. (2016). A high fat diet alters metabolic and bioenergetic function in the brain: a magnetic resonance spectroscopy study. *Neurochem. Int.* 97, 172–180. doi: 10.1016/j.neuint.2016.04.008

Ribeiro, M., Castelhano, J., Petrella, L. I., Sereno, J., Rodrigues, T., Neves, C., et al. (2018). High-fat diet induces a neurometabolic state characterized by changes in glutamate and *N*-acetylaspartate pools associated with early glucose intolerance: an in vivo multimodal MRI study. *J. Magn. Reson. Imaging* doi: 10.1002/jmri.25942 [Epub ahead of print]. doi: 10.1002/jmri.25942

Sager, T. N., Fink-Jensen, A., and Hansen, A. J. (1997). Transient elevation of interstitial *N*-acetylaspartate in reversible global brain ischemia. *J. Neurochem.* 68, 675–682. doi: 10.1046/j.1471-4159.1997.68020675.x

Saravia, F. E., Revsin, Y., Deniselle, M. C. G., Gonzalez, S. L., Roig, P., Lima, A., et al. (2002). Increased astrocyte reactivity in the hippocampus of murine models of type 1 diabetes: the nonobese diabetic (NOD) and streptozotocin-treated mice. *Brain Res.* 957, 345–353. doi: 10.1016/S0006-8993(02)03675-2

Schubert, V., Bouvier, D., and Volterra, A. (2011). SNARE protein expression in synaptic terminals and astrocytes in the adult hippocampus: a comparative analysis. *Glia* 59, 1472–1488. doi: 10.1002/glia.21190

Soares, A. F., Duarte, J. M. N., and Gruetter, R. (2018). Increased hepatic fatty acid polyunsaturation precedes ectopic lipid deposition in the liver in adaptation to high-fat diets in mice. *MAGMA* 31, 341–354. doi: 10.1007/s10334-017-0654-8

Söllner, T., Whiteheart, S. W., Brunner, M., Erdjument-Bromage, H., Geromanos, S., Tempst, P., et al. (1993). SNAP receptors implicated in vesicle targeting and fusion. *Nature* 362, 318–324. doi: 10.1038/362318a0

Sonnay, S., Gruetter, R., and Duarte, J. M. N. (2017). How energy metabolism supports cerebral function: insights from 13C magnetic resonance studies *in vivo*. *Front. Neurosci.* 11:288. doi: 10.3389/fnins.2017.00288

Soontornniyomkij, V., Kesby, J. P., Soontornniyomkij, B., Kim, J. J., Kisseleva, T., Achim, C. L., et al. (2016). Age and high-fat diet effects on glutamine synthetase immunoreactivity in liver and hippocampus and recognition memory in mice. *Curr. Aging. Sci.* 9, 301–309. doi: 10.2174/1874609809666160413113311

Steculorum, S. M., Solas, M., and Brüning, J. C. (2014). The paradox of neuronal insulin action and resistance in the development of aging-associated diseases. *Alzheimers Dement* 10(1 Suppl.), S3–S11. doi: 10.1016/j.jalz.2013.12.008

Tao-Cheng, J. H., Pham, A., Yang, Y., Winters, C. A., Gallant, P. E., and Reese, T. S. (2015). Syntaxin 4 is concentrated on plasma membrane of astrocytes. *Neuroscience* 286, 264–271. doi: 10.1016/j.neuroscience.2014.11.054

Tarantini, S., Valcarcel-Ares, M. N., Yabluchanskiy, A., Tucsek, Z., Hertelendy, P., Kiss, T., et al. (2018). Nrf2 deficiency exacerbates obesity-induced oxidative stress, neurovascular dysfunction, blood-brain barrier disruption, neuroinflammation, amyloidogenic gene expression, and cognitive decline in mice, mimicking the aging phenotype. *J. Gerontol. A Biol. Sci. Med. Sci.* 73, 853–863. doi: 10.1093/gerona/glx177

Taylor, D. L., Davies, S. E., Obrenovitch, T. P., Urenjak, J., Richards, D. A., Clark, J. B., et al. (1994). Extracellular *N*-acetylaspartate in the rat brain: *in vivo* determination of basal levels and changes evoked by high K+. *J. Neurochem.* 62, 2349–2355. doi: 10.1046/j.1471-4159.1994.62062349.x

Thaler, J. P., Yi, C. X., Schur, E. A., Guyenet, S. J., Hwang, B. H., Dietrich, M. O., et al. (2012). Obesity is associated with hypothalamic injury in rodents and humans. *J. Clin. Invest.* 122, 153–162. doi: 10.1172/JCI59660

Tsai, S. F., Wu, H. T., Chen, P. C., Chen, Y. W., Yu, M., Wang, T. F., et al. (2018). High-fat diet suppresses the astrocytic process arborization and downregulates the glial glutamate transporters in the hippocampus of mice. *Brain Res.* 1700, 66–77. doi: 10.1016/j.brainres.2018.07.017

Valladolid-Acebes, I., Merino, B., Principato, A., Fole, A., Barbas, C., Lorenzo, M. P., et al. (2012). High-fat diets induce changes in hippocampal glutamate metabolism and neurotransmission. *Am. J. Physiol. Endocrinol. Metab.* 302, E396–E402. doi: 10.1152/ajpendo.00343.2011

Valtorta, F., Pennuto, M., Bonanomi, D., and Benfenati, F. (2004). Synaptophysin: leading actor or walk-on role in synaptic vesicle exocytosis? *Bioessays* 26, 445–453.

van der Graaf, M., Janssen, S. W., van Asten, J. J., Hermus, A. R., Sweep, C. G., Pikkemaat, J. A., et al. (2004). Metabolic profile of the hippocampus of Zucker Diabetic Fatty rats assessed by *in vivo* 1H magnetic resonance spectroscopy. *NMR Biomed.* 17, 405–410. doi: 10.1002/nbm.896

van Echten-Deckert, G., and Alam, S. (2018). Sphingolipid metabolism - an ambiguous regulator of autophagy in the brain. *Biol. Chem.* 399, 837–850. doi: 10.1515/hsz-2018-0237

Waise, T. M. Z., Toshinai, K., Naznin, F., NamKoong, C., Md Moin, A. S., Sakoda, H., et al. (2015). One-day high-fat diet induces inflammation in the nodose ganglion and hypothalamus of mice. *Biochem. Biophys. Res. Commun.* 464, 1157–1162. doi: 10.1016/j.bbrc.2015.07.097

Wang, W. T., Lee, P., Yeh, H. W., Smirnova, I. V., and Choi, I. Y. (2012). Effects of acute and chronic hyperglycemia on the neurochemical profiles in the rat brain with streptozotocin-induced diabetes detected using *in vivo* ^{1}H MR spectroscopy at 9.4 *T. J. Neurochem.* 121, 407–417. doi: 10.1111/j.1471-4159.2012.07698.x

Yoon, H., Kleven, A., Paulsen, A., Kleppe, L., Wu, J., Ying, Z., et al. (2016). Interplay between exercise and dietary fat modulates myelinogenesis in the central nervous system. *Biochim. Biophys. Acta* 1862, 545–555. doi: 10.1016/j.bbadis.2016.01.019

Zahr, N. M., Mayer, D., Rohlfing, T., Sullivan, E. V., and Pfefferbaum, A. (2014). Imaging neuroinflammation? A perspective from MR spectroscopy. *Brain Pathol.* 24, 654–664. doi: 10.1111/bpa.12197

13

The Role of PGC-1α/UCP2 Signaling in the Beneficial Effects of Physical Exercise on the Brain

Viviane José de Oliveira Bristot[1], *Ana Cristina de Bem Alves*[1,2], *Liziane Rosa Cardoso*[1], *Débora da Luz Scheffer*[1,2] *and Aderbal Silva Aguiar Jr.*[1,2*]

[1] *Research Group on Biology of Exercise, Department of Health Sciences, Centro Araranguá, Federal University of Santa Catarina, Araranguá, Brazil,* [2] *Laboratório de Bioenergética e Estresse Oxidativo, Departamento de Bioquímica, Centro de Ciências Biológicas, Universidade Federal de Santa Catarina, Florianópolis, Brazil*

Correspondence:
Aderbal Silva Aguiar Jr.
aderbal.aguiar@ufsc.br;
aderbalaguiar@gmail.com

In understanding the pathology of neurological diseases, the role played by brain energy metabolism is gaining prominence. Animal models have demonstrated that regular physical exercise improves brain energy metabolism while also providing antidepressant, anxiolytic, antioxidant and neuroprotective functions. This review summarizes the latest evidence on the roles played by peroxisome proliferator-activated receptor gamma (PPAR-γ) coactivator 1-alpha (PGC-1α) and mitochondrial uncoupling protein (UCP) in this scenario. The beneficial effects of exercise seem to depend on crosstalk between muscles and nervous tissue through the increased release of muscle irisin during exercise.

Keywords: physical exercise, mitochondria, irisin, FNDC5, PGC-1α, UCP2

INTRODUCTION

A physically inactive lifestyle is associated with the development of non-communicable diseases (NCD), such as cardiovascular diseases, type 2 diabetes, some cancers, and an overall increased mortality rate (Booth et al., 2012; Koster et al., 2012; Biswas et al., 2015; Same et al., 2016; Patterson et al., 2018). Physical inactivity is also considered a risk factor for abdominal obesity, high serum triglyceride levels, low-density lipoprotein, cholesterol, hypertension, and hyperglycemia, which together characterize metabolic syndrome (Bankoski et al., 2011). Physical exercise has several benefits for physical and mental health (Aguiar et al., 2008; Garber et al., 2011; Esteban-Cornejo et al., 2015; Loprinzi, 2015), including increased physical and cardiorespiratory capacity (or fitness), improved body composition and balance (or fatness), and greater muscle strength and flexibility (Garber et al., 2011; Geneen et al., 2017). Physical exercise also improves the serum lipid profile, decreases glucose intolerance, and attenuates insulin resistance (Lin et al., 2015; Brymer and Davids, 2016; Qiu et al., 2018). The literature supports the fitness-fatness hypothesis, which suggests that a higher level of cardiorespiratory fitness will reduce the adverse effects of obesity on morbidity and mortality, making obesity a much less important factor for health than is generally believed (Hainer et al., 2009; Fogelholm, 2010; Barry et al., 2014). The data are mixed, but for many authors, fitness is more important than fatness for early mortality (Blair et al., 1989; Wei et al., 1999; McAuley et al., 2009; Barry et al., 2014). This is important for individuals who are unable to lose weight but are able to engage in a regular physical activity program.

The American College of Sports Medicine (ACSM) recommends increasing total energy expenditure (TEE; kcal/day) for health, with a minimum of 30 min of moderate physical exercise 5 days/week or 20 min of vigorous exercise 3 days/week (Haskell et al., 2007). The ACSM also recommends combining moderate (3–6 MET) and vigorous activities (>6 MET) (Haskell et al., 2007). The World Health Organization (2000) recommends that individuals participate in at least 150 or 75 min/week of moderate or vigorous physical activities, respectively (World Health Organization, 2010). For overweight and obesity, the ACSM recommends increased physical activity, between 150 and 250 min/week to prevent weight gain or provide modest weight loss (Donnelly et al., 2009). Larger amounts of exercise (>250 min/week) are needed for clinically significant weight loss (Donnelly et al., 2009). However, physical activity for weight loss is controversial; the amount of weight lost due to an exercise intervention is often less than what is predicted to be lost based on the exercise workload, suggesting a smaller increase in TEE (and smaller energy imbalance) than expected (Thomas et al., 2012; Melanson et al., 2013; Flack et al., 2018). This reduced energy imbalance occurs through metabolic and behavioral modifications in humans (Pontzer, 2018) and reinforces the hypothesis that fitness is more important than fatness for health. In general, the 150 min/week of moderate physical activity or 60–75 min/week of vigorous activity recommendations of ACSM and WHO is effective for overall health.

Even single exercise sessions, which increases the production of endogenous opioids (Geneen et al., 2017), angiogenesis factors (such as vascular endothelial growth factor [VEGF], hypoxia-induced 1 alpha factor [HIF-1α] and erythropoietin [EPO]) (Ribeiro et al., 2017) appear to be healthy, and they protect against hyperglycemia peaks (Lang Lehrskov et al., 2018) in humans. A single exercise session increases the plasma endocannabinoid levels in mice (Fuss et al., 2015), which is a possible mechanism for the euphoric state (runner's high) that occurs after long runs (Boecker et al., 2008).

The central nervous system (CNS) was the last physiological system approached by the exercise sciences. Lack of exercise is a major cause of chronic diseases (Booth et al., 2012), including brain diseases, such as depression (Farmer et al., 1988; Aguiar et al., 2014), and neurodegenerative diseases (Radak et al., 2010; Xu et al., 2010; Aguiar et al., 2016). However, physical exercise is a neuroprotective agent against depression (Schuch et al., 2017), anxiety disorders (Jayakody et al., 2014), cognitive decline/dementia in elderly people (Aguiar et al., 2011; Shen et al., 2016), Parkinson's disease (Chen et al., 2018), and Alzheimer's disease (Aguiar et al., 2016; Law et al., 2018). Animal studies have shown that physical exercise increases neuronal survival, cerebral vascularization, neurogenesis, and mitochondrial metabolism, while it decreases the effects of neurotoxins on the CNS (Aguiar et al., 2014; Zhang and Zhang, 2016). Iris and uncoupling proteins (U) are candidate mechanisms for these exercise-induced changes.

In mammals, transcriptional peroxisome proliferator-activated receptor gamma (PPAR-γ) coactivator 1-alpha (PGC-1α)/fibronectin type III domain-containing protein 5 (FNDC5, the precursor of irisin), which is secreted during exercise, promotes the browning of beige fat cells in white adipose tissue (**Figure 1**), resulting in enhanced thermogenesis and increased energy expenditure (Hofmann et al., 2014). In the CNS (**Figure 2**), FCDN5/irisin regulates central mechanisms that mediate adaptive responses by (a) improving neuronal mitochondrial decoupling and (b) increasing the expression of neurotrophins and neuroprotective proteins such as neuronal PAS domain protein 4 (NPAS4), cFOS, activity-regulated cytoskeleton-associated protein (ARC), and zinc finger protein 268 (ZIF268) (**Figure 1**; Wrann et al., 2013; Wrann, 2015). In brown adipose tissue, mitochondrial uncoupling is effected by a specific protein, referred to as uncoupling protein-1 (UCP1), in the inner mitochondrial membrane (Ricquier and Bouillaud, 2000). The cloning of UCP2 and UCP3, two homologs of UCP1, has boosted research into the importance of respiration control in metabolic processes, metabolic diseases and energy balance (Ricquier and Bouillaud, 2000). PPAR-γ/PGC-1α expression also improves mitochondrial decoupling, which reduces mitochondrial membrane potential and reactive oxygen species (ROS) production, oxidative damage, mitochondrial calcium overload and potential apoptotic events through the induction of uncoupling protein 2 (UCP2) (Andrews et al., 2005). Therefore, FND5/irisin is essential for processes involving neurotrophins and synaptic plasticity, mitochondrial biogenesis, and resistance to neuronal stress (Wrann et al., 2013; Marosi and Mattson, 2014; Raefsky and Mattson, 2017).

The purpose of this manuscript is to review the roles played by FND5/irisin and UCP2, which are important for energy metabolism, in the neuroprotective and antioxidant effects of physical activity in the CNS.

THE EXERCISE-INDUCED RELEASE OF IRISIN AND ITS NEUROPROTECTIVE EFFECTS

Because irisin is an exercise induced hormone (or myokine), it is unclear whether the physical exercise-related CNS benefits are attributable to irisin. Irisin is a 112 amino acid peptide that is cleaved (by an unknown protease) from the glycosylated type I membrane protein FNDC5 and released into the bloodstream in a PGC-1α-dependent manner through a muscle contraction-mediated transcription mechanism (Bostrom et al., 2012). PGC-1α is a transcriptional coactivator and does not bind to DNA directly; it needs to interact with another transcription factor to induce neuronal FNDC5 gene expression (Xu, 2013). Several clues indicate that the PGC-1α binding partner is orphan nuclear estrogen-related receptor alpha (ERRα) (Kamei et al., 2003; Xu, 2013). Moreover, irisin enhances PGC-1α expression in the hippocampus and prefrontal cortex of mice in a positive feedback loop (Siteneski et al., 2018). The irisin released from muscles is a myokine that acts preferentially on the subcutaneous 'beige' fat and causes it to 'brown' by increasing the expression of UCP1 and other thermogenic genes (Bostrom et al., 2012). Irisin is involved in human biological adaptations such as increased muscle strength, decreased obesity and insulin resistance, and also has physical and psychological benefits (Bostrom et al., 2012;

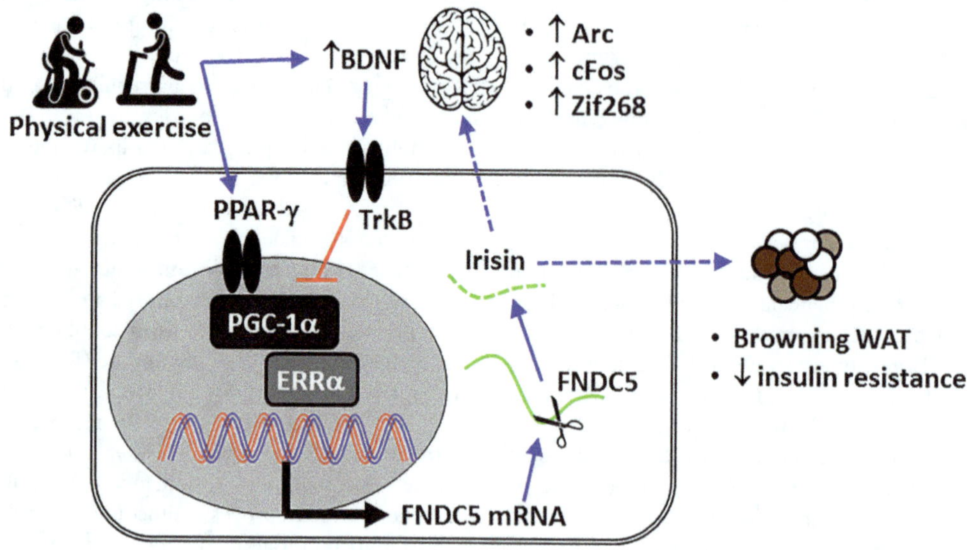

FIGURE 1 | The mechanism of action of irisin in metabolism-associated health issues or metabolic diseases. The expression of Arc, cFos, and Zif268 is induced by neuronal activity. BDNF, brain-derived neurotrophic factor; ERRα, estrogen-related receptor alpha; FNDC5, fibronectin domain-containing protein 5; PGC-1α, peroxisome proliferator-activated receptor gamma coactivator-1-alpha; TrkB, tyrosine receptor kinase B; WAT, white adipose tissue.

Ghahrizjani et al., 2015). Currently, it is hypothesized that irisin circulates in the blood in vesicles containing other molecules, such as proteins, miRNA and nucleic acids, until reaching the target tissues, which include adipose tissue and the brain (Safdar et al., 2016). The exercise-induced release of peptides and nucleic acids from skeletal muscle (collectively termed 'exerkines') has been implicated in mediating systemic biological adaptations (Safdar et al., 2016).

The contraction of large muscle groups increases the muscle-specific expression of PGC1-α and FNDC5 and consequent release of irisin (Bostrom et al., 2012). In humans, blood irisin levels reach approximately 3.6 ng/ml in sedentary individuals and 4.3 ng/ml in active individuals after 12 weeks of regular aerobic exercise (Jedrychowski et al., 2015). Irisin contributes to exercise-induced physiological adaptations in the cardiovascular, immune, digestive, and adipose systems (Bostrom et al., 2012; Zhang et al., 2015; Mazur-Bialy et al., 2017). In obese adult humans, exercise combined with caloric restriction improves health (Mozaffarian et al., 2011) and increases concentrations of circulating irisin (Huang et al., 2017). Although skeletal muscle is the major source of exercise-induced irisin that is released into the plasma (Roca-Rivada et al., 2013), it remains unclear whether neuronal irisin is derived from muscles or is produced in neurons. In neurons, PGC-1α interacts with estrogen-related receptor alpha (ERRα) to regulate the expression of FNDC5 (**Figure 1**; Wrann et al., 2013). Moreover, the increased expression of FNDC5 promotes neuronal development and differentiation (Forouzanfar et al., 2015; Ghahrizjani et al., 2015). FNDC5 can be found in the cerebrospinal fluid, cortical neurons, paraventricular neurons in the hippocampus, Purkinje cells in the cerebellum, hypothalamus, multipolar neurons in the anterior nerve of the spinal cord, and in astrocytes and microglia in the cerebral tissue (Dun et al., 2013; Moon et al., 2013; Piya et al., 2014; Albayrak et al., 2015). In the rat H19-7HN cell line, irisin (50–100 nmol/l) increased the proliferation of hippocampal cells, thus reinforcing its role in neurogenesis (Moon et al., 2013).

Wrann et al. (2013) demonstrated that the expression of PGC-1α and FNDC5 in the hippocampal neurons was enhanced after the mice spent 2 weeks running in exercise wheels. Higher FNDC5 expression also increased the expression of the genes BDNF, Arc, cFos, and Zif268, which is induced by neuronal activity. FNDC5 expression is counterbalanced by BDNF expression in a negative feedback mechanism (**Figure 1**; Wrann et al., 2013). It is possible that this feedback loop is a CNS detraining mechanism that requires regular exercise to maintain its neurological benefits. This evidence suggests that the induction of FNDC5 is part of the transcriptional response to exercise, including neuroplasticity and neuroprotection, in the CNS. Exercise-induced PGC-1α and irisin reduced ischemia-induced neuronal injury (Zhang et al., 2012) via activation of the Akt and ERK1/2 signaling pathways in mice (Li et al., 2017). Exercise-induced irisin also reduced the brain infarct volume, neurological deficits, brain edema and the body weight decline of mice subjected to middle cerebral artery occlusion (MCAO) (Li et al., 2017). Since BDNF is a critical regulator of neural plasticity, irisin may act as a key regulator of neuronal survival following cerebral ischemia. Physical activity (running wheel, 12 weeks) increases levels of circulating irisin and BDNF even in 20-month-old female rats (Belviranli and Okudan, 2018), increases the expression of BDNF and decreases neuroinflammation in the hippocampus of aged rats and mice, and has motor and cognitive benefits (Aguiar et al., 2011; Dallagnol et al., 2017).

Exercise is an antidepressant (Blumenthal et al., 1999; Cunha et al., 2013), and irisin has been linked to the antidepressant effects of exercise. Reduced irisin levels are associated with

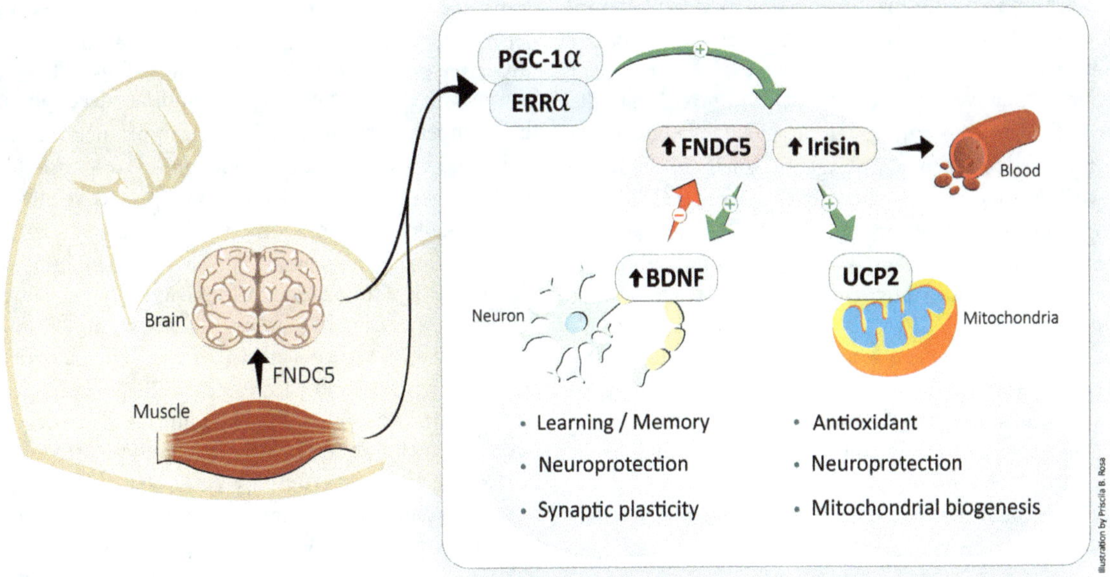

FIGURE 2 | The exercise-increased circulating protein irisin links structural and functional modifications in muscle and brain. BDNF, brain-derived neurotrophic factor; FNDC5, fibronectin type III domain-containing protein 5; UCP2, uncoupling protein 2.

mood impairment and reduced BDNF levels in humans (Papp et al., 2017; Szilasi et al., 2017), and increased circulating concentrations of irisin have been shown to have antidepressant effects in mice (Siteneski et al., 2018). A possible mechanism for the antidepressant effect is the activation of the PGC-1α/BDNF pathway by irisin after exercise (Wrann et al., 2013). As previously mentioned, BDNF is a critical neurotrophin involved in the differentiation, survival, maintenance, and function of neurons; it is also involved in learning and memory processes (Wrann et al., 2013). Torma et al. (2014) demonstrated that the neurotrophic role of BDNF is dependent on PGC-1α.

In humans, the increased plasma levels of FNDC-5, irisin and BDNF seem to depend on exercising large muscle groups, as can be achieved with regular Nordic walking training (Gmiat et al., 2018), aquarobics (16 weeks) (Kim and Kim, 2018), and CrossFit training (12 weeks) (Murawska-Cialowicz et al., 2015). The electrical stimulation of small muscle groups increases BDNF but not irisin in the hippocampus of rats (Maekawa et al., 2018). In healthy elderly women, Nordic walking training improved body composition, anaerobic capacity and cardiovascular fitness (Gmiat et al., 2018), and CrossFit training improved psychological (Quality-of-Life Assessment and The Beck Depression Inventory-2) and cognitive functions (D2 test of attention and Trail Making Test A&B).

NEURONAL UCP2 –AN ANTIOXIDANT MECHANISM OF EXERCISE

The expression of neuronal uncoupling proteins (UCP) is induced by metabolic and oxidative challenges such as physical exercise and caloric restriction (Liu et al., 2015). UCP facilitates proton flux through the internal mitochondrial membrane, thereby dissociating the oxidative phosphorylation of ATP synthesis (Wei et al., 2009). The enhanced proton flux process reduces the mitochondrial membrane potential, increases mitochondrial respiration, decreases the ATP/ADP ratio, and dissipates chemical energy in the form of heat (Chu et al., 2009). Acute mitochondrial decoupling reduces mitochondrial ATP production; however, chronic mitochondrial decoupling promotes an increase in the number of mitochondria and an increased level of ATP production (Coppola et al., 2007).

Initially, UCP1, which functions in heat production, was identified in brown adipose tissue (Geisler et al., 2017). UCP2 is found in organs and tissues such as the liver, kidney, pancreas, endothelium, immune cells, and the CNS (Pecqueur et al., 2001; Chu et al., 2009). UCP2, UCP4, and UCP5 are expressed in the CNS, are referred to as neuronal U, and are involved in the adaptation to cellular stress (Chu et al., 2009). The distribution of neuronal UCPs demonstrates the relevance of mitochondrial decoupling in the CNS to the control of neuronal, neuroendocrine, and autonomic responses (Richard et al., 1998). UCP2 is expressed in the hypothalamus, especially in the arcuate nucleus, limbic system, cerebellum, choroid plexus, and encephalic trunk (Richard et al., 1998; Arsenijevic et al., 2000). UCP4 is detected in most brain tissues, but it is expressed at lower levels in the spinal cord and *Substantia nigra* (Mao et al., 1999). UCP5 is expressed in the cerebral cortex, hippocampus, thalamus, hypothalamus, amygdala, basal ganglia, and spinal cord (Kwok et al., 2010).

Neuronal UCPs influence the regulation of mitochondrial biogenesis, calcium flux, ROS production, and local temperature (Teshima et al., 2003). Neuronal UCPs play an important role in the reduction of ROS production and consequent reduction in oxidative stress without compromising the production of ATP (Arsenijevic et al., 2000). Exposure of cultured neurons to decoupling agents, such as carbonyl cyanide-4-(trifluoromethoxy) phenylhydrazone (FCCP) or 2,4-dinitrophenol (2,4-DNP or simply DNP), reduces the mitochondrial membrane potential and inhibits mitochondrial calcium absorption, and thus prevents cell death (Stout et al., 1998). Neuronal UCPs also influence the temperature of neuronal microenvironments and thus contribute to the dynamics of neuronal activity through greater synaptic plasticity and neuronal transmission (Arsenijevic et al., 2000). Some studies have suggested that mitochondrial decoupling is linked to neuroprotection against physiological processes and pathological mechanisms including aging, Alzheimer's and Parkinson's diseases, neuronal hypoxia and ischemia, and epilepsy (Bechmann et al., 2002; Dietrich et al., 2008).

Among the neuronal UCPs, UCP2 is involved in central autonomic, endocrine, and metabolic regulation and is thus associated with cognition, mood, and behavior (Diano et al., 2000; Wang et al., 2014). UCP2 in the ventromedial nucleus restores glucose tolerance and regulates insulin sensitivity mediated by glucose-excited neurons, which is important for the physiological control of systemic glucose metabolism (Toda et al., 2016). In the arcuate nucleus, UCP2 is associated with mitochondrial fission, increased mitochondrial density and diminished mitochondrial size (Toda et al., 2016). UCP2 shows increased expression after neuronal injury (Bechmann et al., 2002). UCP2 induces mitochondrial decoupling in nigral neurons of the substantia nigra pars compacta (SNpc) and can prevent the loss of dopaminergic cells after 1-methyl-4-phenyl-1,2,5,6-tetrahydropyridine (MPTP)-induced toxicity, which is an essential effect to delay Parkinson's disease pathophysiology (Echtay et al., 2001; Horvath et al., 2003). The relation of UCP2 to exercise occurs through the PGC-1α/PPARα pathway, which can regulate neuronal UCP2 (Wu et al., 2014) and BDNF (Gomez-Pinilla et al., 2008). Physical activity (running wheel, 4 weeks) increased UCP2 expression and mitochondrial oxygen consumption in coupled and uncoupled mitochondria in the hippocampus of mice (Dietrich et al., 2008). Moreover, physical activity (running wheel, 1 week) and exercise (treadmill, 12 weeks) increased UCP2 levels in the hippocampus, cerebellum and brain cortex mitochondria of adult rats (Gomez-Pinilla et al., 2008; Marques-Aleixo et al., 2015). The exercise-induced (running wheel, 1 week) increase in UCP2 correlated with increased BDNF in the hippocampus of rats (Gomez-Pinilla et al., 2008). These changes in BDNF content and mitochondrial metabolism (Vaynman et al., 2006; Aguiar et al., 2007, 2014) coincided with an increase in the number of mitochondria and dendritic spine synapses in the granule cells of the dentate gyrus and the stratum radiatum of the CA1 region and were dependent on UCP2 expression because such changes were not observed in UCP2 knockout mice (Dietrich et al., 2008). The absence of proper mitochondrial decoupling reduced the number of synapses in hippocampal neurons due to the increase in free radical production in response to exercise, thus demonstrating the characteristic protective effect of UCP2 in this knockout mouse model (Dietrich et al., 2008). For example, doxorubicin is an effective antineoplastic agent that is limited by mitochondrial toxicity in non-target tissues, including the brain (Marques-Aleixo et al., 2016; Flanigan et al., 2018). Doxorubicin (2 mg/kg, i.p.) impaired spatial learning/memory and decreased UCP2 protein content in cerebellum and brain cortex mitochondria of adult rats, both of which were prevented by physical activity (treadmill, 12 weeks) (Marques-Aleixo et al., 2016). The UCP2-related nuclear respiration factor 1 (NRF1) and mitochondrial transcription factor A (TFAM) genes, which are involved in mitochondrial biogenesis, are associated with synaptic plasticity and decreased neuronal vulnerability to cellular stress Simon-Areces et al., 2012). In an animal model of Parkinson's disease, 8 weeks of treadmill exercise stimulated mitochondrial biogenesis and increased NRF2 and TFAM expression in the striatum of mice, which protected against neuronal death caused by the neurotoxin 6-OHDA (Aguiar et al., 2016). The mitochondrial mechanism related to UCP2 function is essential for the appropriate bioenergetic adaptation of neurons to increased neuronal activity and synaptic plasticity in response to physical activity.

CONCLUSION

Exercise improves the PGC-1α/BDNF pathway (muscle/brain) through the signaling of circulating irisin, which strengthens synapses and exhibits neuroprotective and antidepressant effects. These neuroprotective effects of exercise are enhanced by the antioxidant effects of UCP2, which is expressed at increased levels in neurons in response to exercise. Therefore, the evidence suggests a role for irisin/UCP2 in the mechanism underlying the benefits of physical exercise on the CNS. Consequently, irisin/UCP2 might be a potential therapeutic target to improve brain function and prevent or treat neurological and neurodegenerative diseases.

AUTHOR CONTRIBUTIONS

All authors listed have made a substantial, direct and intellectual contribution to the work, and approved it for publication.

REFERENCES

Aguiar, A. S. Jr., Castro, A. A., Moreira, E. L., Glaser, V., Santos, A. R., Tasca, C. I., et al. (2011). Short bouts of mild-intensity physical exercise improve spatial learning and memory in aging rats: involvement of hippocampal plasticity via AKT, CREB and BDNF signaling. *Mech. Ageing Dev.* 132, 560–567. doi: 10.1016/j.mad.2011.09.005

Aguiar, A. S. Jr., Duzzioni, M., Remor, A. P., Tristao, F. S., Matheus, F. C., Raisman-Vozari, R., et al. (2016). Moderate-intensity physical exercise protects against experimental 6-hydroxydopamine-induced hemiparkinsonism through Nrf2-antioxidant response element pathway. *Neurochem. Res.* 41, 64–72. doi: 10.1007/s11064-015-1709-8

Aguiar, A. S. Jr., Stragier, E., da Luz, Scheffer, D., Remor, A. P., Oliveira, P. A., et al. (2014). Effects of exercise on mitochondrial function, neuroplasticity and anxio-depressive behavior of mice. *Neuroscience* 271, 56–63. doi: 10.1016/j.neuroscience.2014.04.027

Aguiar, A. S. Jr., Tuon, T., Albuquerque, M. M., Rocha, G. S., Speck, A. E., Araujo, J. C., et al. (2008). The exercise redox paradigm in the Down's syndrome: improvements in motor function and increases in blood oxidative status in young adults. *J. Neural Transm.* 115, 1643–1650. doi: 10.1007/s00702-008-0120-x

Aguiar, A. S. Jr., Tuon, T., Pinho, C. A., Silva, L. A., Andreazza, A. C., Kapczinski, F., et al. (2007). Mitochondrial IV complex and brain neurothrophic derived factor responses of mice brain cortex after downhill training. *Neurosci. Lett.* 426, 171–174. doi: 10.1016/j.neulet.2007.08.058

Albayrak, S., Atci, I. B., Kalayci, M., Yilmaz, M., Kuloglu, T., Aydin, S., et al. (2015). Effect of carnosine, methylprednisolone and their combined application on irisin levels in the plasma and brain of rats with acute spinal cord injury. *Neuropeptides* 52, 47–54. doi: 10.1016/j.npep.2015.06.004

Andrews, Z. B., Diano, S., and Horvath, T. L. (2005). Mitochondrial uncoupling proteins in the CNS: in support of function and survival. *Nat. Rev. Neurosci.* 6, 829–840. doi: 10.1038/nrn1767

Arsenijevic, D., Onuma, H., Pecqueur, C., Raimbault, S., Manning, B. S., Miroux, B., et al. (2000). Disruption of the uncoupling protein-2 gene in mice reveals a role in immunity and reactive oxygen species production. *Nat. Genet.* 26, 435–439. doi: 10.1038/82565

Bankoski, A., Harris, T. B., McClain, J. J., Brychta, R. J., Caserotti, P., Chen, K. Y., et al. (2011). Sedentary activity associated with metabolic syndrome independent of physical activity. *Diabetes Care* 34, 497–503. doi: 10.2337/dc10-0987

Barry, V. W., Baruth, M., Beets, M. W., Durstine, J. L., Liu, J., and Blair, S. N. (2014). Fitness vs. fatness on all-cause mortality: a meta-analysis. *Prog. Cardiovasc. Dis.* 56, 382–390. doi: 10.1016/j.pcad.2013.09.002

Bechmann, I., Diano, S., Warden, C. H., Bartfai, T., Nitsch, R., and Horvath, T. L. (2002). Brain mitochondrial uncoupling protein 2 (UCP2): a protective stress signal in neuronal injury. *Biochem. Pharmacol.* 64, 363–367. doi: 10.1016/S0006-2952(02)01166-8

Belviranli, M., and Okudan, N. (2018). Exercise training increases cardiac, hepatic and circulating levels of brain-derived neurotrophic factor and irisin in young and aged rats. *Horm. Mol. Biol. Clin. Investig.* 36:20180053. doi: 10.1515/hmbci-2018-0053

Biswas, A., Oh, P. I., Faulkner, G. E., Bajaj, R. R., Silver, M. A., Mitchell, M. S., et al. (2015). Sedentary time and its association with risk for disease incidence, mortality, and hospitalization in adults: a systematic review and meta-analysis. *Ann. Intern. Med.* 162, 123–132. doi: 10.7326/M14-1651

Blair, S. N., Kohl, H. W. III, Paffenbarger, R. S. Jr., Clark, D. G., Cooper, K. H., and Gibbons, L. W. (1989). Physical fitness and all-cause mortality. A prospective study of healthy men and women. *JAMA* 262, 2395–2401. doi: 10.1001/jama.1989.03430170057028

Blumenthal, J. A., Babyak, M. A., Moore, K. A., Craighead, W. E., Herman, S., Khatri, P., et al. (1999). Effects of exercise training on older patients with major depression. *Arch. Intern. Med.* 159, 2349–2356. doi: 10.1001/archinte.159.19.2349

Boecker, H., Sprenger, T., Spilker, M. E., Henriksen, G., Koppenhoefer, M., Wagner, K. J., et al. (2008). The runner's high: opioidergic mechanisms in the human brain. *Cereb. Cortex* 18, 2523–2531. doi: 10.1093/cercor/bhn013

Booth, F. W., Roberts, C. K., and Laye, M. J. (2012). Lack of exercise is a major cause of chronic diseases. *Compr. Physiol.* 2, 1143–1211. doi: 10.1002/cphy.c110025

Bostrom, P., Wu, J., Jedrychowski, M. P., Korde, A., Ye, L., Lo, J. C., et al. (2012). A PGC1-alpha-dependent myokine that drives brown-fat-like development of white fat and thermogenesis. *Nature* 11, 463–468. doi: 10.1038/nature10777

Brymer, E., and Davids, K. (2016). Designing environments to enhance physical and psychological benefits of physical activity: a multidisciplinary perspective. *Sports Med.* 46, 925–926. doi: 10.1007/s40279-016-0535-8

Chen, Y. H., Kuo, T. T., Kao, J. H., Huang, E. Y., Hsieh, T. H., Chou, Y. C., et al. (2018). Exercise ameliorates motor deficits and improves dopaminergic functions in the rat hemi-Parkinson's model. *Sci. Rep.* 8:3973. doi: 10.1038/s41598-018-22462-y

Chu, A. C., Ho, P. W., Kwok, K. H., Ho, J. W., Chan, K. H., Liu, H. F., et al. (2009). Mitochondrial UCP4 attenuates MPP+ - and dopamine-induced oxidative stress, mitochondrial depolarization, and ATP deficiency in neurons and is interlinked with UCP2 expression. *Free Radic. Biol. Med.* 46, 810–820. doi: 10.1016/j.freeradbiomed.2008.12.015

Coppola, A., Liu, Z. W., Andrews, Z. B., Paradis, E., Roy, M. C., Friedman, J. M., et al. (2007). A central thermogenic-like mechanism in feeding regulation: an interplay between arcuate nucleus T3 and UCP2. *Cell Metab.* 5, 21–33. doi: 10.1016/j.cmet.2006.12.002

Cunha, M. P., Oliveira, A., Pazini, F. L., Machado, D. G., Bettio, L. E., Budni, J., et al. (2013). The antidepressant-like effect of physical activity on a voluntary running wheel. *Med. Sci. Sports Exerc.* 45, 851–859. doi: 10.1249/MSS.0b013e31827b23e6

Dallagnol, K. M. C., Remor, A. P., da Silva, R. A., Prediger, R. D., Latini, A., and Aguiar, A. S. Jr. (2017). Running for REST: physical activity attenuates neuroinflammation in the hippocampus of aged mice. *Brain Behav. Immun.* 61, 31–35. doi: 10.1016/j.bbi.2016.07.159

Diano, S., Urbanski, H. F., Horvath, B., Bechmann, I., Kagiya, A., Nemeth, G., et al. (2000). Mitochondrial uncoupling protein 2 (UCP2) in the nonhuman primate brain and pituitary. *Endocrinology* 141, 4226–4238. doi: 10.1210/endo.141.11.7740

Dietrich, M. O., Andrews, Z. B., and Horvath, T. L. (2008). Exercise-induced synaptogenesis in the hippocampus is dependent on UCP2-regulated mitochondrial adaptation. *J. Neurosci.* 28, 10766–10771. doi: 10.1523/JNEUROSCI.2744-08.2008

Donnelly, J. E., Blair, S. N., Jakicic, J. M., Manore, M. M., Rankin, J. W., and Smith, B. K. (2009). American college of sports medicine position stand. Appropriate physical activity intervention strategies for weight loss and prevention of weight regain for adults. *Med. Sci. Sports Exerc.* 41, 459–471. doi: 10.1249/MSS.0b013e3181949333

Dun, S. L., Lyu, R. M., Chen, Y. H., Chang, J. K., Luo, J. J., and Dun, N. J. (2013). Irisin-immunoreactivity in neural and non-neural cells of the rodent. *Neuroscience* 240, 155–162. doi: 10.1016/j.neuroscience.2013.02.050

Echtay, K. S., Winkler, E., Frischmuth, K., and Klingenberg, M. (2001). Uncoupling proteins 2 and 3 are highly active H(+) transporters and highly nucleotide sensitive when activated by coenzyme Q (ubiquinone). *Proc. Natl. Acad. Sci. U.S.A.* 98, 1416–1421. doi: 10.1073/pnas.98.4.1416

Esteban-Cornejo, I., Tejero-Gonzalez, C. M., Sallis, J. F., and Veiga, O. L. (2015). Physical activity and cognition in adolescents: a systematic review. *J. Sci. Med. Sport* 18, 534–539. doi: 10.1016/j.jsams.2014.07.007

Farmer, M. E., Locke, B. Z., Moscicki, E. K., Dannenberg, A. L., Larson, D. B., and Radloff, L. S. (1988). Physical activity and depressive symptoms: the NHANES I epidemiologic follow up study. *Am. J. Epidemiol.* 128, 1340–1351. doi: 10.1093/oxfordjournals.aje.a115087

Flack, K. D., Ufholz, K., Johnson, L., Fitzgerald, J. S., and Roemmich, J. N. (2018). Energy compensation in response to aerobic exercise training in overweight adults. *Am. J. Physiol. Regul. Integr. Comp. Physiol.* 315, R619–R626. doi: 10.1152/ajpregu.00071.2018

Flanigan, T. J., Anderson, J. E., Elayan, I., Allen, A. R., and Ferguson, S. A. (2018). Effects of cyclophosphamide and/or doxorubicin in a murine model of postchemotherapy cognitive impairment. *Toxicol. Sci.* 162, 462–474. doi: 10.1093/toxsci/kfx267

Fogelholm, M. (2010). Physical activity, fitness and fatness: relations to mortality, morbidity and disease risk factors. A systematic review. *Obes. Rev.* 11, 202–221. doi: 10.1111/j.1467-789X.2009.00653.x

Forouzanfar, M., Rabiee, F., Ghaedi, K., Beheshti, S., Tanhaei, S., Shoaraye Nejati, A., et al. (2015). Fndc5 overexpression facilitated neural differentiation of mouse embryonic stem cells. *Cell Biol. Int.* 39, 629–637. doi: 10.1002/cbin.10427

Fuss, J., Steinle, J., Bindila, L., Auer, M. K., Kirchherr, H., Lutz, B., et al. (2015). A runner's high depends on cannabinoid receptors in mice. *Proc. Natl. Acad. Sci. U.S.A.* 112, 13105–13108. doi: 10.1073/pnas.1514996112

Garber, C. E., Blissmer, B., Deschenes, M. R., Franklin, B. A., Lamonte, M. J., Lee, I. M., et al. (2011). American college of sports medicine position stand. Quantity and quality of exercise for developing and maintaining cardiorespiratory, musculoskeletal, and neuromotor fitness in apparently healthy adults: guidance for prescribing exercise. *Med. Sci. Sports Exerc.* 43, 1334–1359. doi: 10.1249/MSS.0b013e318213fefb

Geisler, J. G., Marosi, K., Halpern, J., and Mattson, M. P. (2017). DNP, mitochondrial uncoupling, and neuroprotection: a little dab'll do ya. *Alzheimers Dement.* 13, 582–591. doi: 10.1016/j.jalz.2016.08.001

Geneen, L. J., Moore, R. A., Clarke, C., Martin, D., Colvin, L. A., and Smith, B. H. (2017). Physical activity and exercise for chronic pain in adults: an overview of cochrane reviews. *Cochrane Database Syst. Rev.* 1:CD011279. doi: 10.1002/14651858.CD011279.pub3

Ghahrizjani, F. A., Ghaedi, K., Salamian, A., Tanhaei, S., Nejati, A. S., Salehi, H., et al. (2015). Enhanced expression of FNDC5 in human embryonic stem cell-derived neural cells along with relevant embryonic neural tissues. *Gene* 557, 123–129. doi: 10.1016/j.gene.2014.12.010

Gmiat, A., Jaworska, J., Micielska, K., Kortas, J., Prusik, K., Lipowski, M., et al. (2018). Improvement of cognitive functions in response to a regular Nordic walking training in elderly women - a change dependent on the training experience. *Exp. Gerontol.* 104, 105–112. doi: 10.1016/j.exger.2018.02.006

Gomez-Pinilla, F., Vaynman, S., and Ying, Z. (2008). Brain-derived neurotrophic factor functions as a metabotrophin to mediate the effects of exercise on cognition. *Eur. J. Neurosci.* 28, 2278–2287. doi: 10.1111/j.1460-9568.2008.06524.x

Hainer, V., Toplak, H., and Stich, V. (2009). Fat or fit: what is more important? *Diabetes Care* 32(Suppl. 2), S392–S397. doi: 10.2337/dc09-S346

Haskell, W. L., Lee, I. M., Pate, R. R., Powell, K. E., Blair, S. N., Franklin, B. A., et al. (2007). Physical activity and public health: updated recommendation for adults from the American college of sports medicine and the American heart association. *Med. Sci. Sports Exerc.* 39, 1423–1434. doi: 10.1249/mss.0b013e3180616b27

Hofmann, T., Elbelt, U., and Stengel, A. (2014). Irisin as a muscle-derived hormone stimulating thermogenesis–a critical update. *Peptides* 54, 89–100. doi: 10.1016/j.peptides.2014.01.016

Horvath, T. L., Diano, S., Leranth, C., Garcia-Segura, L. M., Cowley, M. A., Shanabrough, M., et al. (2003). Coenzyme Q induces nigral mitochondrial uncoupling and prevents dopamine cell loss in a primate model of Parkinson's disease. *Endocrinology* 144, 2757–2760. doi: 10.1210/en.2003-0163

Huang, J., Wang, S., Xu, F., Wang, D., Yin, H., Lai, Q., et al. (2017). Exercise training with dietary restriction enhances circulating irisin level associated with increasing endothelial progenitor cell number in obese adults: an intervention study. *PeerJ* 5:e3669. doi: 10.7717/peerj.3669

Jayakody, K., Gunadasa, S., and Hosker, C. (2014). Exercise for anxiety disorders: systematic review. *Br. J. Sports Med.* 48, 187–196. doi: 10.1136/bjsports-2012-091287

Jedrychowski, M. P., Wrann, C. D., Paulo, J. A., Gerber, K. K., Szpyt, J., Robinson, M. M., et al. (2015). Detection and quantitation of circulating human irisin by tandem mass spectrometry. *Cell Metab.* 22, 734–740. doi: 10.1016/j.cmet.2015.08.001

Kamei, Y., Ohizumi, H., Fujitani, Y., Nemoto, T., Tanaka, T., Takahashi, N., et al. (2003). PPARgamma coactivator 1beta/ERR ligand 1 is an ERR protein ligand, whose expression induces a high-energy expenditure and antagonizes obesity. *Proc. Natl. Acad. Sci. U.S.A.* 100, 12378–12383. doi: 10.1073/pnas.2135217100

Kim, J. H., and Kim, D. Y. (2018). Aquarobic exercises improve the serum blood irisin and brain-derived neurotrophic factor levels in elderly women. *Exp. Gerontol.* 104, 60–65. doi: 10.1016/j.exger.2018.01.024

Koster, A., Caserotti, P., Patel, K. V., Matthews, C. E., Berrigan, D., Van Domelen, D. R., et al. (2012). Association of sedentary time with mortality independent of moderate to vigorous physical activity. *PLoS One* 7:e37696. doi: 10.1371/journal.pone.0037696

Kwok, K. H., Ho, P. W., Chu, A. C., Ho, J. W., Liu, H. F., Yiu, D. C., et al. (2010). Mitochondrial UCP5 is neuroprotective by preserving mitochondrial membrane potential, ATP levels, and reducing oxidative stress in MPP+ and dopamine toxicity. *Free Radic. Biol. Med.* 49, 1023–1035. doi: 10.1016/j.freeradbiomed.2010.06.017

Lang Lehrskov, L., Lyngbaek, M. P., Soederlund, L., Legaard, G. E., Ehses, J. A., Heywood, S. E., et al. (2018). Interleukin-6 delays gastric emptying in humans with direct effects on glycemic control. *Cell Metab.* 27, 1201.e3–1211.e3. doi: 10.1016/j.cmet.2018.04.008

Law, L. L., Rol, R. N., Schultz, S. A., Dougherty, R. J., Edwards, D. F., Koscik, R. L., et al. (2018). Moderate intensity physical activity associates with CSF biomarkers in a cohort at risk for Alzheimer's disease. *Alzheimers Dement.* 10, 188–195. doi: 10.1016/j.dadm.2018.01.001

Li, D. J., Li, Y. H., Yuan, H. B., Qu, L. F., and Wang, P. (2017). The el exercise-induced hormone irisin protects against neuronal injury via activation of the Akt and ERK1/2 signaling pathways and contributes to the neuroprotection of physical exercise in cerebral ischemia. *Metabolism* 68, 31–42. doi: 10.1016/j.metabol.2016.12.003

Lin, X., Zhang, X., Guo, J., Roberts, C. K., McKenzie, S., Wu, W. C., et al. (2015). Effects of exercise training on cardiorespiratory fitness and biomarkers of cardiometabolic health: a systematic review and meta-analysis of randomized controlled trials. *J. Am. Heart Assoc.* 4:e002014. doi: 10.1161/JAHA.115.002014

Liu, D., Zhang, Y., Gharavi, R., Park, H. R., Lee, J., Siddiqui, S., et al. (2015). The mitochondrial uncoupler DNP triggers brain cell mTOR signaling network reprogramming and CREB pathway up-regulation. *J. Neurochem.* 134, 677–692. doi: 10.1111/jnc.13176

Loprinzi, P. D. (2015). Dose-response association of moderate-to-vigorous physical activity with cardiovascular biomarkers and all-cause mortality: considerations by individual sports, exercise and recreational physical activities. *Prev. Med.* 81, 73–77. doi: 10.1016/j.ypmed.2015.08.014

Maekawa, T., Ogasawara, R., Tsutaki, A., Lee, K., Nakada, S., Nakazato, K., et al. (2018). Electrically evoked local muscle contractions cause an increase in hippocampal BDNF. *Appl. Physiol. Nutr. Metab.* 43, 491–496. doi: 10.1139/apnm-2017-0536

Mao, W., Yu, X. X., Zhong, A., Li, W., Brush, J., Sherwood, S. W., et al. (1999). UCP4, a el brain-specific mitochondrial protein that reduces membrane potential in mammalian cells. *FEBS Lett.* 443, 326–330. doi: 10.1016/S0014-5793(98)01713-X

Marosi, K., and Mattson, M. P. (2014). BDNF mediates adaptive brain and body responses to energetic challenges. *Trends Endocrinol. Metab.* 25, 89–98. doi: 10.1016/j.tem.2013.10.006

Marques-Aleixo, I., Santos-Alves, E., Balca, M. M., Moreira, P. I., Oliveira, P. J., Magalhaes, J., et al. (2016). Physical exercise mitigates doxorubicin-induced brain cortex and cerebellum mitochondrial alterations and cellular quality control signaling. *Mitochondrion* 26, 43–57. doi: 10.1016/j.mito.2015.12.002

Marques-Aleixo, I., Santos-Alves, E., Balca, M. M., Rizo-Roca, D., Moreira, P. I., Oliveira, P. J., et al. (2015). Physical exercise improves brain cortex and cerebellum mitochondrial bioenergetics and alters apoptotic, dynamic and auto(mito)phagy markers. *Neuroscience* 301, 480–495. doi: 10.1016/j.neuroscience.2015.06.027

Mazur-Bialy, A. I., Pochec, E., and Zarawski, M. (2017). Anti-inflammatory properties of irisin, mediator of physical activity, are connected with TLR4/MyD88 signaling pathway activation. *Int. J. Mol. Sci.* 18:E701. doi: 10.3390/ijms18040701

McAuley, P., Pittsley, J., Myers, J., Abella, J., and Froelicher, V. F. (2009). Fitness and fatness as mortality predictors in healthy older men: the veterans exercise testing study. *J. Gerontol. A Biol. Sci. Med. Sci.* 64, 695–699. doi: 10.1093/gerona/gln039

Melanson, E. L., Keadle, S. K., Donnelly, J. E., Braun, B., and King, N. A. (2013). Resistance to exercise-induced weight loss: compensatory behavioral adaptations. *Med. Sci. Sports Exerc.* 45, 1600–1609. doi: 10.1249/MSS.0b013e31828ba942

Moon, H. S., Dincer, F., and Mantzoros, C. S. (2013). Pharmacological concentrations of irisin increase cell proliferation without influencing markers of neurite outgrowth and synaptogenesis in mouse H19-7 hippocampal cell lines. *Metabolism* 62, 1131–1136. doi: 10.1016/j.metabol.2013.04.007

Mozaffarian, D., Hao, T., Rimm, E. B., Willett, W. C., and Hu, F. B. (2011). Changes in diet and lifestyle and long-term weight gain in women and men. *N. Engl. J. Med.* 364, 2392–2404. doi: 10.1056/NEJMoa1014296

Murawska-Cialowicz, E., Wojna, J., and Zuwala-Jagiello, J. (2015). Crossfit training changes brain-derived neurotrophic factor and irisin levels at rest, after wingate and progressive tests, and improves aerobic capacity and body composition of young physically active men and women. *J. Physiol. Pharmacol.* 66, 811–821.

Papp, C., Pak, K., Erdei, T., Juhasz, B., Seres, I., Szentpeteri, A., et al. (2017). Alteration of the irisin-brain-derived neurotrophic factor axis contributes to disturbance of mood in COPD patients. *Int. J. Chron. Obstruct. Pulmon. Dis.* 12, 2023–2033. doi: 10.2147/COPD.S135701

Patterson, R., McNamara, E., Tainio, M., de Sá, T. H., Smith, A. D., Sharp, S. J., et al. (2018). Sedentary behaviour and risk of all-cause, cardiovascular and cancer mortality, and incident type 2 diabetes: a systematic review and dose response meta-analysis. *Eur. J. Epidemiol.* 33, 811–829. doi: 10.1007/s10654-018-0380-1

Pecqueur, C., Alves-Guerra, M. C., Gelly, C., Levi-Meyrueis, C., Couplan, E., Collins, S., et al. (2001). Uncoupling protein 2, in vivo distribution, induction upon oxidative stress, and evidence for translational regulation. *J. Biol. Chem.* 276, 8705–8712. doi: 10.1074/jbc.M006938200

Piya, M. K., Harte, A. L., Sivakumar, K., Tripathi, G., Voyias, P. D., James, S., et al. (2014). The identification of irisin in human cerebrospinal fluid: influence of adiposity, metabolic markers, and gestational diabetes. *Am. J. Physiol. Endocrinol. Metab.* 306, E512–E518. doi: 10.1152/ajpendo.00308.2013

Pontzer, H. (2018). Energy constraint as a el mechanism linking exercise and health. *Physiology* 33, 384–393. doi: 10.1152/physiol.00027.2018

Qiu, S., Cai, X., Yin, H., Sun, Z., Zügel, M., Steinacker, J. M., et al. (2018). Exercise training and endothelial function in patients with type 2 diabetes: a meta-analysis. *Cardiovasc. Diabetol.* 17:64. doi: 10.1186/s12933-018-0711-2

Radak, Z., Hart, N., Sarga, L., Koltai, E., Atalay, M., Ohno, H., et al. (2010). Exercise plays a preventive role against Alzheimer's disease. *J. Alzheimers Dis.* 20, 777–783. doi: 10.3233/JAD-2010-091531

Raefsky, S. M., and Mattson, M. P. (2017). Adaptive responses of neuronal mitochondria to bioenergetic challenges: roles in neuroplasticity and disease resistance. *Free Radic. Biol. Med.* 102, 203–216. doi: 10.1016/j.freeradbiomed.2016.11.045

Ribeiro, F., Ribeiro, I. P., Gonçalves, A. C., Alves, A. J., Melo, E., Fernandes, R., et al. (2017). Effects of resistance exercise on endothelial progenitor cell mobilization in women. *Sci. Rep.* 7:17880. doi: 10.1038/s41598-017-18156-6

Richard, D., Rivest, R., Huang, Q., Bouillaud, F., Sanchis, D., Champigny, O., et al. (1998). Distribution of the uncoupling protein 2 mRNA in the mouse brain. *J. Comp. Neurol.* 397, 549–560. doi: 10.1002/(SICI)1096-9861(19980810)397:4<549::AID-CNE7>3.0.CO;2-1

Ricquier, D., and Bouillaud, F. (2000). Mitochondrial uncoupling proteins: from mitochondria to the regulation of energy balance. *J. Physiol.* 529(Pt 1), 3–10. doi: 10.1111/j.1469-7793.2000.00003.x

Roca-Rivada, A., Castelao, C., Senin, L. L., Landrove, M. O., Baltar, J., Belen Crujeiras, A., et al. (2013). FNDC5/irisin is not only a myokine but also an adipokine. *PLoS One* 8:e60563. doi: 10.1371/journal.pone.0060563

Safdar, A., Saleem, A., and Tarnopolsky, M. A. (2016). The potential of endurance exercise-derived exosomes to treat metabolic diseases. *Nat. Rev. Endocrinol.* 12, 504–517. doi: 10.1038/nrendo.2016.76

Same, R. V., Feldman, D. I., Shah, N., Martin, S. S., Al Rifai, M., Blaha, M. J., et al. (2016). Relationship between sedentary behavior and cardiovascular risk. *Curr. Cardiol. Rep.* 18:6. doi: 10.1007/s11886-015-0678-5

Schuch, F., Vancampfort, D., Firth, J., Rosenbaum, S., Ward, P., Reichert, T., et al. (2017). Physical activity and sedentary behavior in people with major depressive disorder: a systematic review and meta-analysis. *J. Affect. Disord.* 210, 139–150. doi: 10.1016/j.jad.2016.10.050

Shen, X., Wong-Yu, I. S., and Mak, M. K. (2016). Effects of exercise on falls, balance, and gait ability in Parkinson's disease: a meta-analysis. *Neurorehabil. Neural Repair* 30, 512–527. doi: 10.1177/1545968315613447

Simon-Areces, J., Dietrich, M. O., Hermes, G., Garcia-Segura, L. M., Arevalo, M. A., and Horvath, T. L. (2012). UCP2 induced by natural birth regulates neuronal differentiation of the hippocampus and related adult behavior. *PLoS One* 7:e42911. doi: 10.1371/journal.pone.0042911

Siteneski, A., Cunha, M. P., Lieberknecht, V., Pazini, F. L., Gruhn, K., Brocardo, P. S., et al. (2018). Central irisin administration affords antidepressant-like effect and modulates neuroplasticity-related genes in the hippocampus and prefrontal cortex of mice. *Prog. Neuropsychopharmacol. Biol. Psychiatry* 84, 294–303. doi: 10.1016/j.pnpbp.2018.03.004

Stout, A. K., Raphael, H. M., Kanterewicz, B. I., Klann, E., and Reynolds, I. J. (1998). Glutamate-induced neuron death requires mitochondrial calcium uptake. *Nat. Neurosci.* 1, 366–373. doi: 10.1038/1577

Szilasi, M. E., Pak, K., Kardos, L., Varga, V. E., Seres, I., Mikaczo, A., et al. (2017). The alteration of irisin-brain-derived neurotrophic factor axis parallels severity of distress disorder in bronchial asthma patients. *Front. Neurosci.* 11:653. doi: 10.3389/fnins.2017.00653

Teshima, Y., Akao, M., Jones, S. P., and Marbán, E. (2003). Uncoupling protein-2 overexpression inhibits mitochondrial death pathway in cardiomyocytes. *Circ. Res.* 93, 192–200. doi: 10.1161/01.RES.0000085581.60197.4D

Thomas, D. M., Bouchard, C., Church, T., Slentz, C., Kraus, W. E., Redman, L. M., et al. (2012). Why do individuals not lose more weight from an exercise intervention at a defined dose? An energy balance analysis. *Obes. Rev.* 13, 835–847. doi: 10.1111/j.1467-789X.2012.01012.x

Toda, C., Kim, J. D., Impellizzeri, D., Cuzzocrea, S., Liu, Z. W., and Diano, S. (2016). UCP2 regulates mitochondrial fission and ventromedial nucleus control of glucose responsiveness. *Cell* 164, 872–883. doi: 10.1016/j.cell.2016.02.010

Torma, F., Bori, Z., Koltai, E., Felszeghy, K., Vacz, G., Koch, L., et al. (2014). Eating habits modulate short term memory and epigenetical regulation of brain derived neurotrophic factor in hippocampus of low- and high running capacity rats. *Brain Res. Bull.* 107, 54–60. doi: 10.1016/j.brainresbull.2014.07.003

Vaynman, S., Ying, Z., Wu, A., and Gomez-Pinilla, F. (2006). Coupling energy metabolism with a mechanism to support brain-derived neurotrophic factor-mediated synaptic plasticity. *Neuroscience* 139, 1221–1234. doi: 10.1016/j.neuroscience.2006.01.062

Wang, D., Zhai, X., Chen, P., Yang, M., Zhao, J., Dong, J., et al. (2014). Hippocampal UCP2 is essential for cognition and resistance to anxiety but not required for the benefits of exercise. *Neuroscience* 277, 36–44. doi: 10.1016/j.neuroscience.2014.06.060

Wei, M., Kampert, J. B., Barlow, C. E., Nichaman, M. Z., Gibbons, L. W., Paffenbarger, R. S. Jr., et al. (1999). Relationship between low cardiorespiratory fitness and mortality in normal-weight, overweight, and obese men. *JAMA* 282, 1547–1553. doi: 10.1001/jama.282.16.1547

Wei, Z., Chigurupati, S., Bagsiyao, P., Henriquez, A., and Chan, S. L. (2009). The brain uncoupling protein UCP4 attenuates mitochondrial toxin-induced cell death: role of extracellular signal-regulated kinases in bioenergetics adaptation and cell survival. *Neurotox. Res.* 16, 14–29. doi: 10.1007/s12640-009-9039-8

World Health Organization (2010). *Global Recommendations on Physical Activity for Health*. Available at: http://whqlibdoc.who.int/publications/2010/9789241599979_eng.pdf

World Health Organization (2000). Obesity: Preventing and Managing the Global Epidemic: Report of a WHO Consultation. World Health Organ Tech Rep Ser. 894. Geneva: World Health Organization, 1–253.

Wrann, C. D. (2015). FNDC5/irisin - their role in the nervous system and as a mediator for beneficial effects of exercise on the brain. *Brain Plast.* 1, 55–61. doi: 10.3233/BPL-150019

Wrann, C. D., White, J. P., Salogiannnis, J., Laznik Bogoslavski, D., Wu, J., Ma, D., et al. (2013). Exercise induces hippocampal BDNF through a PGC-1alpha/FNDC5 pathway. *Cell Metab.* 18, 649–659. doi: 10.1016/j.cmet.2013.09.008

Wu, R. M., Sun, Y. Y., Zhou, T. T., Zhu, Z. Y., Zhuang, J. J., Tang, X., et al. (2014). Arctigenin enhances swimming endurance of sedentary rats partially by regulation of antioxidant pathways. *Acta Pharmacol. Sin.* 35, 1274–1284. doi: 10.1038/aps.2014.70

Xu, B. (2013). BDNF (I)rising from exercise. *Cell Metab.* 18, 612–614. doi: 10.1016/j.cmet.2013.10.008

Xu, Q., Park, Y., Huang, X., Hollenbeck, A., Blair, A., Schatzkin, A., et al. (2010). Physical activities and future risk of Parkinson disease. *Neurology* 75, 341–348. doi: 10.1212/WNL.0b013e3181ea1597

Zhang, J., and Zhang, W. (2016). Can irisin be a linker between physical activity and brain function? *Biomol. Concepts* 7, 253–258. doi: 10.1515/bmc-2016-0012

Zhang, Q., Wu, Y., Sha, H., Zhang, P., Jia, J., Hu, Y., et al. (2012). Early exercise affects mitochondrial transcription factors expression after cerebral ischemia in rats. *Int. J. Mol. Sci.* 13, 1670–1679. doi: 10.3390/ijms13021670

Zhang, W., Chang, L., Zhang, C., Zhang, R., Li, Z., Chai, B., et al. (2015). Central and peripheral irisin differentially regulate blood pressure. *Cardiovasc. Drugs Ther.* 29, 121–127. doi: 10.1007/s10557-015-6580-y

14

Neurons and Microglia: A Sickly-Sweet Duo in Diabetic Pain Neuropathy

Trevor Rajchgot[1]*, Sini Christine Thomas*[1]*, Jo-Chiao Wang*[2]*, Maryam Ahmadi*[1]*, Mohammad Balood*[1]*, Théo Crosson*[1]*, Jenny Pena Dias*[3]*, Réjean Couture*[1]*, Audrey Claing*[1] *and Sébastien Talbot*[1*]

[1] *Département de Pharmacologie et Physiologie, Faculté de Médecine, Université de Montréal, Montréal, QC, Canada,* [2] *Graduate Institute of Microbiology, College of Medicine, National Taiwan University, Taipei, Taiwan,* [3] *Johns Hopkins University School of Medicine, Division of Endocrinology, Diabetes and Metabolism, Baltimore, MD, United States*

Correspondence:
Sébastien Talbot
Sebastien.talbot@umontreal.ca

Diabetes is a common condition characterized by persistent hyperglycemia. High blood sugar primarily affects cells that have a limited capacity to regulate their glucose intake. These cells include capillary endothelial cells in the retina, mesangial cells in the renal glomerulus, Schwann cells, and neurons of the peripheral and central nervous systems. As a result, hyperglycemia leads to largely intractable complications such as retinopathy, nephropathy, hypertension, and neuropathy. Diabetic pain neuropathy is a complex and multifactorial disease that has been associated with poor glycemic control, longer diabetes duration, hypertension, advanced age, smoking status, hypoinsulinemia, and dyslipidemia. While many of the driving factors involved in diabetic pain are still being investigated, they can be broadly classified as either neuron -intrinsic or -extrinsic. In neurons, hyperglycemia impairs the polyol pathway, leading to an overproduction of reactive oxygen species and reactive nitrogen species, an enhanced formation of advanced glycation end products, and a disruption in Na^+/K^+ ATPase pump function. In terms of the extrinsic pathway, hyperglycemia leads to the generation of both overactive microglia and microangiopathy. The former incites a feed-forward inflammatory loop that hypersensitizes nociceptor neurons, as observed at the onset of diabetic pain neuropathy. The latter reduces neurons' access to oxygen, glucose and nutrients, prompting reductions in nociceptor terminal expression and losses in sensation, as observed in the later stages of diabetic pain neuropathy. Overall, microglia can be seen as potent and long-lasting amplifiers of nociceptor neuron activity, and may therefore constitute a potential therapeutic target in the treatment of diabetic pain neuropathy.

Keywords: pain, diabetes, neuropathy, neurons, microglia, oxidative stress, hyperglycemia

INTRODUCTION

Pain is defined as an unpleasant sensation triggered by noxious stimuli, inflammation, or damage to the nervous system. It is an evolutionarily-conserved defensive mechanism that prevents excessive tissue damage and preserves homeostasis by generating defensive withdrawal reflexes (Scholz and Woolf, 2002). Nociception is initiated by the detection of mechanical, chemical, or thermal noxious stimuli by specialized ion channel receptors present on sensory neurons (Scholz and Woolf, 2002).

The activation of these ion channels triggers an influx of various cations, depolarizing the neurons' membrane potentials, which, in turn, activate voltage-gated sodium channels (Na_Vs). This leads to an influx of sodium, and the subsequent firing of action potentials. In the peripheral nervous system (first order fiber), painful sensations are relayed by small, myelinated Aδ-fibers (fast pain transmission) and unmyelinated C-fibers (slow pain transmission) to the spinal cord (second order fiber) (Tesfaye and Kempler, 2005). These action potentials then trigger defensive reflexes, and travel up to the brain (third order fiber) where pain information is integrated and its emotional perception occurs.

Chronic Pain

Chronic pain is a highly debilitating condition and it is the most common reasons for visits to health care providers (Scholz and Woolf, 2002). The most incapacitating type of chronic pain is peripheral neuropathic pain. This pain is unique in regard to its constancy, the severity of its symptoms, and its resistance to current pharmacological treatment (Zimmermann, 2001; Woolf, 2004). Neuropathic pain is usually generated by peripheral nerve damage resulting from neuronal or spinal cord injuries, surgery, cancer, infection, or diabetes (Scholz and Woolf, 2002; Woolf, 2004; Tsuda et al., 2005). In pathological states, this pain often persists after the disappearance of its causal stimulus. In some cases, pain can be perceived more severely, a phenomenon known as hyperalgesia, or can be generated by normally innocuous stimuli, a condition known as allodynia. Tactile allodynia originates from afferent Aβ fibers (light touch/pressure transmission) that gain the ability to release pro-inflammatory neuropeptides (SP and CGRP) in the synaptic cleft, and/or the sprouting of these fibers to the dorsal superficial laminae IIb, a zone normally restricted to the projection of C fibers (Woolf et al., 1992; Miki et al., 1998). In the CNS, thalamic higher-order neurons often become hyperexcitable and act as pain generators or amplifiers (Fischer and Waxman, 2010). For example, increasing N-Methyl-D-Aspartate receptor (NMDAR) phosphorylation reduces its endogenous blockade by magnesium, thereby enhancing calcium (Ca^{+2}) and sodium (Na^{+}) influx. This ultimately promotes the establishment of spinal windup, which is an increase in the excitability of spinal neurons (Haigh and Blake, 2001).

Sensitization of Sensory Neurons

Most drugs targeted to alleviate neuropathic pain are designed to block neurotransmission, and as such, only bring temporary relief (Ji and Suter, 2007). Neuropathic pain is often accompanied by persistent inflammation, as evidenced by the high levels of oxidative substances (Pabreja et al., 2011), inflammatory cytokines (Pabreja et al., 2011), and mediators (Tsuda et al., 2005) present in the neuronal micro-environment. Unlike classical neurotransmitters, these inflammatory molecules are mainly produced by peripheral immunocytes and central glial cells (Marchand et al., 2005; Tsuda et al., 2005). The transcriptomic data of nociceptor neurons notably revealed the expression of specific receptors for immunoglobulins, cytokines and chemokines (Chiu et al., 2014). This evidences the role of nociceptors in directly detecting and responding to interleukins (IL)-1β (Samad et al., 2001; Binshtok et al., 2008) and IL-6 (Opree and Kress, 2000), activin (TGFβ member) (Zhu et al., 2007), TNF-α (Wagner and Myers, 1996), CCL3 (Zhang et al., 2005), GDNF (Malin et al., 2006), histamine (Shim et al., 2007), kinin (Talbot et al., 2012; De Brito Gariepy et al., 2013), and PGE_2 (Samad et al., 2001, 2002) released in the context of pain. Nociceptors can also sense IL-5 produced during allergic airway inflammation (Talbot et al., 2015), IL-31 produced during lymphoma-associated itch (Cevikbas et al., 2014), thymic stromal lymphopoietin (TSLP) and IL-4 produced during atopic dermatitis (Wilson et al., 2013; Oetjen et al., 2017), and IL-33 derived from contact with poison ivy (Liu et al., 2016). Additionally, nociceptors can drive IL-23 production during psoriasis (Riol-Blanco et al., 2014). Intracellular kinases and transcription factors downstream of these tyrosine kinase receptors, include PI3K (Pereira et al., 2015), MAP kinases (Ji et al., 2002a), p38 (Ji et al., 2002b), JAK1 (Ludbrook et al., 2016; Oetjen et al., 2017), and STAT3 (Mori et al., 2011) and their activation can lead to pain. Thus, these kinases lead to the post-translational modifications of ion channel transducers or voltage gated sodium channels (Julius, 2013). Nociceptor sensitization is thereby largely due to a decrease in the activation threshold of transient receptor potential vannilloid-1 (TRPV1) or transient receptor potential ankyrin-1 (TRPA1) (Davis et al., 2000; Bautista et al., 2006), and $Na_V1.7$, $Na_V1.8$, and $Na_V1.9$ (Kerr et al., 2001; Nassar et al., 2004). In short, lowering the activation threshold of nociceptors results in pain hypersensitivity. For example, prostaglandin PGE_2 is a well-known neuron sensitizer (Samad et al., 2001), which partly explains why non-steroidal anti-inflammatory drugs exhibit analgesic effects in inflammatory conditions (Vardeh et al., 2009). Nerve growth factor (NGF) has also been recognized as a major neuronal sensitizer (Ji et al., 2002b), which has led to the development of neutralizing monoclonal anti-NGF antibodies as a treatment for chronic inflammatory pain conditions (Hefti et al., 2006). These changes in hypersensitivity are limited to sites where sensitizing mediators are produced, which are known as zones of primary hyperalgesia. Outside of these zones, pain hypersensitivity usually results from central sensitization, which involves changes in the CNS (Woolf et al., 1992; Woolf, 2007; von Hehn et al., 2012). During inflammation, many sensitizing mediators are likely to be released simultaneously; therefore, the targeted pharmacological blockade of only one of these agents will have a limited effect. Conversely, targeting the sensitized nerve or convergent signaling mediators or enzymes may have broader and more durable effects as to treating inflammatory pain by stopping it at its source (Khoutorsky and Price, 2017).

DIABETES

Diabetes, derived from the Greek word *diabanein*, means "to pass through," in reference to the symptomatic excessive urine production observed in patients (Kumar et al., 2005). The term diabetes, without qualification, usually refers to *diabetes mellitus*, which roughly translates to "excessive production of sweet urine," known clinically as glycosuria (Kumar et al., 2005). According to the World Health Organization, at least 422 million people worldwide suffered from diabetes in 2014, representing 8.5% of the world's adult population (WHO, 2016). In 2012, diabetes was responsible for 1.5 million deaths, and its incidence is increasing by more than 8% per year (WHO, 2016). In some regions, such as in Eastern Mediterranean countries, prevalence is increasing by nearly 14%. The National Diabetes Information Clearinghouse estimates the yearly costs of diabetes to more than $132 billion in the United States. In terms of pathology, diabetes is the result of chronic high blood sugar stemming from either low insulin production, as observed in type 1 diabetes; or to a severe reduction in the response of insulin receptors (IR) to insulin, as observed in type 2 diabetes (Kumar et al., 2005). Chronic hyperglycemia causes the classical symptoms of diabetes, including polyuria (frequent urination), polydipsia and polyphagia (Kumar et al., 2005). While both types of diabetes share similar symptoms, they can be distinguished by measuring endogenous insulin production (Kumar et al., 2005).

Type 1 Diabetes

Formerly known as juvenile diabetes, type 1 diabetes (T1D) represents approximately 10% of diabetes cases in North America and Europe. There is currently no known preventive measure against type 1 diabetes, which is considered immune-mediated or idiopathic (Kumar et al., 2005). Insulin-dependent diabetes mellitus is characterized by the auto-immune, T-cell mediated (Rother, 2007) destruction of insulin-producing beta cells of the pancreatic islets of Langerhans. The destruction of β cells triggers insulin deficiency, which leads to increases of glucose in the patient's blood and urine. Evidence indicates that type I diabetes is induced by a combination of genetic susceptibility [mutation(s) to *iddm1*, *drb1*, *dqa*, and *dqb1* gene locus], environmental factors [diet, vitamin D deficiency (Mathieu et al., 2005)], or exposure to a driving antigen (exposure to wheat protein (Knip and Siljander, 2008), antibody from cow's milk protein (Virtanen et al., 1994). There is no current preventive measure against T1D, which can be highly pathogenic, or even fatal, if left untreated. Emerging treatments such as pancreas (Noguchi, 2010) and islet transplants (Noguchi, 2009) have shown relatively positive outcomes in pre-clinical models, and are currently being studied in clinical trials. However, drawbacks to implantation include the necessity for immunosuppressant administration, which increased susceptibility to infection and cancer, graft rejection of the implanted pancreas/islets, hypoglycemia, and a current lack of suitable donors (Balamurugan et al., 2014).

Type 2 Diabetes

Type 2 diabetes (T2D), also known as non-insulin dependent diabetes mellitus, is a metabolic disorder characterized by chronic high blood glycemia and insulin receptor resistance, sometimes in combination with relative insulin deficiency (Kumar et al., 2005). This type of diabetes can be initially managed by increasing exercise and dietary modification. It represents almost 90% of Western countries' diabetic populations (Kumar et al., 2005). The onset of T2D is related to genetic and environmental factors. The environmental detrimental factors can include smoking, obesity, diet, alcoholism, low physical activity, high cholesterol, hypertension, metabolic syndrome, and Cushing syndrome (Kumar et al., 2005). In recent years, compelling research and efforts have been made to genetically identify mutant or polymorphic genes that predispose individuals to develop type 2 diabetes. These have been found to include *tcf7l2, pparγ, fto, kcnj11, notch2, wfs1, cdkal1, igf2bp2, slc30a8, jazf1, hhex* (Groop and Lyssenko, 2008; Lyssenko, 2008) and *mody* genes, which themselves can account for up to 5% of T2D cases (Billings and Florez, 2010). Mutations in both human leptin production and the human leptin receptor gene can cause severe obesity and pituitary dysfunction, which can in turn engender T2D (Clement et al., 1998; Wabitsch et al., 2015).

Complications of Diabetes

The chronic impairment of glucose metabolism associated with both types of diabetes has been associated with severe macrovascular (cardiovascular) disease and microvascular complications including retinopathy, nephropathy and sensory poly-neuropathy (Schemmel et al., 2009). Neuropathy is the most common complication seen in ambulatory care of type 2 diabetes patients (Schemmel et al., 2009). Overall, the aforementioned complications can result in debilitating and/or life-threatening conditions such as renal failure, erectile dysfunction, blindness, macular edema, impaired wound healing, hypertension, obesity, coronary artery disease, cerebrovascular accidents, heart failure, allodynia, hyperalgesia, nerve degeneration, insensitivity, and limb amputation.

Diabetic Pain Neuropathy

Diabetic pain neuropathy (DPN) is defined as the presence of signs and symptoms of peripheral nerve dysfunction in people with diabetes after having excluded other potential causes (Crofford, 1995). DPN is considered the principal cause of mortality, morbidity (Ziegler, 2008), and amputation (Molines et al., 2010) in diabetic patients, as well as the most common cause of neuropathy (Obrosova, 2009). The prevalence of DPN is thought to be proportional to disease duration and seems to be potentiated by an improper control of blood glycemia (Kumar et al., 2005). Ten percentage of 1-year diabetes patients suffer from neuropathy; this number increases to 50% amongst 25-year diabetes patients. Overall, 30% of diabetic patients suffer from DPN (Guastella and Mick, 2009). Interestingly, 39% of diabetic patients either receive no treatment for their symptoms or remain unmanaged (Daousi et al., 2004). While the prevalence of poorly-managed blood glycemia makes a significant proportion of diabetic patients highly susceptible to developing DPN, glycemic management in clinical care is slowly improving (Aschner et al., 2018). There is emerging evidence that genetic factors may play an important role in DPN pathogenesis (Prabodha et al., 2018).

DPN symptoms include paresthesia, numbness, and burning (Schemmel et al., 2009), which vary in nature and severity depending on the particular subpopulation of neurons being affected (Kumar et al., 2005). Certain patients with DPN do not present any symptoms; however, most report pain and/or loss of function in distal regions such as in their toes, feet, fingers, hands, or arms (Ziegler, 2008). Thus, at the onset of DPN, peripheral nerves often act as pulse generators, maintaining distal terminals of sensory nerve fibers in a state of hyperexcitability (Obrosova, 2009). When these fibers undergo active degeneration or impaired regeneration, they can begin to generate ectopic discharges, which induce positive pain symptoms. Later stages of DPN are characterized by a progressive loss of neuronal fibers, which is associated with a loss of sensation, and can ultimately cause diabetic foot syndrome (Yagihashi et al., 2007). The specific clinical diagnosis of DPN involves both electrophysiological and electromyography testing, respectively, assessing nerve conduction and muscular responses to electric stimulation (Kumar et al., 2005; Guastella and Mick, 2009). The metrics of blood glycemia, arterial pressure, heart rate, muscle force, reflex quality, and sensitivity to spatiotemporal changes can be used to indirectly help diagnose diabetic neuropathy in a more general sense (Guastella and Mick, 2009).

A FOCUS ON THE MOLECULAR DRIVERS OF DIABETIC PAIN NEUROPATHY

The origins of DPN are multifactorial (**Figure 1**), and result from neuron intrinsic (**Figure 2**) and extrinsic factors (**Figure 3**). This review will examine pre-clinical evidence supporting how chronic hyperglycemia dysregulate neurons' biochemical pathways, activates glia and how such impairments trigger DPN. Current theories (Brownlee, 2001, 2005) regarding neurons intrinsic factor driving the development of DPN include: uncontrolled oxidative stress (section Reactive Oxygen Species) (Nishikawa et al., 2000; Pop-Busui et al., 2006), the formation of reactive nitrogen species (section Reactive Nitrogen Species) (Zochodne and Levy, 2005), the formation of advanced glycation end products (section Advanced Glycation End Products) (Brownlee, 2005; Sugimoto et al., 2008), impaired Na^+/K^+ ATPase activity (section Ion Imbalance) (Vague et al., 1997; Gerbi et al., 1998; Raccah, 1998), an imbalance in the polyol pathway (section Polyol Pathway) and/or to the activity of the aldol reductase (section Aldose Reductase) (Oates, 2002). Extrinsically, it is believed that, at the spinal synapse, the neuro-immune interplay occurring between activated microglia and pain-sensing neurons maintains DPN (section Painful Glia to Microglia, an Emerging Target in DPN). The neuronal loss of energy supply occurring through microangiopathy (see Microangiopathy section) appears to be responsible for the loss of sensation observed in later stages of DPN. Finally, future therapeutic avenues will be discussed in the Conclusion and Future Therapeutic Directions section.

NEURON INTRINSIC FACTORS DRIVING DIABETIC PAIN NEUROPATHY

Reactive Oxygen Species

Cellular aerobic respiration generates the majority of intracellular free radicals (Kumar et al., 2005; Marieb et al., 2009), which are implicated in normal aging processes (Kumar et al., 2005). Cells are said to be in an oxidative stress state when their levels of reactive oxygen species (ROS) exceed their antioxidant capacity (Kumar et al., 2005). ROS are characterized by their high reactivity stemming from their unpaired valance electrons. These electrons can damage or modify the function of RNA, DNA and proteins. Given that neurons are unable to limit their glucose uptake (Brownlee, 2001), possess numerous mitochondria and long axons make them highly sensitive to oxidative damage. Excessive glucose metabolism by the mitochondrial respiratory chains increases the generation of superoxide anions (Nishikawa et al., 2000).

As seen in **Figure 2**, mitochondrial superoxide anions reduce glyceraldehyde-3-phosphate dehydrogenase (GAPDH) activity, which in turn reduces cells' anti-oxidative capacity (Du et al., 2000). The exposure of mitochondria to ROS progressively induces mitochondrial dysfunction, which in turn promotes energy deficiency, axonal degeneration and DPN. Mitochondria are key regulators of cell survival and apoptosis. Damaged mitochondria trigger axon degeneration through caspase activation and cycles of fusion and fission (Green and Reed, 1998). The fission of mitochondria is partly regulated by dynamin related protein 1 (DRP1) (Twig et al., 2008). Increased DRP1 levels have been associated with mitochondria dysfunction, reduced ATP production, and axonal degeneration (Leinninger et al., 2006). DRP1 is notably upregulated in the axons of diabetic patients (Leinninger et al., 2006). Overall, an excess of ROS generation along with the inability of neurons to metabolize free radicals can promote the progressive loss of organelles and dysfunction in nuclear cell membranes (Figueroa-Romero et al., 2008).

ROS also reduce axon neurotrophic factor (IGF-1, IGF-II, NGF, and NT-3) production levels, thereby impairing neurons' ability to regenerate (Ishii, 1995; Tomlinson et al., 1997). High glucose levels stimulate the generation of pro-oxidant and highly reactive advanced glycation end products (AGE; section Advanced Glycation End Products) (Baynes and Thorpe, 1999). AGEs and ROS appear to be interdependent (Metz et al., 2003; Monnier, 2003), and central to the etiology of neurovascular dysfunction (Cameron et al., 2001). AGE generation is enhanced by oxygen and ROS; AGE formation can trigger ROS generation and oxidative damage (Monnier, 2003). Finally, hyperglycemia promotes the over-activation of polyol pathways (section Polyol Pathway), reducing cells' $NADPH/NADP^+$ ratios and neurons' antioxidant capacities (Figueroa-Romero et al., 2008). Chronic hyperglycemia also enhances PKC activity, either through PLC-DAG pathways, or by reducing DAG-kinase activity (Xia et al., 1994) (King and Loeken, 2004). Enhanced PKC activity also increases mitochondrial NADPH oxidase activity (Inoguchi et al., 2000), further enhancing ROS levels (Balbi et al., 2018). A visual summary of ROS effects on neurons and glia can be found in **Figures 2, 3**.

ROS are normally metabolized by endogenous antioxidant enzymes such as superoxide dismutase, catalase and glutathione peroxidase, and by certain vitamins such as A, C (ascorbic acid) and E (tocopherol) (Figueroa-Romero et al., 2008; Midaoui et al., 2015; Talbot et al., 2016a). Nutritional supplementation with antioxidants was shown to reduce DPN in rodents (Pop-Busui et al., 2006). While alpha-lipoic acid and superoxide dismutase improved symptoms and electroneurographic parameters among subjects with diabetic neuropathy (Bertolotto and Massone, 2012), clinical studies generally have shown mixed results in terms of antioxidant efficacy (Oyenihi et al., 2015). Overall, it is

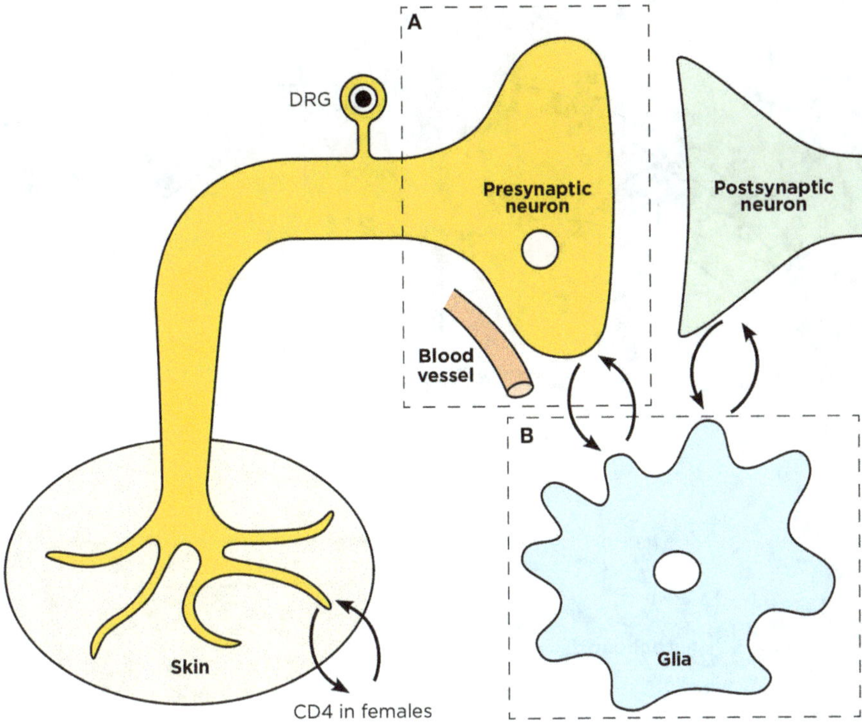

FIGURE 1 | Schematic representation of a spinal dorsal horn tripartite synapse. Overview of the pre **(A)** and post- synaptic neurons interplay with microglia **(B)** in the spinal cord dorsal horn.

believed that increasing the bioavailability of antioxidant, as well as associated reductive stress, have limited impact on the patients' health outcome.

Reactive Nitrogen Species

Nitric oxide (NO) is a potent vasoactive gas formed by three nitric oxide synthase (NOS) isoenzymes: neuronal (nNOS), endothelial (eNOS), and inducible (iNOS) (Kumar et al., 2005). In physiology, eNOS releases NO, which dilates vascular endothelial cells (Kumar et al., 2005) and reduces platelet aggregation (Riddell and Owen, 1999). In the context of inflammation, as is seen in diabetes, iNOS is overexpressed/activated, producing large amounts of NO (~100-fold than other NOS) (Vareniuk et al., 2008; Haddad and Couture, 2016). In DPN, iNOS hyperactivation is found in keratinocytes, macrophages, leukocytes, sensory neurons, and microglia (Zochodne et al., 2000). Excess NO from nNOS acts as a pro-nociceptive mediator in sensory C fibers (Matsui et al., 2010). It can also overactivate neuronal NADPH oxidase and mitochondrial xanthine oxidase. These effects reduce the antioxidant capacity of cells and contribute to ROS overproduction. Hyperglycemia-induced ROS react with cellular and/or circulating NO to form reactive nitrogen species (RNS) and peroxynitrite (Zochodne et al., 2000). RNS react with the thiol groups of SNAP proteins (Di Stasi et al., 2002), impairing the formation of neuronal regeneration cones. Consequently, RNS severely impact the capacity of neurons to repair themselves after oxidative damage (Kennedy and Zochodne, 2005). Currently, no therapy aims to reduce RNS generation, as it is still considered to be a contributing factor to DPN rather than an inducer. Please refer to **Figures 2**, **3** for visual summaries of NO interactions with neurons and glia.

Advanced Glycation end Products

Advanced glycation end products (AGE) comprise a heterogeneous group of molecules formed by the non-enzymatic reaction of a sugar with an amino acid, a protein, a lipid, or a nucleic acid (Marieb et al., 2009). AGE precursors pass through several dehydration and redox reactions and molecular rearrangements to form AGEs (Sugimoto et al., 2008). The initial reaction leading to AGE formation is reversible, and depends on the available quantity of substrate (glucose) (Brownlee, 2005). However, in cases of chronic hyperglycemia (diabetes), AGE precursors are not degraded, but rather build in numbers, thereby generating AGEs (Sugimoto et al., 2008). As seen in **Figure 2**, AGEs are highly reactive, and can affect any type of protein, including matrix, basal membrane and structural proteins (Sugimoto et al., 2008). For example, AGEs bind to and modify the myelin of nervous fibers, prompting their phagocytosis by circulating macrophages or microglia (Bruck and Friede, 1990). This process contributes to classical DPN segmental demyelination (Said, 2007). AGEs can also directly interact with tubulin and actin neurofilaments found in neurons' axonal cytoskeletons (Sugimoto et al., 2008). AGE-directed modification of these proteins impairs axonal transport, and promotes axonal atrophy and/or degeneration (Sugimoto et al., 2008). The glycation of extracellular matrix (laminin)

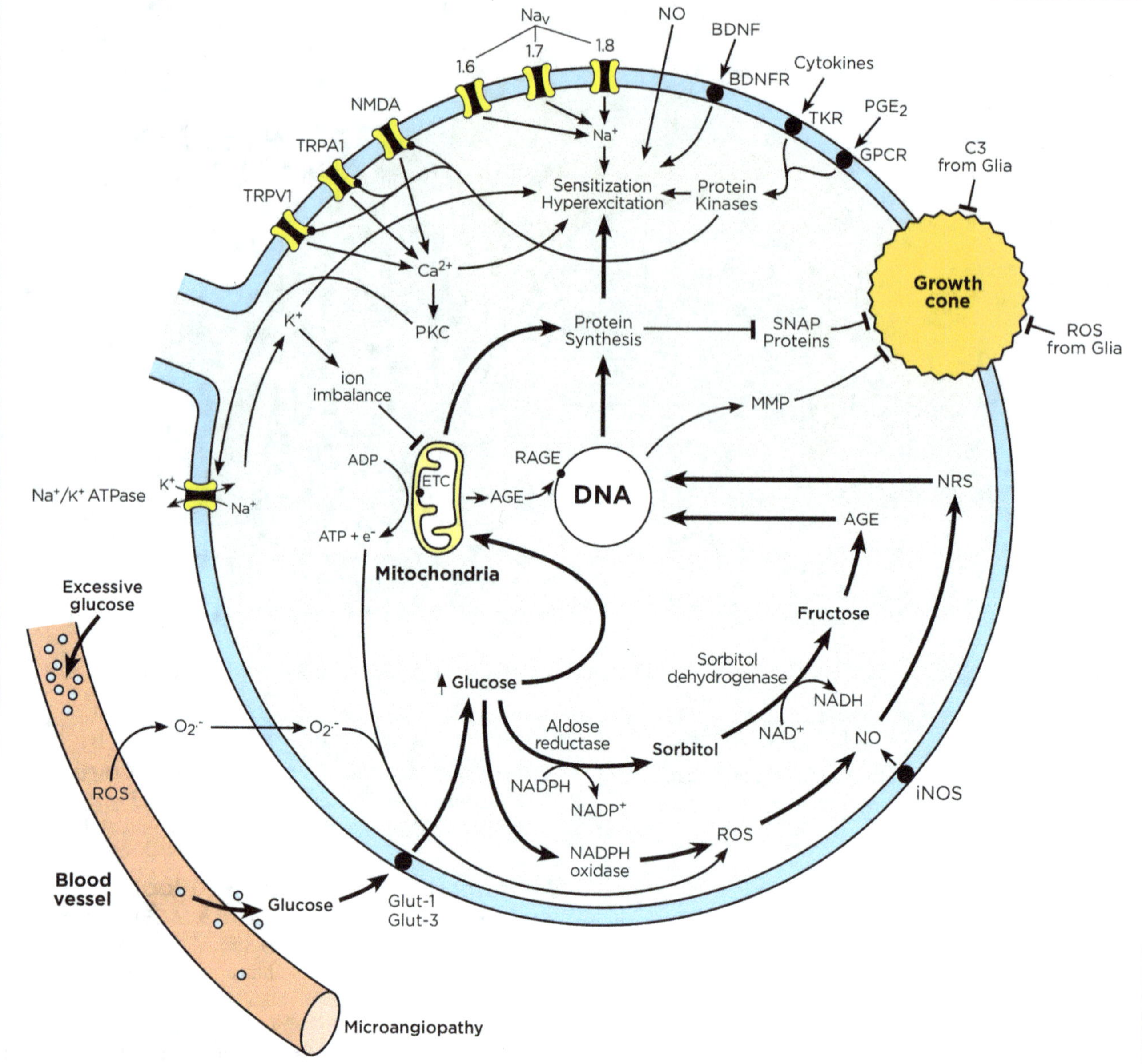

FIGURE 2 | Chronic hyperglycemia impairs neuron function. Sensory neurons have a limited capacity to regulate their uptake of glucose. In the context of chronic hyperglycemia, such as in diabetes, high glucose concentrations drive mitochondria to produce ATP and transfer electrons. Excess glucose is also metabolized through the polyol pathway, leading to the production of advanced glycation end products. The electrons from the mitochondrial respiratory chain combine with intracellular oxygen and nitric oxide to produce ROS and RNS. Consequently, RNS, ROS, and AGE activate nuclear transcription factors, which enhance the expression of ion channel transducers (TRP and Na_V channels) in addition to impairing neurons' capacity to self-repair. At the same time, microglia-released mediators (cytokines, ATP, BDNF, NO) stimulate GPCR and tyrosine kinase receptors, triggering downstream signaling cascades, which lead to the phosphorylation of TRP and Na_V channels. A decrease in the activation threshold of these ion channel transducers can augment the influx of cations, which ultimately results in action potential firing and ectopic discharges. These effects enhance pain perception and signaling to the CNS. Chronic hyperglycemia also increases oxidative stress in the blood vessels that supply oxygen and nutrients to neuron terminals. This oxidative stress can cause microangiopathy, a phenomenon characterized by the loss of capillaries, which starves neuronal energy supplies. These phenomena are responsible for the loss of neuron terminals and pain insensitivity, as typically observed in later stage of DPN.

membranes is AGE-mediated and can counteract the innate ability of neurons to self-repair (Duran-Jimenez et al., 2009; Singh et al., 2014). AGE additionally binds to specific membrane receptors known as RAGE (Haslbeck et al., 2005), driving the transcription of pro-inflammatory mediators (Brownlee, 2005). RAGE stimulation increases matrix metalloproteinase production, which can further exacerbate nerve fiber damage (King, 2001). AGEs demonstrably accumulate in hyperglycemic patients experiencing retinopathy, nephropathy, hypertension and neuropathy (Brownlee, 2005). Environmental pollutants,

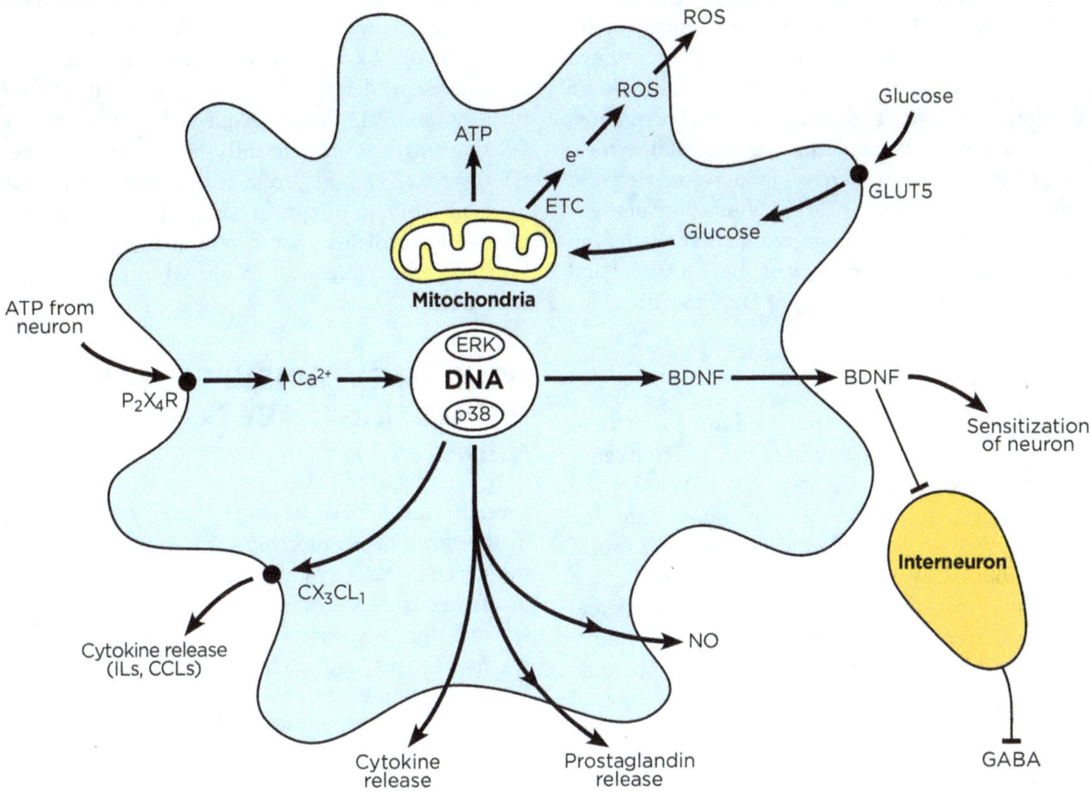

FIGURE 3 | Chronic hyperglycemia impairs microglial function. Circulating glucose is taken up by microglia, which enhances mitochondrial ATP production and electron transfer. The released electrons combine with intracellular oxygen to produce reactive oxygen species. Sensory neurons release ATP, which in turn activates microglial P_2X_4R; this drives microglial calcium influx, MAPK activation, receptor phosphorylation and protein transduction (cytokines, prostaglandins, BDNF) as well as NO production. These mediators are subsequently released by microglia, and either block inhibitory interneurons or enhance neuronal activation.

smoking, and poor nutrition also enhance AGE formation (Sugimoto et al., 2008). Avoiding these factors can help control AGE formation and its associated damage (Sugimoto et al., 2008; Singh et al., 2014). Specific inhibitors such as aminoguanidine improve patients' nerve conduction velocity and neuronal blood flow, in addition to mitigating apoptosis and oxidative stress (Sugimoto et al., 2008; Orman et al., 2015).

Ion Imbalance

Na^+/K^+ ATPase Pump

The Na^+/K^+ ATPase pump is a ubiquitous, energy-dependent enzyme implicated in the cellular membrane transport of ions. Using ATP, it transfers three sodium ions outside the cell in exchange for two potassium ions transported into the cell (Kumar et al., 2005). In doing so, it maintains the membrane's electric potential and nerve conductance (Creange et al., 2006). During hyperglycemia, impairments to polyol pathways (section Polyol Pathway) and PKC activity alter the function of the Na^+/K^+ ATPase pump leading to faulty nerve conduction (Creange et al., 2006). Reduced intracellular potassium levels curbed nodal potassium conductance, thereby affecting axonal excitability (Misawa et al., 2005). Hypokalemia can also alter Ca^{2+}/K^+ pump function, leading to neuronal hypocalcaemia.

Calcium

In early stages of DPN, the elevated levels of intracellular calcium disrupt nerve conductance (Kostyuk et al., 2001) and can, through calcium cytotoxicity, cause irreversible damage to the nerve fibers (Creange et al., 2006). Conversely, the hypocalcaemia observed in later stages of DPN mediates axonal degeneration, as seen in **Figure 2** (Gispen and Hamers, 1994). Overall, impaired neurotrophic factor levels in DPN-afflicted neurons drive mitochondrial depolarization and Ca^{2+} concentration impairment, which in turn negatively impacts the TCA cycle and ATP production (Fernyhough and Calcutt, 2010). ATP dysregulation impairs cellular calcium homeostasis, reducing levels of endoplasmic reticulum (ER) and plasma membrane Ca^{2+} pumps (PMCA), as evidenced in streptozotocin (STZ)-treated rats. The impairment of ER calcium homeostasis disrupts protein synthesis, post-translational modification, and trafficking, all of which may contribute to distal axonal degeneration (Fernyhough and Calcutt, 2010). T-type calcium channel blockers notably improve thermal and mechanical hypersensitivity in T2D mice (Misawa et al., 2009).

Sodium

The DRG neurons of STZ-treated rats show an increased expression of sodium channels ($Na_V1.3$, $Na_V1.6$, and $Na_V1.9$) (Craner et al., 2002; Hong et al., 2004), which contributes to ectopic impulse generation and neuronal hypersensitivity (Fischer and Waxman, 2010). The groups of Howe (Howe et al., 1977) and Wall (Wall and Gutnick, 1974) demonstrated that thermal, mechanical, and chemical stimuli thresholds are reduced following spontaneous electrical activity. Uninjured axons proximal to the affected neurons also exhibit ectopic discharge. Both of these phenomena result in increased electrical impulses in the spinal dorsal horn. The association between ectopic discharges and increased sodium channel expression can partly account for the therapeutic efficacy of anticonvulsant and tricyclic antidepressants in the treatment of DPN (Spruce et al., 2003).

Polyol Pathway

Cellular glucose is converted into pyruvate by the actions of diverse enzymes implicated in glycolysis. In hyperglycemic conditions, excess glucose is not oxidized, but rather directed to the polyol pathway (Oates, 2002). Firstly, aldose reductase (AR) metabolizes glucose into sorbitol, which is later transformed into fructose by sorbitol dehydrogenase. Fructose is, notably, ten times more potent than glucose in generating AGE (Oka and Kato, 2001) (section Advanced Glycation End Products). Aldose reductase and sorbitol dehydrogenase are characterized by their lowered substrate affinity (elevated Km); the concentration of available substrate is therefore the limiting factor of this reaction (Oates, 2002).

Elevated sorbitol levels have been associated with cellular and organ damage (Oyama et al., 2006). It is believed that sorbitol directly depletes bioavailable myoinositol (MI) and increases its expulsion from the cell (Oka and Kato, 2001; Oates, 2002). Elevated blood sugar also prevents sorbitol's cellular reuptake by saturating its membrane transporter. A deficit in MI alters the metabolism of phospho-inositides, reducing diacylglycerol (DAG) and inositol triphosphate (IP_3) production. This results in a lesser activation of PKC, which is itself a key activator of the Na^+/K^+ ATPase pump (Oka and Kato, 2001). A reduction in Na^+/K^+ ATPase pump activity triggers an intracellular reduction in K^+, combined with increases in the concentration of Na^+. In neurons, imbalances in ionic charges directly contribute to DPN by generating conductance anomalies (Oka and Kato, 2001). In this context, decreases in intracellular sodium concentrations affect sodium-dependent membrane transport. This transport is implicated in the reuptake of several amino acids and MI, contributing to a retro-positive feedback loop (Das Evcimen and King, 2007; Oates, 2008). Disruptions in the polyol pathway also increase ROS levels (section Reactive Oxygen Species) by reducing the production of glutathione, in addition to intracellular levels of antioxidants (NADPH). Polyol pathway pathologies also reduce the production of NO, which can in turn enhance vessel constriction. This impairs endothelial cell function can lead to the onset of microangiopathy (section Microangiopathy) (Oka and Kato, 2001); the effects of polyol pathways in DPN can be seen in **Figure 1**.

Aldose Reductase

In patients with T1D, polymorphisms in the genes coding for aldose reductase (AR) can impair thermal nociceptive thresholds (Thamotharampillai et al., 2006). Higher AR levels also correlate with a higher severity of intra-epidermal nerve fiber loss (Hirai et al., 2000). AR specific inhibitors (ARi) have been shown to reverse or delay the onset of DPN in diabetic animals (Schemmel et al., 2009). While ARis are unavailable on the US market, they are currently being used clinically in Japan (Hotta et al., 1996). Epalrestat is currently the only commercially available inhibitor (Singh Grewal et al., 2016); and prevented the progression of diabetic neuropathy and retinopathy/nephropathy in neuropathic patients as compared to a control group (Hotta et al., 2012).

NEURON EXTRINSIC FACTORS PROMOTING DIABETIC PAIN NEUROPATHY

Several neuron-extrinsic factors contribute to the onset and maintenance of neuropathic pain. Recent data has highlighted the key contribution of immune cells, acting as extrinsic factors, in driving DPN. Normally, the immune and sensory nervous systems work in concert to preserve homeostasis. They do so via interactions and exchanges between receptors, cytokines and neuropeptides (Talbot et al., 2016b; Veiga-Fernandes and Mucida, 2016). While this bidirectional communication helps to protect humans from danger, it can also contribute to disease pathophysiology (Chiu et al., 2013; Wilson et al., 2013; Talbot et al., 2015, 2016b; Foster et al., 2017). In fact, the somatosensory nervous system is anatomically positioned within primary and secondary lymphoid tissues and mucosa so as to interact with the cells of the immune system (Downing and Miyan, 2000; Rosas-Ballina et al., 2011; McMahon et al., 2015; Talbot et al., 2015; Veiga-Fernandes and Mucida, 2016; HD iPSC Consortium., 2017). Nociceptors, when sensing immunocyte-released cytokines, lower their firing thresholds; in doing so, they incite pain hypersensitivity (Wilson et al., 2013). While various immunocytes contribute to this phenomenon, this review will focus on the crucial role of microglia. Finally, we will review the role of blood vessels, which supply oxygen and glucose to the nerve, in generating DPN.

Microglia

The central nervous system (CNS) is primarily composed of afferent and efferent neuron fibers that transport electrical signals to and from the periphery, oligodendrocytes that form and repair myelin, and astrocytes and microglia that support and protect neurons (Marieb et al., 2009). Microglial cells represent 10–15% of all cells found within the human brain (Foster et al., 2015). Glia act as resident macrophage-related cells of the CNS, comprising the first line of defense against pathogen invasion, generating innate immune responses by recognizing, sequestering and processing antigens (Lawson et al., 1992). While there are two major types of microglia: resident, and perivascular (Gosselin et al., 2010), which express receptors for most inflammatory neurotransmitters (Hickey and Kimura, 1988), it seems that glia exists in nine distinct subtypes with different functions, appearance, and presence. Resident microglial cells are bone marrow-derived hematopoietic cells that invade the CNS during embryonic development (Pocock and Kettenmann, 2007). These are very rarely replaced, and rapidly proliferate while activated (Milligan and Watkins, 2009). Conversely, perivascular microglial cells are continuously replenished by bone marrow-derived hematopoietic precursors (Gosselin et al., 2010), particularly during CNS inflammation (Romero-Sandoval et al., 2008). Perivascular microglia can alter the blood-brain barrier's permeability, and exert anti-inflammatory effects, while resident microglial cells exert both pro- and anti-inflammatory effects (Milligan and Watkins, 2009).

While on a polarization continuum, microglia activation can be classified as either resting or activated. A resting microglial cell possesses a small soma with thin and ramified processes (Tsuda et al., 2005), express immunoreceptors (Lawson et al., 1992), and perform immune roles to maintain CNS homeostasis (Tsuda et al., 2005). Upon activation due to trauma, inflammation, or infection, microglia undergo several stereotypic changes in morphology, gene expression, function, and number (Tsuda et al., 2005). They upregulate various transmitters and receptors, including the complement receptor 3 (CR3) (Eriksson et al., 1993; Lassmann et al., 1993), major histocompatibility complex 2 (MHC2) (Shi et al., 2017), TLR4 (Sweitzer et al., 2002), and CD14 (Sweitzer et al., 2002). The intracellular events promoting glial cell activation remain unclear, but are known to involve the activation of cannabinoid CB2 receptors (Tanga et al., 2004), kinin B1 receptors (Li and Kim, 2017), P_2X_4R (Noda et al., 2007), NK-1R (Inoue, 2008), CX3CR-1 (Abbadie et al., 2009; Gao and Ji, 2010; Zhou et al., 2010), CCR-2 (Zhang and De Koninck, 2006; Milligan et al., 2008), MMP9 (Thacker et al., 2009), BDNF-R (Kawasaki et al., 2008), TLR3 (Tender et al., 2010) and TLR4 (Kim et al., 2007); leading to the phosphorylation of p38 MAPK (Jin et al., 2003; Tsuda et al., 2004; Tanga et al., 2005; Daulhac et al., 2006; Ji et al., 2009). For more information on microglia intracellular signaling refer to Popiolek-Barczyk and Mika (Chang et al., 2010). Furthermore, microglial activation can occur via endogenous pro-inflammatory signals (IL-1β, TNFα, IL-6, and NO), opioids (Popiolek-Barczyk and Mika, 2016) or heat shock protein (Hutchinson et al., 2008). Activated microglial soma increase in size and their long and thin ramifications withdraw, ultimately resulting in an amoeboid shape with few ramifications (Tsuda et al., 2005). They have implicated microglia in reward behavior (Costigan et al., 1998) as well as in the onset of chronic neurodegenerative diseases (Taylor et al., 2015; Hammond et al., 2018), such as lupus erythematosus (Salter and Stevens, 2017), Huntington's chorea (Nestor et al., 2018), and Alzheimer's disease (Eriksson et al., 1993).

Painful Glia

Microglial cells produce and release various excitatory peptides, including PG, SP, EAA, NO, and ATP, and express selective receptors for immunomodulatory neurotransmitters. Both peptides and receptors allow microglia to detect, and respond to, neuronal signals, thereby generating autocrine or paracrine feed forward inflammatory loops (McMahon et al., 2005). For example, TNFα and MMPs activate microglial p38 MAPK in the spinal cord dorsal horn during peripheral neuropathic pain (Svensson et al., 2005). MMP9-induced pro-IL-1β cleavage leads to p38 MAPK phosphorylation in microglia during the onset and early stages of neuropathic pain. MMP2-induced pro-IL-1β cleavage leads to astrocyte activation in later disease stages (Kawasaki et al., 2008). ATP-stimulated microglial P_2X_4R enhances the levels of intracellular Ca^{2+}. Such influx activates various transcription factors, including NF-κB, p38, and ERK-MAPK (Tsuda et al., 2005), leading to the synthesis of pro-inflammatory cytokines (IL-1β, TNFα, and IL-6) (Watkins et al., 2001a; Marchand et al., 2005) or neuroexcitatory substances such as D-serine (Petrenko et al., 2003). This transcriptomic profile can initiate and maintain neuropathic pain by facilitating neuron-glial interactions (Hickey and Kimura, 1988; Abbadie et al., 2009). The interplay between neurons and glia can therefore sustain neuronal stimulation and sensitization by increasing glutamatergic stimulation and by reducing GABAergic inhibitory signals (Tsuda et al., 2005; Inoue, 2006; Scholz and Woolf, 2007; Biggs et al., 2010); the process can be seen in **Figure 3.**

In current pre-clinical literature, activated microglia have emerged as key drivers of pathological pain in chemotherapy-induced neuropathy and peripheral nerve and spinal cord injuries (Watkins et al., 2001b; Marchand et al., 2005; Tsuda et al., 2005; Daulhac et al., 2006; Pocock and Kettenmann, 2007; Gadani et al., 2015; McMahon et al., 2015). For example, CB2 receptor agonists dramatically attenuate iNOS induction and ROS generation in LPS-activated microglia (Ribeiro et al., 2013). The incitement of inflammation signals microglia to migrate, proliferate, synthesize and release pro-inflammatory mediators that maintain neuron activation. In keeping with the fact that an intrathecal injection of activated microglia induces both thermal hyperalgesia and tactile allodynia (Tsuda et al., 2003; Narita et al., 2006), while resting microglia or activated astrocytes are without effect (Narita et al., 2006). Blockades of p38 MAPK (Tanga et al., 2005; Ji et al., 2009), CX3CR-1 (Milligan et al., 2004; Verge et al., 2004; Sun et al., 2007) or P_2X_4R (Tsuda et al., 2003) have been shown to alleviate chronic pain in rodents. Other chemokines, such as RANTES, IP-10, and SDF1 are also implicated in enhanced microglia migration, infiltration, phagocytosis; they are therefore contributors to microglia-induced neuropathic pain (White et al., 2007).

Salter and Beggs have made several discoveries linking neuronal hypersensitivity to overactive microglia (Beggs and Salter, 2016). Firstly, they were able to show that nerve injury activates microglia and causes them to express P_2X_4R. They demonstrated that the IRF-8/IRF-5 transcriptional cascade clearly regulates the expression of P_2X_4R gene. Additionally, they showed that external stimulation (CCL2 and LPS) leads to the translocation of P_2X_4R protein from lysosome to cell surface (Tsuda and Inoue, 2016). A targeted silencing of P_2X_4R suppressed injury-induced tactile allodynia, while an intraspinal administration of P_2X_4R-expressing glia had the opposite effect (Tsuda et al., 2003). They also identified spinal dorsal horn neurons as a source of ATP (Masuda et al., 2016), and that ATP-stimulated microglia release brain derived neurotrophic factor (BDNF). BDNF limits GABAergic inhibitory signals sent to afferent nociceptor neurons (Torsney and MacDermott, 2005);

this enhances their activity by uncoupling the transmembrane anion gradient (Coull et al., 2005). A disruption of chloride transport changed spinal lamina I neurons' phenotype, causing them to (i) increase nociceptive responsiveness, (ii) relay innocuous mechanical inputs, and (iii) generate spontaneous bursts of activity; respectively, accounting for (a) hyperalgesia, (b) mechanical allodynia, and (c) spontaneous pain (Keller et al., 2007). The microglia-to-neuron P_2X_4R -BDNF-KCC2 axis was also found to drive opioid-induced thermal hyperalgesia. Interestingly, Salter and Beggs found that this hyperalgesia mechanistically differs from opioid-induced tolerance (Beggs and Salter, 2016). Microglia-derived BDNF also emerged in their research as a negative regulator of reward in opioid-dependent states (Taylor et al., 2016), while the Panx1-mediated release of microglial ATP controls morphine withdrawal without affecting opiate-induced analgesia (Burma et al., 2017).

Peripheral tissue injury was found to increase the intensity, spatial distribution, and persistence of Iba-1^+ microglial activity within the spinal dorsal horn, resulting in a long-lasting priming of withdrawal reflex sensitivity and microglial responsiveness (Beggs et al., 2012). MCP-1^+ neurons drive the bone marrow-derived microglial infiltration of injured spinal cords. These neurons also facilitate glial activation and drive mechanical allodynia (Zhang et al., 2007). CCL21, a microglial activator, is also found to be upregulated in the cell bodies of spinothalamic tract neurons following nerve injury. This molecule is transported rostrally to the thalamus, where it activates microglia and drives neuron hyperexcitability (Zhao et al., 2007b). Spinal microglia consequently remain activated for more than 3 months following nerve injury in rodents, thereby maintaining chronic pain (Echeverry et al., 2017). Newly-generated microglia also appear to be coded with an inherent "memory" of previous injuries, contributing to long-lasting neuropathic pain (Yao et al., 2016).

Following a spinal cord injury, microglial ERK kinases are activated, prompting the intraspinal release of PGE_2, which results in spinal cord dorsal horn neuron hyperresponsiveness (Zhao et al., 2007a). Following the spinal release of IL-1β and IL-6, fractalkine triggers pain by activating microglia expressing CX3CR1 (Milligan et al., 2004, 2005). IL-1β upregulates both neuronal NMDAR phosphorylation and expression. These effects enhance NMDAR conductivity (Zhang et al., 2008) and calcium influx (Viviani et al., 2003), increasing neuronal excitability and synaptic strength (Beattie et al., 2002; Stellwagen and Malenka, 2006). Microglial NO and PGE_2 can also increase the excitability of pain-projecting neurons (Besson, 1999). Overall, a modulation of microglial polarization was shown to alleviate neuropathic pain (Chang et al., 2010; Piotrowska et al., 2016; Xu et al., 2018). Intriguingly, microglia only induce mechanical pain hypersensitivity in male rodents (Mapplebeck et al., 2018), as T-lymphocytes appear to be responsible for this mechanism in females (Sorge et al., 2015).

Microglia, an Emerging Target in DPN

Given that db/db mice and T2D patients show increased levels of activated microglia (Arroba and Valverde, 2017), and that the pharmacological inhibition of spinal resident microglia reverses painful neuropathy (Wodarski et al., 2009; Sun et al., 2015; Lin, 2017; Zhang et al., 2018), we take the overall view that microglia may drive DPN (**Figure 1**). Activated microglia levels have been found to correlate with thalamus hyperresponsiveness (Fischer and Waxman, 2010), and the brain thalami of DPN patients demonstrate increases in blood flow (Paulson et al., 2007), spontaneous neuronal activity (Fischer et al., 2009), receptive field size enhancement (Fischer et al., 2009), and alterations in neuronal connectivity (Cauda et al., 2010). Additionally, activated microglia drive DPN in STZ-treated rats (Wodarski et al., 2009; Talbot et al., 2010); this process can successfully be reversed by gabapentin (Wodarski et al., 2009) or minocycline treatment (Talbot et al., 2010).

Additionally, diabetes-induced hyperglycemia enhances microglial NADPH oxidase and iNOS activation (**Figure 3**), promoting the production of ROS (Quan et al., 2007, 2011) and peroxynitrite (Li et al., 2005). As a result of the iNOS-NO-NRS axis, activated microglia are a major source of free radicals in the spinal cords of animals with DPN (Li et al., 2005; Candelario-Jalil et al., 2007). Glial-released NO inhibits neuronal cytochrome oxidase, blocking mitochondrial respiration, which in turn depletes the production of ATP (Brown and Bal-Price, 2003). Moreover, ROS and RNS deplete endothelial cell NO levels, contributing to the generation of microangiopathy (section Microangiopathy). A reduction in neuronal blood supply leads to hypoxia and mitochondrial dysfunction; this results in cellular energy deficits, and ultimately, neuron death. Finally, elevated ROS levels also impair axonal transport (Larsen and Sidenius, 1989) and the capacity of the nerve to repair itself (Longo et al., 1986), further worsening nerve health in DPN patients.

Microglia exposed to high glucose levels show increases in mRNA expression, and secrete TNFα and MCP-1, leading to neuronal activation (Quan et al., 2011). The spinal microglia's activation of P2Y12 and P2Y13 receptors triggers the production of IL-1β and IL-6 in a rat model of DPN (Liu et al., 2017; Zhou et al., 2018). The activation of microglial RAGE (Thornalley, 1998) leads to the release of chemokines CCL3, CCL5, and CXCL12, which activate microglia (Bianchi et al., 2011). The resulting activated microglia actively phagocyte neuronal myelin, thereby promoting DPN (Mosley and Cuzner, 1996).

Microangiopathy

Microangiopathy is characterized by the shrinking and weakening of small blood vessels. This pathology leads to a reduction in blood flow, protein leakage, and bleeding. In diabetic states, endothelial cells take up excessively large quantities of circulating glucose, raising the production of AGE (section Advanced Glycation End Products). These AGEs enhance the proliferation of endothelial cells, which leads to a thickening of basal membranes and progressive vessel occlusion, which are associated with reduced neuronal blood flow (Tuck et al., 1984; Cameron et al., 1991) and ischemia. In turn, the ischemia reduces neuronal oxygen and nutrient supplies, triggering nerve fiber loss (Yagihashi et al., 2007). Microangiopathy in neuron-irrigating vessels also impairs their capacity to regenerate and repair (Kennedy and Zochodne, 2005). A thickening of basement membranes and endothelial cell swelling thereby positively correlates with reduced nerve fiber myelin densities (Yagihashi et al., 2007). The occlusion of neuronal capillaries promotes axonal degeneration and a dysfunctional loss of sensory perception, as typically observed in the later stages of DPN.

Multifocal nerve lesions and alterations in endoneurial capillaries indicate a role for circulatory factors in the symmetrical form of DPN (Dyck et al., 1986; King et al., 1989). Peripheral nerve fiber loss in DPN is well-associated with the increased migration and infiltration of inflammatory cytokines released by T-lymphocytes and macrophages (Said et al., 2003; Said, 2007). These cytokines increase vessel damage and promote microangiopathy (Said, 2007). Considering that microglia and macrophages share similar roles and inflammatory characteristics, it is probable that microglia may also promote microangiopathy within the CNS (**Figure 3**).

CONCLUSION AND FUTURE THERAPEUTIC DIRECTIONS

Multiple molecular mechanisms generate and amplify hyperglycemia-induced neuropathic pain. This collaboration involves voltage-gated ion channels, ligand-gated channels, cytokine receptors, direct myelin damage (Edwards et al., 2008; Vincent et al., 2008), neuronal depolarization (Abbadie et al., 2009), conduction impairment (Kramer et al., 2004), a loss of interneuron inhibitory input (Wood, 2008), Aβ-fiber sprouting (Yasuda et al., 2003), and neuronal death (Inoue, 2006). This multicentric view accounts for why hyperglycemia-induced DPN remains highly refractory to treatment paradigms. Given such potential heterogeneity amongst patients, personalizing of DPN management may prove useful. This will necessitate improved diagnostic methods and personalized medicine tailored to the specific pathology in question.

While design, safety and drug efficacy often vary between rodent and clinical models of disease, calcium channel α2-delta ligands (pregabalin, gabapentin), antidepressants (TCA and SSRI), and opioid-like drugs as well as topical agents including capsaicin, lidocaine, or botulinum toxin A can help alleviate patients' DPN (Finnerup et al., 2015). The long-term efficacies of these approaches have yet to be demonstrated. Overall, the high plasticity of microglial phenotypic and transcriptomic changes persists even after glycemic control, inciting and maintaining neuron sensitization (Milligan et al., 2008). Therefore, the microglia, which potentially act upstream of pain neurons, should rightly be considered as a crucial therapeutic target in the treatment of diabetic pain neuropathy. Future therapies may therefore involve targeting specific receptors and signaling cascades which engage such deleterious neuro-immune crosstalk.

AUTHOR CONTRIBUTIONS

TR, RC, AC, and ST conceived the study and wrote the manuscript while SCT, J-CW, MA, MB, TC, and JD contributed to its design.

REFERENCES

Abbadie, C., Bhangoo, S., De Koninck, Y., Malcangio, M., Melik-Parsadaniantz, S., and White, F. A. (2009). Chemokines and pain mechanisms. *Brain Res. Rev.* 60, 125–134. doi: 10.1016/j.brainresrev.2008.12.002

Arroba, A. I., and Valverde, A. M. (2017). Modulation of microglia in the retina: new insights into diabetic retinopathy. *Acta Diabetol.* 54, 527–533. doi: 10.1007/s00592-017-0984-z

Aschner, P., Gagliardino, J. J., Ilkova, H. M., Lavalle-Gonzalez, F. J., Ramachandran, A., Kaddaha, G., et al. (2018). No improvement in glycemic control or rates of diabetes-related complications for people with type 2 diabetes—results from 10 years of the international diabetes management practices study (IDMPS). *Am. Diabetes Assoc.* 67 (Suppl. 1):1583-P. doi: 10.2337/db18-1583-P

Balamurugan, A. N., Naziruddin, B., Lockridge, A., Tiwari, M., Loganathan, G., Takita, M., et al. (2014). Islet product characteristics and factors related to successful human islet transplantation from the Collaborative Islet Transplant Registry (CITR) 1999-2010. *Am. J. Transl.* 14, 2595–2606. doi: 10.1111/ajt.12872

Balbi, M. E., Tonin, F. S., Mendes, A. M., Borba, H. H., Wiens, A., Fernandez-Llimos, F., et al. (2018). Antioxidant effects of vitamins in type 2 diabetes: a meta-analysis of randomized controlled trials. *Diabetol. Metab. Syndr.* 10:18. doi: 10.1186/s13098-018-0318-5

Bautista, D. M., Jordt, S. E., Nikai, T., Tsuruda, P. R., Read, A. J., Poblete, J., et al. (2006). TRPA1 mediates the inflammatory actions of environmental irritants and proalgesic agents. *Cell* 124, 1269–1282. doi: 10.1016/j.cell.2006.02.023

Baynes, J. W., and Thorpe, S. R. (1999). Role of oxidative stress in diabetic complications: a new perspective on an old paradigm. *Diabetes* 48, 1–9. doi: 10.2337/diabetes.48.1.1

Beattie, E. C., Stellwagen, D., Morishita, W., Bresnahan, J. C., Ha, B. K., Von Zastrow, M., et al. (2002). Control of synaptic strength by glial TNFalpha. *Science* 295, 2282–2285. doi: 10.1126/science.1067859

Beggs, S., Currie, G., Salter, M. W., Fitzgerald, M., and Walker, S. M. (2012). Priming of adult pain responses by neonatal pain experience: maintenance by central neuroimmune activity. *Brain* 135, 404–417. doi: 10.1093/brain/awr288

Beggs, S., and Salter, M. W. (2016). SnapShot: microglia in disease. *Cell* 165, 1294–1294.e1. doi: 10.1016/j.cell.2016.05.036

Bertolotto, F., and Massone, A. (2012). Combination of alpha lipoic acid and superoxide dismutase leads to physiological and symptomatic improvements in diabetic neuropathy. *Drugs R D* 12, 29–34. doi: 10.2165/11599200-000000000-00000

Besson, J. M. (1999). The neurobiology of pain. *Lancet* 353, 1610–1615. doi: 10.1016/S0140-6736(99)01313-6

Bianchi, R., Kastrisianaki, E., Giambanco, I., and Donato, R. (2011). S100B protein stimulates microglia migration via RAGE-dependent up-regulation of chemokine expression and release. *J. Biol. Chem.* 286, 7214–7226. doi: 10.1074/jbc.M110.169342

Biggs, J. E., Lu, V. B., Stebbing, M. J., Balasubramanyan, S., and Smith, P. A. (2010). Is BDNF sufficient for information transfer between microglia and dorsal horn neurons during the onset of central sensitization? *Mol. Pain* 6:44. doi: 10.1186/1744-8069-6-44

Billings, L. K., and Florez, J. C. (2010). The genetics of type 2 diabetes: what have we learned from GWAS? *Ann. N. Y. Acad. Sci.* 1212, 59–77. doi: 10.1111/j.1749-6632.2010.05838.x

Binshtok, A. M., Wang, H., Zimmermann, K., Amaya, F., Vardeh, D., Shi, L., et al. (2008). Nociceptors are interleukin-1beta sensors. *J. Neurosci.* 28, 14062–14073. doi: 10.1523/JNEUROSCI.3795-08.2008

Brown, G. C., and Bal-Price, A. (2003). Inflammatory neurodegeneration mediated by nitric oxide, glutamate, and mitochondria. *Mol. Neurobiol.* 27, 325–355. doi: 10.1385/MN:27:3:325

Brownlee, M. (2001). Biochemistry and molecular cell biology of diabetic complications. *Nature* 414, 813–820. doi: 10.1038/414813a

Brownlee, M. (2005). The pathobiology of diabetic complications: a unifying mechanism. *Diabetes* 54, 1615–1625. doi: 10.2337/diabetes.54.6.1615

Bruck, W., and Friede, R. L. (1990). L-fucosidase treatment blocks myelin phagocytosis by macrophages *in vitro*. *J. Neuroimmunol.* 27, 217–227. doi: 10.1016/0165-5728(90)90072-U

Burma, N. E., Bonin, R. P., Leduc-Pessah, H., Baimel, C., Cairncross, Z. F., Mousseau, M., et al. (2017). Blocking microglial pannexin-1 channels alleviates morphine withdrawal in rodents. *Nat. Med.* 23, 355–360. doi: 10.1038/nm.4281

Cameron, N. E., Cotter, M. A., and Low, P. A. (1991). Nerve blood flow in early experimental diabetes in rats: relation to conduction deficits. *Am. J. Physiol.* 261, E1–E8. doi: 10.1152/ajpendo.1991.261.1.E1

Cameron, N. E., Eaton, S. E., Cotter, M. A., and Tesfaye, S. (2001). Vascular factors and metabolic interactions in the pathogenesis of diabetic neuropathy. *Diabetologia* 44, 1973–1988. doi: 10.1007/s001250100001

Candelario-Jalil, E., de Oliveira, A. C., Graf, S., Bhatia, H. S., Hull, M., Munoz, E., et al. (2007). Resveratrol potently reduces prostaglandin E2 production and free radical formation in lipopolysaccharide-activated primary rat microglia. *J. Neuroinflammation* 4:25. doi: 10.1186/1742-2094-4-25

Cauda, F., D'Agata, F., Sacco, K., Duca, S., Cocito, D., Paolasso, I., et al. (2010). Altered resting state attentional networks in diabetic neuropathic pain. *J. Neurol. Neurosurg. Psychiatry* 81, 806–811. doi: 10.1136/jnnp.2009.188631

Cevikbas, F., Kempkes, C., Buhl, T., Mess, C., Buddenkotte, J., and Steinhoff, M. (2014). "Role of interleukin-31 and oncostatin M in itch and neuroimmune communication," in *Itch: Mechanisms and Treatment*, eds E. Carstens and T. Akiyama (Boca Raton, FL: CRC Press/Taylor & Francis), 237–256.

Chang, K. H., de Pablo, Y., Lee, H. P., Lee, H. G., Smith, M. A., and Shah, K. (2010). Cdk5 is a major regulator of p38 cascade: relevance to neurotoxicity in Alzheimer's disease. *J. Neurochem.* 113, 1221–1229. doi: 10.1111/j.1471-4159.2010.06687.x

Chiu, I. M., Barrett, L. B., Williams, E. K., Strochlic, D. E., Lee, S., Weyer, A. D., et al. (2014). Transcriptional profiling at whole population and single cell levels reveals somatosensory neuron molecular diversity. *Elife* 3:e04660. doi: 10.7554/eLife.04660

Chiu, I. M., Heesters, B. A., Ghasemlou, N., Von Hehn, C. A., Zhao, F., Tran, J., et al. (2013). Bacteria activate sensory neurons that modulate pain and inflammation. *Nature* 501, 52–57. doi: 10.1038/nature12479

Clement, K., Vaisse, C., Lahlou, N., Cabrol, S., Pelloux, V., Cassuto, D., et al. (1998). A mutation in the human leptin receptor gene causes obesity and pituitary dysfunction. *Nature* 392, 398–401. doi: 10.1038/32911

Costigan, M., Mannion, R. J., Kendall, G., Lewis, S. E., Campagna, J. A., Coggeshall, R. E., et al. (1998). Heat shock protein 27: developmental regulation and expression after peripheral nerve injury. *J. Neurosci.* 18, 5891–5900. doi: 10.1523/JNEUROSCI.18-15-05891.1998

Coull, J. A., Beggs, S., Boudreau, D., Boivin, D., Tsuda, M., Inoue, K., et al. (2005). BDNF from microglia causes the shift in neuronal anion gradient underlying neuropathic pain. *Nature* 438, 1017–1021. doi: 10.1038/nature 04223

Craner, M. J., Klein, J. P., Renganathan, M., Black, J. A., and Waxman, S. G. (2002). Changes of sodium channel expression in experimental painful diabetic neuropathy. *Ann. Neurol.* 52, 786–792. doi: 10.1002/ana.10364

Creange, A., Boerio, D., and Lefaucheur, J. P. (2006). Inflammatory demyelinating neuropathies: classification, evolution and prognosis. *J. Soc. Biol.* 200, 301–306. doi: 10.1051/jbio:2006035

Crofford, O. B. (1995). Diabetes control and complications. *Annu. Rev. Med.* 46, 267–279. doi: 10.1146/annurev.med.46.1.267

Daousi, C., MacFarlane, I. A., Woodward, A., Nurmikko, T. J., Bundred, P. E., and Benbow, S. J. (2004). Chronic painful peripheral neuropathy in an urban community: a controlled comparison of people with and without diabetes. *Diabet. Med.* 21, 976–982. doi: 10.1111/j.1464-5491.2004.01271.x

Das Evcimen, N., and King, G. L. (2007). The role of protein kinase C activation and the vascular complications of diabetes. *Pharmacol. Res.* 55, 498–510. doi: 10.1016/j.phrs.2007.04.016

Daulhac, L., Mallet, C., Courteix, C., Etienne, M., Duroux, E., Privat, A. M., et al. (2006). Diabetes-induced mechanical hyperalgesia involves spinal mitogen-activated protein kinase activation in neurons and microglia via N-methyl-D-aspartate-dependent mechanisms. *Mol. Pharmacol.* 70, 1246–1254. doi: 10.1124/mol.106.025478

Davis, J. B., Gray, J., Gunthorpe, M. J., Hatcher, J. P., Davey, P. T., Overend, P., et al. (2000). Vanilloid receptor-1 is essential for inflammatory thermal hyperalgesia. *Nature* 405, 183–187. doi: 10.1038/35012076

De Brito Gariepy, H., Talbot, S., Senecal, J., and Couture, R. (2013). Brain kinin B(1) receptor contributes to the onset of stereotypic nocifensive behavior in rat. *Behav. Brain Res.* 241, 17–26. doi: 10.1016/j.bbr.2012.11.032

Di Stasi, A. M., Mallozzi, C., Macchia, G., Maura, G., Petrucci, T. C., and Minetti, M. (2002). Peroxynitrite affects exocytosis and SNARE complex formation and induces tyrosine nitration of synaptic proteins. *J. Neurochem.* 82, 420–429. doi: 10.1046/j.1471-4159.2002.00980.x

Downing, J. E., and Miyan, J. A. (2000). Neural immunoregulation: emerging roles for nerves in immune homeostasis and disease. *Immunol. Today* 21, 281–289. doi: 10.1016/S0167-5699(00)01635-2

Du, X. L., Edelstein, D., Rossetti, L., Fantus, I. G., Goldberg, H., Ziyadeh, F., et al. (2000). Hyperglycemia-induced mitochondrial superoxide overproduction activates the hexosamine pathway and induces plasminogen activator inhibitor-1 expression by increasing Sp1 glycosylation. *Proc. Natl. Acad. Sci. U.S.A.* 97, 12222–12226. doi: 10.1073/pnas.97.22.12222

Duran-Jimenez, B., Dobler, D., Moffatt, S., Rabbani, N., Streuli, C. H., Thornalley, P. J., et al. (2009). Advanced glycation end products in extracellular matrix proteins contribute to the failure of sensory nerve regeneration in diabetes. *Diabetes* 58, 2893–2903. doi: 10.2337/db09-0320

Dyck, P. J., Lais, A., Karnes, J. L., O'Brien, P., and Rizza, R. (1986). Fiber loss is primary and multifocal in sural nerves in diabetic polyneuropathy. *Ann. Neurol.* 19, 425–439. doi: 10.1002/ana.410190503

Echeverry, S., Shi, X. Q., Yang, M., Huang, H., Wu, Y., Lorenzo, L. E., et al. (2017). Spinal microglia are required for long-term maintenance of neuropathic pain. *Pain* 158, 1792–1801. doi: 10.1097/j.pain.0000000000000982

Edwards, J. L., Vincent, A. M., Cheng, H. T., and Feldman, E. L. (2008). Diabetic neuropathy: mechanisms to management. *Pharmacol. Ther.* 120, 1–34. doi: 10.1016/j.pharmthera.2008.05.005

Eriksson, N. P., Persson, J. K., Svensson, M., Arvidsson, J., Molander, C., and Aldskogius, H. (1993). A quantitative analysis of the microglial cell reaction in central primary sensory projection territories following peripheral nerve injury in the adult rat. *Exp. Brain Res.* 96, 19–27. doi: 10.1007/BF00230435

Fernyhough, P., and Calcutt, N. A. (2010). Abnormal calcium homeostasis in peripheral neuropathies. *Cell Calcium* 47, 130–139. doi: 10.1016/j.ceca.2009.11.008

Figueroa-Romero, C., Sadidi, M., and Feldman, E. L. (2008). Mechanisms of disease: the oxidative stress theory of diabetic neuropathy. *Rev. Endocr. Metab. Disord.* 9, 301–314. doi: 10.1007/s11154-008-9104-2

Finnerup, N. B., Attal, N., Haroutounian, S., McNicol, E., Baron, R., Dworkin, R. H., et al. (2015). Pharmacotherapy for neuropathic pain in adults: a systematic review and meta-analysis. *Lancet Neurol.* 14, 162–173. doi: 10.1016/S1474-4422(14)70251-0

Fischer, T. Z., Tan, A. M., and Waxman, S. G. (2009). Thalamic neuron hyperexcitability and enlarged receptive fields in the STZ model of diabetic pain. *Brain Res.* 1268, 154–161. doi: 10.1016/j.brainres.2009.02.063

Fischer, T. Z., and Waxman, S. G. (2010). Neuropathic pain in diabetes–evidence for a central mechanism. *Nat. Rev. Neurol.* 6, 462–466. doi: 10.1038/nrneurol.2010.90

Foster, S. L., Seehus, C. R., Woolf, C. J., and Talbot, S. (2017). Sense and immunity: context-dependent neuro-immune interplay. *Front. Immunol.* 8:1463. doi: 10.3389/fimmu.2017.01463

Foster, S. L., Talbot, S., and Woolf, C. J. (2015). CNS injury: IL-33 sounds the alarm. *Immunity* 42, 403–405. doi: 10.1016/j.immuni.2015.02.019

Gadani, S. P., Walsh, J. T., Smirnov, I., Zheng, J., and Kipnis, J. (2015). The glia-derived alarmin IL-33 orchestrates the immune response and promotes recovery following CNS injury. *Neuron* 85, 703–709. doi: 10.1016/j.neuron.2015.01.013

Gao, Y. J., and Ji, R. R. (2010). Chemokines, neuronal-glial interactions, and central processing of neuropathic pain. *Pharmacol. Ther.* 126, 56–68. doi: 10.1016/j.pharmthera.2010.01.002

Gerbi, A., Maixent, J. M., Barbey, O., Jamme, I., Pierlovisi, M., Coste, T., et al. (1998). Alterations of Na,K-ATPase isoenzymes in the rat diabetic neuropathy: protective effect of dietary supplementation with n-3 fatty acids. *J. Neurochem.* 71, 732–740. doi: 10.1046/j.1471-4159.1998.71020732.x

Gispen, W. H., and Hamers, F. P. (1994). Calcium and neuronal dysfunction in peripheral nervous system. *Ann. N. Y. Acad. Sci.* 747, 419–430. doi: 10.1111/j.1749-6632.1994.tb44426.x

Gosselin, R. D., Suter, M. R., Ji, R. R., and Decosterd, I. (2010). Glial cells and chronic pain. *Neuroscientist* 16, 519–531. doi: 10.1177/1073858409360822

Green, D. R., and Reed, J. C. (1998). Mitochondria and apoptosis. *Science* 281, 1309–1312. doi: 10.1126/science.281.5381.1309

Groop, L., and Lyssenko, V. (2008). Genes and type 2 diabetes mellitus. *Curr. Diabetes Rep.* 8, 192–197. doi: 10.1007/s11892-008-0033-y

Guastella, V., and Mick, G. (2009). Strategies for the diagnosis and treatment of neuropathic pain secondary to diabetic peripheral sensory polyneuropathy. *Diabetes Metab.* 35, 12–19. doi: 10.1016/j.diabet.2008.09.003

Haddad, Y., and Couture, R. (2016). Interplay between the kinin B1 receptor and inducible nitric oxide synthase in insulin resistance. *Br. J. Pharmacol.* 173, 1988–2000. doi: 10.1111/bph.13491

Haigh, R. C., and Blake, D. R. (2001). Understanding pain. *Clin. Med.* 1, 44–48. doi: 10.7861/clinmedicine.1-1-44

Hammond, T. R., Robinton, D., and Stevens, B. (2018). Microglia and the brain: complementary partners in development and disease. *Annu. Rev. Cell Dev. Biol.* 34, 523–544. doi: 10.1146/annurev-cellbio-100616-060509

Haslbeck, K. M., Schleicher, E., Bierhaus, A., Nawroth, P., Haslbeck, M., Neundorfer, B., et al. (2005). The AGE/RAGE/NF-(kappa)B pathway may contribute to the pathogenesis of polyneuropathy in impaired glucose tolerance (IGT). *Exp. Clin. Endocrinol. Diabetes* 113, 288–291. doi: 10.1055/s-2005-865600

HD iPSC Consortium. (2017). Developmental alterations in Huntington's disease neural cells and pharmacological rescue in cells and mice. *Nat. Neurosci.* 20, 648–660. doi: 10.1038/nn.4532

Hefti, F. F., Rosenthal, A., Walicke, P. A., Wyatt, S., Vergara, G., Shelton, D. L., et al. (2006). Novel class of pain drugs based on antagonism of NGF. *Trends Pharmacol. Sci.* 27, 85–91. doi: 10.1016/j.tips.2005.12.001

Hickey, W. F., and Kimura, H. (1988). Perivascular microglial cells of the CNS are bone marrow-derived and present antigen *in vivo*. *Science* 239, 290–292. doi: 10.1126/science.3276004

Hirai, A., Yasuda, H., Joko, M., Maeda, T., and Kikkawa, R. (2000). Evaluation of diabetic neuropathy through the quantitation of cutaneous nerves. *J. Neurol. Sci.* 172, 55–62. doi: 10.1016/S0022-510X(99)00290-7

Hong, S., Morrow, T. J., Paulson, P. E., Isom, L. L., and Wiley, J. W. (2004). Early painful diabetic neuropathy is associated with differential changes in tetrodotoxin-sensitive and -resistant sodium channels in dorsal root ganglion neurons in the rat. *Biol. Chem.* 279, 29341–29350. doi: 10.1074/jbc.M4041 67200

Hotta, N., Kawamori, R., Fukuda, M., Shigeta, Y., and Aldose Reductase Inhibitor-Diabetes Complications Trial Study Group. (2012). Long-term clinical effects of epalrestat, an aldose reductase inhibitor, on progression of diabetic neuropathy and other microvascular complications: multivariate epidemiological analysis based on patient background factors and severity of diabetic neuropathy. *Diabetes Med.* 29, 1529–1533. doi: 10.1111/j.1464-5491.2012.03684.x

Hotta, N., Sakamoto, N., Shigeta, Y., Kikkawa, R., and Goto, Y. (1996). Clinical investigation of epalrestat, an aldose reductase inhibitor, on diabetic neuropathy in Japan: multicenter study. Diabetic Neuropathy Study Group in Japan. *J. Diabetes Complications* 10, 168–172. doi: 10.1016/1056-8727(96)00113-4

Howe, J. F., Loeser, J. D., and Calvin, W. H. (1977). Mechanosensitivity of dorsal root ganglia and chronically injured axons: a physiological basis for the radicular pain of nerve root compression. *Pain* 3, 25–41. doi: 10.1016/0304-3959(77)90033-1

Hutchinson, M. R., Zhang, Y., Brown, K., Coats, B. D., Shridhar, M., Sholar, P. W., et al. (2008). Non-stereoselective reversal of neuropathic pain by naloxone and naltrexone: involvement of toll-like receptor 4 (TLR4). *Eur. J. Neurosci.* 28, 20–29. doi: 10.1111/j.1460-9568.2008.06321.x

Inoguchi, T., Li, P., Umeda, F., Yu, H. Y., Kakimoto, M., Imamura, M., et al. (2000). High glucose level and free fatty acid stimulate reactive oxygen species production through protein kinase C-dependent activation of NAD(P)H oxidase in cultured vascular cells. *Diabetes* 49, 1939–1945. doi: 10.2337/diabetes.49.11.1939

Inoue, K. (2006). The function of microglia through purinergic receptors: neuropathic pain and cytokine release. *Pharmacol. Ther.* 109, 210–226. doi: 10.1016/j.pharmthera.2005.07.001

Inoue, K. (2008). Purinergic systems in microglia. *Cell Mol. Life Sci.* 65, 3074–3080. doi: 10.1007/s00018-008-8210-3

Ishii, D. N. (1995). Implication of insulin-like growth factors in the pathogenesis of diabetic neuropathy. *Brain Res. Rev.* 20, 47–67. doi: 10.1016/0165-0173(94)00005-A

Ji, R. R., Befort, K., Brenner, G. J., and Woolf, C. J. (2002a). ERK MAP kinase activation in superficial spinal cord neurons induces prodynorphin and NK-1 upregulation and contributes to persistent inflammatory pain hypersensitivity. *J. Neurosci.* 22, 478–485. doi: 10.1523/JNEUROSCI.22-02-00478.2002

Ji, R. R., Gereau, R. W. IV, Malcangio, M., and Strichartz, G. R. (2009). MAP kinase and pain. *Brain Res. Rev.* 60, 135–148. doi: 10.1016/j.brainresrev.2008.12.011

Ji, R. R., Samad, T. A., Jin, S. X., Schmoll, R., and Woolf, C. J. (2002b). p38 MAPK activation by NGF in primary sensory neurons after inflammation increases TRPV1 levels and maintains heat hyperalgesia. *Neuron* 36, 57–68. doi: 10.1016/S0896-6273(02)00908-X

Ji, R. R., and Suter, M. R. (2007). p38 MAPK, microglial signaling, and neuropathic pain. *Mol. Pain* 3:33. doi: 10.1186/1744-8069-3-33

Jin, S. X., Zhuang, Z. Y., Woolf, C. J., and Ji, R. R. (2003). p38 mitogen-activated protein kinase is activated after a spinal nerve ligation in spinal cord microglia and dorsal root ganglion neurons and contributes to the generation of neuropathic pain. *J. Neurosci.* 23, 4017–4022. doi: 10.1523/JNEUROSCI.23-10-04017.2003

Julius, D. (2013). TRP channels and pain. *Annu. Rev. Cell Dev. Biol.* 29, 355–384. doi: 10.1146/annurev-cellbio-101011-155833

Kawasaki, Y., Xu, Z. Z., Wang, X., Park, J. Y., Zhuang, Z. Y., Tan, P. H., et al. (2008). Distinct roles of matrix metalloproteases in the early- and late-phase development of neuropathic pain. *Nat. Med.* 14, 331–336. doi: 10.1038/nm1723

Keller, A. F., Beggs, S., Salter, M. W., and De Koninck, Y. (2007). Transformation of the output of spinal lamina I neurons after nerve injury and microglia stimulation underlying neuropathic pain. *Mol. Pain* 3:27. doi: 10.1186/1744-8069-3-27

Kennedy, J. M., and Zochodne, D. W. (2005). Impaired peripheral nerve regeneration in diabetes mellitus. *J. Peripher. Nerv. Syst.* 10, 144–157. doi: 10.1111/j.1085-9489.2005.0010205.x

Kerr, B. J., Souslova, V., McMahon, S. B., and Wood, J. N. (2001). A role for the TTX-resistant sodium channel Nav 1.8 in NGF-induced hyperalgesia, but not neuropathic pain. *Neuroreport* 12, 3077–3080. doi: 10.1097/00001756-200110080-00019

Khoutorsky, A., and Price, T. J. (2017). Translational control mechanisms in persistent pain. *Trends Neurosci.* 41, 100–114. doi: 10.1016/j.tins.2017.11.006

Kim, D., Kim, M. A., Cho, I. H., Kim, M. S., Lee, S., Jo, E. K., et al. (2007). A critical role of toll-like receptor 2 in nerve injury-induced spinal cord glial cell activation and pain hypersensitivity. *J. Biol. Chem.* 282, 14975–14983. doi: 10.1074/jbc.M607277200

King, G. L., and Loeken, M. R. (2004). Hyperglycemia-induced oxidative stress in diabetic complications. *Histochem. Cell Biol.* 122, 333–338. doi: 10.1007/s00418-004-0678-9

King, R. H. (2001). The role of glycation in the pathogenesis of diabetic polyneuropathy. *Mol. Pathol.* 54, 400–408. doi: 10.1136/mp.54.6.400

King, R. H., Llewelyn, J. G., Thomas, P. K., Gilbey, S. G., and Watkins, P. J. (1989). Diabetic neuropathy: abnormalities of Schwann cell and perineurial basal laminae. Implications for diabetic vasculopathy. *Neuropathol. Appl. Neurobiol.* 15, 339–355. doi: 10.1111/j.1365-2990.1989.tb01234.x

Knip, M., and Siljander, H. (2008). Autoimmune mechanisms in type 1 diabetes. *Autoimmun. Rev.* 7, 550–557. doi: 10.1016/j.autrev.2008.04.008

Kostyuk, E., Voitenko, N., Kruglikov, I., Shmigol, A., Shishkin, V., Efimov, A., et al. (2001). Diabetes-induced changes in calcium homeostasis and the effects of calcium channel blockers in rat and mice nociceptive neurons. *Diabetologia* 44, 1302–1309. doi: 10.1007/s001250100642

Kramer, H. H., Schmelz, M., Birklein, F., and Bickel, A. (2004). Electrically stimulated axon reflexes are diminished in diabetic small fiber neuropathies. *Diabetes* 53, 769–774. doi: 10.2337/diabetes.53.3.769

Kumar, V., Abbas, A. K., Fausto, N., Robbins, S. L., and Cotran, R. S. (2005). *Robbins and Cotran Pathologic Basis of Disease*. Philadelphia, PA: Elsevier Saunders.

Larsen, J. R., and Sidenius, P. (1989). Slow axonal transport of structural polypeptides in rat, early changes in streptozocin diabetes, and effect of insulin treatment. *J. Neurochem.* 52, 390–401. doi: 10.1111/j.1471-4159.1989.tb09134.x

Lassmann, H., Schmied, M., Vass, K., and Hickey, W. F. (1993). Bone marrow derived elements and resident microglia in brain inflammation. *Glia* 7, 19–24. doi: 10.1002/glia.440070106

Lawson, L. J., Perry, V. H., and Gordon, S. (1992). Turnover of resident microglia in the normal adult mouse brain. *Neuroscience* 48, 405–415. doi: 10.1016/0306-4522(92)90500-2

Leinninger, G. M., Backus, C., Sastry, A. M., Yi, Y. B., Wang, C. W., and Feldman, E. L. (2006). Mitochondria in DRG neurons undergo hyperglycemic mediated injury through Bim, Bax and the fission protein Drp1. *Neurobiol. Dis.* 23, 11–22. doi: 10.1016/j.nbd.2006.01.017

Li, J., Baud, O., Vartanian, T., Volpe, J. J., and Rosenberg, P. A. (2005). Peroxynitrite generated by inducible nitric oxide synthase and NADPH oxidase mediates microglial toxicity to oligodendrocytes. *Proc. Natl. Acad. Sci. U.S.A.* 102, 9936–9941. doi: 10.1073/pnas.0502552102

Li, Y., and Kim, J. (2017). Distinct roles of neuronal and microglial CB2 cannabinoid receptors in the mouse hippocampus. *Neuroscience* 363, 11–25. doi: 10.1016/j.neuroscience.2017.08.053

Lin, W.-W. (2017). Trehalose-6, 6′-dibehenate inhibits lipopolysaccharide-induced NF-κB activation via PLC-γ1-PKC-ERK signaling and promotes M2 microglial polarization. *Am. Assoc. Immnol.* 198 (Suppl. 1), 129.14.

Liu, B., Tai, Y., Achanta, S., Kaelberer, M. M., Caceres, A. I., Shao, X., et al. (2016). IL-33/ST2 signaling excites sensory neurons and mediates itch response in a mouse model of poison ivy contact allergy. *Proc. Natl. Acad. Sci. U.S.A.* 113, E7572–E7579. doi: 10.1073/pnas.1606608113

Liu, X. S., Fan, B., Szalad, A., Jia, L., Wang, L., Wang, X., et al. (2017). MicroRNA-146a mimics reduce the peripheral neuropathy in type 2 diabetic mice. *Diabetes* 66, 3111–3121. doi: 10.2337/db16-1182

Longo, F. M., Powell, H. C., Lebeau, J., Gerrero, M. R., Heckman, H., and Myers, R. R. (1986). Delayed nerve regeneration in streptozotocin diabetic rats. *Muscle Nerve* 9, 385–393. doi: 10.1002/mus.880090502

Ludbrook, V. J., Hicks, K. J., Hanrott, K. E., Patel, J. S., Binks, M. H., Wyres, M. R., et al. (2016). Investigation of selective JAK1 inhibitor GSK2586184 for the treatment of psoriasis in a randomized placebo-controlled phase IIa study. *Br. J. Dermatol.* 174, 985–995. doi: 10.1111/bjd.14399

Lyssenko, V. (2008). The transcription factor 7-like 2 gene and increased risk of type 2 diabetes: an update. *Curr. Opin. Clin. Nutr. Metab. Care* 11, 385–392. doi: 10.1097/MCO.0b013e328304d970

Malin, S. A., Molliver, D. C., Koerber, H. R., Cornuet, P., Frye, R., Albers, K. M., et al. (2006). Glial cell line-derived neurotrophic factor family members sensitize nociceptors *in vitro* and produce thermal hyperalgesia *in vivo*. *J. Neurosci.* 26, 8588–8599. doi: 10.1523/JNEUROSCI.1726-06.2006

Mapplebeck, J. C. S., Dalgarno, R., Tu, Y., Moriarty, O., Beggs, S., Kwok, C. H. T., et al. (2018). Microglial P2X4R-evoked pain hypersensitivity is sexually dimorphic in rats. *Pain* 159, 1752–1763. doi: 10.1097/j.pain.0000000000001265

Marchand, F., Perretti, M., and McMahon, S. B. (2005). Role of the immune system in chronic pain. *Nat. Rev. Neurosci.* 6, 521–532. doi: 10.1038/nrn1700

Marieb, E. N., Kollett, L. S., and Zao, P. Z. (2009). *Human Anatomy & Physiology Laboratory Manual*. San Francisco, CA: Pearson/Benjamin Cummings.

Masuda, T., Ozono, Y., Mikuriya, S., Kohro, Y., Tozaki-Saitoh, H., Iwatsuki, K., et al. (2016). Dorsal horn neurons release extracellular ATP in a VNUT-dependent manner that underlies neuropathic pain. *Nat. Commun.* 7:12529. doi: 10.1038/ncomms12529

Mathieu, C., Gysemans, C., Giulietti, A., and Bouillon, R. (2005). Vitamin D and diabetes. *Diabetologia* 48, 1247–1257. doi: 10.1007/s00125-005-1802-7

Matsui, T., Svensson, C. I., Hirata, Y., Mizobata, K., Hua, X. Y., and Yaksh, T. L. (2010). Release of prostaglandin E(2) and nitric oxide from spinal microglia is dependent on activation of p38 mitogen-activated protein kinase. *Anesth. Analg.* 111, 554–560. doi: 10.1213/ANE.0b013e3181e3a2a2

McMahon, S. B., Cafferty, W. B., and Marchand, F. (2005). Immune and glial cell factors as pain mediators and modulators. *Exp. Neurol.* 192, 444–462. doi: 10.1016/j.expneurol.2004.11.001

McMahon, S. B., La Russa, F., and Bennett, D. L. (2015). Crosstalk between the nociceptive and immune systems in host defence and disease. *Nat. Rev. Neurosci.* 16, 389–402. doi: 10.1038/nrn3946

Metz, T. O., Alderson, N. L., Thorpe, S. R., and Baynes, J. W. (2003). Pyridoxamine, an inhibitor of advanced glycation and lipoxidation reactions: a novel therapy for treatment of diabetic complications. *Arch. Biochem. Biophys.* 419, 41–49. doi: 10.1016/j.abb.2003.08.021

Midaoui, A. E., Talbot, S., Lahjouji, K., Dias, J. P., Fantus, I. G., and Couture, R. (2015). Effects of alpha-lipoic acid on oxidative stress and kinin receptor expression in obese zucker diabetic fatty rats. *J. Diabetes Metab.* 6, 1–7. doi: 10.4172/2155-6156.1000556

Miki, K., Fukuoka, T., Tokunaga, A., and Noguchi, K. (1998). Calcitonin gene-related peptide increase in the rat spinal dorsal horn and dorsal column nucleus following peripheral nerve injury: up-regulation in a subpopulation of primary afferent sensory neurons. *Neuroscience* 82, 1243–1252. doi: 10.1016/S0306-4522(97)00258-3

Milligan, E., Zapata, V., Schoeniger, D., Chacur, M., Green, P., Poole, S., et al. (2005). An initial investigation of spinal mechanisms underlying pain enhancement induced by fractalkine, a neuronally released chemokine. *Eur. J. Neurosci.* 22, 2775–2782. doi: 10.1111/j.1460-9568.2005.04470.x

Milligan, E. D., Sloane, E. M., and Watkins, L. R. (2008). Glia in pathological pain: a role for fractalkine. *J. Neuroimmunol.* 198, 113–120. doi: 10.1016/j.jneuroim.2008.04.011

Milligan, E. D., and Watkins, L. R. (2009). Pathological and protective roles of glia in chronic pain. *Nat. Rev. Neurosci.* 10, 23–36. doi: 10.1038/nrn2533

Milligan, E. D., Zapata, V., Chacur, M., Schoeniger, D., Biedenkapp, J., O'Connor, K. A., et al. (2004). Evidence that exogenous and endogenous fractalkine can induce spinal nociceptive facilitation in rats. *Eur. J. Neurosci.* 20, 2294–2302. doi: 10.1111/j.1460-9568.2004.03709.x

Misawa, S., Kuwabara, S., Kanai, K., Tamura, N., Hiraga, A., Nakata, M., et al. (2005). Axonal potassium conductance and glycemic control in human diabetic nerves. *Clin. Neurophysiol.* 116, 1181–1187. doi: 10.1016/j.clinph.2004.12.019

Misawa, S., Sakurai, K., Shibuya, K., Isose, S., Kanai, K., Ogino, J., et al. (2009). Neuropathic pain is associated with increased nodal persistent Na(+) currents in human diabetic neuropathy. *J. Peripher. Nerv. Syst.* 14, 279–284. doi: 10.1111/j.1529-8027.2009.00239.x

Molines, L., Darmon, P., and Raccah, D. (2010). Charcot's foot: newest findings on its pathophysiology, diagnosis and treatment. *Diabetes Metab.* 36, 251–255. doi: 10.1016/j.diabet.2010.04.002

Monnier, V. M. (2003). Intervention against the Maillard reaction *in vivo*. *Arch. Biochem. Biophys.* 419, 1–15. doi: 10.1016/j.abb.2003.08.014

Mori, T., Miyamoto, T., Yoshida, H., Asakawa, M., Kawasumi, M., Kobayashi, T., et al. (2011). IL-1beta and TNFalpha-initiated IL-6-STAT3 pathway is critical in mediating inflammatory cytokines and RANKL expression in inflammatory arthritis. *Int. Immunol.* 23, 701–712. doi: 10.1093/intimm/dxr077

Mosley, K., and Cuzner, M. L. (1996). Receptor-mediated phagocytosis of myelin by macrophages and microglia: effect of opsonization and receptor blocking agents. *Neurochem. Res.* 21, 481–487. doi: 10.1007/BF02527713

Narita, M., Yoshida, T., Nakajima, M., Miyatake, M., Takagi, T., Yajima, Y., et al. (2006). Direct evidence for spinal cord microglia in the development of a neuropathic pain-like state in mice. *J. Neurochem.* 97, 1337–1348. doi: 10.1111/j.1471-4159.2006.03808.x

Nassar, M. A., Stirling, L. C., Forlani, G., Baker, M. D., Matthews, E. A., Dickenson, A. H., et al. (2004). Nociceptor-specific gene deletion reveals a major role for Nav1.7 (PN1) in acute and inflammatory pain. *Proc. Natl. Acad. Sci. U.S.A.* 101, 12706–12711. doi: 10.1073/pnas.0404915101

Nestor, J., Arinuma, Y., Huerta, T. S., Kowal, C., Nasiri, E., Kello, N., et al. (2018). Lupus antibodies induce behavioral changes mediated by microglia and blocked by ACE inhibitors. *J. Exp. Med.* 215, 2554–2566. doi: 10.1084/jem.20180776

Nishikawa, T., Edelstein, D., Du, X. L., Yamagishi, S., Matsumura, T., Kaneda, Y., et al. (2000). Normalizing mitochondrial superoxide production blocks three pathways of hyperglycaemic damage. *Nature* 404, 787–790. doi: 10.1038/35008121

Noda, M., Kariura, Y., Pannasch, U., Nishikawa, K., Wang, L., Seike, T., et al. (2007). Neuroprotective role of bradykinin because of the attenuation of pro-inflammatory cytokine release from activated microglia. *J. Neurochem.* 101, 397–410. doi: 10.1111/j.1471-4159.2006.04339.x

Noguchi, H. (2009). Pancreatic islet transplantation. *World J. Gastrointest. Surg.* 1, 16–20. doi: 10.4240/wjgs.v1.i1.16

Noguchi, H. (2010). Pancreatic stem/progenitor cells for the treatment of diabetes. *Rev. Diabet. Stud.* 7, 105–111. doi: 10.1900/RDS.2010.7.105

Oates, P. J. (2002). Polyol pathway and diabetic peripheral neuropathy. *Int. Rev. Neurobiol.* 50, 325–392. doi: 10.1016/S0074-7742(02)50082-9

Oates, P. J. (2008). Aldose reductase, still a compelling target for diabetic neuropathy. *Curr. Drug Targets* 9, 14–36. doi: 10.2174/138945008783431781

Obrosova, I. G. (2009). Diabetic painful and insensate neuropathy: pathogenesis and potential treatments. *Neurotherapeutics* 6, 638–647. doi: 10.1016/j.nurt.2009.07.004

Oetjen, L. K., Mack, M. R., Feng, J., Whelan, T. M., Niu, H., Guo, C. J., et al. (2017). Sensory neurons Co-opt classical immune signaling pathways to mediate chronic itch. *Cell* 171, 217–228 e13. doi: 10.1016/j.cell.2017.08.006

Oka, M., and Kato, N. (2001). Aldose reductase inhibitors. *J. Enzym. Inhib.* 16, 465–473. doi: 10.1080/14756360127568

Opree, A., and Kress, M. (2000). Involvement of the proinflammatory cytokines tumor necrosis factor-alpha, IL-1 beta, and IL-6 but not IL-8 in the development of heat hyperalgesia: effects on heat-evoked calcitonin gene-related peptide release from rat skin. *J. Neurosci.* 20, 6289–6293. doi: 10.1523/JNEUROSCI.20-16-06289.2000

Orman, D., Vardi, N., Ates, B., Taslidere, E., and Elbe, H. (2015). Aminoguanidine mitigates apoptosis, testicular seminiferous tubules damage, and oxidative stress in streptozotocin-induced diabetic rats. *Tissue Cell.* 47, 284–290. doi: 10.1016/j.tice.2015.03.006

Oyama, T., Miyasita, Y., Watanabe, H., and Shirai, K. (2006). The role of polyol pathway in high glucose-induced endothelial cell damages. *Diabetes Res. Clin Pract.* 73, 227–234. doi: 10.1016/j.diabres.2006.02.010

Oyenihi, A. B., Ayeleso, A. O., Mukwevho, E., and Masola, B. (2015). Antioxidant strategies in the management of diabetic neuropathy. *Biomed. Res. Int.* 2015:515042. doi: 10.1155/2015/515042

Pabreja, K., Dua, K., Sharma, S., Padi, S. S., and Kulkarni, S. K. (2011). Minocycline attenuates the development of diabetic neuropathic pain: possible anti inflammatory and anti-oxidant mechanisms. *Eur. J. Pharmacol.* 661, 15–21. doi: 10.1016/j.ejphar.2011.04.014

Paulson, P. E., Wiley, J. W., and Morrow, T. J. (2007). Concurrent activation of the somatosensory forebrain and deactivation of periaqueductal gray associated with diabetes-induced neuropathic pain. *Exp. Neurol.* 208, 305–313. doi: 10.1016/j.expneurol.2007.09.001

Pereira, P. J., Machado, G. D., Danesi, G. M., Canevese, F. F., Reddy, V. B., Pereira, T. C., et al. (2015). GRPR/PI3Kgamma: partners in central transmission of itch. *J. Neurosci.* 35, 16272–16281. doi: 10.1523/JNEUROSCI.2310-15.2015

Petrenko, A. B., Yamakura, T., Baba, H., and Shimoji, K. (2003). The role of N-methyl-D-aspartate (NMDA) receptors in pain: a review. *Anesth. Analg.* 97, 1108–1116. doi: 10.1213/01.ANE.0000081061.12235.55

Piotrowska, A., Kwiatkowski, K., Rojewska, E., Makuch, W., and Mika, J. (2016). Maraviroc reduces neuropathic pain through polarization of microglia and astroglia - Evidence from *in vivo* and *in vitro* studies. *Neuropharmacology* 108, 207–219. doi: 10.1016/j.neuropharm.2016.04.024

Pocock, J. M., and Kettenmann, H. (2007). Neurotransmitter receptors on microglia. *Trends Neurosci.* 30, 527–535. doi: 10.1016/j.tins.2007.07.007

Pop-Busui, R., Sima, A., and Stevens, M. (2006). Diabetic neuropathy and oxidative stress. *Diabetes Metab. Res. Rev.* 22, 257–273. doi: 10.1002/dmrr.625

Popiolek-Barczyk, K., and Mika, J. (2016). Targeting the microglial signaling pathways: new insights in the modulation of neuropathic pain. *Curr. Med. Chem.* 23, 2908–2928. doi: 10.2174/0929867323666160607120124

Prabodha, L. B. L., Sirisena, N. D., and Dissanayake, V. H. W. (2018). Susceptible and prognostic genetic factors associated with diabetic peripheral neuropathy: a comprehensive literature review. *Int. J. Endocrinol.* 2018:8641942. doi: 10.1155/2018/8641942

Quan, X., Lim, S. O., and Jung, G. (2011). Reactive oxygen species downregulate catalase expression via methylation of a CpG Island in the Oct-1 promoter. *FEBS Lett.* 585, 3436–3441. doi: 10.1016/j.febslet.2011.09.035

Quan, Y., Du, J., and Wang, X. (2007). High glucose stimulates GRO secretion from rat microglia via ROS, PKC, and NF-kappaB pathways. *J. Neurosci. Res.* 85, 3150–3159. doi: 10.1002/jnr.21421

Raccah, D. (1998). Physiopathology of diabetic neuropathies. Functional exploration of peripheral involvement. *Diabetes Metab.* 24 (Suppl. 3), 73–78.

Ribeiro, R., Wen, J., Li, S., and Zhang, Y. (2013). Involvement of ERK1/2, cPLA2 and NF-kappaB in microglia suppression by cannabinoid receptor agonists and antagonists. *Prostaglandins Other Lipid Mediat.* 100–101, 1–14. doi: 10.1016/j.prostaglandins.2012.11.003

Riddell, D. R., and Owen, J. S. (1999). Nitric oxide and platelet aggregation. *Vitam. Horm.* 57, 25–48. doi: 10.1016/S0083-6729(08)60639-1

Riol-Blanco, L., Ordovas-Montanes, J., Perro, M., Naval, E., Thiriot, A., Alvarez, D., et al. (2014). Nociceptive sensory neurons drive interleukin-23-mediated psoriasiform skin inflammation. *Nature* 510, 157–161. doi: 10.1038/nature13199

Romero-Sandoval, E. A., Horvath, R. J., and DeLeo, J. A. (2008). Neuroimmune interactions and pain: focus on glial-modulating targets. *Curr. Opin. Investig. Drugs* 9, 726–734.

Rosas-Ballina, M., Olofsson, P. S., Ochani, M., Valdes-Ferrer, S. I., Levine, Y. A., Reardon, C., et al. (2011). Acetylcholine-synthesizing T cells relay neural signals in a vagus nerve circuit. *Science* 334, 98–101. doi: 10.1126/science.1209985

Rother, K. I. (2007). Diabetes treatment–bridging the divide. *N. Engl. J. Med.* 356, 1499–1501. doi: 10.1056/NEJMp078030

Said, G. (2007). Diabetic neuropathy–a review. *Nat. Clin. Pract. Neurol.* 3, 331–340. doi: 10.1038/ncpneuro0504

Said, G., Lacroix, C., Lozeron, P., Ropert, A., Plante, V., and Adams, D. (2003). Inflammatory vasculopathy in multifocal diabetic neuropathy. *Brain* 126, 376–385. doi: 10.1093/brain/awg029

Salter, M. W., and Stevens, B. (2017). Microglia emerge as central players in brain disease. *Nat. Med.* 23, 1018–1027. doi: 10.1038/nm.4397

Samad, T. A., Moore, K. A., Sapirstein, A., Billet, S., Allchorne, A., Poole, S., et al. (2001). Interleukin-1beta-mediated induction of Cox-2 in the CNS contributes to inflammatory pain hypersensitivity. *Nature* 410, 471–475. doi: 10.1038/35068566

Samad, T. A., Sapirstein, A., and Woolf, C. J. (2002). Prostanoids and pain: unraveling mechanisms and revealing therapeutic targets. *Trends Mol. Med.* 8, 390–396. doi: 10.1016/S1471-4914(02)02383-3

Schemmel, K. E., Padiyara, R. S., and D'Souza, J. J. (2009). Aldose reductase inhibitors in the treatment of diabetic peripheral neuropathy: a review. *J. Diabetes Complications* 24, 354–360. doi: 10.1016/j.jdiacomp.2009.07.005

Scholz, J., and Woolf, C. J. (2002). Can we conquer pain? *Nat. Neurosci.* 5 (Suppl.), 1062–1067. doi: 10.1038/nn942

Scholz, J., and Woolf, C. J. (2007). The neuropathic pain triad: neurons, immune cells and glia. *Nat. Neurosci.* 10, 1361–1368. doi: 10.1038/nn1992

Shi, Q., Chowdhury, S., Ma, R., Le, K. X., Hong, S., Caldarone, B. J., et al. (2017). Complement C3 deficiency protects against neurodegeneration in aged plaque-rich APP/PS1 mice. *Sci. Transl. Med.* 9:eaaf6295. doi: 10.1126/scitranslmed.aaf6295

Shim, W. S., Tak, M. H., Lee, M. H., Kim, M., Kim, M., Koo, J. Y., et al. (2007). TRPV1 mediates histamine-induced itching via the activation of phospholipase A2 and 12-lipoxygenase. *J. Neurosci.* 27, 2331–2337. doi: 10.1523/JNEUROSCI.4643-06.2007

Singh Grewal, A., Bhardwaj, S., Pandita, D., Lather, V., and Sekhon, B. S. (2016). Updates on aldose reductase inhibitors for management of diabetic complications and non-diabetic diseases. *Mini. Rev. Med. Chem.* 16, 120–162. doi: 10.2174/1389557515666150909143737

Singh, V. P., Bali, A., Singh, N., Jaggi, A. S. (2014). Advanced glycation end products and diabetic complications. *Korean J. Physiol. Pharmacol.* 18, 1–14. doi: 10.4196/kjpp.2014.18.1.1

Sorge, R. E., Mapplebeck, J. C., Rosen, S., Beggs, S., Taves, S., Alexander, J. K., et al. (2015). Different immune cells mediate mechanical pain hypersensitivity in male and female mice. *Nat. Neurosci.* 18, 1081–1083. doi: 10.1038/nn.4053

Spruce, M. C., Potter, J., and Coppini, D. V. (2003). The pathogenesis and management of painful diabetic neuropathy: a review. *Diabet. Med.* 20, 88–98. doi: 10.1046/j.1464-5491.2003.00852.x

Stellwagen, D., and Malenka, R. C. (2006). Synaptic scaling mediated by glial TNF-alpha. *Nature* 440, 1054–1059. doi: 10.1038/nature04671

Sugimoto, K., Yasujima, M., and Yagihashi, S. (2008). Role of advanced glycation end products in diabetic neuropathy. *Curr. Pharm. Des.* 14, 953–961. doi: 10.2174/138161208784139774

Sun, J. S., Yang, Y. J., Zhang, Y. Z., Huang, W., Li, Z. S., and Zhang, Y. (2015). Minocycline attenuates pain by inhibiting spinal microglia activation in diabetic rats. *Mol. Med. Rep.* 12, 2677–2682. doi: 10.3892/mmr.2015.3735

Sun, S., Cao, H., Han, M., Li, T. T., Pan, H. L., Zhao, Z. Q., et al. (2007). New evidence for the involvement of spinal fractalkine receptor in pain facilitation and spinal glial activation in rat model of monoarthritis. *Pain* 129, 64–75. doi: 10.1016/j.pain.2006.09.035

Svensson, C. I., Fitzsimmons, B., Azizi, S., Powell, H. C., Hua, X. Y., and Yaksh, T. L. (2005). Spinal p38beta isoform mediates tissue injury-induced hyperalgesia and spinal sensitization. *J. Neurochem.* 92, 1508–1520. doi: 10.1111/j.1471-4159.2004.02996.x

Sweitzer, S. M., White, K. A., Dutta, C., and DeLeo, J. A. (2002). The differential role of spinal MHC class II and cellular adhesion molecules in peripheral inflammatory versus neuropathic pain in rodents. *J. Neuroimmunol.* 125, 82–93. doi: 10.1016/S0165-5728(02)00036-X

Talbot, S., Abdulnour, R. E., Burkett, P. R., Lee, S., Cronin, S. J., Pascal, M. A., et al. (2015). Silencing nociceptor neurons reduces allergic airway inflammation. *Neuron* 87, 341–354. doi: 10.1016/j.neuron.2015.06.007

Talbot, S., Chahmi, E., Dias, J. P., and Couture, R. (2010). Key role for spinal dorsal horn microglial kinin B1 receptor in early diabetic pain neuropathy. *J. Neuroinflamm.* 7:36. doi: 10.1186/1742-2094-7-36

Talbot, S., De Brito Gariepy, H., Saint-Denis, J., and Couture, R. (2012). Activation of kinin B1 receptor evokes hyperthermia through a vagal sensory mechanism in the rat. *J. Neuroinflamm.* 9:214. doi: 10.1186/1742-2094-9-214

Talbot, S., Dias, J. P., El Midaoui, A., and Couture, R. (2016a). Beneficial effects of kinin B1 receptor antagonism on plasma fatty acid alterations and obesity in Zucker diabetic fatty rats. *Can. J. Physiol. Pharmacol.* 94, 752–757. doi: 10.1139/cjpp-2016-0063

Talbot, S., Foster, S. L., and Woolf, C. J. (2016b). Neuroimmunity: physiology and pathology. *Annu. Rev. Immunol.* 34, 421–447. doi: 10.1146/annurev-immunol-041015-055340

Tanga, F. Y., Nutile-McMenemy, N., and DeLeo, J. A. (2005). The CNS role of Toll-like receptor 4 in innate neuroimmunity and painful neuropathy. *Proc. Natl. Acad. Sci. U.S.A.* 102, 5856–5861. doi: 10.1073/pnas.0501634102

Tanga, F. Y., Raghavendra, V., and DeLeo, J. A. (2004). Quantitative real-time RT-PCR assessment of spinal microglial and astrocytic activation markers in a rat model of neuropathic pain. *Neurochem. Int.* 45, 397–407. doi: 10.1016/j.neuint.2003.06.002

Taylor, A. M., Castonguay, A., Ghogha, A., Vayssiere, P., Pradhan, A. A., Xue, L., et al. (2016). Neuroimmune regulation of GABAergic neurons within the ventral tegmental area during withdrawal from chronic morphine. *Neuropsychopharmacology* 41, 949–959. doi: 10.1038/npp.2015.221

Taylor, A. M., Castonguay, A., Taylor, A. J., Murphy, N. P., Ghogha, A., Cook, C., et al. (2015). Microglia disrupt mesolimbic reward circuitry in chronic pain. *J. Neurosci.* 35, 8442–8450. doi: 10.1523/JNEUROSCI.4036-14.2015

Tender, G. C., Li, Y. Y., and Cui, J. G. (2010). Brain-derived neurotrophic factor redistribution in the dorsal root ganglia correlates with neuropathic pain inhibition after resiniferatoxin treatment. *Spine J.* 10, 715–720. doi: 10.1016/j.spinee.2010.03.029

Tesfaye, S., and Kempler, P. (2005). Painful diabetic neuropathy. *Diabetologia* 48, 805–807. doi: 10.1007/s00125-005-1721-7

Thacker, M. A., Clark, A. K., Bishop, T., Grist, J., Yip, P. K., Moon, L. D., et al. (2009). CCL2 is a key mediator of microglia activation in neuropathic pain states. *Eur. J. Pain* 13, 263–272. doi: 10.1016/j.ejpain.2008.04.017

Thamotharampillai, K., Chan, A. K., Bennetts, B., Craig, M. E., Cusumano, J., Silink, M., et al. (2006). Decline in neurophysiological function after 7 years in an adolescent diabetic cohort and the role of aldose reductase gene polymorphisms. *Diabetes Care* 29, 2053–2057. doi: 10.2337/dc06-0678

Thornalley, P. J. (1998). Cell activation by glycated proteins. AGE receptors, receptor recognition factors and functional classification of AGEs. *Cell Mol. Biol.* 44, 1013–1023.

Tomlinson, D. R., Fernyhough, P., and Diemel, L. T. (1997). Role of neurotrophins in diabetic neuropathy and treatment with nerve growth factors. *Diabetes* 46 (Suppl. 2), S43–S49. doi: 10.2337/diab.46.2.S43

Torsney, C., and MacDermott, A. B. (2005). Neuroscience: a painful factor. *Nature* 438, 923–925. doi: 10.1038/438923a

Tsuda, M., and Inoue, K. (2016). Neuron-microglia interaction by purinergic signaling in neuropathic pain following neurodegeneration. *Neuropharmacology* 104, 76–81. doi: 10.1016/j.neuropharm.2015.08.042

Tsuda, M., Inoue, K., and Salter, M. W. (2005). Neuropathic pain and spinal microglia: a big problem from molecules in "small" glia. *Trends Neurosci.* 28, 101–107. doi: 10.1016/j.tins.2004.12.002

Tsuda, M., Mizokoshi, A., Shigemoto-Mogami, Y., Koizumi, S., and Inoue, K. (2004). Activation of p38 mitogen-activated protein kinase in spinal hyperactive microglia contributes to pain hypersensitivity following peripheral nerve injury. *Glia* 45, 89–95. doi: 10.1002/glia.10308

Tsuda, M., Shigemoto-Mogami, Y., Koizumi, S., Mizokoshi, A., Kohsaka, S., Salter, M. W., et al. (2003). P2X4 receptors induced in spinal microglia gate tactile allodynia after nerve injury. *Nature* 424, 778–783. doi: 10.1038/nature01786

Tuck, R. R., Schmelzer, J. D., and Low, P. A. (1984). Endoneurial blood flow and oxygen tension in the sciatic nerves of rats with experimental diabetic neuropathy. *Brain* 107(Pt 3), 935–950.

Twig, G., Elorza, A., Molina, A. J., Mohamed, H., Wikstrom, J. D., Walzer, G., et al. (2008). Fission and selective fusion govern mitochondrial segregation and elimination by autophagy. *EMBO J.* 27, 433–446. doi: 10.1038/sj.emboj.7601963

Vague, P., Dufayet, D., Lamotte, M. F., Mouchot, C., and Raccah, D. (1997). Genetic factors, Na K ATPase activity and neuropathy in diabetics. *Bull. Acad. Natl. Med.* 181, 1811–1821; discussion 1821–1823.

Vardeh, D., Wang, D., Costigan, M., Lazarus, M., Saper, C. B., Woolf, C. J., et al. (2009). COX2 in CNS neural cells mediates mechanical inflammatory pain hypersensitivity in mice. *J. Clin. Invest.* 119, 287–294. doi: 10.1172/JCI37098

Vareniuk, I., Pavlov, I. A., and Obrosova, I. G. (2008). Inducible nitric oxide synthase gene deficiency counteracts multiple manifestations of peripheral neuropathy in a streptozotocin-induced mouse model of diabetes. *Diabetologia* 51, 2126–2133. doi: 10.1007/s00125-008-1136-3

Veiga-Fernandes, H., and Mucida, D. (2016). Neuro-immune interactions at barrier surfaces. *Cell* 165, 801–811. doi: 10.1016/j.cell.2016.04.041

Verge, G. M., Milligan, E. D., Maier, S. F., Watkins, L. R., Naeve, G. S., and Foster, A. C. (2004). Fractalkine (CX3CL1) and fractalkine receptor (CX3CR1) distribution in spinal cord and dorsal root ganglia under basal and neuropathic pain conditions. *Eur. J. Neurosci.* 20, 1150–1160. doi: 10.1111/j.1460-9568.2004.03593.x

Vincent, A. M., Edwards, J. L., Sadidi, M., and Feldman, E. L. (2008). The antioxidant response as a drug target in diabetic neuropathy. *Curr. Drug Targets* 9, 94–100. doi: 10.2174/138945008783431754

Virtanen, S. M., Saukkonen, T., Savilahti, E., Ylonen, K., Rasanen, L., Aro, A., et al. (1994). Diet, cow's milk protein antibodies and the risk of IDDM in Finnish children. Childhood diabetes in finland study group. *Diabetologia* 37, 381–387. doi: 10.1007/BF00408475

Viviani, B., Bartesaghi, S., Gardoni, F., Vezzani, A., Behrens, M. M., Bartfai, T., et al. (2003). Interleukin-1beta enhances NMDA receptor-mediated intracellular calcium increase through activation of the Src family of kinases. *J. Neurosci.* 23, 8692–8700. doi: 10.1523/JNEUROSCI.23-25-08692.2003

von Hehn, C. A., Baron, R., and C.,Woolf, J. J. N. (2012). Deconstructing the neuropathic pain phenotype to reveal neural mechanisms. *Neuron* 73, 638–652. doi: 10.1016/j.neuron.2012.02.008

Wabitsch, M., Funcke, J. B., von Schnurbein, J., Denzer, F., Lahr, G., Mazen, I., et al. (2015). Severe early-onset obesity due to bioinactive leptin caused by a p.N103K mutation in the leptin gene. *J. Clin. Endocrinol. Metab.* 100, 3227–3230. doi: 10.1210/jc.2015-2263

Wagner, R., and Myers, R. R. (1996). Endoneurial injection of TNF-alpha produces neuropathic pain behaviors. *Neuroreport* 7, 2897–2901. doi: 10.1097/00001756-199611250-00018

Wall, P. D., and Gutnick, M. (1974). Ongoing activity in peripheral nerves: the physiology and pharmacology of impulses originating from a neuroma. *Exp. Neurol.* 43, 580–593. doi: 10.1016/0014-4886(74)90197-6

Watkins, L. R., Milligan, E. D., and Maier, S. F. (2001a). Glial activation: a driving force for pathological pain. *Trends Neurosci.* 24, 450–455. doi: 10.1016/S0166-2236(00)01854-3

Watkins, L. R., Milligan, E. D., and Maier, S. F. (2001b). Spinal cord glia: new players in pain. *Pain* 93, 201–205. doi: 10.1016/S0304-3959(01)00359-1

White, F. A., Jung, H., and Miller, R. J. (2007). Chemokines and the pathophysiology of neuropathic pain. *Proc. Natl. Acad. Sci. U.S.A.* 104, 20151–20158. doi: 10.1073/pnas.0709250104

WHO (2016). *Global Report on Diabetes*. Geneva: World Health Organization.

Wilson, S. R., The, L., Batia, L. M., Beattie, K., Katibah, G. E., McClain, S. P., et al. (2013). The epithelial cell-derived atopic dermatitis cytokine TSLP activates neurons to induce itch. *Cell* 155, 285–295. doi: 10.1016/j.cell.2013.08.057

Wodarski, R., Clark, A. K., Grist, J., Marchand, F., and Malcangio, M. (2009). Gabapentin reverses microglial activation in the spinal cord of streptozotocin-induced diabetic rats. *Eur. J. Pain* 13, 807–811. doi: 10.1016/j.ejpain.2008.09.010

Wood, P. B. (2008). Role of central dopamine in pain and analgesia. *Expert Rev. Neurother.* 8, 781–797. doi: 10.1586/14737175.8.5.781

Woolf, C. J. (2004). Dissecting out mechanisms responsible for peripheral neuropathic pain: implications for diagnosis and therapy. *Life Sci.* 74, 2605–2610. doi: 10.1016/j.lfs.2004.01.003

Woolf, C. J. (2007). Central sensitization. *Anesthesiology* 106, 864–867. doi: 10.1097/01.anes.0000264769.87038.55

Woolf, C. J., Shortland, P., and Coggeshall, R. E. (1992). Peripheral nerve injury triggers central sprouting of myelinated afferents. *Nature* 355, 75–78. doi: 10.1038/355075a0

Xia, P., Inoguchi, T., Kern, T. S., Engerman, R. L., Oates, P. J., and King, G. L. (1994). Characterization of the mechanism for the chronic activation of diacylglycerol-protein kinase C pathway in diabetes and hypergalactosemia. *Diabetes* 43, 1122–1129. doi: 10.2337/diab.43.9.1122

Xu, J., Zhang, L., Xie, M., Li, Y., Huang, P., Saunders, T. L., et al. (2018). Role of complement in a rat model of paclitaxel induced peripheral neuropathy. *J. Immunol.* 200, 4094–4101. doi: 10.4049/jimmunol.1701716

Yagihashi, S., Yamagishi, S., and Wada, R. (2007). Pathology and pathogenetic mechanisms of diabetic neuropathy: correlation with clinical signs and symptoms. *Diabetes Res. Clin. Pract.* 77 (Suppl. 1), S184 S189. doi: 10.1016/j.diabres.2007.01.054

Yao, Y., Echeverry, S., Shi, X. Q., Yang, M., Yang, Q. Z., Wang, G. Y., et al. (2016). Dynamics of spinal microglia repopulation following an acute depletion. *Sci. Rep.* 6:22839. doi: 10.1038/srep22839

Yasuda, H., Terada, M., Maeda, K., Kogawa, S., Sanada, M., Haneda, M., et al. (2003). Diabetic neuropathy and nerve regeneration. *Prog. Neurobiol.* 69, 229–285. doi: 10.1016/S0301-0082(03)00034-0

Zhang, B., Yu, Y., Aori, G., Wang, Q., Kong, D., Yang, W., et al. (2018). Tanshinone IIA attenuates diabetic peripheral neuropathic pain in experimental rats via inhibiting inflammation. *J. Evidence Based Complementary Alter. Med.* 8:2789847. doi: 10.1155/2018/2789847

Zhang, J., and De Koninck, Y. (2006). Spatial and temporal relationship between monocyte chemoattractant protein-1 expression and spinal glial activation following peripheral nerve injury. *J. Neurochem.* 97, 772–783. doi: 10.1111/j.1471-4159.2006.03746.x

Zhang, J., Shi, X. Q., Echeverry, S., Mogil, J. S., De Koninck, Y., and Rivest, S. (2007). Expression of CCR2 in both resident and bonemarrow-derived microglia plays a critical role in neuropathic pain. *J. Neurosci.* 27, 12396–12406. doi: 10.1523/JNEUROSCI.3016-07.2007

Zhang, N., Inan, S., Cowan, A., Sun, R., Wang, J. M., Rogers, T. J., et al. (2005). A proinflammatory chemokine, CCL3, sensitizes the heat- and capsaicin-gated ion channel TRPV1. *Proc. Natl. Acad. Sci. U.S.A.* 102, 4536–4541. doi: 10.1073/pnas.0406030102

Zhang, R. X., Li, A., Liu, B., Wang, L., Ren, K., Zhang, H., et al. (2008). IL-1ra alleviates inflammatory hyperalgesia through preventing phosphorylation of NMDA receptor NR-1 subunit in rats. *Pain* 135, 232–239. doi: 10.1016/j.pain.2007.05.023

Zhao, P., Waxman, S. G., and Hains, B. C. (2007a). Extracellular signal-regulated kinase-regulated microglia-neuron signaling by prostaglandin E2 contributes to pain after spinal cord injury. *J. Neurosci.* 27, 2357–2368. doi: 10.1523/JNEUROSCI.0138-07.2007

Zhao, P., Waxman, S. G., and Hains, B. C. (2007b). Modulation of thalamic nociceptive processing after spinal cord injury through remote activation of thalamic microglia by cysteine cysteine chemokine ligand 21. *J. Neurosci.* 27, 8893–8902. doi: 10.1523/JNEUROSCI.2209-07.2007

Zhou, R., Xu, T., Liu, X., Chen, Y., Kong, D., Tian, H., et al. (2018). Activation of spinal dorsal horn P2Y13 receptors can promote the expression of IL-1beta and IL-6 in rats with diabetic neuropathic pain. *J. Pain Res.* 11, 615–628. doi: 10.2147/JPR.S154437

Zhou, Z., Peng, X., Hagshenas, J., Insolera, R., Fink, D. J., and Mata, M. (2010). A novel cell-cell signaling by microglial transmembrane TNFalpha with implications for neuropathic pain. *Pain* 151, 296–306. doi: 10.1016/j.pain.2010.06.017

Zhu, W., Xu, P., Cuascut, F. X., Hall, A. K., and Oxford, G. S. (2007). Activin acutely sensitizes dorsal root ganglion neurons and induces hyperalgesia via PKC-mediated potentiation of transient receptor potential vanilloid I. *J. Neurosci.* 27, 13770–13780. doi: 10.1523/JNEUROSCI.3822-07.2007

Ziegler, D. (2008). Painful diabetic neuropathy: treatment and future aspects. *Diabetes Metab. Res. Rev.* 24 (Suppl. 1), S52–S57. doi: 10.1002/dmrr.817

Zimmermann, M. (2001). Pathobiology of neuropathic pain. *Eur. J. Pharmacol.* 429, 23–37. doi: 10.1016/S0014-2999(01)01303-6

Zochodne, D. W., and Levy, D. (2005). Nitric oxide in damage, disease and repair of the peripheral nervous system. *Cell Mol. Biol.* 51, 255–267. doi: 10.117 0/T626

Zochodne, D. W., Verge, V. M., Cheng, C., Hoke, A., Jolley, C., Thomsen, K., et al. (2000). Nitric oxide synthase activity and expression in experimental diabetic neuropathy. *J. Neuropathol. Exp. Neurol.* 59, 798–807. doi: 10.1093/jnen/59.9.798

15

Interglial Crosstalk in Obesity-Induced Hypothalamic Inflammation

Md Habibur Rahman[1], Min-Seon Kim[2], In-Kyu Lee[3], Rina Yu[4] and Kyoungho Suk[1]**

[1] Department of Pharmacology, Brain Science and Engineering Institute, BK21 Plus KNU Biomedical Convergence Program, School of Medicine, Kyungpook National University, Daegu, South Korea, [2] Division of Endocrinology and Metabolism, University of Ulsan College of Medicine, Seoul, South Korea, [3] Department of Internal Medicine, Division of Endocrinology and Metabolism, School of Medicine, Kyungpook National University, Daegu, South Korea, [4] Department of Food Science and Nutrition, University of Ulsan, Ulsan, South Korea

***Correspondence:**
Kyoungho Suk
ksuk@knu.ac.kr
Rina Yu
rinayu@ulsan.ac.kr

Glial cells have recently gained particular attention for their close involvement in neuroinflammation and metabolic disorders including obesity and diabetes. In the central nervous system (CNS), different types of resident glial cells have been documented to express several signaling molecules and related receptors, and their crosstalks have been implicated in physiology and pathology of the CNS. Emerging evidence illustrates that malfunctioning glia and their products are an important component of hypothalamic inflammation. Recent studies have suggested that glia–glia crosstalk is a pivotal mechanism of overnutrition-induced chronic hypothalamic inflammation, which might be intrinsically associated with obesity/diabetes and their pathological consequences. This review covers the recent advances in the molecular aspects of interglial crosstalk in hypothalamic inflammation, proposing a central role of such a crosstalk in the development of obesity, diabetes, and related complications. Finally, we discuss the possibilities and challenges of targeting glial cells and their crosstalk for a better understanding of hypothalamic inflammation and related metabolic dysfunctions.

Keywords: obesity, diabetes, hypothalamus, inflammation, glia, chemokine, metabolism

INTRODUCTION

The hypothalamus is a critical brain structure and consists of three major areas such as the periventricular, the medial, and the lateral hypothalamic area. The median eminence (ME) is located in the middle–basal hypothalamus and the dorsal side of the third ventricle, and has blood vessels without barrier, which act as a window to release hypothalamic metabolic signals (Peruzzo et al., 2000; Elizondo-Vega et al., 2015). Nuclei of each area are metabolically important and play crucial roles in diverse functions including nutrient sensing, appetite control, and energy metabolism (Coll and Yeo, 2013; Elizondo-Vega et al., 2015). The hypothalamus receives metabolic signals from periphery through hormonal and cellular communication, letting the hypothalamus to control whole-body metabolism (Alquier and Kahn, 2004). However, disturbance of this mechanism is a major concern in a broad range of metabolic diseases including obesity and diabetes. Rising evidence suggests that hypothalamic inflammation particularly in the arcuate nucleus (ARC), a part of periventricular area, is a common pathological feature related with obesity and diabetes (Valdearcos et al., 2015). It affects the endocrine system and disturbs nutritional homeostasis, which causes metabolic alterations and subsequent pathologies. In animal experiments, high-fat diet (HFD)-induced chronic inflammation in the hypothalamus has been documented to modulate feeding behavior, energy expenditure, insulin secretion, and hepatic glucose production, all of which have been associated with dysregulation of glucose and fatty acid (FA) metabolism in obesity and diabetes (Cai and Liu, 2011). It has been reported that hypothalamic inflammation is observed within first 3 days of HFD onset with increased level of inflammatory markers (Thaler et al., 2012; Baufeld et al., 2016). An animal study of neonatal overnutrition revealed that hypothalamic inflammation is age- and sex-dependent, which is observed only in male animals with significant weight gain at postnatal day 150 (Argente-Arizon et al., 2018). The possible reason of such differences is the elevated level of circulating estrogens in female animals, probably inhibiting the effects of FAs on inflammation. As in other brain regions, the hypothalamus also contains various types of non-neuronal cells such as microglia, astrocytes, tanycytes, and NG2-positive glial cells (oligodendrocyte progenitor cells), which all play important physiological roles as metabolic sensors in the hypothalamus (Garcia-Caceres et al., 2012; Elizondo-Vega et al., 2015; Djogo et al., 2016; Freire-Regatillo et al., 2017). Emerging evidence suggests that glial cells may be a key component of pathological hypothalamic inflammation as well. Notably, wide structural changes have been observed in hypothalamic astrocytes in animal models of obesity and type 2 diabetes (Horvath et al., 2010). This study suggests that astrocytes contribute to synaptic rewiring by altering the glial ensheathment of neurons, which may disturb the ability of neurons to receive direct nutritional signals from the periphery. In line with this thought, it has been proposed that hypothalamic inflammation is a potential cause of leptin and insulin resistance in the hypothalamus of rodents (Thaler et al., 2012; Andre et al., 2017) and patients with obesity and diabetes (Schur et al., 2015; Kreutzer et al., 2017).

In recent years, glial cells have become a focus of modern neuroscience research, for instance, with respect to neurodevelopment and brain health/disease (Barres, 2008). They are homeostatic regulators in the central nervous system (CNS) and play a critical role by providing metabolic support for neurons. In addition, they maintain extracellular pH, protect neurons from any insults, as well as participate in neurovascular coupling, neurotransmitter uptake, synaptic formation and pruning, and phagocytosis (Jha and Suk, 2013; Jha et al., 2014). Moreover, glial cells participate in these functions by communicating with and influencing other glial cell types in a mutual manner, ultimately playing a crucial role in brain development, function, and diseases (Jha et al., 2018). This interglial communication occurs through various cell surface molecules and the release of signaling molecules such as cytokines, chemokines, adenosine triphosphate, and growth factors (Tanuma et al., 2006; Pascual et al., 2012; Rocha et al., 2012; Liddelow et al., 2017). It has been reported that glial crosstalk plays a crucial role in the development and progression of neuropathologies depending on the level of their secreted molecules following various CNS insults (Tian et al., 2012). Among different glial cell types, microglia and astrocytes are the primary innate immune cells and key responders to a variety of CNS insults such as pathogens, ischemia, and chemogenic factors, which further lead to the activation of these glial cells and ensue the production of increased levels of proinflammatory mediators, for example, cytokines, chemokines, reactive oxygen species, and nitric oxide (NO) (Tanuma et al., 2006; Iizumi et al., 2016; Hou et al., 2017; Liddelow et al., 2017). These mediators are responsible for chronic inflammation and resultant pathologies in the CNS. However, several molecular targets such as anti-inflammatory cytokines and neurotrophic factors have been identified in other brain areas where the inflammatory response due to microglia and astrocytic activation has been reduced in Alzheimer's disease (Mandrekar-Colucci et al., 2012), Parkinson disease (PD) (Subramaniam and Federoff, 2017), and epilepsy (Benson et al., 2015). It has been reported that activated microglia-derived IL-10 reduces inflammatory responses in the stratum, which has been proposed as a crucial target to enhance the neuroprotection in an experimental model of PD (Schwenkgrub et al., 2013; Joniec-Maciejak et al., 2014).

Emerging evidence highlights that microglia, astrocytes, and their interaction play an important role in the regulation of immune and inflammatory responses in the CNS (Farina et al., 2007; Ransohoff and Brown, 2012; Kirkley et al., 2017). In the context of metabolic inflammation in the hypothalamus, the interaction between these glial cell types has been reported to be a decisive contributor to progression and severity of neurometabolic diseases (Kim et al., 2018). In addition, glial interaction modulates their activation states, particularly through the expression of cell surface receptors including cytokine and chemokine receptors, and activation of intracellular signaling pathways (Zhang et al., 2017; Kim et al., 2018; Valdearcos et al., 2018), potentially amplifying the inflammatory activation in the hypothalamus under diabetes and obesity conditions (Rahman et al., 2018). A recent study has revealed that inflammatory activation of astrocytes by lipid droplets and the potential crosstalk of these astrocytes with microglia in free FA (FFA)-rich environments might be implicated in the obesity-induced pathological hypothalamic inflammation and subsequent metabolic complications (Kwon et al., 2017).

This review discusses the recent advances in the molecular aspects of interglial crosstalk in hypothalamic inflammation, particularly astrocyte–microglia crosstalk, with extended discussion on the potential crosstalks between microglia–astrocyte and tanycyte–astrocyte, suggesting a central role of the interglial crosstalk in the development of obesity, diabetes, and their complications, based on the data currently available in the literatures (**Figure 1**). Finally, we also discuss the possibilities and challenges of targeting glial cells and their crosstalk for a better understanding

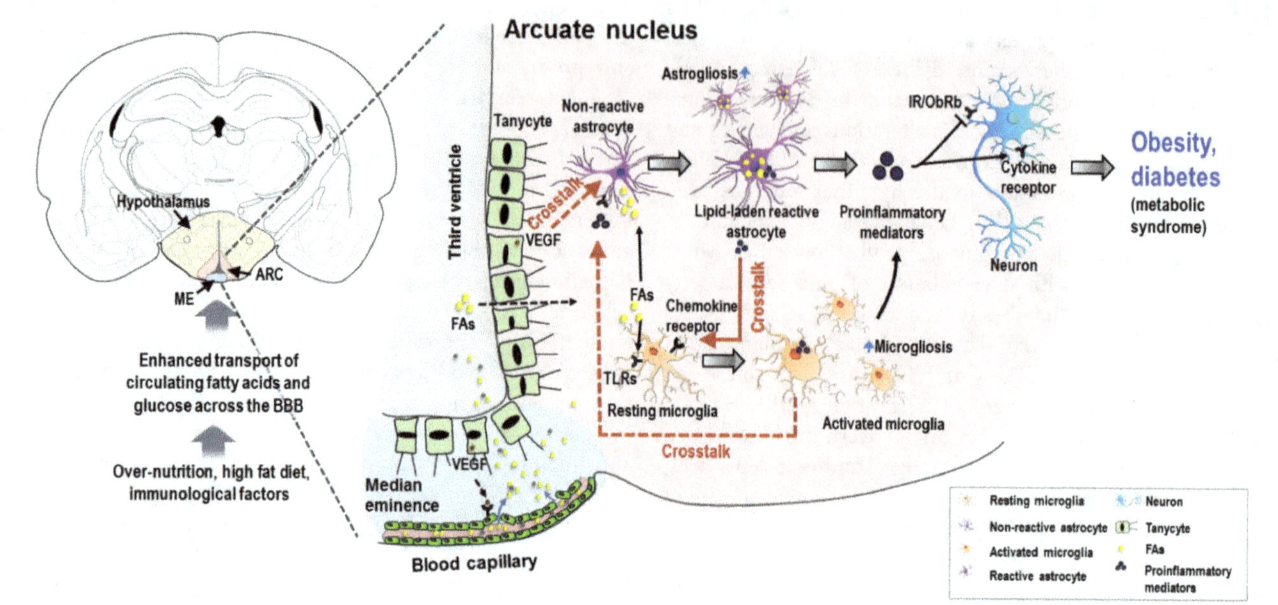

FIGURE 1 | Schematic representation of potential interglial crosstalk in hypothalamic inflammation and the ontology of obesity and diabetes. Overnutrition, HFD, immunological factors, and increased circulating nutrients (FAs and glucose), arising in a temporal sequence, appear to induce glial malfunctions and pathological hypothalamic inflammation. The excessive circulating nutrients are transported into the hypothalamus through the permeable blood capillaries. Tanycytes, a specialized ependymal cell type located in the lateral walls and surface of the third ventricle, allow the passage of these excessive nutrients particularly FAs from the circulation to the hypothalamic ARC. This may be due to the expression of VEGF in tanycytes, which targets microvessel loops and promotes microvessel permeability. FAs can activate both microglia and astrocytes, primarily by binding to TLRs expressed in microglia. Similarly, FAs cause accumulation of lipid droplets in astrocytes, leading to inflammatory activation of astrocytes and release of proinflammatory mediators, which may further activate microglia by molecular interaction enhancing the inflammatory processes. In addition, activated microglia and VEGF-rich tanycytes may also contribute to chronic hypothalamic inflammation by their secreted molecules and subsequent crosstalk with astrocytes. This proinflammatory mechanism impairs insulin and leptin signaling in neurons, leading to cellular stress responses. This condition negatively affects the proper functioning of hypothalamic neuronal circuits, which leads to metabolic dysregulation associated with obesity and diabetes. Solid red arrows, reported glial crosstalk; dotted red arrows, possible crosstalk. BBB, blood–brain barrier; ARC, arcuate nucleus; FA, fatty acid; TLR, toll-like receptor; VEGF, vascular endothelial growth factor; IR, insulin receptor; ObRb, leptin receptor b.

of hypothalamic inflammation and its related metabolic dysfunctions.

CHEMOKINE-MEDIATED ASTROCYTE–MICROGLIA CROSSTALK

Chemokines are a superfamily of structurally related small (most of them between 8 and 14 kDa) chemotactic cytokines, i.e., they promote leukocyte migration, and are implicated in various inflammatory pathological processes and infectious diseases. In the healthy brain, different cell types including glial cells or neurons constitutively express many chemokines and their receptors, and their expression levels are found to be increased in activated astrocytes and microglia (Le Thuc et al., 2017). Among those, some chemokines such as monocyte chemoattractant protein-1 (MCP-1/CCL2), stromal cell-derived factor (SDF-1/CXCL12), and fractalkine/CX3CL1 and their receptors have been shown to be expressed in the hypothalamus (Banisadr et al., 2005), and their association with obesity-induced inflammatory responses and metabolic complications have been reported (Morari et al., 2014; Poon et al., 2016).

The chemokine MCP-1/CCL2 is expressed in glial cells such as astrocytes and microglia, and central delivery of MCP-1 has been shown to promote hypothalamic inflammation and metabolic dysregulation as well (Le Thuc et al., 2016). Intriguingly, a recent study has demonstrated that astrocyte-derived MCP-1 is crucial for the onset and/or progress of the obesity-induced glial cell-mediated hypothalamic inflammation (Kwon et al., 2017). *In vitro* experiment using primary hypothalamic astrocytes has revealed that the cells accumulate lipid droplets under FFA-rich conditions with their increased inflammatory reactivity, mimicking obese conditions. The lipid-laden astrocytes produce large amounts of proinflammatory mediators such as tumor necrosis factor (TNF)-α, interleukin (IL)-1β, IL-6, and MCP-1, suggesting that under obese conditions these lipid-laden astrocytes may trigger the onset of hypothalamic inflammation. Of note, treatment of microglia with fatty astrocytes-conditioned medium markedly increased the chemotactic activity of microglia with upregulation of CCR2 (receptor for MCP-1/CCL2), and treatment of anti-MCP-1 antibody diminished the chemotactic activity. These results indicate that the fatty astrocytes-derived inflammatory chemokine MCP-1 enhances microglial chemotactic activity by binding to its receptor, and the recruited microglia may interact with the neighboring astrocytes, amplifying the hypothalamic inflammatory responses (**Figure 2**). It has been reported that mice fed with HFD show the increased number of microglia in ARC region of the hypothalamus.

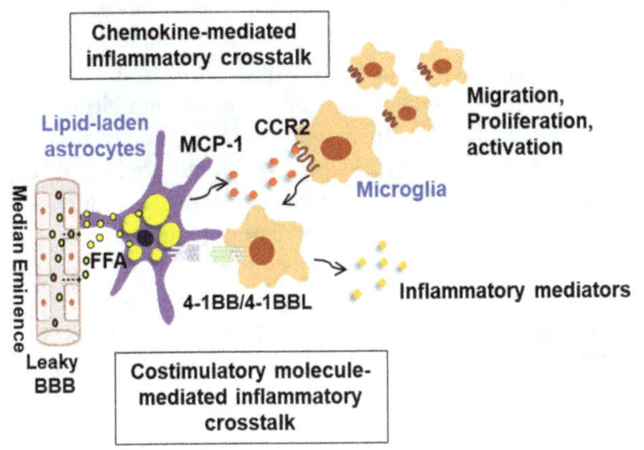

FIGURE 2 | Schematic representation of interglial crosstalk via chemokines and costimulatory molecules in hypothalamic inflammation under obese conditions. In the hypothalamus, glial cells such as astrocytes and microglia can directly respond to peripheral excess nutrient signals, such as FAs, through a unique vascular system (fenestrated capillaries) and damaged BBB and these glial cells become reactive to release inflammatory mediators. In obese environments rich in FAs, astrocytes accumulate lipid droplets, and they release the proinflammatory chemokine MCP-1, which promotes microglia migration, proliferation, and activation. The lipid-laden astrocytes can also directly interact with the migrated microglia through membrane-bound costimulatory receptors/ligands such as 4-1BB/4-1BBL, thus reinforcing the inflammation. This glial cell-mediated inflammatory crosstalk may be crucial for obesity-induced hypothalamic inflammation. BBB, blood–brain barrier; FFA, free fatty acid; MCP-1, monocyte chemoattractant protein-1; CCR2, C–C chemokine receptor type 2.

The study suggested that the increased number of microglia in the ARC might be due to increased infiltration of bone marrow-derived monocytes/macrophages into the CNS (Thaler et al., 2012; Buckman et al., 2014; Valdearcos et al., 2014). Given that the chemokine MCP-1 disrupts the integrity of the blood–brain barrier (BBB) (Yao and Tsirka, 2014), the chemokine MCP-1 may also act in obesity as a signal to recruit bone marrow-derived monocytes/macrophages into the hypothalamus.

In recent years, chemokines such as SDF-1/CXCL12 and fractalkine/CX3CL1 have been shown to be associated with obesity-induced hypothalamic inflammation. SDF-1 is constitutively expressed in hypothalamic astrocytes, microglia, as well as in neurons (Banisadr et al., 2003). SDF-1 and its receptors CXCR4 and CXCR7 have been shown to be upregulated in the hypothalamic nuclei by HFD intake, which is accompanied by an increase of orexigenic neuropeptides (Poon et al., 2016). Moreover, central administration of CXCL12 increases caloric intake, stimulates the expression of orexigenic neuropeptides, and reduces novelty-induced locomotor activity, suggesting that SDF-1 might have an important role in mediating the HFD-induced neuronal and behavioral effects. The crosstalk between astrocytic SDF-1 and microglial CXCR4 has been shown to participate in the development of neuroinflammation and the pathogenesis of neuropathic pain hypersensitivity (Luo et al., 2016). Fractalkine/CX3CL1 is predominantly expressed and released by neurons, and its receptor CX3CR1 is expressed in microglia (Tian et al., 2012). Fractalkine and its receptor play a pivotal role in the recruitment, infiltration, and proinflammatory polarization of leukocytes and microglial cells that are involved in the regulation of neuroinflammatory conditions (Cardona et al., 2006; Cardona et al., 2008), indicating that the chemokine acts as a mediator in the crosstalk between leukocytes and microglia. Fractalkine has been shown to exert both anti-inflammatory (Zujovic et al., 2000) and proinflammatory properties (Huang et al., 2006; Denes et al., 2008), however, recent studies support the proinflammatory role of fractalkine in obesity-induced hypothalamic inflammation. In obesity-prone mice, the inhibition of hypothalamic fractalkine reduces obesity-related inflammatory activity as demonstrated by the reduction of TNF-α and IL-1β levels and the decreased recruitment of bone marrow-derived cells to the hypothalamus. This model also prevents the development of obesity and glucose intolerance (Morari et al., 2014), indicating that fractalkine is a key player in diet-induced early hypothalamic inflammation. Chemokines such as SDF-1 and fractalkine are considered interesting therapeutic targets to fight against obesity-induced inflammatory complications; however, detailed molecular mechanisms underlying the chemokine-mediated interglial crosstalk in obesity-induced hypothalamic inflammation remain to be further investigated.

INTERGLIAL CROSSTALK MEDIATED BY COSTIMULATORY MOLECULES

The contribution of glia–glia interaction to hypothalamic inflammation is strongly influenced by their potential for mutual interaction with the inflammatory microenvironment. Substantial evidence points to reactive glia as a pivotal factor during the obesity-induced hypothalamic inflammation process. As mentioned earlier, astrocytes and microglia in the hypothalamus are often found in close proximity to each other, indicating a potential reciprocal contact-dependent communication between them, facilitating their inflammatory crosstalk.

Several immune signaling costimulatory molecules (ligands/their receptors, membrane-bound proteins), which are mostly expressed in immune cells, glial cells, and neurons, and their crosstalk has been implicated in CNS inflammatory pathologies. For instance, different TNF receptor superfamily (TNFRSF) members and their ligands such as TWEAK/FN14 and CD40/CD40L contribute to the pathogenesis of Alzheimer's disease and multiple sclerosis, which have a strong inflammatory component and glia involvement (Aarts et al., 2017). CD40/CD40L interaction has been reported to enhance the inflammatory response in multiple sclerosis, and genetic ablation or antibody-mediated inhibition of the CD40/CD40L interaction reduces the severity of experimental autoimmune encephalomyelitis (EAE), a murine model for multiple sclerosis (Gerritse et al., 1996; Grewal et al., 1996; Aarts et al., 2017). The 4-1BB (also known as TNFRSF9 or

CD137) receptor/ligand system may be another potent mediator in controlling neuroinflammatory pathologies. It has been reported that mice with 4-1BB ligand (4-1BBL) deficiency display profoundly less microglial activation following EAE induction compared with wild-type animals, and, thus, the gene deficiency reduces the severity of this neuroinflammatory pathology (Yeo et al., 2012). These costimulatory receptors/ligands are, therefore, considered to be attractive therapeutic candidates for diverse neuroinflammatory diseases. However, studies on the association of these receptors/ligands system with obesity-induced hypothalamic inflammation are currently limited.

Nonetheless, there is recent evidence supporting the occurrence of interglial crosstalk through 4-1BB/4-1BBL interaction in the hypothalamus under obese conditions (Kim et al., 2018). 4-1BB is a member of the TNFRSF and a membrane-bound costimulatory protein, which is highly expressed in activated T cells as well as NK cells (Vinay and Kwon, 2011). It has also been reported to be expressed by some nonimmune cells such as adipocytes and endothelial cells (Drenkard et al., 2007; Kim et al., 2011) and delivers potent costimulatory or inflammatory signals upon activation. 4-1BB binds to its ligand 4-1BBL, which is highly expressed in antigen-presenting cells such as macrophages. In addition, the 4-1BB receptor/ligand system can transmit bidirectional signals between two interacting cells, a process referred to as forward and reverse signaling (Shao and Schwarz, 2011). Although most studies are focused on 4-1BB/4-1BBL-mediated immune regulations, a few recent studies have shown that the 4-1BB/4-1BBL-mediated bidirectional signal can promote obesity-induced adipose tissue inflammation by the recruitment of adipocytes/macrophages and inflammation in skeletal muscle by myotubes/macrophages recruitment (Tu et al., 2012; Le et al., 2013). Intriguingly, astrocytes express 4-1BB, whereas microglia express 4-1BBL (Reali et al., 2003; Yeo et al., 2012), and these molecules are likely to have the potential to mediate the crosstalk between astrocytes and microglia. Indeed, it has been shown that mice fed with HFD display an increased expression of 4-1BB and 4-1BBL transcripts in the hypothalamus when compared with lean controls (Kim et al., 2018), supporting the idea that these molecules may be responsible for the crosstalk between astrocytes and microglia in obese conditions. Using mouse primary astrocytes and BV-2 mouse microglial cells *in vitro*, the involvement of these molecules in glial cells-mediated hypothalamic inflammatory responses was assessed in a recent study (Kim et al., 2018). First, obesity-related factors such as lipopolysaccharide, FFA, glucose, and adipose tissue-conditioned medium treatment increased the transcript levels of 4-1BB in astrocytes and 4-1BBL in microglia, mimicking the conditions of obesity. Second, stimulation of 4-1BB on astrocytes delivered an inflammatory signal to increase astrocyte reactivity, leading to an increased production of proinflammatory mediators such as TNF-α, IL-6, and MCP-1 at the levels of mRNA and protein. Third, 4-BBL stimulation of microglial cells increased microglial activation, enhanced the release of proinflammatory mediators such as MCP-1 and ICL-6, and decreased the level of an anti-inflammatory cytokine IL-10. This was mediated through activation of the mitogen-activated protein kinase pathway. Fourth, an increased production of inflammatory cytokines was observed in the co-culture of glial cells with augmented glial activation markers. More importantly, inhibition of 4-1BB/4-1BBL crosstalk with a neutralizing antibody decreased the inflammatory responses in the co-cultured glial cells. Moreover, 4-1BB-deficient astrocytes revealed a reduction in the inflammatory responses when co-cultured with microglia, compared with those astrocytes/microglia isolated from wild-type animals. Finally, consistent with these findings, an *in vivo* study revealed that 4-1BB deficiency reduces HFD-induced hypothalamic inflammation, which is accompanied by the reduction of glial activation markers and the level of inflammatory cytokines. Taken all together, these findings suggest that 4-1BB and/or 4-1BBL signaling plays a crucial role in the interglial crosstalk in hypothalamic inflammatory responses under obese conditions (**Figure 2**) and might be a potential therapeutic target for the inhibition of obesity-induced hypothalamic inflammation and associated metabolic complications.

TANYCYTES AND THEIR POTENTIAL CROSSTALK

Tanycytes are specialized ependymal cells. Anatomically, this cell type is located in the lateral walls and surface of the third ventricle. Tanycytes maintain the nutrient transport from the circulation to the energy-sensing ARC of the hypothalamus (Mullier et al., 2010; Rahman et al., 2018). According to their location and morphological distribution, tanycytes are classified as two major subtypes (α- and β-tanycytes), which are further subdivided into α1-, α2-, β1-, and β2-tanycytes (Rizzoti and Lovell-Badge, 2017). Specifically, α-tanycytes reside dorsally, while β-tanycytes occupy the ventral side wall and surface of the third ventricle in the ME. Previous studies revealed that HFD increases the proliferation of β2-tanycytes with postnatal neurogenesis in the ME. It is also found that the new born neurons are derived from the β2-tanycytes, and inhibition of tanycyte division and differentiation decreases the HFD-induced body weight gain (Lee and Blackshaw, 2012; Lee et al., 2012). These findings suggest that β2-tanycytes-derived neurogenesis might contribute to energy homeostasis in response to HFD. In the hypothalamus, tanycytes are a source of vascular endothelial growth factor (VEGF) (Langlet, 2014). It has been reported that in mice under food deprivation condition, tanycytes express VEGF-A, which targets microvessel loops to promote microvessel permeability and to reorganize tight junction complexes in the ME and ARC (Langlet et al., 2013). This, in turn, may facilitate the communication between circulating metabolites and brain parenchyma. In a previous study, microglia-secreted VEGF has been shown to regulate the pathogenic activities of astrocytes in an EAE mouse model of multiple sclerosis (Rothhammer et al., 2018). In line with this thought, tanycytes-derived VEGF can be a potential contributor to overnutrition-induced hypothalamic inflammation by interacting with astrocytes. It has been reported that mice fed a HFD show an early loss of the structural organization of β1-tanycytes (Ramalho et al., 2018) in the ME. In this study, immunofluorescence analyses revealed that consumption of an HFD alters the expression and spatial distribution of different proteins including insulin-like growth factor-binding protein 2, the most specific marker of β1-tanycytes, involved in the organization of the BBB. This may facilitate the transport of excess lipid-rich nutrients into the hypothalamus. A previous animal study revealed that hypothalamic tanycytes also accumulate lipid droplets in normal condition (Brion et al., 1982). A recent study using a microscopy analysis of the lipid droplet distribution in the hypothalamus has demonstrated numerous lipid droplets in tanycytes in response to HFD or obese condition (Hofmann et al., 2017). Further research is required to better understand the acute and chronic effects of HFD on tanycyte characteristics in energy metabolism and the role of tanycyte interaction with other glial cells in hypothalamic inflammation and subsequent pathologies.

CONCLUSION AND FUTURE PERSPECTIVES

Accumulating evidence suggests that hypothalamic glial cells respond to diet rich in FAs. In particular, long-chain FAs, such as palmitic acid, have been implicated in microglial activation and subsequent initiation of intracellular inflammatory pathways through toll-like receptors (Milanski et al., 2009; Valdearcos et al., 2014). It has been reported that mice fed with HFD show an activation and proliferation of both microglia and astrocytes in the hypothalamus, and activation of these glial cells play a crucial role in the alteration of local neuronal circuits, which has been suggested to promote obesity (Horvath et al., 2010; Andre et al., 2017). An *in vitro* study using primary microglia and astrocytes isolated from mice brains have revealed that only microglia, but not astrocytes, respond to FAs (Valdearcos et al., 2014). Indeed, FA-mediated inflammatory activation of primary microglia cultures isolated from whole mouse brains or of BV-2 mouse microglial cells is associated with an increased release of proinflammatory mediators, such as TNF-α, IL-1β, and IL-6 (Wang et al., 2012). These findings suggest that HFD-induced inflammatory activation of astrocytes in the hypothalamus might be due to microglial crosstalk with astrocytes through interaction between microglia-secreted proinflammatory mediators and related receptors expressed in astrocytes. In contrast, a previous study reported that FAs, such as palmitic acid, stearic acid, and lauric acid, can activate inflammatory signaling leading to the release of cytokines in cultured astrocytes isolated from rat brain (Gupta et al., 2012). These previous findings suggest that HFD-induced hypothalamic inflammation might be mediated by both glial cell types through their direct or indirect molecular interaction. The contrast in the data in the literature might be due to differences in experimental conditions or species. Further studies are required to explain these discrepancies.

Several *in vivo* and *in vitro* studies provided in the last few years a new view on the roles of microglia–astrocyte interaction involved in the pathogenesis of neuroinflammatory and degenerative diseases (Jha et al., 2018). In addition, bidirectional communication between microglia and astrocytes has been reported to mediate prolonged inflammation via their released molecules such as TNF-α, NO, nicotinamide adenine dinucleotide phosphate (NADPH) oxidase-derived hydrogen peroxide (H_2O_2), and transforming growth factors following CNS insults (Jha et al., 2018). Similarly, in the context of metabolic inflammation in the hypothalamus, several animal studies have revealed an increased level of such molecules in the hypothalamus and their role in pathological hypothalamic inflammation associated with obesity and diabetes (Duparc et al., 2011; Dalvi et al., 2017; Katashima et al., 2017; Mendes et al., 2018), but the molecular mechanisms underlying the interglial crosstalk in relation to chronic inflammation in the hypothalamus need to be further highlighted in future research. Glial cells and their inflammatory activation in response to fat-rich diet are closely involved in chronic hypothalamic inflammation and leptin/insulin resistance, which have drawn growing attention to the role of these glial cells in metabolic dysregulation associated with obesity and diabetes. Various secreted molecules from malfunctioning glia and signaling from cell surface receptors have been proposed as a potential mechanism of hypothalamic inflammation. Recent studies have provided a significant insight into our understanding of the complex roles of glial cells and their crosstalk in overnutrition-induced chronic hypothalamic inflammation and its pathological consequences. The complex heterogeneous nature of each glial cell type has made a challenging task to gain a clear insight into the interglial crosstalk in CNS physiology as well as pathologies. Further investigations will be needed for a better understanding regarding the functional significance of the interglial crosstalk in such pathological hypothalamic inflammation. Recently established innovative tools, such as isolation technique of high-purity glial cell populations from rodents and humans, optogenetics, chemogenetics, nanotechnology, single-cell multi-omics, induced pluripotent stem cells, and organoids may accelerate preclinical research.

Diverse glia-secreted molecules including cytokines, chemokines, and gliotransmitters, as well as related receptors expressed in specific glial cell types, can be possible targets for a further clarification of the interglial crosstalk in chronic hypothalamic inflammation. A recent study has demonstrated that restoring the feeding pattern by blocking gap-junction hemichannels in the CNS prevents HFD-induced obesity in mice (Sasaki et al., 2018). It has been suggested that blockade of hemichannels inhibits microglial release of small molecules, without attenuating acute inflammatory cytokine induction. In line with these findings, the authors speculated that HFD-induced obesity can be mediated via the gap junction hemichannel pathway, which affects the timing of meal and the inflammatory cytokine signaling pathway, thereby revealing a new therapeutic target in the CNS for the treatment of obesity. As gap-junction hemichannels control the release of diverse microglial molecules, it is important to understand their association with interglial crosstalk in both acute and chronic phase of obesity. Current and future research may boost the feasibility of glia-based therapeutic strategies targeting the interglial crosstalk and related molecules (either secreted or cell surface molecules) to prevent and alleviate hypothalamic inflammation and metabolic diseases.

AUTHOR CONTRIBUTIONS

All authors have made a substantial intellectual contribution to this work, and approved submission of the manuscript. RY and KS formulated the focus of this review. MR, M-SK, and I-KL conducted the literature review and participated in the discussion. MR, RY, and KS wrote the manuscript.

REFERENCES

Aarts, S. A., Seijkens, T. T., van Dorst, K. J., Dijkstra, C. D., Kooij, G., and Lutgens, E. (2017). The CD40-CD40L dyad in experimental autoimmune encephalomyelitis and multiple sclerosis. *Front. Immunol.* 8:1791. doi: 10.3389/fimmu.2017.01791

Alquier, T., and Kahn, B. B. (2004). Peripheral signals set the tone for central regulation of metabolism. *Endocrinology* 145, 4022–4024. doi: 10.1210/en.2004-0861

Andre, C., Guzman-Quevedo, O., Rey, C., Remus-Borel, J., Clark, S., Castellanos-Jankiewicz, A., et al. (2017). Inhibiting microglia expansion prevents diet-induced hypothalamic and peripheral inflammation. *Diabetes Metab. Res. Rev.* 66, 908–919. doi: 10.2337/db16-0586

Argente-Arizon, P., Diaz, F., Ros, P., Barrios, V., Tena-Sempere, M., Garcia-Segura, L. M., et al. (2018). The hypothalamic inflammatory/gliosis response to neonatal overnutrition is sex and age dependent. *Endocrinology* 159, 368–387. doi: 10.1210/en.2017-00539

Banisadr, G., Rostene, W., Kitabgi, P., and Parsadaniantz, S. M. (2005). Chemokines and brain functions. *Curr. Drug Targets Inflamm. Allergy* 4, 387–399. doi: 10.2174/1568010054022097

Banisadr, G., Skrzydelski, D., Kitabgi, P., Rostene, W., and Parsadaniantz, S. M. (2003). Highly regionalized distribution of stromal cell-derived factor-1/CXCL12 in adult rat brain: constitutive expression in cholinergic, dopaminergic and vasopressinergic neurons. *Eur. J. Neurosci.* 18, 1593–1606. doi: 10.1046/j.1460-9568.2003.02893.x

Barres, B. A. (2008). The mystery and magic of glia: a perspective on their roles in health and disease. *Neuron* 60, 430–440. doi: 10.1016/j.neuron.2008.10.013

Baufeld, C., Osterloh, A., Prokop, S., Miller, K. R., and Heppner, F. L. (2016). High-fat diet-induced brain region-specific phenotypic spectrum of CNS resident microglia. *Acta Neuropathol.* 132, 361–375. doi: 10.1007/s00401-016-1595-4

Benson, M. J., Manzanero, S., and Borges, K. (2015). Complex alterations in microglial M1/M2 markers during the development of epilepsy in two mouse models. *Epilepsia* 56, 895–905. doi: 10.1111/epi.12960

Brion, J. P., Depierreux, M., Couck, A. M., and Flament-Durand, J. (1982). Transmission and scanning electron-microscopic observations on tanycytes in the mediobasal hypothalamus and the median eminence of adrenalectomized rats. *Cell Tissue Res.* 221, 643–655. doi: 10.1007/BF00215708

Buckman, L. B., Hasty, A. H., Flaherty, D. K., Buckman, C. T., Thompson, M. M., Matlock, B. K., et al. (2014). Obesity induced by a high-fat diet is associated with increased immune cell entry into the central nervous system. *Brain Behav. Immun.* 35, 33–42. doi: 10.1016/j.bbi.2013.06.007

Cai, D., and Liu, T. (2011). Hypothalamic inflammation: a double-edged sword to nutritional diseases. *Ann. N. Y. Acad. Sci.* 1243, E1–E39. doi: 10.1111/j.1749-6632.2011.06388.x

Cardona, A. E., Li, M., Liu, L., Savarin, C., and Ransohoff, R. M. (2008). Chemokines in and out of the central nervous system: much more than chemotaxis and inflammation. *J. Leukoc. Biol.* 84, 587–594. doi: 10.1189/jlb.1107763

Cardona, A. E., Pioro, E. P., Sasse, M. E., Kostenko, V., Cardona, S. M., Dijkstra, I. M., et al. (2006). Control of microglial neurotoxicity by the fractalkine receptor. *Nat. Neurosci.* 9, 917–924. doi: 10.1038/nn1715

Coll, A. P., and Yeo, G. S. (2013). The hypothalamus and metabolism: integrating signals to control energy and glucose homeostasis. *Curr. Opin. Pharmacol* 13, 970–976. doi: 10.1016/j.coph.2013.09.010

Dalvi, P. S., Chalmers, J. A., Luo, V., Han, D. Y., Wellhauser, L., Liu, Y., et al. (2017). High fat induces acute and chronic inflammation in the hypothalamus: effect of high-fat diet, palmitate and TNF-alpha on appetite-regulating NPY neurons. *Int. J. Obes.* 41, 149–158. doi: 10.1038/ijo.2016.183

Denes, A., Ferenczi, S., Halasz, J., Kornyei, Z., and Kovacs, K. J. (2008). Role of CX3CR1 (fractalkine receptor) in brain damage and inflammation induced by focal cerebral ischemia in mouse. *J. Cereb. Blood Flow Metab.* 28, 1707–1721. doi: 10.1038/jcbfm.2008.64

Djogo, T., Robins, S. C., Schneider, S., Kryzskaya, D., Liu, X., Mingay, A., et al. (2016). Adult NG2-glia are required for median eminence-mediated leptin sensing and body weight control. *Cell Metab.* 23, 797–810. doi: 10.1016/j.cmet.2016.04.013

Drenkard, D., Becke, F. M., Langstein, J., Spruss, T., Kunz-Schughart, L. A., Tan, T. E., et al. (2007). CD137 is expressed on blood vessel walls at sites of inflammation and enhances monocyte migratory activity. *FASEB J.* 21, 456–463. doi: 10.1096/fj.05-4739com

Duparc, T., Colom, A., Cani, P. D., Massaly, N., Rastrelli, S., Drougard, A., et al. (2011). Central apelin controls glucose homeostasis via a nitric oxide-dependent pathway in mice. *Antioxid. Redox Signal.* 15, 1477–1496. doi: 10.1089/ars.2010.3454

Elizondo-Vega, R., Cortes-Campos, C., Barahona, M. J., Oyarce, K. A., Carril, C. A., and Garcia-Robles, M. A. (2015). The role of tanycytes in hypothalamic glucosensing. *J. Cell Mol. Med.* 19, 1471–1482. doi: 10.1111/jcmm.12590

Farina, C., Aloisi, F., and Meinl, E. (2007). Astrocytes are active players in cerebral innate immunity. *Trends Immunol.* 28, 138–145. doi: 10.1016/j.it.2007.01.005

Freire-Regatillo, A., Argente-Arizon, P., Argente, J., Garcia-Segura, L. M., and Chowen, J. A. (2017). Non-neuronal cells in the hypothalamic adaptation to metabolic signals. *Front. Endocrinol.* 8:51. doi: 10.3389/fendo.2017.00051

Garcia-Caceres, C., Fuente-Martin, E., Argente, J., and Chowen, J. A. (2012). Emerging role of glial cells in the control of body weight. *Mol. Metab.* 1, 37–46. doi: 10.1016/j.molmet.2012.07.001

Gerritse, K., Laman, J. D., Noelle, R. J., Aruffo, A., Ledbetter, J. A., Boersma, W., et al. (1996). CD40-CD40 ligand interactions in experimental allergic encephalomyelitis and multiple sclerosis. *Proc. Natl. Acad. Sci. U.S.A.* 93, 2499–2504. doi: 10.1073/pnas.93.6.2499

Grewal, I. S., Foellmer, H. G., Grewal, K. D., Xu, J., Hardardottir, F., Baron, J. L., et al. (1996). Requirement for CD40 ligand in costimulation induction, T cell activation, and experimental allergic encephalomyelitis. *Science* 273, 1864–1867. doi: 10.1126/science.273.5283.1864

Gupta, S., Knight, A. G., Gupta, S., Keller, J. N., and Bruce-Keller, A. J. (2012). Saturated long-chain fatty acids activate inflammatory signaling in astrocytes. *J. Neurochem.* 120, 1060–1071. doi: 10.1111/j.1471-4159.2012.07660.x

Hofmann, K., Lamberz, C., Piotrowitz, K., Offermann, N., But, D., Scheller, A., et al. (2017). Tanycytes and a differential fatty acid metabolism in the hypothalamus. *Glia* 65, 231–249. doi: 10.1002/glia.23088

Horvath, T. L., Sarman, B., Garcia-Caceres, C., Enriori, P. J., Sotonyi, P., Shanabrough, M., et al. (2010). Synaptic input organization of the melanocortin system predicts diet-induced hypothalamic reactive gliosis and obesity. *Proc. Natl. Acad. Sci. U.S.A.* 107, 14875–14880. doi: 10.1073/pnas.1004282107

Hou, L., Zhou, X., Zhang, C., Wang, K., Liu, X., Che, Y., et al. (2017). NADPH oxidase-derived H2O2 mediates the regulatory effects of microglia on astrogliosis in experimental models of Parkinson's disease. *Redox Biol.* 12, 162–170. doi: 10.1016/j.redox.2017.02.016

Huang, D., Shi, F. D., Jung, S., Pien, G. C., Wang, J., Salazar-Mather, T. P., et al. (2006). The neuronal chemokine CX3CL1/fractalkine selectively recruits NK cells that modify experimental autoimmune encephalomyelitis within the central nervous system. *FASEB J.* 20, 896–905. doi: 10.1096/fj.05-5465com

Iizumi, T., Takahashi, S., Mashima, K., Minami, K., Izawa, Y., Abe, T., et al. (2016). A possible role of microglia-derived nitric oxide by lipopolysaccharide in activation of astroglial pentose-phosphate pathway via the Keap1/Nrf2 system. *J. Neuroinflammation* 13:99. doi: 10.1186/s12974-016-0564-0

Jha, M. K., Jo, M., Kim, J. H., and Suk, K. (2018). Microglia-astrocyte crosstalk: an intimate molecular conversation. *Neuroscientist* doi: 10.1177/1073858418783959 [Epub ahead of print].

Jha, M. K., Kim, J. H., and Suk, K. (2014). Proteome of brain glia: the molecular basis of diverse glial phenotypes. *Proteomics* 14, 378–398. doi: 10.1002/pmic.201300236

Jha, M. K., and Suk, K. (2013). Glia-based biomarkers and their functional role in the CNS. *Expert Rev. Proteomics* 10, 43–63. doi: 10.1586/epr.12.70

Joniec-Maciejak, I., Ciesielska, A., Wawer, A., Sznejder-Pacholek, A., Schwenkgrub, J., Cudna, A., et al. (2014). The influence of AAV2-mediated gene transfer of human IL-10 on neurodegeneration and immune response in a murine model of Parkinson's disease. *Pharmacol. Rep.* 66, 660–669. doi: 10.1016/j.pharep.2014.03.008

Katashima, C. K., Silva, V. R. R., Lenhare, L., Marin, R. M., and Carvalheira, J. B. C. (2017). iNOS promotes hypothalamic insulin resistance associated with deregulation of energy balance and obesity in rodents. *Sci. Rep.* 7:9265. doi: 10.1038/s41598-017-08920-z

Kim, C. S., Kim, J. G., Lee, B. J., Choi, M. S., Choi, H. S., Kawada, T., et al. (2011). Deficiency for costimulatory receptor 4-1BB protects against obesity-induced inflammation and metabolic disorders. *Diabetes Metab. Res. Rev.* 60, 3159–3168. doi: 10.2337/db10-1805

Kim, J., Kwon, Y. H., Kim, C. S., Tu, T. H., Kim, B. S., Joe, Y., et al. (2018). The involvement of 4-1BB/4-1BBL signaling in glial cell-mediated hypothalamic inflammation in obesity. *FEBS Open Bio.* 8, 843–853. doi: 10.1002/2211-5463.12426

Kirkley, K. S., Popichak, K. A., Afzali, M. F., Legare, M. E., and Tjalkens, R. B. (2017). Microglia amplify inflammatory activation of astrocytes in manganese neurotoxicity. *J. Neuroinflammation* 14:99. doi: 10.1186/s12974-017-0871-0

Kreutzer, C., Peters, S., Schulte, D. M., Fangmann, D., Turk, K., Wolff, S., et al. (2017). Hypothalamic inflammation in human obesity is mediated by environmental and genetic factors. *Diabetes Metab. Res. Rev.* 66, 2407–2415. doi: 10.2337/db17-0067

Kwon, Y. H., Kim, J., Kim, C. S., Tu, T. H., Kim, M. S., Suk, K., et al. (2017). Hypothalamic lipid-laden astrocytes induce microglia migration and activation. *FEBS Lett.* 591, 1742–1751. doi: 10.1002/1873-3468.12691

Langlet, F. (2014). Tanycytes: a gateway to the metabolic hypothalamus. *J. Neuroendocrinol.* 26, 753–760. doi: 10.1111/jne.12191

Langlet, F., Levin, B. E., Luquet, S., Mazzone, M., Messina, A., Dunn-Meynell, A. A., et al. (2013). Tanycytic VEGF-A boosts blood-hypothalamus barrier plasticity and access of metabolic signals to the arcuate nucleus in response to fasting. *Cell Metab.* 17, 607–617. doi: 10.1016/j.cmet.2013.03.004

Le, N. H., Kim, C. S., Tu, T. H., Choi, H. S., Kim, B. S., Kawada, T., et al. (2013). Blockade of 4-1BB and 4-1BBL interaction reduces obesity-induced skeletal muscle inflammation. *Mediators Inflamm.* 2013:865159. doi: 10.1155/2013/865159

Le Thuc, O., Cansell, C., Bourourou, M., Denis, R. G., Stobbe, K., Devaux, N., et al. (2016). Central CCL2 signaling onto MCH neurons mediates metabolic and behavioral adaptation to inflammation. *EMBO Rep.* 17, 1738–1752. doi: 10.15252/embr.201541499

Le Thuc, O., Stobbe, K., Cansell, C., Nahon, J. L., Blondeau, N., and Rovere, C. (2017). Hypothalamic inflammation and energy balance disruptions: spotlight on chemokines. *Front. Endocrinol.* 8:197. doi: 10.3389/fendo.2017.00197

Lee, D. A., Bedont, J. L., Pak, T., Wang, H., Song, J., Miranda-Angulo, A., et al. (2012). Tanycytes of the hypothalamic median eminence form a diet-responsive neurogenic niche. *Nat. Neurosci.* 15, 700–702. doi: 10.1038/nn.3079

Lee, D. A., and Blackshaw, S. (2012). Functional implications of hypothalamic neurogenesis in the adult mammalian brain. *Int. J. Dev. Neurosci.* 30, 615–621. doi: 10.1016/j.ijdevneu.2012.07.003

Liddelow, S. A., Guttenplan, K. A., Clarke, L. E., Bennett, F. C., Bohlen, C. J., Schirmer, L., et al. (2017). Neurotoxic reactive astrocytes are induced by activated microglia. *Nature* 541, 481–487. doi: 10.1038/nature21029

Luo, X., Tai, W. L., Sun, L., Pan, Z., Xia, Z., Chung, S. K., et al. (2016). Crosstalk between astrocytic CXCL12 and microglial CXCR4 contributes to the development of neuropathic pain. *Mol. Pain* 12:1744806916636385. doi: 10.1177/1744806916636385

Mandrekar-Colucci, S., Karlo, J. C., and Landreth, G. E. (2012). Mechanisms underlying the rapid peroxisome proliferator-activated receptor-gamma-mediated amyloid clearance and reversal of cognitive deficits in a murine model of Alzheimer's disease. *J. Neurosci.* 32, 10117–10128. doi: 10.1523/JNEUROSCI.5268-11.2012

Mendes, N. F., Gaspar, J. M., Lima-Júnior, J. C., Donato, J. Jr., Velloso, L. A., and Araújo, E. P. (2018). TGF-beta1 down-regulation in the mediobasal hypothalamus attenuates hypothalamic inflammation and protects against diet-induced obesity. *Metabolism* 85, 171–182. doi: 10.1016/j.metabol.2018.04.005

Milanski, M., Degasperi, G., Coope, A., Morari, J., Denis, R., Cintra, D. E., et al. (2009). Saturated fatty acids produce an inflammatory response predominantly through the activation of TLR4 signaling in hypothalamus: implications for the pathogenesis of obesity. *J. Neurosci.* 29, 359–370. doi: 10.1523/JNEUROSCI.2760-08.2009

Morari, J., Anhe, G. F., Nascimento, L. F., de Moura, R. F., Razolli, D., Solon, C., et al. (2014). Fractalkine (CX3CL1) is involved in the early activation of hypothalamic inflammation in experimental obesity. *Diabetes Metab. Res. Rev.* 63, 3770–3784. doi: 10.2337/db13-1495

Mullier, A., Bouret, S. G., Prevot, V., and Dehouck, B. (2010). Differential distribution of tight junction proteins suggests a role for tanycytes in blood-hypothalamus barrier regulation in the adult mouse brain. *J. Comp. Neurol.* 518, 943–962. doi: 10.1002/cne.22273

Pascual, O., Ben Achour, S., Rostaing, P., Triller, A., and Bessis, A. (2012). Microglia activation triggers astrocyte-mediated modulation of excitatory neurotransmission. *Proc. Natl. Acad. Sci. U.S.A.* 109, E197–E205. doi: 10.1073/pnas.1111098109

Peruzzo, B., Pastor, F. E., Blazquez, J. L., Schobitz, K., Pelaez, B., Amat, P., et al. (2000). A second look at the barriers of the medial basal hypothalamus. *Exp. Brain. Res.* 132, 10–26. doi: 10.1007/s002219900289

Poon, K., Barson, J. R., Ho, H. T., and Leibowitz, S. F. (2016). Relationship of the chemokine, CXCL12, to effects of dietary fat on feeding-related behaviors and hypothalamic neuropeptide systems. *Front. Behav. Neurosci.* 10:51. doi: 10.3389/fnbeh.2016.00051

Rahman, M. H., Bhusal, A., Lee, W. H., Lee, I. K., and Suk, K. (2018). Hypothalamic inflammation and malfunctioning glia in the pathophysiology of obesity and diabetes: translational significance. *Biochem. Pharmacol.* 153, 123–133. doi: 10.1016/j.bcp.2018.01.024

Ramalho, A. F., Bombassaro, B., Dragano, N. R., Solon, C., Morari, J., Fioravante, M., et al. (2018). Dietary fats promote functional and structural changes in the median eminence blood/spinal fluid interface-the protective role for BDNF. *J. Neuroinflammation* 15:10. doi: 10.1186/s12974-017-1046-8

Ransohoff, R. M., and Brown, M. A. (2012). Innate immunity in the central nervous system. *J. Clin. Invest.* 122, 1164–1171. doi: 10.1172/JCI58644

Reali, C., Curto, M., Sogos, V., Scintu, F., Pauly, S., Schwarz, H., et al. (2003). Expression of CD137 and its ligand in human neurons, astrocytes, and microglia: modulation by FGF-2. *J. Neurosci. Res.* 74, 67–73. doi: 10.1002/jnr.10727

Rizzoti, K., and Lovell-Badge, R. (2017). Pivotal role of median eminence tanycytes for hypothalamic function and neurogenesis. *Mol. Cell Endocrinol.* 445, 7–13. doi: 10.1016/j.mce.2016.08.020

Rocha, S. M., Cristovao, A. C., Campos, F. L., Fonseca, C. P., and Baltazar, G. (2012). Astrocyte-derived GDNF is a potent inhibitor of microglial activation. *Neurobiol. Dis.* 47, 407–415. doi: 10.1016/j.nbd.2012.04.014

Rothhammer, V., Borucki, D. M., Tjon, E. C., Takenaka, M. C., Chao, C. C., Ardura-Fabregat, A., et al. (2018). Microglial control of astrocytes in response to microbial metabolites. *Nature* 557, 724–728. doi: 10.1038/s41586-018-0119-x

Sasaki, T., Numano, R., Yokota-Hashimoto, H., Matsui, S., Kimura, N., Takeuchi, H., et al. (2018). A central-acting connexin inhibitor, INI-0602, prevents high-fat diet-induced feeding pattern disturbances and obesity in mice. *Mol. Brain* 11:28. doi: 10.1186/s13041-018-0372-9

Schur, E. A., Melhorn, S. J., Oh, S. K., Lacy, J. M., Berkseth, K. E., Guyenet, S. J., et al. (2015). Radiologic evidence that hypothalamic gliosis is associated with obesity and insulin resistance in humans. *Obesity* 23, 2142–2148. doi: 10.1002/oby.21248

Schwenkgrub, J., Joniec-Maciejak, I., Sznejder-Pacholek, A., Wawer, A., Ciesielska, A., Bankiewicz, K., et al. (2013). Effect of human interleukin-10 on the expression of nitric oxide synthases in the MPTP-based model of Parkinson's disease. *Pharmacol. Rep.* 65, 44–49. doi: 10.1016/S1734-1140(13)70962-9

Shao, Z., and Schwarz, H. (2011). CD137 ligand, a member of the tumor necrosis factor family, regulates immune responses via reverse signal transduction. *J. Leukoc. Biol.* 89, 21–29. doi: 10.1189/jlb.0510315

Subramaniam, S. R., and Federoff, H. J. (2017). Targeting microglial activation states as a therapeutic avenue in Parkinson's Disease. *Front. Aging Neurosci.* 9:176. doi: 10.3389/fnagi.2017.00176

Tanuma, N., Sakuma, H., Sasaki, A., and Matsumoto, Y. (2006). Chemokine expression by astrocytes plays a role in microglia/macrophage activation and subsequent neurodegeneration in secondary progressive multiple sclerosis. *Acta Neuropathol.* 112, 195–204. doi: 10.1007/s00401-006-0083-7

Thaler, J. P., Yi, C. X., Schur, E. A., Guyenet, S. J., Hwang, B. H., Dietrich, M. O., et al. (2012). Obesity is associated with hypothalamic injury in rodents and humans. *J. Clin. Invest.* 122, 153–162. doi: 10.1172/JCI59660

Tian, L., Ma, L., Kaarela, T., and Li, Z. (2012). Neuroimmune crosstalk in the central nervous system and its significance for neurological diseases. *J. Neuroinflammation* 9, 155. doi: 10.1186/1742-2094-9-155

Tu, T. H., Kim, C. S., Goto, T., Kawada, T., Kim, B. S., and Yu, R. (2012). 4-1BB/4-1BBL interaction promotes obesity-induced adipose inflammation by triggering bidirectional inflammatory signaling in adipocytes/macrophages. *Mediators Inflamm.* 2012:972629. doi: 10.1155/2012/972629

Valdearcos, M., Douglass, J. D., Robblee, M. M., Dorfman, M. D., Stifler, D. R., Bennett, M. L., et al. (2018). Microglial inflammatory signaling orchestrates the hypothalamic immune response to dietary excess and mediates obesity susceptibility. *Cell Metab.* 27, 185–197.e3. doi: 10.1016/j.cmet.2018.04.019

Valdearcos, M., Robblee, M. M., Benjamin, D. I., Nomura, D. K., Xu, A. W., and Koliwad, S. K. (2014). Microglia dictate the impact of saturated fat consumption on hypothalamic inflammation and neuronal function. *Cell Rep.* 9, 2124–2138. doi: 10.1016/j.celrep.2014.11.018

Valdearcos, M., Xu, A. W., and Koliwad, S. K. (2015). Hypothalamic inflammation in the control of metabolic function. *Annu. Rev. Physiol.* 77, 131–160. doi: 10.1146/annurev-physiol-021014-071656

Vinay, D. S., and Kwon, B. S. (2011). 4-1BB signaling beyond T cells. *Cell Mol. Immunol.* 8, 281–284. doi: 10.1038/cmi.2010.82

Wang, Z., Liu, D., Wang, F., Liu, S., Zhao, S., Ling, E. A., et al. (2012). Saturated fatty acids activate microglia via Toll-like receptor 4/NF-kappaB signalling. *Br. J. Nutr.* 107, 229–241. doi: 10.1017/S0007114511002868

Yao, Y., and Tsirka, S. E. (2014). Monocyte chemoattractant protein-1 and the blood-brain barrier. *Cell Mol. Life Sci.* 71, 683–697. doi: 10.1007/s00018-013-1459-1

Yeo, Y. A., Martinez Gomez, J. M., Croxford, J. L., Gasser, S., Ling, E. A., and Schwarz, H. (2012). CD137 ligand activated microglia induces oligodendrocyte apoptosis via reactive oxygen species. *J. Neuroinflammation* 9:173. doi: 10.1186/1742-2094-9-173

Zhang, Y., Reichel, J. M., Han, C., Zuniga-Hertz, J. P., and Cai, D. (2017). Astrocytic process plasticity and IKKbeta/NF-kappaB in central control of blood glucose, blood pressure, and body weight. *Cell Metab.* 25, 1091–1102.e4. doi: 10.1016/j.cmet.2017.04.002

Zujovic, V., Benavides, J., Vige, X., Carter, C., and Taupin, V. (2000). Fractalkine modulates TNF-alpha secretion and neurotoxicity induced by microglial activation. *Glia* 29, 305–315. doi: 10.1002/(SICI)1098-1136(20000215)29:4<305::AID-GLIA2>3.0.CO;2-V

16

Animal Foetal Models of Obesity and Diabetes – From Laboratory to Clinical Settings

Emilia Grzęda[1], *Julia Matuszewska*[1], *Kamil Ziarniak*[1,2], *Anna Gertig-Kolasa*[3], *Izabela Krzyśko-Pieczka*[3], *Bogda Skowrońska*[3] *and Joanna H. Sliwowska*[1*]

[1] Laboratory of Neurobiology, Faculty of Veterinary Medicine and Animal Science, Poznań University of Life Sciences, Poznań, Poland, [2] Molecular and Cell Biology Unit, Poznań University of Medical Sciences, Poznań, Poland, [3] Department of Paediatric Diabetes and Obesity, Poznań University of Medical Sciences, Poznań, Poland

***Correspondence:**
Joanna H. Sliwowska
joanna.sliwowska@up.poznan.pl

The prenatal period, during which a fully formed newborn capable of surviving outside its mother's body is built from a single cell, is critical for human development. It is also the time when the foetus is particularly vulnerable to environmental factors, which may modulate the course of its development. Both epidemiological and animal studies have shown that foetal programming of physiological systems may alter the growth and function of organs and lead to pathology in adulthood. Nutrition is a particularly important environmental factor for the pregnant mother as it affects the condition of offspring. Numerous studies have shown that an unbalanced maternal metabolic status (under- or overnutrition) may cause long-lasting physiological and behavioural alterations, resulting in metabolic disorders, such as obesity and type 2 diabetes (T2DM). Various diets are used in laboratory settings in order to induce maternal obesity and metabolic disorders, and to alter the offspring development. The most popular models are: high-fat, high-sugar, high-fat-high-sugar, and cafeteria diets. Maternal undernutrition models are also used, which results in metabolic problems in offspring. Similarly to animal data, human studies have shown the influence of mothers' diets on the development of children. There is a strong link between the maternal diet and the birth weight, metabolic state, changes in the cardiovascular and central nervous system of the offspring. The mechanisms linking impaired foetal development and adult diseases remain under discussion. Epigenetic mechanisms are believed to play a major role in prenatal programming. Additionally, sexually dimorphic effects on offspring are observed. Therefore, further research on both sexes is necessary.

Keywords: obesity, diabetes, brain, sex differences, behaviour, cardiovascular system, prenatal programming

INTRODUCTION: WE ARE WHAT OUR MOTHERS EAT

Over the years numerous epidemiological findings and data from animal studies revealed the effects of mother's nutrition on the development of offspring. Researchers proposed the concept of foetal/early programming, according to which early environmental factors can permanently organise or imprint physiological and behavioural systems. Programming is defined as the process in which environmental factor(s), acting during the sensitive period, affect the structure and functions of tissues and organs, leading to lifelong effects (1, 2). Accordingly, researchers suggested redirecting investigations towards the intrauterine environment rather than the environment in later childhood and indicated that the womb may be more important than home (1).

Although hunger is still common nowadays, especially in Africa, paradoxically, all over the world more people are dying of the health problems caused by overeating rather than malnutrition. This subject is particularly interesting at the time when obesity is a worldwide problem, and it is even greater due to the COVID-19 pandemic. As pandemic-related lockdowns reduced people's physical activity and increased overeating (the factors contributing to the development of obesity), the rates of these metabolic problems are expected to increase rapidly in our society in the future, also among mothers-to-be and their offspring. It is a well-known fact that the Western pattern diet (WPD), which is common in the US and other developed countries, may chronically activate the innate immune system and inhibit the adaptive immune system. Thus, the WPD impairs adaptive immunity while ramping up innate immunity. This leads to chronic inflammation and severely impairs the host's defence against viral pathogens, including COVID-19 (3). A report on 4,103 patients with COVID-19 disease in New York City showed that the most important clinical features leading to hospital admission were age >65 years and obesity (4). The author of another study on critically ill adults with COVID-19 admitted to two hospitals in New York City reported that the majority were men aged over 60 years and nearly half of them were obese (5). These findings were also confirmed by the authors of European studies on 165 adult patients with a mean BMI 26, who found that severe forms of COVID-19 were associated with high visceral adiposity (6).

According to the findings of studies on animals and humans, both maternal under and overnutrition/obesity affects the cognitive function and the development of neurological and psychiatric disorders in offspring.

The foetal programming concept suggests that maternal nutritional imbalance (both under- and overnutrition) have a long-term effect on the health of offspring and on the risk of diseases such as diabetes (7). The mechanisms responsible for the effects of maternal undernutrition and obesity on the increased risk of future metabolic disease have not been thoroughly investigated. They include changes in the foetal supply of nutrients, genetic and epigenetic factors. Moreover, as results from animal studies on perinatal high-fat diet (HFD) programming, the potential mechanisms of neural pathways include circulating factors, such as hormones (leptin, insulin), nutrients (fatty acids, triglycerides (TG) and glucose), and inflammatory cytokines.

The aim of this paper was to review the data on maternal undernutrition, obesity, and diabetes provided by the authors of research on humans and animals, and to discuss the potential mechanisms underlying the foetal metabolic programming. The main focus of this review is the foetal metabolic system and central nervous system (CNS), because they seem to be the most vulnerable to the harmful effects of programming (8). The mechanism(s) contributing to the sexual dimorphism of metabolic diseases were also investigated. The detailed analysis of data concerning sexual differences observed in the offspring of malnourished and overnourished mothers is shown in the **Table 1**. The understanding of these mechanisms could provide useful tools for the prevention and treatment of these diseases in offspring.

ANIMAL MODELS OF OBESITY WITH SPECIAL EMPHASIS ON DIET-INDUCED OBESITY

Studies on different animal species, mostly mice, rats, and sheep, allow us to understand the mechanisms responsible for the development of obesity and diabetes, and search for intervention strategies. Obesity can be induced in animals chemically (with drugs), surgically, genetically, or through diet (57–61). Obesity has multifactorial aetiology and in the light of the increasing occurrence of unhealthy nutrition (e.g. the consumption of fast food), the rising prevalence of obesity suggests that it is caused by environmental factors. The authors of this review focused mostly on diet-induced obesity in rodents and made references to numerous excellent comprehensive reviews of other models of animal obesity (59, 60).

The most popular models of diet-induced obesity are: high-fat (HFD), high-sugar (HSD), high-fat-high-sugar (HFHSD), and cafeteria (CAF) diets. High-fat diets caused metabolic imbalance, decreased energy expenditure and, as a result, increased the body weight of laboratory animals (62, 63). However, there are differences between species and even strains of rodents. Both Wistar and Sprague-Dawley rats can be used as models of HFD-induced obesity (64), although the metabolic effects caused by this type of dietary regimen are more pronounced in Wistar rats. In recent decades the HFD has been most widely applied in experiments on rodents, but there were significant differences in the composition and fat content of the diets provided to animals to induce obesity. The fat in these diets came from multiple sources, including animals (lard, tallow), plants (olive oil, sunflower, corn, coconut), and fish. The fat composition seems to have a major role in obesity because saturated fats cause more deleterious effects than unsaturated fats (63, 65). Another important factor is the concentration of fat in the diet, which usually ranges from 30% to 60%. The diet-feeding period also differed between studies – it usually ranged from 4 to 16 weeks (62, 63).

Similarly to the situation observed in highly developed countries, a high-sugar diet also contributed to the development of obesity in laboratory animals. In experimental models, sucrose was fed separately from the standard feed, as a superadditive or mixed with drinking water (61). The HSD negatively influenced the glycaemic control in rodents. These effects were similar to those observed after feeding an HFD.

TABLE 1 | Maternal under- and overnutrition induce sex-specific differences in body weight, fat content, metabolic and hormonal status, cardiovascular system and brain and behavioural outcomes in offspring; ↑ - increase; ↓ decrease; - no change.

Outcomes	Species	Maternal undernutrition effects on offspring outcomes	Maternal overnutrition effects on offspring outcomes
BODY WEIGHT	Mice	Food restricted diet (FR/50%) ↓males and females birth weight (9) FR/70% ↓males and females birth weight (10)	High fat diet (HFD) – males birth weight ↓females birth weight (11) High fat high sugar diet (HFHSD) ↑adult males body weight > ↑ adult females body weight (12)
	Rats	FR/70% ↓males and females birth weight (13) Protein restricted diet (PR/9%) ↓adult males body weight (14) PR/9% ↓females birth weight – males birth weight (15) PR/5% ↓adult males and females body weight (16)	HFHSD ↓males and females birth weight ↑adult males body weight > ↑ adult females body weight (17) Cafeteria diet (CAF) – males and females birth weight ↓adult males body weight < ↓ adult females body weight (18) CAF ↑ body weight (adult females) (19)
	Human	Maternal undernutrition ↓ females birth weight > ↓males birth weight (20) ↓ females birth weight < ↓ males birth weight (21) ↓ females birth weight <↓ males birth weight (22)	Maternal gestational diabetes mellitus (GDM) and/or obesity ↑males BMI ↑males - risk of the obesity development in adulthood (23)
FAT CONTENT	Mice	PR/6% ↑ adiposity in males and females which fed HFD (24)	HFD ↑ adult males body fat content ↓ adult females body fat content (25) HFD ↑adult males body fat content > adult females body fat content (26) HFHSD ↑ adult males and females - inguinal fat pad mass (12)
	Rats	PR/10% ↑ adult males deposits of abdominal fat – adult females deposits of abdominal fat ↓ adult males deposits of gonadal fat – adult females deposits of gonadal fat (14) PR/10% ↑ young females body fat content – young males body fat content (27)	CAF ↑adult males perirenal fat mass > ↑ female perirenal fat mass ↑adult males gonadal fat content < ↑ females gonadal fat content (28) CAF ↓adult males fat content < ↓ adult females fat content (18) CAF ↑ abdominal fat in adult males and females (19)
	Sheep	FR ↑ fat mass in adult males – fat mass in adult females (29)	
	Human	Maternal uandernutrition ↓ lean and fat mass in females and males at birth ↑ fat mass in girls > ↑ fat mass in boys (30)	Maternal pre-pregnancy BMI ↑ adult females fat mass (31) ↑ young females fat mass (32)
METABOLIC AND HORMONAL STATUS	Rats	PR/10% ↑ insulin and leptin levels in young males and females ↑ TG levels in young males – TG levels in young females (27)	CAF ↑glucose levels in young females ↑insulin levels in young males < ↑ insulin levels in young females (18) CAF ↑glucose levels in adult females ↑leptin levels in adult females (33) HSD ↑ insulin resistance and oxidative stress in adult males – insulin resistance and oxidative stress in adult females (34) HFD ↑glucose levels in adult females – glucose levels in adult males ↑TG levels in adult females – TG levels in adult males (35) CAF ↑ plasma leptin, insulin and TG levels in adult males and females (19)
	Sheep	FR ↓ POMC expression in adult males – POMC expression in adult females (29)	
	Humans	Maternal undernutrition ↑ LDL level in adults males and females	Maternal obesity ↑ blood insulin concentration at birth in boys < ↑ blood insulin concentration at birth in girls

(Continued)

TABLE 1 | Continued

Outcomes	Species	Maternal undernutrition effects on offspring outcomes	Maternal overnutrition effects on offspring outcomes
		↓ glucose tolerance in adult males and females ↑ insulin resistance in adult males and females (36)	↑insulin resistance in girls adult life (37) Maternal diabetes ↑insulin resistance in girls adult life (38)
CARDIOVASCULAR SYSTEM	Mice	FR ↑ mean arterial pressure (MAP) in adult males - MAP in adult females (39)	HFHSD ↑ diastolic blood pressure (DBP) in adult males ↑ systolic blood pressure (SBP) in adult males ↑ DBP, SBP in adult females > ↑ DBP, SBP in adult males ↑ Heart rate (HR) in adult males and females (12)
	Rats	PR ↑ risk of hypertension in young males > ↑ risk of hypertension in young females (40) PR ↑ risk of hypertension develops in young males and females (41)	HFD ↑ DBP, SBP in adult females – DBP, SBP in adult males (35)
	Humans	Maternal undernutrition ↑ risk of coronary heart disease in adult females ↑ risk of coronary heart disease in adult males (42) ↑ risk of hypertension in adult females ↑ risk of hypertension in adult males (36)	Maternal obesity ↑ risk of stroke in adult females – risk of stroke in adult males (43) Maternal diabetes ↑ blood pressure during childhood in the males – blood pressure during childhood in the females (44)
BRAIN AND BEHAVIOURAL OUTCOMES	Baboons	FR ↓ working memory in adolescent females – working memory in adolescent males ↑impulsivity in adolescent males – impulsivity in adolescent females (45)	
	Mice	FR/70% ↓ locomotor activity in males and females ↓ recognition memory (NOR) in males and females ↓ synaptophysin level in the female hippocampus (10) PR/8% ↑ anxiety- and depression-like behaviours in males – anxiety- and depression-like behaviours in females (46)	HFD ↓ myelination in the medial cortex in young males – myelination in the medial cortex in young females ↓ memory parameters assessed in the NOR in young males – memory parameters assessed in the NOR in young females (47) HFD ↑ anxiety-like behaviours in adult males – anxiety-like behaviours in adult females (48)
	Rats	LP/9% ↓ locomotor activity in males – locomotor activity in females ↓ feeding behaviour in females – feeding behaviour in males (14)	HFD ↓ memory parameters assessed in the MWM in adolescent males – memory parameters assessed in the MWM in adolescent females (49) HFD ↑ depression-like symptoms in adult males – depression-like symptoms in adult females (50) HFD ↑ anxiety in adult males < ↑anxiety in adult females (51) HFD ↑ anxiety in young females – anxiety in young males ↓ sociability in young females – sociability in young males (52) HFD ↑ anxiety in male and female neonates (53)
	Humans	Maternal undernutrition ↓ total brain volume in boys/men – total brain volume in girls/women ↓ volumes of grey and white matter in boys/men – volumes of grey and white matter in girls/women (54) ↑ ASD, ADHD and schizophrenia in boys > ↑ ASD, ADHD and schizophrenia in girls (55)	Maternal obesity ↓ hippocampal development/volume in boys – hippocampal development/volume in girls (56)

ASD, autism spectrum disorder; ADHD, attention deficit hyperactivity disorder; CAF, cafeteria diet; DBP, diastolic blood pressure; FR, food restricted diet; GDM, gestational diabetes mellitus; HFD, high-fat diet; HR, heart rate; HSHFD, high-fat high sugar diet; LDL, low-density lipoprotein; MAP, mean arterial pressure; MWM, Morris water maze; NOR, novel object recognition; POMC, pro-opiomelanocortin; PR, protein restricted diet; SBP, systolic blood pressure; TG, triglycerides.

However, the body weight gain and adiposity in HSD-fed animals were lesser than after feeding an HFD (59).

A combination of HFD and HSD better imitates human characteristics. The HFHSD has widely been used in studies on rodents as a Western pattern diet. However, Omar et al. showed that the HFHSD was not as effective as the HFD in C57BL/6J mice (66).

The CAF diet is employed in laboratory settings, where animals receive a mix of high-fat and high-sugar food products, which are commonly consumed by people (e.g. cake, biscuits, crisps, processed meat, peanut butter, chocolate, cheese, dried fruit) (60, 61, 65). The components of the CAF diet have a high energy value and are highly palatable, which increases animals' tendency to overconsumption (60, 61, 65). This model mimics the occurrence of obesity in humans as a consequence of a tasty but unbalanced diet. However, this diet varies in the number and type of products used and its energy value [for more details see (67)].

Experimental paradigms may also vary in terms of exposure to these diets, i.e. the length of food consumption before and/or during pregnancy and/or lactation, which may also influence the results. Among the environmental factors influencing the programming of the foetal phenotype, particular attention is paid to disturbed maternal nutrition. Animal and epidemiological studies have indicated that foetal nutritional deprivation is a strong programming stimulus. On the other hand experimental evidence suggests that maternal overnutrition can result in a phenotype of the offspring characteristic of metabolic syndrome. Moreover, both in humans and animal studies, it has been confirmed that prenatal, perinatal and postnatal factors that are associated with disturbed maternal and offspring nutrition are additive (28, 68–71). In consequence, they lead to unfavourable changes in metabolism in adulthood, and induce diabetes. *In utero*, epigenetic changes exacerbate the negative effects associated with the influence of environmental factors throughout life (68–71).

ANIMAL MODELS OF DIABETES

There are two major types of diabetes, i.e. type 1 (T1DM) and type 2 (T2DM). The latter is the most common, as it represents more than 90% of all cases. T1DM is caused by an autoimmune destruction of the insulin-producing β-cells in the pancreas (72). Due to the pathophysiology of T1DM, insulin therapy is implemented at the onset of this disease. On the other hand, T2DM can be associated with elevated, normal, or low insulin levels, depending on the stage at which the levels of this hormone are measured. This is a progressive disorder, which is manifested by diminishing pancreatic function over time. The authors of this review mostly focused on T2DM occurring during gestation, as it is often associated with obesity and more prevalent than T1DM. Gestational diabetes mellitus (GDM) is an issue of particular interest in this review. This is a heterogeneous entity and affects mostly insulin-resistant overweight and obese women. It is also a strong female risk factor for the progression of T2DM (73).

There are multiple animal models used for the induction of diabetes – mostly rodents (mice and rats) as well as sheep, dogs, cats, and other animals. Diabetes can be induced surgically, chemically or genetically. The surgical method requires pancreatectomy, i.e. removal of most of the pancreatic tissue. Diabetes can be induced non-surgically through damage to the pancreatic cells. This effect can be obtained through the administration of drugs such as alloxan and streptozotocin (STZ, toxins destroying β-cells of the pancreas), which cause insulin deficiency and hyperglycaemia in animals. Alloxan diabetogenicity occurs through the rapid uptake of the drug by insulin-secreting cells, the formation of reactive oxygen species, and disturbances in intracellular calcium homeostasis. It is also necessary to remember that the range of the diabetogenic dose of alloxan is quite narrow and even a small overdose may be generally toxic and kill animals due to kidney failure (74).

Like alloxan, the dose range of STZ is narrow. To date researchers have applied single or multiple injections in experimental paradigms with different animal species and strains (75–78). STZ is taken up by pancreatic β-cells *via* the glucose transporter GLUT2, which changes the DNA in these cells and provokes its fragmentation. For more detailed information on the mechanisms of alloxan and STZ action see Szkudelski (74).

A combination of HFD and STZ is often employed in laboratory settings. These two stressors mimic the pathology of T2DM, though on a shorter timescale than the one observed in humans. The use of HFD causes insulin resistance and/or glucose intolerance, while the administration of STZ reduces functional β-cell mass (79). Another advantage of this model is that it mimics the slow pathogenesis of T2DM occurring in most humans, which progresses from the slow development of an adult-onset diet-induced obesity to glucose intolerance, insulin resistance (and the resulting compensatory insulin release) and, finally, STZ-induced partial β-cell death. Despite its limitations, e.g. the use of two stressors – HFD and STZ, the HFD/STZ is a reasonable animal model of T2DM and represents the late stage of the disease (80).

Sex-dependent differences in the induction of T2DM by STZ are also of particular interest in this review because, according to scientific reports, males are more prone to develop diabetes (81, 82). There are also sex-specific differences in the development and complications of diabetes in humans. For example, diabetes is considered a stronger risk factor for cardiovascular diseases in women than men (81). Women tend to store the fat tissue, whereas men tend to mobilise adipose tissue burning (83). Women exhibit greater insulin sensitivity than men. There are sex-specific differences in body fat distribution, which point to the crucial role of sex hormones (84).

There are also various genetic models of diabetes, but they will not be discussed here because they do not fall within the scope of this review [e.g. see (85)].

Animal models of T2DM provide not only an opportunity to investigate the pathophysiology underlying this disorder, but also enable the assessment of potential strategies for the treatment and prevention of the disease and related complications.

ANIMAL MODELS OF UNDERNUTRITION

To date research on undernutrition has been successfully conducted on various species of animals, such as laboratory rodents (rats, mice), sheep, pigs, and primates. Due to the fact that rodents and sheep are the most commonly used species in this research area, they will be henceforth discussed in this review. For more information on the advantages and disadvantages of other species see the review by Swanson (86).

Perinatal undernutrition can be induced in rodents through either maternal underfeeding (general food restriction or protein content restriction) during gestation or the modification of the offspring's energy intake during the suckling period. Rodents have been used in numerous studies to examine different degrees of dietary restriction during gestation - from mild (30%), through moderate (50%), up to severe (70%) protein restriction (PR) or food restriction (FR) [for reviews see (87, 88)]. Postnatal manipulations usually include various forms of maternal milk restriction, e.g. maternal deprivation (which promotes perinatal stress) (89–91), early weaning induced with pharmacological compounds such as bromocriptine a drug inhibiting lactation (92)], non-pharmacological early weaning (in the last three days of the suckling period, when nipple suction can be interrupted with a physical barrier, e.g. by wrapping the breast area with a bandage (93–95) or rearing pups in large litters (96, 97). Maternal undernutrition in sheep is usually induced through FR [30-50% of the control feed allowance (98)]. However, there are some changes in the time of nutritional insult.

In conclusion, researchers interested in studying the effects of the maternal diet on offspring in laboratory settings have a variety of options, but due caution is necessary to ensure proper dietary controls and provide a detailed description of the diets used during the experiment, including the time of exposure and considering possible sex differences. The choice of a suitable animal model is a key point affecting the translational potential of the results.

EFFECTS OF MATERNAL OVERNUTRITION ON BODY WEIGHT AND FAT CONTENT: ANIMAL STUDIES

Maternal overnutrition and/or obesity affect the weight of rodent offspring in a time-dependent manner (**Figure 1**). White et al. conducted a study on rats in which they investigated the relationship between the effects of maternal obesity and an HFD of the offspring on their body weight. They observed that these effects were independent and additive (99). Maternal obesity induced by an HFD caused a significantly lower birth weight of rats (17, 100, 101) and mice (102, 103). Similarly, the offspring of the female rats receiving a CAF diet before and during pregnancy were lighter (28, 104–106). However, other studies showed that the birth weights of the mice delivered by dams exposed to an HFD were significantly greater than those of the control offspring (25, 107). Similarly, the maternal consumption of a CAF diet resulted in a greater body weight of neonatal rats (19). Additionally, several experiments showed that the administration of a CAF diet (70) and an HFD (108, 109) before and during pregnancy did not influence the birth weight of rat and mice pups (110). The differences in the results of various studies may have been caused by the use of different sources of fat and the duration of feeding the diets to the dams and/or offspring (before pregnancy, and/or during pregnancy, and/or lactation), as well as the different effect of obese pregnancies on placental functions. Obesity may increase the placental growth and cause foetal overgrowth or reduce the placental blood flow and limit the foetal growth (111).

Thus, pre-gestational and/or gestational overnutrition of female rodents resulted in a heavier weight of adult offspring, which led to obesity. This effect was observed when: i) the birth weight was significantly lower [rats/HFHSD (17)], ii) the birth weight was not affected (mice/male/HFHCD) (11), and iii) the birth weight was significantly greater [mice/HFD (25, 107)]. Sasson et al. observed that pre-gestational exposure of mice to an HFD restricted the growth of newborn pups, but there was no effect on the weight of adult animals (103). Importantly, studies also revealed a catch-up in the body weight of offspring. The birth weight of the offspring of the female rats fed a CAF diet was either smaller or greater than the weight of the animals in the control group. However, the differences in the body weight disappeared during further development (19, 106).

There is not much data on the sex-specific differences in the effects of maternal diet on the weight of offspring. King et al. found that the maternal HFD did not affect the birth weight of male mice offspring, but reduced the birth weight of females (11). Nivoit et al. found that the offspring of obese rat dams had lower birth weights than the offspring of the animals in the control group. However, when the rats matured, the adult offspring of the HFHSD females became heavier than those in the control group, and these differences were less pronounced in the females (17). Similarly, Samuelsson et al. have found that in the offspring of HFHSD mothers, adult male mice were heavier than females (12). Matuszewska et al. (18) observed that on postnatal day (PND) 25 both male and female offspring of the dams fed a CAF diet had lower body weights than the animals in the control group. However, there was no difference in this parameter on PND 3. Moreover, on PND 25 the CAF females were lighter than the CAF males. On the contrary, in a study conducted by Jacobs et al., feeding mothers the CAF diet resulted in an increase in body weight of adult female rat offspring (19).

As numerous studies on rodents showed, changes in the body weight of the offspring of obese dams seem to be caused by an increase in the body fat content. Increased proportions of the body fat content (112) were described in the rat offspring of females fed HFD (99, 112), HFHSD (17), and CAF diets (18, 28, 70). The authors of the aforementioned studies with the CAF diet observed an increase in the fat content, but there was no change (70) or a decrease in the body weight of the offspring receiving the other two protocols of dietary regime (18, 28). The authors of studies on mice also observed that the fat content in the offspring was influenced by the HFD provided to their mothers (25, 103, 113).

Researchers also observed sex-specific changes in the fat content in offspring. Dahlhoff et al. found that the male offspring of HFD mice had more fat than the animals in the control group, but the

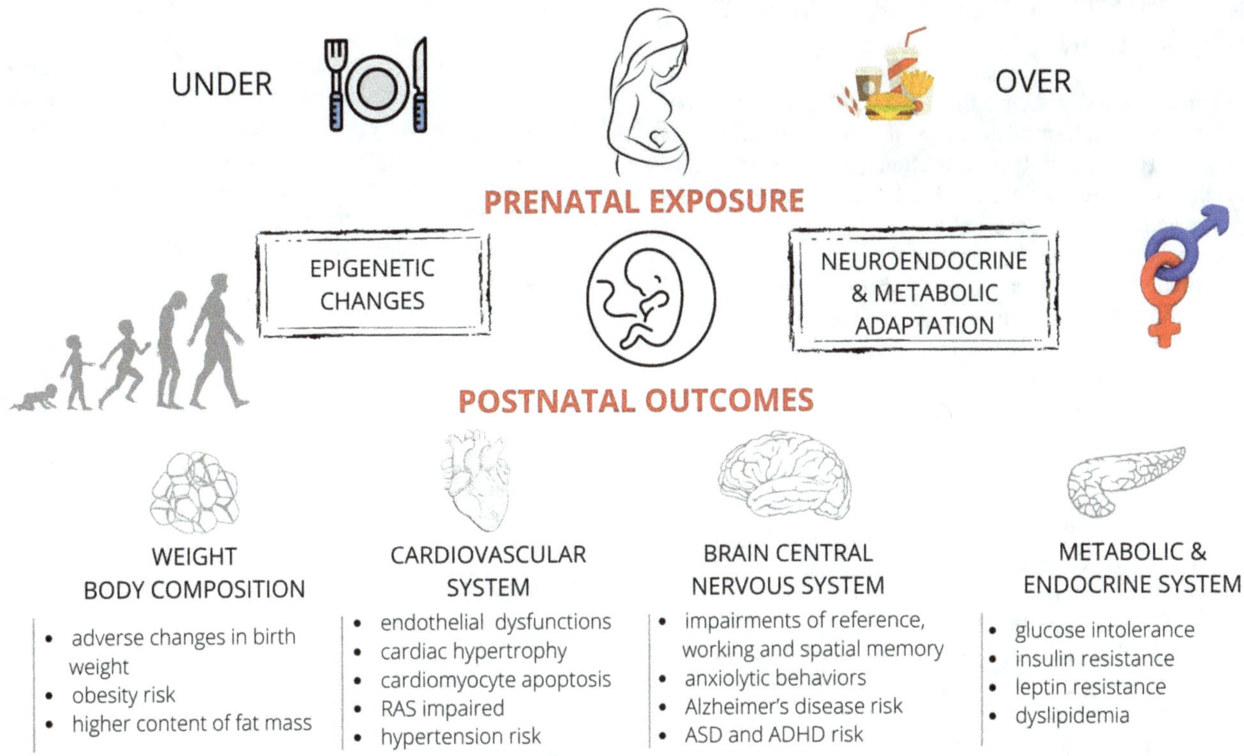

FIGURE 1 | The effects of maternal nutritional imbalance (under- and overnutrition) on offspring during foetal development. Short and long-term negative outcomes (observed both in humans and laboratory animals) include the adverse effects of unbalanced diet on offspring's metabolism, hormonal state, changes in the body weight and fat content, and abnormal function of the nervous and cardiovascular systems. These effects appear to be sex-specific. ASD, autism spectrum disorder; ADHD, attention deficit hyperactivity disorder; RAS, the renin-angiotensin system.

female offspring had a lower body fat content than the animals in the control group (25). Masuyama and Hiramatsu (26) observed that maternal obesity induced by an HFD caused an increased fat mass gain in the male and female offspring at 14 weeks of age, but this effect was less pronounced in the females. However, in a mouse model of HFHSD, both adult male and female offspring had increased inguinal fat pad mass (12). Similarly, male and female offspring of rats exposed to CAF diet had higher abdominal fat content (19). Moreover, among the four-week offspring of CAF mothers the males had a higher perirenal fat mass than the females, whereas the females had a greater gonadal fat content than the males (28). Matuszewska et al. (18) observed that both the male and female offspring of mothers receiving a CAF diet for four weeks before pregnancy, and then during pregnancy and lactation, had a lower fat content on PND 25, but these changes were more pronounced in the female CAF offspring.

EFFECTS OF MATERNAL OVERNUTRITION ON BODY WEIGHT AND FAT CONTENT: HUMAN STUDIES

Maternal overweight is a risk factor for foetal macrosomia and it increases the risk of development of obesity throughout childhood and adolescence (114–117). High maternal weight during all three trimesters of pregnancy increases the risk of elevated birth weight of offspring (118, 119). The meta-analysis of clinical studies showed that excessive gestational weight gain increased the risk of childhood obesity by 33% (120). The proposed mechanisms underlying these associations include abnormal placental transfer, epigenetic mechanisms, and altered peripheral and central metabolic profile in offspring (114, 115).

A higher pre-pregnancy BMI also increases the total body fat mass during childhood, and abdominal subcutaneous and preperitoneal fat mass (121, 122). Eshrigui et al. (31) indicated a direct linkage between the maternal pre-pregnancy BMI and the fat mass index, the percentage of body fat, the visceral adipose tissue, and the android-to-gynoid fat ratio of offspring.

Cohort clinical studies showed that metabolic disorders resulting from the obesity of offspring were sex-specific (23). The male but not female offspring exposed to gestational diabetes mellitus (GDM) and/or obesity had a higher BMI and were more likely to develop obesity from late childhood to early adulthood (123). Maternal glycaemia appears to be a major factor initiating adiposity in male infants, whereas the maternal BMI is the main predictor in female infants (23). Moreover, Chaparo et al. and Eshriqui et al. found that the maternal pre-pregnancy BMI was directly associated with a greater fat mass in daughters, but not sons (31, 32).

EFFECTS OF MATERNAL UNDERNUTRITION ON BODY WEIGHT AND FAT CONTENT: ANIMAL STUDIES

Numerous studies assessing the effects of malnutrition on a number of animal models have shown that either food restriction (FR) or protein restriction (PR) can programme offspring to altered adiposity and body weight at different stages of gestation and postnatal life.

In rats both paradigms of maternal malnutrition (regardless of the timeframe of undernutrition, whether energy restriction lasted throughout gestation or only part of this period) often resulted in a lower birth weight (up to ~40%) (124–127). However, most of these studies showed that despite the lower birth weight observed in the offspring, these animals were often characterised by increased adiposity, gain of the adipose tissue or adipocyte size at later stages of life (124, 128, 129). Few studies showed that a lower body weight could persist for several days, weeks (126, 127, 130) or even for up to ten months, especially when the dam's age was taken into consideration, as Ware et al. (131) observed. In their experiment dams were mated at different ages, i.e. at 2 and 4 months of age (the young maternal group), and at 6 and 9 months of age (the old maternal group). The animals in both age groups were fed a low protein (LP) diet (50% restriction) or a control diet throughout gestation. After weaning both the male and female offspring of these dams were fed a control diet until 9 months of age. After this period the offspring were fed either the control diet or an HFD (40% of fat) for 9 weeks. In general, at 10 months of age the male offspring of the animals fed the LP diet were smaller than the control counterparts. However, the male offspring of the older LP dams had over a 50% lower weight gain than the male offspring of the young LP mothers. The male offspring of the LP females also had less fat and a smaller adipocyte diameter than the animals in the control group, regardless of the dams' age. On the other hand, although the female offspring exhibited similar changes in adiposity, the maternal diet had no effect on their body weight or weight gain at 10 months of age (131). The offspring of PR mothers also seemed to be more sensitive to the deleterious effects of the HFD as they exhibited apparent catch-up growth to match the body weight of the control counterparts fed the hypercaloric diet (125).

Available data also suggest that the detrimental *in utero* effects of maternal malnutrition can be transmitted transgenerationally, with altered glucose homeostasis (132), number of larger adipocytes (subcutaneous white adipose tissue on the abdomen) in generation F2 (males), as well as an increased area of GFAP-immunoreactive astrocytes, which is a marker of neuroinflammation (124). Importantly, these effects seem to be transmitted mainly through the maternal rather than paternal line (132).

It is also noteworthy that the majority of experiments on maternal malnutrition focused on male offspring. There is also some evidence [e.g. (14, 15, 131, 133)] that exposure to maternal undernutrition programmes the adipose tissue in a sex-dependent manner, as it seems to be the case in humans. Recently Christians et al. published a systematic review and meta-analysis, in which they analysed the effects of PR and FR on the physiological traits of offspring (e.g. body weight, body fat percentage, fat pad weight, concentration of blood lipids), and checked if any of these traits were more severely affected in either sex. In general, the meta-analysis showed that the birth weight of offspring was consistently reduced in both sexes, regardless of the stage of gestation when the PR or FR occurred. The authors also concluded that less than a half of the studies they analysed tested the interaction between the sex of the offspring and the maternal diet, which may have resulted in a higher incidence of false-positive sex-specific effects (87). However, a maternal FR diet in murine (9, 10): and rat (13) models resulted in a decrease in birth weight in both male and female offspring. Zambardo et al. have found that in the rat offspring of PR mothers, females after birth were lighter than males (15). Weight loss has also been reported in the adult rat offspring of PR mothers of both sexes (16), or in males only (14). Bellinger et al. have described that abdominal fat deposits increased only in rat males, but when it comes to gonadal fat – fat content increased only in females (14). Furthermore, Vega et al. have found that body fat content increased in juvenile rat females only (27), while Begum et al. showed that fat content increased in adult sheep males (29).

EFFECTS OF MATERNAL UNDERNUTRITION ON BODY WEIGHT AND FAT CONTENT: HUMAN STUDIES

World human conflicts and socio-geographical conditions resulted in times of famine and provided unique opportunities to study the influence of undernourishment during pregnancy on the health of offspring in childhood and adulthood (134, 135). Maternal malnutrition during pregnancy results in a small size of offspring at birth, and the low birth weight is interpreted as an indicator of foetal malnutrition (134–136). However, Roseboom et al., who analysed the children of the mothers who were pregnant during the Dutch famine, observed that the babies whose mothers were caught by famine in the first trimester of gestation, were heavier at birth than the population average before and after the period of starvation. On the other hand, the birth weights of the babies affected by the famine in late gestation were usually lower than the birth weights of the babies who were born before or conceived after the famine (137). Additionally, the exposure to the Dutch famine during gestation affected the sex ratio of liveborn babies. The percentage of boys born alive was lower, especially after the exposure to famine during late gestation (137). Interestingly, the offspring of prenatally undernourished fathers, but not mothers during the Dutch famine were heavier and more obese than the offspring of the fathers and mothers who had not been undernourished prenatally (138).

Researchers also observed that malnutrition during the first and second trimesters of pregnancy was associated with an increased prevalence of obesity (regardless of the birth weight) (137), whereas malnutrition in the third trimester correlated with a lower to normal weight in adult life (139, 140). Hence, exposure to famine in early gestation was associated with greater prevalence of obesity in adult life.

The aforementioned human studies showed that maternal overnutrition was associated with macrosomia and increased fat content in progeny, which predisposed them to metabolic imbalance later in life. There were sex-specific differences in these results. On the other hand, studies on humans showed that although the children of malnourished mothers had lower birth weights, they tended to be overweight and obese later in life. This relationship could be explained by the so-called 'thrifty phenotype' hypothesis, which proposes epidemiological associations between poor foetal and infant growth, and the subsequent development of T2DM and the metabolic syndrome. This stems from the effects of poor nutrition in early life, which leads to permanent changes in glucose-insulin metabolism (2, 141–143).

The sex-specific birth weight changes in human offspring of children of malnourished mothers have been also reported. Ntenda et al. (21) and Thurstans et al. (22) have found that boys developed greater decrease in body weight than girls after birth, while Sakisaka et al. (20) described the opposite effect where the lower birth weight was more pronounced in girls than in boys compared to the control groups. Andersen et al. have described that along with the decrease in weight in newborns, fat mass decreased in both sexes, however, later in life, fat mass increased and this effect was more pronounced in girls (30).

EFFECTS OF MATERNAL OVERNUTRITION ON METABOLIC AND HORMONAL STATUS OF OFFSPRING: ANIMAL STUDIES

Maternal overnutrition also affects the metabolic status of animals. The murine and rat offspring of HFD dams had higher blood glucose, TG and/or cholesterol levels (33, 144–147). Moreover, the offspring of obese rat dams fed an HFD, CAF or HSD had higher insulin, leptin, and adiposity levels (145, 146, 148, 149). Research showed that a CAF diet induced obesity more effectively and resulted in a more pronounced increase in the plasma leptin, TG, and cholesterol levels than the HFD protocol (150, 151). Moreover, the maternal HFD, HSD, and CAF diets resulted in a low-grade inflammatory phenotype in the rat offspring. They had higher levels of pro-inflammatory cytokines such as interleukins: IL-1β, IL-6, and tumour necrosis factor α (TNF-α), which mimics the situation observed in obese patients (152–154).

Overnutrition and/or obesity lead to a combination of peripheral and central nervous system alterations and affect the brain circuitry controlling energy homeostasis and adverse programming of central appetite regulators (149). Central leptin and insulin resistance is commonly observed in the offspring of obese HFD-fed rat females (149). Researchers observed changes in the brain appetite regulators, such as downregulated hypothalamic neuropeptide Y (NPY) and upregulated hypothalamic proopiomelanocortin POMC receptor expression in the offspring of HFD-fed rat females (149). Moreover, epigenetic markers at POMC are influenced by both maternal food excess and restriction [for a review see (155)].

Recently researchers have paid more attention to sex-specific differences in the offspring's response to mother's overnutrition. For example, there were sex-specific differences in the blood glucose levels of 25-day-old female offspring of dams fed a CAF diet. These animals had higher glucose levels than those in the control group (18). The concentration of insulin was elevated both in the male and female CAF offspring on postnatal day 25 (PND 25), but this rise in insulin levels was more pronounced in the females (18). Similarly, Bayol et al. observed that feeding rats a CAF diet during pregnancy, lactation, and post-weaning period resulted in sex-specific differences in the glucose and insulin levels in the offspring (33). The concentration of glucose in the ten-week-old female offspring of the rats fed a CAF diet was higher than in the control animals. However, in the studies conducted by Bayol and Matuszewska there was no difference in the glucose levels between the male offspring of the CAF rats and the animals in the control group. Khan et al. have shown that glucose and TG levels were raised only in female rat offspring of HFD mothers (35). Another study revealed sex-specific differences in insulin secretion and leptin transcription – the males had a higher circulating insulin level, whereas the females had an elevated leptin transcript level (33). Rodriguez et al. also observed maternal HSD-induced insulin resistance and oxidative stress in the male but not in the female rat offspring (34). Chowen et al. (156) also noted differences between the males and females in their response to obesogenic diets/environments and the possible implication of hypothalamic astrocytes.

Sanchez-Garrido et al. observed that obesity was transmitted to offspring in a sex-specific manner by the paternal line. The male, but not female offspring of rat fathers with HFD-induced obesity had higher body weights and leptin levels. However, these animals did not exhibit glucose intolerance. Moreover, the authors noted a decrease in the luteinising hormone (LH) levels and an exacerbated drop in the testosterone levels in the male offspring. On the other hand, the female offspring exhibited reduced LH response to kisspeptin-10 (157).

EFFECTS OF MATERNAL OVERNUTRITION ON METABOLIC AND HORMONAL STATUS OF OFFSPRING: HUMAN STUDIES

The children of obese mothers (BMI > 30 kg/m^2) had higher percentage of body fat, systolic blood pressure, TG, and leptin levels, and developed insulin resistance at the age of 8 (121). An interim analysis of 898 obese and normal weight mothers and their offspring from the Programming of Enhanced Adiposity Risk in Childhood-Early Screening (PEACHES) (158) cohort study showed that the children of obese, GDM-negative mothers with late-pregnancy dysglycaemia had a worse outcome with higher weight gain (150–154) and a higher BMI in early childhood than the children of obese mothers treated for GDM (158). Furthermore, the Helsinki birth cohort study showed not only a positive correlation between the BMI of the mothers and offspring, but also a higher body fat percentage in the children of the mothers with a higher BMI (159). The study also showed that the higher maternal BMI increased the risk of the offspring's death, cancer, stroke, coronary heart disease, and T2DM, with the latter two being the most strongly correlated. Apart from that, the risk of developing TDM2 was higher in women than men, while the incidence of coronary heart disease was greater in men (43).

Moreover, exposure to endocrine disruptors (EDs), which becomes increasingly widespread in the environment, influences weight regulation and has obesogenic effects on humans (160–163). EDs act as hormones at low but persistent doses and mostly mimic oestrogen properties. They activate or inactivate cellular receptors, cell responses, and other targets, and lead to higher insulin resistance and hyperinsulinaemia. EDs also change the adipokine level in a sex-specific way. For example, in the Canadian Maternal-Infant Research on Environmental Chemicals Study, newborns exhibited sex-specific differences in the leptin and adiponectin levels, caused by the maternal exposure to bisphenol A (BPA) *in utero*. The female offspring had higher leptin levels than males. By contrast, adiponectin did not differ between the sexes, but was inversely related to the BPA level in the males (164). The topic of environmental chemicals in the context of parental/early exposure to them and programming of obesity and diabetes type 2 is of great importance, but beyond the scope of this review. For reviews on this subject, see e.g. (165–167). Moreover, the concept of transgenerational inheritance – an endocrine of an adverse outcome after a chemical exposure was proposed in 2005 and discussed later by other researchers [e.g. (165, 168, 169)].

The risk factors leading to the development of T2DM also include sugar-sweetened beverages (SSBs). The meta-analysis of prospective cohort studies showed that the men and women drinking SSBs in the highest quantile had a 26% excess risk of developing T2DM than those in the lowest quantile (170).

Male and female offspring seem to adapt differently to the milieu created by maternal obesity and diabetes during pregnancy (171), which may be connected to the sex hormone regulation of several genes involved in both the physiological control of metabolism and the pathophysiological background of cardiometabolic diseases (172, 173). Shields et al. (37) and Krishnaveni et al. (38, 174) noted that girls not only had a higher cord blood insulin concentration at birth than their male peers, but when exposed to GDM *in utero*, they were more likely to develop insulin resistance later in life. Studies also suggest that androgen excess during pregnancy may play a crucial role in insulin resistance programming in female offspring (175). The teenage daughters of mothers with polycystic ovarian syndrome (PCOS) or congenital adrenal hyperplasia (CAH) had hyperinsulinaemia (176, 177).

EFFECTS OF MATERNAL UNDERNUTRITION ON METABOLIC AND HORMONAL STATUS OF OFFSPRING: ANIMAL STUDIES

The offspring of undernourished rat dams tend to exhibit numerous metabolic and hormonal changes in the postnatal period. There are relatively frequent alterations in insulin signalling and glucose tolerance, transcriptional and protein changes in the adipose tissue, liver, and pancreas, as well as inflammatory markers. Changes in insulin signalling and glucose tolerance involve hyperglycaemia (either after fasting or in non-fasted animals), lower insulin sensitivity, as well as higher insulin increment during glucose tolerance test (GTT) (126, 128, 178). This metabolic imbalance can be accompanied by increased blood concentrations of TG and low-density lipoproteins (LDL), as well as decreased concentration of high-density lipoproteins (HDL) (128, 130). Moreover, there was a strong positive correlation between the plasma TG concentration and the body weight of the offspring of the dams fed a diet with 70% FR throughout the gestation (130).

According to data, the livers of the offspring of malnourished mothers are also highly affected, but the results vary across studies. On the one hand, the male offspring of rat dams subjected to severe PR in a diet (80% restriction in the diet protein content) during the second half of gestation exhibited hepatic steatosis at the age of 90 days (128), whereas Lecoutre et al. observed that 70% FR during gestation and lactation did not affect the liver mass or the content of liver lipids (also in male offspring, aged 4 months) (179). This observation is consistent with the results of the study conducted by Morris et al. on the male offspring (aged 110 days) of FR dams (70% FR throughout gestation), whose liver weight did not change, either. Interestingly, a lower liver weight was observed in a group of younger rats (aged 55 days). Transcriptional liver profiling in the group of younger animals revealed that although these individuals did not yet exhibit the characteristics of the metabolic syndrome phenotype that was observed in older rats, the results suggest that these animals might exhibit metabolic abnormalities in advance of the full metabolic syndrome phenotype observed later in life (i.e. at 110 days of age) (180). The effects of maternal malnutrition during pregnancy on the liver may also be transgenerational and transmitted mainly through the maternal line, as described by Hanafi et al. The F2 foetuses of F1 females fed an LP diet for 2 months after weaning (60% PR) exhibited an overexpression of GLUT2 and glucokinase (GK) in the liver. Moreover, these genes as well as UCP2 were also overexpressed in the pancreas, which suggests that these F2 offspring might be predisposed to diabetes later in life. Indeed, higher postnatal levels of fasting blood glucose, insulin, and HOMA-IR later in life (at the age of 20 and 30 weeks) indicated that maternal undernutrition significantly altered glucose tolerance in generation F2 (132).

Research has shown that maternal malnutrition highly affects the adipose tissue function. Guan et al. observed changes in 650 genes in the visceral adipose tissue in the male offspring of dams subjected to 60% PR throughout pregnancy and lactation. The analysis of the results revealed a global upregulation of the genes involved in carbohydrate, lipid, and protein metabolism, as well as adipocyte differentiation and angiogenesis. This suggests that maternal PR during gestation and lactation programmes the susceptibility to visceral adiposity later in life (181). Importantly, research findings also indicate that the restriction of the mother's calorie intake (20% restriction, gestational days 1-12) significantly affects the function of the brown adipose tissue (BAT) in the offspring of both sexes (aged 25 days) (182). Maternal malnutrition may also induce epigenetic changes in the adipose tissue of the offspring, e.g. in the means of programming changes in the miRNA or CpG site methylation [for a review see (179)]. Sex-specific alterations (e.g. in the POMC expression) were observed in the offspring of food-restricted sheep. Begum et al. noted a lower POMC expression (accompanied by increased fat mass in adulthood) in the male adult sheep which had been undernourished during early pregnancy, but there was no difference in the females (29). In rats, offspring of PR mothers (both juvenile males and females) had elevated insulin and leptin levels, but TG levels were elevated only in males.

EFFECTS OF MATERNAL UNDERNUTRITION ON METABOLIC AND HORMONAL STATUS OF OFFSPRING: HUMAN STUDIES

The spectrum of maternal malnutrition spans undernutrition with caloric and/or macro- and micronutrient restrictions during pregnancy. Research has shown that the timing of nutritional restriction seems to play an important role on the health of offspring later in life. Studies on the offspring of the mothers who were pregnant during the Dutch famine (183), Biafran (184), and Chinese (185) provided data on the consequences of maternal caloric restriction in offspring, who developed glucose intolerance, microalbuminuria, an atherogenic lipid profile with a higher LDL/HDL ratio, and hypercholesterolaemia (186). Roseboom et al. indicated that the exposure to the famine at an early gestational age was correlated with an increased risk of coronary heart disease, atherogenic lipid profiles, and higher adiposity (187). Painter et al. (188) observed that the exposure to the famine in the middle of gestation was related to microalbuminuria and impaired renal function. The children whose mothers were malnourished during pregnancy had lower insulin levels and insulin-like growth factor 1 (IGF-1) concentrations, but higher proteolytic activity of the insulin-like growth factor binding protein (the protein binding and regulating the IGF activity) immediately after birth. This may have affected the growth of the foetus (189–191). The proper nutrition of children after birth causes a rapid increase in the insulin and IGF-1 levels, which may result in a rapid weight gain, insulin resistance, and T2DM in adulthood (referred to a as the catch up growth hypothesis) (189, 191).

Researchers found a correlation between the low birth weight and increased risk of developing overweight and obesity, altered body composition, T2DM, hypertension, and cardiovascular disease (24). This evidence is in line with the data from the aforementioned epidemiological studies on individuals exposed to the Dutch famine *in utero*. There was a correlation between the exposure to famine *in utero* and the development of diabetes (192), high blood pressure (193), and impaired body composition of the offspring later in life (24, 139).

Similar data were presented by Finer et al., who researched the metabolic outcomes of exposure to famine during developmental life in rural Bangladesh. Their research additionally showed that gestational and postnatal windows of exposure had variable effects on the offspring's phenotype (194).

These data could be explained by the thrifty phenotype hypothesis, first described by Hales and Baker. According to the hypothesis, suboptimal nutrition *in utero* may result not only in impaired growth of the foetus and children being born small for gestational age/with intrauterine growth retardation (SGA/IUGR), but also in the reprogramming of metabolic pathways to ensure foetal survival in the challenging *in utero* milieu. However, when these individuals experience the postnatal environment with excessive or normal nutrition, they are more prone to develop impaired glucose tolerance (2, 141–143).

In summary, similarly to the animal data, the studies on humans showed marked alterations in the metabolic and hormonal profiles of the offspring of obese, diabetic, and undernourished mothers. There are emerging reports suggesting that female offspring (animal studies on overnutrition) and girls (human studies; exposure to GDM *in utero*) may be more vulnerable to insulin resistance later in life (36). However, further research on sex-specific differences needs to be conducted, especially to reveal the underlying mechanisms. Studies also have shown that the timing of nutritional restriction seems to play an important role on the health of offspring later in life.

EFFECTS OF MATERNAL OVERNUTRITION ON OFFSPRING CARDIOVASCULAR SYSTEM: ANIMAL STUDIES

Animal studies, mainly on rodents (rats and mice) (12, 195), but also on sheep (196–198) and non-human primates showed that maternal overnutrition affects the cardiovascular system (199) (**Figure 1**). The maternal HFD caused cardiac hypertrophy and reduced the vascular density of the cardiac muscle in rodents (200, 201) and primates (199). Moreover, lactational overnutrition (resulting from the reduced litter size) altered the cardiac gene expression in rodents. This may impair cardiac anatomy/metabolism and increase the susceptibility to myocardial injury after an ischaemic insult (202). The potential mechanisms related to myocardial dysfunction include impaired cardiac insulin signalling, metabolic status, increased oxidative stress, inflammation, and mitochondrial dysfunction (200, 201). In the sheep model of maternal obesity, in which the offspring's entire heart function was evaluated in the Langendorff model (an *in vitro* system), the contractile function of the heart was impaired (198). Moreover, the phosphorylation of AMP-activated protein kinase (a cardioprotective signalling pathway) was reduced in the hearts of the foetuses of obese mothers, but the stress-signalling pathway p38 MAPK was upregulated. This indicated impaired cardiac insulin signalling, as compared with the animals in the control group (198). In animal models (especially mice and rats) maternal obesity altered DNA methylation, which was responsible for the abnormal fat metabolism (203, 204), and histone acetylation in the promoter regions of adiponectin and leptin (107). These changes had the atherogenic effect because they increased the adhesion of particles circulating in the blood vessels. In consequence of these epigenetic changes the levels of LDL and free fatty acids increased and altered the nitric oxide synthase (NOS) function, which is a well-known factor in the development of hypertension (205). Maternal overnutrition may also alter specific gene expression and result in cardiomyocyte hypertrophy and abnormal heart development (206, 207).

The exposure of developing mouse and rat offspring to maternal obesity led to their hypertension in adulthood, which deteriorated with age (12, 208, 209). Maternal obesity also programmes the vascular system in offspring. Endothelial dysfunction was observed in the small mesenteric arteries of all offspring whose mothers consumed a fat-rich diet. This showed that this disorder commonly occurs with elevated blood pressure. Endothelial dysfunction may be a consequence of insulin resistance and could reflect the activation of inflammatory pathways as a result of increased adiposity (210).

Sex-specific differences were observed in the offspring of obese mice and rats. Both male and female offspring had elevated blood pressure, but it was more pronounced in the females (12, 35). These studies suggested that female offspring exhibited greater sensitivity to overnutritional insults during foetal life and the cardiovascular development. The following factors influence the development of hypertension in offspring: increased sympathetic activity, increased renal norepinephrine concentration and renin expression, as well as vascular conditions (12, 209, 211).

EFFECTS OF MATERNAL OVERNUTRITION ON OFFSPRING CARDIOVASCULAR SYSTEM: HUMAN STUDIES

Multiple observational studies on humans revealed a correlation between maternal obesity before and during pregnancy and an increased risk of cardiovascular anomalies (114, 115, 212, 213). The exposure of the foetus to maternal obesity increased its blood pressure, altered the vascular system (endothelial function), and myocardial function (199, 214). Researchers observed a positive correlation between maternal obesity and/or gestational weight gain and higher systolic blood pressure in the offspring (114, 215-217). Moreover, a cohort study showed that a higher maternal BMI increased the risk of hospital admissions of adult offspring due to cardiovascular events (43, 213). Additionally, the vascular markers of endothelial dysfunction were increased in the children exposed to maternal diabetes and obesity during foetal life (218). Atherosclerosis may also be influenced by the maternal diet and/or maternal hypercholesterolaemia, which may cause the development of this disease in offspring (219). The inherent risk of hypertension and vascular dysfunction resulting from maternal obesity, cardiac hypertrophy, and contractile dysfunction is also observed in the offspring (200). Epidemiological studies on humans showed that epigenetic mechanisms were involved in the cardiological consequences of maternal obesity and/or diabetes (206). Moreover, the epigenetic mechanisms of altered metabolic control in the offspring of obese mothers may cause abnormal placental function, altered cholesterol circulation, and higher blood pressure in humans (206, 220, 221).

Only a few studies described the influence of sex on the programming of cardiovascular risk, following a pregnancy complicated by obesity and/or diabetes. Ericsson et al. noted a correlation between maternal obesity and stroke only in the female offspring (43). Aceti et al. conducted a systematic review and observed a strong correlation between maternal diabetes and increased blood pressure in the offspring during childhood, with a stronger correlation in the male rather than female offspring (44).

EFFECTS OF MATERNAL UNDERNUTRITION ON OFFSPRING CARDIOVASCULAR SYSTEM: ANIMAL STUDIES

Hypertension (40, 196, 222, 223), coronary heart disease/heart hypertrophy (40, 224), and vascular dysfunction (225) are among the disorders observed in the offspring of undernourished females in experimental animal models. A global restriction of maternal food intake (30-70% food restriction) during pregnancy resulted in arterial hypertension both in murine (222) and rat offspring (40, 226). There were similar observations made on sheep (196) and cows (223). Studies on pregnant rats (227, 228), mice (229), and sheep (230) showed that a reduced maternal dietary protein intake programmed hypertension in offspring. The elevated arterial blood pressure observed in these animals may have been caused by the increased cardiovascular sympathetic tone (227), suppressed activity of the hypothalamic-pituitary adrenal (HPA) axis, impaired function of the renin-angiotensin system (RAS) (231), and/or altered structure and function of the vessels and the cardiac muscle (40, 224). Torrens et al. and Ozaki et al. observed that the dietary protein restriction or global undernutrition in rats compromised the maternal cardiovascular adaptations to pregnancy and led to the endothelial and peripheral artery dysfunction in the offspring (40, 224). The sheep offspring exposed to a maternal LP diet throughout the foetal period developed right and left ventricular hypertrophy (232). Cardiac enlargement was also observed in the offspring of the rats fed an LP diet (233). In addition, they had a lower heart weight, which was associated with an increased rate of cardiomyocyte apoptosis and a lower total number of cardiomyocytes per heart at birth (234). Maternal undernutrition also affects the epigenetic mechanisms that control and change the transcription of genes involved in the cardiovascular homeostasis. A study on rats showed that the offspring of the females which received a LP diet had incorrect histone modifications of a specific enzyme, and these changes were associated with an increase in the blood cholesterol level (235). A study on mice showed that the offspring of the females which received a restricted diet had cardiovascular diseases in adulthood (236). Studies on animals showed that a restrictive diet of rat mothers during pregnancy resulted in significant miRNA dysregulation in the offspring's heart (237). Specific miRNA molecules responsible for maintaining the elasticity of blood vessels were inhibited (238), which reduced vascular contractility. Altered global DNA methylation was observed in the offspring of rodent females receiving a restrictive diet. It caused the dysregulation of the renin-angiotensin system in rats (239) and endothelium-dependent artery vasodilation in mice (225). Few of these epigenetic-dependent changes can induce the development of arterial hypertension in offspring. Barros et al. hypothesised that epigenetic mechanisms were involved in the overactivation of the sympathetic nervous system in the offspring of mothers fed an LP diet (227).

The authors of studies on the functioning of the circulatory system in the offspring of malnourished mothers did not usually describe sex-specific differences. However, Ozaki et al. found that hypertension developed more rapidly and severely in the male rather than female rat offspring exposed to a maternal LP diet during pregnancy (40). Additionally, male, but not the female mice offspring of malnourished mothers had elevated mean arterial pressure (MAP) (39). Elmes et al. observed that the effects of the mother's LP diet on the increased blood pressure of rat offspring were not sex-specific (41).

EFFECTS OF MATERNAL UNDERNUTRITION ON OFFSPRING CARDIOVASCULAR SYSTEM: HUMAN STUDIES

For ethical reasons there is not much data on the influence of maternal malnutrition on cardiac disorders in their children. However, scientists try to analyse the effects of famine in different areas of the world. The analysis of data coming from the offspring of the mothers who starved during pregnancy (e.g. during the Dutch Hunger Winter and during the Second World War) indicate that exposure to famine during foetal life increases the risk of cardiovascular diseases (219, 240). Research has also shown that the people who were exposed to malnutrition *in utero* more often develop coronary heart disease and hypertension (241–243). According to the results of Le Clair et al. (42) and Barker (36), the risk of developing hypertension and coronary heart disease increases in both sexes. Maternal FR causes changes in miRNA, which alters the level of vascular endothelium-derived growth factor involved in the proper maturation and differentiation of the endothelium and its receptors (244).

To sum up, the data presented in the aforementioned animal studies on rodents, sheep, and non-human primates as well as the observations conducted on humans showing the effects of diet on the cardiovascular system clearly indicate that the maternal diet has influence on the cardiovascular system of offspring. Various mechanism responsible for these alterations have been proposed, with a special focus on epigenetic mechanisms. So far the sparse data from animal studies have suggested that female offspring exhibit greater sensitivity to overnutritional insults affecting the development of the cardiovascular system during foetal life. However, it is necessary to conduct further research, especially on animal models of undernutrition as well as the children of undernourished mothers, to analyse sex-specific differences.

EFFECTS OF MATERNAL OVERNUTRITION ON BRAIN AND BEHAVIOURAL OUTCOMES IN OFFSPRING: ANIMAL STUDIES

Animal models of maternal overnutrition have provided evidence of persistent changes in offspring's cognition and behaviour, and complemented human epidemiological data with potential insights into the mechanism linking maternal excessive food intake to adverse neurodevelopmental and psychiatric outcomes in offspring (**Figure 1**). Studies across different animal species indicated effects of maternal overnutrition on memory impairment e.g. working and spatial memory (mice 240, and rats 91, 241, 242).

The study by Robb et al. (49) confirmed a sexually dimorphic effect in the Morris water maze performance, where males performed worse than females. Graf et al. observed that the mice pups whose mothers consumed an HFD exhibited altered myelination and neurobehavioural deficits, and these effects were sex-dependent (47). The disturbed myelination in the medial cortex was observed in the male but not female offspring of HFD-fed dams. These structural changes were correlated with changes in the males' behaviour only (assigned in the novel object recognition test).

Research has also shown the relationship between maternal obesity and depression. Young adult male rodents exposed to an HFD either *in utero* (48) or during lactation (50) exhibited higher rates of depression-like symptoms than the offspring of control group. The rodent offspring of the dams fed an HFD before mating and during gestation and lactation exhibited more anxiolytic behaviours than the control offspring (245, 246). The authors of some studies on animals also suggested that maternal obesity may increase the risk of neurodegenerative diseases such as Alzheimer's disease in offspring (246, 247).

The following mechanisms might be responsible for behavioural alterations in the offspring of dams fed a CAF diet and HFD: reduced expression of neurotrophins, lower concentrations of synaptophysin and BDNF, which are involved in the development of memory (248, 249). Studies on rodents showed that maternal overnutrition hindered the neuronal growth and maturation by altering differentiation, neurogenesis, and disruption in apoptotic processes in such areas of the brain as the hippocampus, hypothalamus, and the cerebral cortex (102, 250, 251). Apart from the impaired neuronal anatomy and function, the offspring of HFD-fed dams exhibit altered neurotransmission (252). Research on rodents showed that the serotonin axon density and embryonic neuronal survival in the brain regions critical for behavioural regulation were reduced (250, 253). The offspring of female mice and rats fed an HFD had impaired mesolimbic dopaminergic signalling, which was associated with impaired reward response to food (254, 255). The levels of expression of the N-methyl-D-aspartate receptor (NMDA) receptor subunit NR2B in the hippocampus of rat offspring were significantly reduced in response to maternal overnutrition (249). The adult offspring of mice exposed to maternal obesity and an HFD during gestation and lactation were also characterised by increased hippocampal expression of $GABA_A$ receptor (256). Increased anxiety in the rat offspring resulted in higher glutamatergic activity in the prefrontal cortex. It was associated with reduced inhibitory input into the glutamate synapses through the cannabinoid/GABA receptors, whose expression decreased. These changes were sex-dependent, and they were more intense in the males than females (51). On the other hand, Kang et al. found that maternal HFD increased anxiety and decreased the sociability of the female offspring only (52). The study on non-human primates (Japanese macaques) showed that the maternal HFD caused behavioural changes in the female offspring, which exhibited higher anxiety. Instead, male exhibited increased aggression (257). On the other hand, the observed increase in the anxiety-like behaviour was not sex-specific in the murine (256) and rat (53) offspring of mothers fed an HFD.

Researchers have suggested multiple mechanisms underlying the effects of maternal HFD on the offspring's brain, e.g. increased hippocampal lipid peroxidation, microglial activation in pups, and increased peripheral and central proinflammatory cytokine expression in the post-weaning and adult life (245). Other suggested mechanisms include: dysregulation of insulin, glucose, and leptin signalling in the developing brain (notably in the regions involved in behavioural regulation such as cortex, amygdala, thalamus, hippocampus and hypothalamus) (250, 258). Animal studies have also corroborated associations between maternal obesity, placental inflammation, foetal brain inflammation, and abnormal neurodevelopment in offspring (259). Moreover, these multidirectional changes associated with long-term effects of poor maternal diet are often accompanied by epigenetic changes [for details see the review by Moody et al. (252)]. It is important to note that there have been few studies on sex-specific differences in early programming of behaviour and brain function (as compared with data on males alone) and further research is necessary.

EFFECTS OF MATERNAL OVERNUTRITION ON BRAIN AND BEHAVIOURAL OUTCOMES IN OFFSPRING: HUMAN STUDIES

According to the findings of recent studies on humans, maternal overnutrition/obesity affects the cognitive function and the development of neurological and psychiatric disorders in offspring (55). Research has provided evidence that there is a correlation between maternal overnutrition and/or obesity and the poorer cognitive performance of offspring, including lower IQ, poorer motor, spatial, and verbal skills (246, 260, 261). Maternal overweight is a predictor of children's poorer psychosocial development, as evidenced by lower social competence and increased risk of depression and anxiety (262–264). Brain imaging techniques are very valuable in this respect, but they are still relatively underrepresented. An MRI study revealed a significant correlation between prenatal exposure to maternal obesity and a smaller hippocampal volume in boys but not girls (56). Moreover, sex-dependent differences were observed across hippocampal subfields (CA1, CA2/3, CA4, dentate gyrus, and subiculum) (56). Thus, the study suggested that boys may be more vulnerable than girls to the negative consequences of exposure to maternal obesity, as manifested by hippocampal development. There are also sex-dependent differences in susceptibility to neurodevelopmental disorders.

Exposure to maternal obesity also induces alterations in the HPA axis of offspring. Prenatal maternal overnutrition exposes offspring to maternal metabolism abnormalities (e.g. high levels of glucose, TG, and total cholesterol), which are associated with increased activity of the HPA axis, for example, in the means of changes in the children's cortisol reactivity (262, 263). This is another possible mechanism through which maternal overnutrition may increase the risk of cognitive decline and anxiety-related disorders in offspring (265).

The authors of studies also suggest that there might be a correlation between maternal obesity and increased symptoms of ADHD (266) and autism spectrum disorder in children (267). The analysis of long-term human studies also showed a correlation between maternal obesity and the increased risk of offspring developing anorexia and/or bulimia later in life (268, 269).

EFFECTS OF MATERNAL UNDERNUTRITION ON BRAIN AND BEHAVIOURAL OUTCOMES IN OFFSPRING: ANIMAL STUDIES

Global caloric and/or protein restriction during gestation is correlated with deficits in exploration, social behaviour, emotionality, avoidance conditioning, learning, and memory in adult life (270–275). Batista et al. observed that maternal protein malnutrition caused autism spectrum disorder in rat offspring (276). Changes in the behaviour of the offspring of malnourished mothers were accompanied by neurochemical and neuroanatomical abnormalities such as: abnormal proliferation, apoptosis, astrogenesis, neuronal differentiation, dendritic arborisation and cerebral astrogliosis in the cortex and hippocampus (277, 278), and lower thickness of the visual cortex, parietal neocortex, dentate gyrus, CA3 region of the hippocampus and cerebellum (276, 279, 280). Experiments on rats also showed that FR during gestation reduced the essential factors enhancing neuronal proliferation, growth, and maintenance, e.g. BDNF and insulin-like growth factor (IGF) (252, 275). Additionally, the offspring of malnourished rats exhibited changes in their central neurochemical profiles, such as altered NMDA transmission and receptor composition, a decrease in the synaptic NO in the hippocampus (252, 281), enhanced GABA-ergic inputs to the hippocampus, and unfavourable changes in the noradrenergic, serotonergic, and dopaminergic transmission (252, 271, 282, 283). Consequently, nutrition-induced deficits in the synaptic transmission impaired memory formation and the LTP (long-term potentiation) (252). Barra et al. suggested that prenatal malnutrition-induced brain disturbances depend on two mechanisms: i) the direct effect of foetal programming on the brain, including negative epigenetic changes in foetal progenitor cells and developing neurons, which will form the cerebral cortex, hippocampus, and other brain regions involved in neuroplasticity, and ii) the indirect effect on the brain mediated by the postnatal development of obesity/metabolic syndrome (271).

Rodriguez et al. conducted research on baboons, which have a similar genetic constitution and developmental trajectory to humans. The researchers observed that moderate global nutrient restriction during pregnancy and lactation affected the development of the offspring brain in a sex-specific manner (45). The baboon offspring exposed to moderate maternal nutrient restriction were less motivated and their working memory was impaired. The female offspring learnt better than the males, whose learning was impaired and they were more impulsive (45).

Natt et al. have described the enhancement of anxiety and depressive behaviour in male, but not female mice offspring from PR mothers (46). However, Akitake et al. have described a decrease in motor activity and recognition memory in male and female mice, while hippocampal synaptophysin level was decreased only in females (10). Additionally, Bellinger et al. in their study on rat offspring of LP mothers, have found that locomotor activity was impaired in males but feeding behaviour was impaired in females (14).

EFFECTS OF MATERNAL UNDERNUTRITION ON BRAIN AND BEHAVIOURAL OUTCOMES IN OFFSPRING: HUMAN STUDIES

Two meta-analyses described the effects of maternal malnutrition on the learning, memory, and behaviour of the schoolchildren who were small for their gestational age. These children exhibited cognitive impairments, lower verbal and performance IQ, and more behavioural disorders than the children in the control group (271, 284, 285).

Researchers also observed that prenatal exposure to famine (during the Dutch famine) permanently affected the size of the brain, and these changes were sex-dependent. A structural magnetic resonance imaging was conducted on the Dutch famine birth cohort members when they were about 67 years old (54). The MRI showed that the total brain volume as well as the volumes of grey and white matter were smaller only in the early exposed males. The intracranial and total brain volumes of the prenatally exposed males were smaller than the volumes of the control subjects. Such changes were not observed in the females (54). Smith and Reyes described that sons of malnourished mothers are more likely to develop ASD and ADHD than daughters (55).

To sum up, the results discussed above showed that multiple animal models of over- and undernutrition as well as the data obtained in human studies provide convincing insight supporting the influence of an unhealthy maternal diet on the development of the brain and behavioural outcomes in offspring. The authors of these studies also suggested sex-specific responses to maternal diets and proposed various mechanisms underlying such divergences, among which the epigenetic ones have been the most explored recently. Imaging techniques, such as MRI, are invaluable for further analysis of subtle differences in the brain structures of the offspring to obese mothers, with emphasis on possible sex-specific differences.

CONCLUSIONS AND FUTURE DIRECTIONS – FROM LABORATORY TO CLINICAL SETTINGS

This review provided the evidence based on epidemiological data and animal models that both maternal over- and undernutrition changes the metabolic profiles, alters the body weight and fat content, and influences the offspring's brain development and behaviour. Moreover, the effects observed in offspring are long-lasting. There is a relatively wide range of scientific publications discussing changes in the peripheral nervous system (i.e. hormones and metabolites), but there is not much data on changes in the central nervous system (i.e. in the brain). Non-invasive imaging techniques such as MRI could help to further and more precisely investigate these changes not only within different brain structures but also in the peripheral organs (e.g. changes in the fat distribution). These techniques could be used to monitor the development of diseases and during treatments.

As results from the studies conducted on animals and humans, there are sex-specific differences in the effects of the maternal diet on numerous physiological and anatomical traits. Therefore, further research should be conducted, especially on the epigenetic mechanisms through which both maternal over- and undernutrition affects offspring. These epigenetic processes, including DNA methylation, histone modification, chromatin remodelling, and RNA-based mechanisms may affect gene expression and change the foetal neuroendocrine system through modification of the brain circuitry (286). Epigenetic testing could be used in clinical settings as a biomarker for early diagnosis of the risk of obesity and as a predictor of response to obesity interventions. However, in epigenetic studies on humans it is a challenge to select relevant tissues accessible to examination such as peripheral blood cells (PBC), buccal epithelial cells (BEC), or hair follicles. As both maternal and paternal history and experiences exert influence through the epigenomic information which is not contained in the DNA sequence, including variations in sperm and oocyte cytosine methylation and chromatin patterning, the influence of non-coding RNAs and mitochondria of both maternal and paternal lines should be considered (287, 288). Currently, very little is known about the effects of the paternal metabolic status on the outcomes of offspring. Moreover, the mechanisms involved in the intergenerational transmission of undernutrition, obesity, and diabetes are difficult to study in humans because of the complex relationships between the maternal and foetal conditions, and the postnatal environmental factors.

Therefore, it is also necessary to continue using relevant animal models of metabolic diseases. As the consumption of SSBs is a high risk factor for the development of T2DM, and due to the fact that endocrine disruptors lead to the development of metabolic diseases, animal models with these variables should be developed and employed. Although animal models will never be able to fully mimic the human situation, they make it possible to study the mechanisms through which the mother's diet programmes the organs and systems of the offspring. Moreover, thanks to animal models of obesity, diabetes, and undernutrition it is possible to search for prevention and treatment strategies, and to increase the awareness of sex-specific risk factors. It is necessary to conduct further research on the sex-dependent pathophysiological mechanisms of undernutrition, obesity, and T2DM, because it could contribute to more personalised care in the future.

The subject of this review seems to be particularly relevant at the time of the pandemic and the post-COVID period, when lockdowns reduce people's physical activity and increase the consumption of unhealthy food products, which results in higher incidence of obesity. Therefore, it is necessary to develop and implement local, national, and international prevention and treatment strategies to slow down the rate of incidence of obesity. These insights compel us to revise generally held notions to accommodate the prospect that biological parenting, including proper diet, commences well before birth, even prior to conception. As the womb may be more important than home, it is also necessary to urgently implement these strategies long before conception as well as during the crucial and vulnerable times of pregnancy and lactation.

AUTHOR CONTRIBUTIONS

EG wrote the draft of the manuscript and especially the following sections: Animal models of obesity with special emphasis on the diet-induced obesity, Effects of maternal overnutrition on body weight and fat content: animal and human studies, Effects of maternal undernutrition on body weight and fat content: human studies, Effects of maternal overnutrition on metabolic and hormonal status of offspring. animal studies, Effects of maternal overnutrition and undermatron on the cardiovascular system in offspring: animal and human studies, Effects of maternal overnutrition and undernutrition on the brain and behavioral outcomes in offspring: animal and human studies. Prepared the figure. JM–collected and formatted literature database. KZ wrote the following sections: Animal models of undernutrition, Effects of maternal undernutrition on body weight and fat content, and metabolic and hormonal status of offspring: animal studies, edited the whole text. AG-K, IK- P, and BS wrote the following sections: Effects of maternal overnutrition on metabolic and hormonal status of offspring: human studies, Effects of maternal undernutrition on metabolic and hormonal status of offspring: human studies and contributed to the Conclusion section; JHS-wrote the following sections: Introduction, Animal models of diabetes, conclusions, overviewed the process of writing the paper. All authors contributed to the article and approved the submitted version.

ACKNOWLEDGMENTS

We would like to thank all the researchers who contributed to this review. Due to the large number of scientific publications on the subject, especially those discussing animals models, we were not able to cite all available studies.

REFERENCES

1. Barker DJ. The Fetal and Infant Origins of Adult Disease. *BMJ* (1990) 301 (6761):1111. doi: 10.1136/bmj.301.6761.1111
2. Barker DJ, Hales CN, Fall CH, Osmond C, Phipps K, Clark PM. Type 2 (Non-Insulin-Dependent) Diabetes Mellitus, Hypertension and Hyperlipidaemia (Syndrome X): Relation to Reduced Fetal Growth. *Diabetologia* (1993) 36(1):62–7. doi: 10.1007/BF00399095
3. Butler MJ, Barrientos RM. The Impact of Nutrition on COVID-19 Susceptibility and Long-Term Consequences. *Brain Behav Immun* (2020) 87:53–4. doi: 10.1016/j.bbi.2020.04.040
4. Petrilli CM, Jones SA, Jeam Y. Factors Associated With Hospitalization and Critical Illness Among 4,103 Patients With COVID-19 Disease in New York. *BMJ* (2020) 369:m1966. doi: 10.1101/2020.04.08.20057794
5. Cummings MJ, Baldwin MR, Abrams D, Jacobson SD, Meyer BJ, Balough EM, et al. Epidemiology, Clinical Course, and Outcomes of Critically Ill Adults With COVID-19 in New York City: A Prospective Cohort Study. *Lancet* (2020) 395(10239):1763–70. doi: 10.1016/S0140-6736(20)31189-2
6. Favre G, Legueult K, Pradier C, Raffaelli C, Ichai C, Iannelli A, et al. Visceral Fat Is Associated to the Severity of COVID-19. *Metabolism* (2021) 115:154440. doi: 10.1016/j.metabol.2020.154440
7. Padmanabhan V, Cardoso RC, Puttabyatappa M. Developmental Programming, a Pathway to Disease. *Endocrinology* (2016) 157(4):1328–40. doi: 10.1210/en.2016-1003
8. Sullivan EL, Smith MS, Grove KL. Perinatal Exposure to High-Fat Diet Programs Energy Balance, Metabolism and Behavior in Adulthood. *Neuroendocrinology* (2011) 93(1):1–8. doi: 10.1159/000322038
9. Jimenez-Chillaron JC, Isganaitis E, Charalambous M, Gesta S, Pentinat-Pelegrin T, Faucette RR, et al. Intergenerational Transmission of Glucose Intolerance and Obesity by *In Utero* Undernutrition in Mice. *Diabetes* (2009) 58(2):460–8. doi: 10.2337/db08-0490
10. Akitake Y, Katsuragi S, Hosokawa M, Mishima K, Ikeda T, Miyazato M, et al. Moderate Maternal Food Restriction in Mice Impairs Physical Growth, Behavior, and Neurodevelopment of Offspring. *Nutr Res* (2015) 35(1):76–87. doi: 10.1016/j.nutres.2014.10.014
11. King V, Dakin RS, Liu L, Hadoke PW, Walker BR, Seckl JR, et al. Maternal Obesity has Little Effect on the Immediate Offspring But Impacts on the Next Generation. *Endocrinology* (2013) 154(7):2514–24. doi: 10.1210/en.2013-1013
12. Samuelsson AM, Matthews PA, Argenton M, Christie MR, McConnell JM, Jansen EH, et al. Diet-Induced Obesity in Female Mice Leads to Offspring Hyperphagia, Adiposity, Hypertension, and Insulin Resistance: A Novel Murine Model of Developmental Programming. *Hypertension* (2008) 51 (2):383–92. doi: 10.1161/HYPERTENSIONAHA.107.101477

13. Sánchez-Garrido MA, Castellano JM, Ruiz-Pino F, Garcia-Galiano D, Manfredi-Lozano M, Leon S, et al. Metabolic Programming of Puberty: Sexually Dimorphic Responses to Early Nutritional Challenges. *Endocrinology* (2013) 154(9):3387–400. doi: 10.1210/en.2012-2157
14. Bellinger L, Sculley DV, Langley-Evans SC. Exposure to Undernutrition in Fetal Life Determines Fat Distribution, Locomotor Activity and Food Intake in Ageing Rats. *Int J Obes (Lond)* (2006) 30(5):729–38. doi: 10.1038/sj.ijo.0803205
15. Zambrano E, Bautista CJ, Deas M, Martinez-Samayoa PM, Gonzalez-Zamorano M, Ledesma H, et al. A Low Maternal Protein Diet During Pregnancy and Lactation has Sex- and Window of Exposure-Specific Effects on Offspring Growth and Food Intake, Glucose Metabolism and Serum Leptin in the Rat. *J Physiol* (2006) 571(Pt 1):221–30. doi: 10.1113/jphysiol.2005.100313
16. Woods LL, Weeks DA, Rasch R. Programming of Adult Blood Pressure by Maternal Protein Restriction: Role of Nephrogenesis. *Kidney Int* (2004) 65 (4):1339–48. doi: 10.1111/j.1523-1755.2004.00511.x
17. Nivoit P, Morens C, Van Assche FA, Jansen E, Poston L, Remacle C, et al. Established Diet-Induced Obesity in Female Rats Leads to Offspring Hyperphagia, Adiposity and Insulin Resistance. *Diabetologia* (2009) 52 (6):1133–42. doi: 10.1007/s00125-009-1316-9
18. Matuszewska J, Zalewski T, Klimaszyk A, Ziarniak K, Jurga S, Chmurzynska A, et al. Mothers' Cafeteria Diet Induced Sex-Specific Changes in Fat Content, Metabolic Profiles, and Inflammation Outcomes in Rat Offspring. *Sci Rep* (2021) 11(1):18573. doi: 10.1038/s41598-021-97487-x
19. Jacobs S, Teixeira DS, Guilherme C, da Rocha CF, Aranda BC, Reis AR, et al. The Impact of Maternal Consumption of Cafeteria Diet on Reproductive Function in the Offspring. *Physiol Behav* (2014) 129:280–6. doi: 10.1016/j.physbeh.2014.03.003
20. Sakisaka K, Wakai S, Kuroiwa C, Cuadra Flores L, Kai I, Mercedes Aragón M, et al. Nutritional Status and Associated Factors in Children Aged 0-23 Months in Granada, Nicaragua. *Public Health* (2006) 120(5):400–11. doi: 10.1016/j.puhe.2005.10.018
21. Ntenda PAM, Chuang YC. Analysis of Individual-Level and Community-Level Effects on Childhood Undernutrition in Malawi. *Pediatr Neonatol* (2018) 59(4):380–9. doi: 10.1016/j.pedneo.2017.11.019
22. Thurstans S, Opondo C, Seal A, Wells J, Khara T, Dolan C, et al. Boys Are More Likely to be Undernourished Than Girls: A Systematic Review and Meta-Analysis of Sex Differences in Undernutrition. *BMJ Glob Health* (2020) 5(12):e004030. doi: 10.1136/bmjgh-2020-004030
23. Lingwood BE, Henry AM, d'Emden MC, Fullerton AM, Mortimer RH, Colditz PB, et al. Determinants of Body Fat in Infants of Women With Gestational Diabetes Mellitus Differ With Fetal Sex. *Diabetes Care* (2011) 34 (12):2581–5. doi: 10.2337/dc11-0728
24. Sutton EF, Gilmore LA, Dunger DB, Heijmans BT, Hivert MF, Ling C, et al. Developmental Programming: State-of-the-Science and Future Directions-Summary From a Pennington Biomedical Symposium. *Obes (Silver Spring)* (2016) 24(5):1018–26. doi: 10.1002/oby.21487
25. Dahlhoff M, Pfister S, Blutke A, Rozman J, Klingenspor M, Deutsch MJ, et al. Peri-Conceptional Obesogenic Exposure Induces Sex-Specific Programming of Disease Susceptibilities in Adult Mouse Offspring. *Biochim Biophys Acta* (2014) 1842(2):304–17. doi: 10.1016/j.bbadis.2013.11.021
26. Masuyama H, Hiramatsu Y. Additive Effects of Maternal High Fat Diet During Lactation on Mouse Offspring. *PloS One* (2014) 9(3):e92805. doi: 10.1371/journal.pone.0092805
27. Vega CC, Reyes-Castro LA, Rodríguez-González GL, Bautista CJ, Vázquez-Martínez M, Larrea F, et al. Resveratrol Partially Prevents Oxidative Stress and Metabolic Dysfunction in Pregnant Rats Fed a Low Protein Diet and Their Offspring. *J Physiol* (2016) 594(5):1483–99. doi: 10.1113/JP271543
28. George G, Draycott SAV, Muir R, Clifford B, Elmes MJ, Langley-Evans SC. Exposure to Maternal Obesity During Suckling Outweighs *In Utero* Exposure in Programming for Post-Weaning Adiposity and Insulin Resistance in Rats. *Sci Rep* (2019) 9(1):10134. doi: 10.1038/s41598-019-46518-9
29. Begum G, Davies A, Stevens A, Oliver M, Jaquiery A, Challis J, et al. Maternal Undernutrition Programs Tissue-Specific Epigenetic Changes in the Glucocorticoid Receptor in Adult Offspring. *Endocrinology* (2013) 154 (12):4560–9. doi: 10.1210/en.2013-1693
30. Andersen GS, Girma T, Wells JC, Kæstel P, Leventi M, Hother AL, et al. Body Composition From Birth to 6 Mo of Age in Ethiopian Infants: Reference Data Obtained by Air-Displacement Plethysmography. *Am J Clin Nutr* (2013) 98(4):885–94. doi: 10.3945/ajcn.113.063032
31. Eshriqui I, Valente AMM, Folchetti LD, de Almeida-Pititto B, Ferreira SRG. Pre-Pregnancy BMI Is Associated With Offspring Body Composition in Adulthood Before Adiposity-Related Disorders: A Retrospective Cohort. *Public Health Nutr* (2021) 24(6):1296–303. doi: 10.1017/S1368980020005285
32. Chaparro MP KI, Byberg L. Maternal Prepregnancy BMI and Offspring Body Composition in Young Adulthood: The Modifying Role of Offspring Sex and Birth Order. *Public Health Nutr* (2018) 20:3084–9. doi: 10.1017/S1368980017002191
33. Bayol SA, Simbi BH, Bertrand JA, Stickland NC. Offspring From Mothers Fed a 'Junk Food' Diet in Pregnancy and Lactation Exhibit Exacerbated Adiposity That Is More Pronounced in Females. *J Physiol* (2008) 586 (13):3219–30. doi: 10.1113/jphysiol.2008.153817
34. Rodriguez L, Otero P, Panadero MI, Rodrigo S, Alvarez-Millan JJ, Bocos C. Maternal Fructose Intake Induces Insulin Resistance and Oxidative Stress in Male, But Not Female, Offspring. *J Nutr Metab* (2015) 2015:158091. doi: 10.1155/2015/158091
35. Khan IY, Taylor PD, Dekou V, Seed PT, Lakasing L, Graham D, et al. Gender-Linked Hypertension in Offspring of Lard-Fed Pregnant Rats. *Hypertension* (2003) 41(1):168–75. doi: 10.1161/01.HYP.0000047511.97879.FC
36. Barker DJ. Fetal Origins of Coronary Heart Disease. *BMJ* (1995) 311 (6998):171–4. doi: 10.1136/bmj.311.6998.171
37. Shields BM, Knight B, Hopper H, Hill A, Powell RJ, Hattersley AT, et al. Measurement of Cord Insulin and Insulin-Related Peptides Suggests That Girls Are More Insulin Resistant Than Boys at Birth. *Diabetes Care* (2007) 30(10):2661–6. doi: 10.2337/dc06-1501
38. Krishnaveni GV, Veena SR, Hill JC, Kehoe S, Karat SC, Fall CH. Intrauterine Exposure to Maternal Diabetes Is Associated With Higher Adiposity and Insulin Resistance and Clustering of Cardiovascular Risk Markers in Indian Children. *Diabetes Care* (2010) 33(2):402–4. doi: 10.2337/dc09-1393
39. Roghair RD, Segar JL, Volk KA, Chapleau MW, Dallas LM, Sorenson AR, et al. Vascular Nitric Oxide and Superoxide Anion Contribute to Sex-Specific Programmed Cardiovascular Physiology in Mice. *Am J Physiol Regul Integr Comp Physiol* (2009) 296(3):R651–62. doi: 10.1152/ajpregu.90756.2008
40. Ozaki T, Nishina H, Hanson MA, Poston L. Dietary Restriction in Pregnant Rats Causes Gender-Related Hypertension and Vascular Dysfunction in Offspring. *J Physiol* (2001) 530(Pt 1):141–52. doi: 10.1111/j.1469-7793.2001.0141m.x
41. Elmes MJ, Gardner DS, Langley-Evans SC. Fetal Exposure to a Maternal Low-Protein Diet Is Associated With Altered Left Ventricular Pressure Response to Ischaemia-Reperfusion Injury. *Br J Nutr* (2007) 98(1):93–100. doi: 10.1017/S000711450769182X
42. Le Clair C, Abbi T, Sandhu H, Tappia PS. Impact of Maternal Undernutrition on Diabetes and Cardiovascular Disease Risk in Adult Offspring. *Can J Physiol Pharmacol* (2009) 87(3):161–79. doi: 10.1139/Y09-006
43. Eriksson JG, Sandboge S, Salonen MK, Kajantie E, Osmond C. Long-Term Consequences of Maternal Overweight in Pregnancy on Offspring Later Health: Findings From the Helsinki Birth Cohort Study. *Ann Med* (2014) 46 (6):434–8. doi: 10.3109/07853890.2014.919728
44. Aceti A, Santhakumaran S, Logan KM, Philipps LH, Prior E, Gale C, et al. The Diabetic Pregnancy and Offspring Blood Pressure in Childhood: A Systematic Review and Meta-Analysis. *Diabetologia* (2012) 55(11):3114–27. doi: 10.1007/s00125-012-2689-8
45. Rodriguez JS, Bartlett TQ, Keenan KE, Nathanielsz PW, Nijland MJ. Sex-Dependent Cognitive Performance in Baboon Offspring Following Maternal Caloric Restriction in Pregnancy and Lactation. *Reprod Sci* (2012) 19 (5):493–504. doi: 10.1177/1933719111424439
46. Nätt D, Barchiesi R, Murad J, Feng J, Nestler EJ, Champagne FA, et al. Perinatal Malnutrition Leads to Sexually Dimorphic Behavioral Responses With Associated Epigenetic Changes in the Mouse Brain. *Sci Rep* (2017) 7 (1):11082. doi: 10.1038/s41598-017-10803-2

47. Graf AE LS, Waidyaratne G, Thompson MD, Tipple TE, Hester ME, Trask AJ, et al. Maternal High Fat Diet Exposure Is Associated With Increased Hepcidin Levels, Decreased Myelination, and Neurobehavioral Changes in Male Offspring. *Brain Behav Immun* (2016) 58:369–78. doi: 10.1016/j.bbi.2016.08.005
48. Balsevich G, Baumann V, Uribe A, Chen A, Schmidt MV. Prenatal Exposure to Maternal Obesity Alters Anxiety and Stress Coping Behaviors in Aged Mice. *Neuroendocrinology* (2016) 103(3-4):354–68. doi: 10.1159/000439087
49. Robb JL, Messa I, Lui E, Yeung D, Thacker J, Satvat E, et al. A Maternal Diet High in Saturated Fat Impairs Offspring Hippocampal Function in a Sex-Specific Manner. *Behav Brain Res* (2017) 326:187–99. doi: 10.1016/j.bbr.2017.02.049
50. Giriko CA, Andreoli CA, Mennitti LV, Hosoume LF, Souto Tdos S, Silva AV, et al. Delayed Physical and Neurobehavioral Development and Increased Aggressive and Depression-Like Behaviors in the Rat Offspring of Dams Fed a High-Fat Diet. *Int J Dev Neurosci* (2013) 31(8):731–9. doi: 10.1016/j.ijdevneu.2013.09.001
51. Rivera P, Tovar R, Ramirez-Lopez MT, Navarro JA, Vargas A, Suarez J, et al. Sex-Specific Anxiety and Prefrontal Cortex Glutamatergic Dysregulation Are Long-Term Consequences of Pre-and Postnatal Exposure to Hypercaloric Diet in a Rat Model. *Nutrients* (2020) 12(6). doi: 10.3390/nu12061829
52. Kang SS, Kurti A, Fair DA, Fryer JD. Dietary Intervention Rescues Maternal Obesity Induced Behavior Deficits and Neuroinflammation in Offspring. *J Neuroinflamm* (2014) 11:156. doi: 10.1186/s12974-014-0156-9
53. Abuaish S, Spinieli RL, McGowan PO. Perinatal High Fat Diet Induces Early Activation of Endocrine Stress Responsivity and Anxiety-Like Behavior in Neonates. *Psychoneuroendocrinology* (2018) 98:11–21. doi: 10.1016/j.psyneuen.2018.08.003
54. de Rooij SR, Caan MW, Swaab DF, Nederveen AJ, Majoie CB, Schwab M, et al. Prenatal Famine Exposure has Sex-Specific Effects on Brain Size. *Brain* (2016) 139(Pt 8):2136–42. doi: 10.1093/brain/aww132
55. Smith BL, Reyes TM. Offspring Neuroimmune Consequences of Maternal Malnutrition: Potential Mechanism for Behavioral Impairments That Underlie Metabolic and Neurodevelopmental Disorders. *Front Neuroendocrinol* (2017) 47:109–22. doi: 10.1016/j.yfrne.2017.07.007
56. Alves JM, Luo S, Chow T, Herting M, Xiang AH, Page KA. Sex Differences in the Association Between Prenatal Exposure to Maternal Obesity and Hippocampal Volume in Children. *Brain Behav* (2020) 10(2):e01522. doi: 10.1002/brb3.1522
57. Barrett P, Mercer JG, Morgan PJ. Preclinical Models for Obesity Research. *Dis Model Mech* (2016) 9(11):1245–55. doi: 10.1242/dmm.026443
58. Bray GA, York DA. Hypothalamic and Genetic Obesity in Experimental Animals: An Autonomic and Endocrine Hypothesis. *Physiol Rev* (1979) 59 (3):719–809. doi: 10.1152/physrev.1979.59.3.719
59. Kleinert M, Clemmensen C, Hofmann SM, Moore MC, Renner S, Woods SC, et al. Animal Models of Obesity and Diabetes Mellitus. *Nat Rev Endocrinol* (2018) 14(3):140–62. doi: 10.1038/nrendo.2017.161
60. Lutz TA, Woods SC. Overview of Animal Models of Obesity. *Curr Protoc Pharmacol* (2012) Chapter 5:Unit5 61.
61. Pinheiro-Castro N, Silva L, Novaes GM, Ong TP. Hypercaloric Diet-Induced Obesity and Obesity-Related Metabolic Disorders in Experimental Models. *Adv Exp Med Biol* (2019) 1134:149–61. doi: 10.1007/978-3-030-12668-1_8
62. de Moura EDM, Dos Reis SA, da Conceicao LL, Sediyama C, Pereira SS, de Oliveira LL, et al. Diet-Induced Obesity in Animal Models: Points to Consider and Influence on Metabolic Markers. *Diabetol Metab Syndr* (2021) 13(1):32. doi: 10.1186/s13098-021-00647-2
63. Hariri N, Thibault L. High-Fat Diet-Induced Obesity in Animal Models. *Nutr Res Rev* (2010) 23(2):270–99. doi: 10.1017/S0954422410000168
64. Marques C, Meireles M, Norberto S, Leite J, Freitas J, Pestana D, et al. High-Fat Diet-Induced Obesity Rat Model: A Comparison Between Wistar and Sprague-Dawley Rat. *Adipocyte* (2016) 5(1):11–21. doi: 10.1080/21623945.2015.1061723
65. Small L, Brandon AE, Turner N, Cooney GJ. Modeling Insulin Resistance in Rodents by Alterations in Diet: What Have High-Fat and High-Calorie Diets Revealed? *Am J Physiol Endocrinol Metab* (2018) 314(3):E251–E65. doi: 10.1152/ajpendo.00337.2017
66. Omar B, Pacini G, Ahren B. Differential Development of Glucose Intolerance and Pancreatic Islet Adaptation in Multiple Diet Induced Obesity Models. *Nutrients* (2012) 4(10):1367–81. doi: 10.3390/nu4101367
67. Lalanza JF, Snoeren EMS. The Cafeteria Diet: A Standardized Protocol and Its Effects on Behavior. *Neurosci Biobehav Rev* (2021) 122:92–119. doi: 10.1016/j.neubiorev.2020.11.003
68. Dyer JS, Rosenfeld CR. Metabolic Imprinting by Prenatal, Perinatal, and Postnatal Overnutrition: A Review. *Semin Reprod Med* (2011) 29(3):266–76. doi: 10.1055/s-0031-1275521
69. Jiang X, Ma H, Wang Y, Liu Y. Early Life Factors and Type 2 Diabetes Mellitus. *J Diabetes Res* (2013) 2013:485082. doi: 10.1155/2013/485082
70. Mucellini AB, Goularte JF, de Araujo da Cunha AC, Caceres RC, Noschang C, da Silva Benetti C, et al. Effects of Exposure to a Cafeteria Diet During Gestation and After Weaning on the Metabolism and Body Weight of Adult Male Offspring in Rats. *Br J Nutr* (2014) 111(8):1499–506. doi: 10.1017/S0007114513003838
71. Tamashiro KL, Moran TH. Perinatal Environment and Its Influences on Metabolic Programming of Offspring. *Physiol Behav* (2010) 100(5):560–6. doi: 10.1016/j.physbeh.2010.04.008
72. Mathis D VL, Benoist C. Beta-Cell Death During Progression to Diabetes. *Nature* (2001) 414:792–8. doi: 10.1038/414792a
73. Bellamy L CJ, Hingorani AD, Williams D. Type 2 Diabetes Mellitus After Gestational Diabetes: A Systematic Review and Meta-Analysis. *Lancet* (2009) 373:1773–9. doi: 10.1016/S0140-6736(09)60731-5
74. Szkudelski T. The Mechanism of Alloxan and Streptozotocin Action in B Cells of the Rat Pancreas. *Physiol Res* (2001) 50(6):537–46.
75. Dickinson JE, Meyer BA, Chmielowiec S, Palmer SM. Streptozocin-Induced Diabetes Mellitus in the Pregnant Ewe. *Am J Obstet Gynecol* (1991) 165(6 Pt 1):1673–7. doi: 10.1016/0002-9378(91)90013-H
76. Junod A, Lambert AE, Stauffacher W, Renold AE. Diabetogenic Action of Streptozotocin: Relationship of Dose to Metabolic Response. *J Clin Invest* (1969) 48(11):2129–39. doi: 10.1172/JCI106180
77. Ramsay TG, Wolverton CK, Steele NC. Alteration in IGF-I Mrna Content of Fetal Swine Tissues in Response to Maternal Diabetes. *Am J Physiol* (1994) 267(5 Pt 2):R1391–6. doi: 10.1152/ajpregu.1994.267.5.R1391
78. Tsai MY, Schallinger LE, Josephson MW, Brown DM. Disturbance of Pulmonary Prostaglandin Metabolism in Fetuses of Alloxan-Diabetic Rabbits. *Biochim Biophys Acta* (1982) 712(2):395–9. doi: 10.1016/0005-2760(82)90358-7
79. Skovso S. Modeling Type 2 Diabetes in Rats Using High Fat Diet and Streptozotocin. *J Diabetes Investig* (2014) 5(4):349–58. doi: 10.1111/jdi.12235
80. Fang J-Y, Lin C-H, Huang T-H, Chuang S-Y. *In Vivo* Rodent Models of Type 2 Diabetes and Their Usefulness for Evaluating Flavonoid Bioactivity. *Nutrients* (2019) 11(530):1–23. doi: 10.3390/nu11030530
81. Peters SAE, Woodward M. Sex Differences in the Burden and Complications of Diabetes. *Curr Diabetes Rep* (2018) 18(6):33. doi: 10.1007/s11892-018-1005-5
82. Rossini AA, Williams RM, Appel MC, Like AA. Sex Differences in the Multiple-Dose Streptozotocin Model of Diabetes. *Endocrinology* (1978) 103 (4):1518–20. doi: 10.1210/endo-103-4-1518
83. Link JC, Reue K. Genetic Basis for Sex Differences in Obesity and Lipid Metabolism. *Annu Rev Nutr* (2017) 37:225–45. doi: 10.1146/annurev-nutr-071816-064827
84. Lovejoy JC, Sainsbury A, Stock Conference Working G. Sex Differences in Obesity and the Regulation of Energy Homeostasis. *Obes Rev* (2009) 10 (2):154–67. doi: 10.1111/j.1467-789X.2008.00529.x
85. Jawerbaum A, White V. Animal Models in Diabetes and Pregnancy. *Endocr Rev* (2010) 31(5):680–701. doi: 10.1210/er.2009-0038
86. Swanson AM, David AL. Animal Models of Fetal Growth Restriction: Considerations for Translational Medicine. *Placenta* (2015) 36(6):623–30. doi: 10.1016/j.placenta.2015.03.003
87. Christians JK, Shergill HK, Albert AYK. Sex-Dependent Effects of Prenatal Food and Protein Restriction on Offspring Physiology in Rats and Mice: Systematic Review and Meta-Analyses. *Biol Sex Differ* (2021) 12(1):21. doi: 10.1186/s13293-021-00365-4
88. Lopes GA, Ribeiro VL, Barbisan LF, Marchesan Rodrigues MA. Fetal Developmental Programing: Insights From Human Studies and Experimental Models. *J Matern Fetal Neonatal Med* (2017) 30(6):722–8. doi: 10.1080/14767058.2016.1183635
89. dos Santos Oliveira L, de Lima DP, da Silva AA, da Silva MC, de Souza SL, Manhaes-de-Castro R. Early Weaning Programs Rats to Have a Dietary

Preference for Fat and Palatable Foods in Adulthood. *Behav Processes* (2011) 86(1):75–80. doi: 10.1016/j.beproc.2010.09.005

90. Ghizoni H, Figueiredo PM, Moisan MP, Ogias D, Osaki LH, Gama P. Regulation of Corticosterone Function During Early Weaning and Effects on Gastric Cell Proliferation. *Nutrition* (2014) 30(3):343–9. doi: 10.1016/j.nut.2013.09.003
91. Kikusui T, Nakamura K, Kakuma Y, Mori Y. Early Weaning Augments Neuroendocrine Stress Responses in Mice. *Behav Brain Res* (2006) 175 (1):96–103. doi: 10.1016/j.bbr.2006.08.007
92. de Moura EG, Bonomo IT, Nogueira-Neto JF, de Oliveira E, Trevenzoli IH, Reis AM, et al. Maternal Prolactin Inhibition During Lactation Programs for Metabolic Syndrome in Adult Progeny. *J Physiol* (2009) 587(Pt 20):4919–29. doi: 10.1113/jphysiol.2009.176289
93. Fraga MC, de Moura EG, da Silva Lima N, Lisboa PC, de Oliveira E, Silva JO, et al. Anxiety-Like, Novelty-Seeking and Memory/Learning Behavioral Traits in Male Wistar Rats Submitted to Early Weaning. *Physiol Behav* (2014) 124:100–6. doi: 10.1016/j.physbeh.2013.11.001
94. Lima NS, Moura EG, Franco JG, Pinheiro CR, Pazos-Moura CC, Cabanelas A, et al. Developmental Plasticity of Endocrine Disorders in Obesity Model Primed by Early Weaning in Dams. *Horm Metab Res* (2013) 45(1):22–30. doi: 10.1055/s-0032-1323703
95. Souza LL, de Moura EG, Lisboa PC. Does Early Weaning Shape Future Endocrine and Metabolic Disorders? Lessons From Animal Models. *J Dev Orig Health Dis* (2020) 11(5):441–51. doi: 10.1017/S2040174420000410
96. Glavas MM, Hui Q, Tuduri E, Erener S, Kasteel NL, Johnson JD, et al. Early Overnutrition Reduces Pdx1 Expression and Induces Beta Cell Failure in Swiss Webster Mice. *Sci Rep* (2019) 9(1):3619. doi: 10.1038/s41598-019-39177-3
97. Patterson CM, Bouret SG, Park S, Irani BG, Dunn-Meynell AA, Levin BE. Large Litter Rearing Enhances Leptin Sensitivity and Protects Selectively Bred Diet-Induced Obese Rats From Becoming Obese. *Endocrinology* (2010) 151(9):4270–9. doi: 10.1210/en.2010-0401
98. Khanal P, Nielsen MO. Impacts of Prenatal Nutrition on Animal Production and Performance: A Focus on Growth and Metabolic and Endocrine Function in Sheep. *J Anim Sci Biotechnol* (2017) 8:75. doi: 10.1186/s40104-017-0205-1
99. White CL, Pistell PJ, Purpera MN, Gupta S, Fernandez-Kim SO, Hise TL, et al. Effects of High Fat Diet on Morris Maze Performance, Oxidative Stress, and Inflammation in Rats: Contributions of Maternal Diet. *Neurobiol Dis* (2009) 35(1):3–13. doi: 10.1016/j.nbd.2009.04.002
100. Christante CM, Taboga SR, Pinto-Fochi ME, Goes RM. Maternal Obesity Disturbs the Postnatal Development of Gonocytes in the Rat Without Impairment of Testis Structure at Prepubertal Age. *Reproduction* (2013) 146(6):549–58. doi: 10.1530/REP-13-0037
101. Reynolds CM, Vickers MH, Harrison CJ, Segovia SA, Gray C. High Fat and/or High Salt Intake During Pregnancy Alters Maternal Meta-Inflammation and Offspring Growth and Metabolic Profiles. *Physiol Rep* (2014) 2(8): e12110. doi: 10.14814/phy2.12110
102. Niculescu MD, Lupu DS. High Fat Diet-Induced Maternal Obesity Alters Fetal Hippocampal Development. *Int J Dev Neurosci* (2009) 27(7):627–33. doi: 10.1016/j.ijdevneu.2009.08.005
103. Sasson IE, Vitins AP, Mainigi MA, Moley KH, Simmons RA. Pre-Gestational vs Gestational Exposure to Maternal Obesity Differentially Programs the Offspring in Mice. *Diabetologia* (2015) 58(3):615–24. doi: 10.1007/s00125-014-3466-7
104. Akyol A, Langley-Evans SC, McMullen S. Obesity Induced by Cafeteria Feeding and Pregnancy Outcome in the Rat. *Br J Nutr* (2009) 102(11):1601–10. doi: 10.1017/S0007114509990961
105. Crew RC, Waddell BJ, Mark PJ. Maternal Obesity Induced by a 'Cafeteria' Diet in the Rat Does Not Increase Inflammation in Maternal, Placental or Fetal Tissues in Late Gestation. *Placenta* (2016) 39:33–40. doi: 10.1016/j.placenta.2016.01.002
106. Sanchez-Blanco C, Amusquivar E, Bispo K, Herrera E. Influence of Cafeteria Diet and Fish Oil in Pregnancy and Lactation on Pups' Body Weight and Fatty Acid Profiles in Rats. *Eur J Nutr* (2016) 55(4):1741–53. doi: 10.1007/s00394-015-0992-0
107. Masuyama H, Hiramatsu Y. Effects of a High-Fat Diet Exposure *In Utero* on the Metabolic Syndrome-Like Phenomenon in Mouse Offspring Through Epigenetic Changes in Adipocytokine Gene Expression. *Endocrinology* (2012) 153(6):2823–30. doi: 10.1210/en.2011-2161
108. Gupta A, Srinivasan M, Thamadilok S, Patel MS. Hypothalamic Alterations in Fetuses of High Fat Diet-Fed Obese Female Rats. *J Endocrinol* (2009) 200 (3):293–300. doi: 10.1677/JOE-08-0429
109. Srinivasan M, Katewa SD, Palaniyappan A, Pandya JD, Patel MS. Maternal High-Fat Diet Consumption Results in Fetal Malprogramming Predisposing to the Onset of Metabolic Syndrome-Like Phenotype in Adulthood. *Am J Physiol Endocrinol Metab* (2006) 291(4):E792–9. doi: 10.1152/ajpendo.00078.2006
110. Murabayashi N, Sugiyama T, Zhang L, Kamimoto Y, Umekawa T, Ma N, et al. Maternal High-Fat Diets Cause Insulin Resistance Through Inflammatory Changes in Fetal Adipose Tissue. *Eur J Obstet Gynecol Reprod Biol* (2013) 169(1):39–44. doi: 10.1016/j.ejogrb.2013.02.003
111. Howell KR, Powell TL. Effects of Maternal Obesity on Placental Function and Fetal Development. *Reproduction* (2017) 153(3):R97–R108. doi: 10.1530/REP-16-0495
112. Buckley AJ, Keseru B, Briody J, Thompson M, Ozanne SE, Thompson CH. Altered Body Composition and Metabolism in the Male Offspring of High Fat-Fed Rats. *Metabolism* (2005) 54(4):500–7. doi: 10.1016/j.metabol.2004.11.003
113. Fante T, Simino LA, Reginato A, Payolla TB, Vitoreli DC, Souza M, et al. Diet-Induced Maternal Obesity Alters Insulin Signalling in Male Mice Offspring Rechallenged With a High-Fat Diet in Adulthood. *PloS One* (2016) 11(8):e0160184. doi: 10.1371/journal.pone.0160184
114. Brunton N DB, Dart A, Azad MB, McGavoc JM. Maternal Obesity Before Pregnancy Predicts Offspring Blood Pressure at 18 Years of Age: A Causal Mediation Analysis. *medRxiv* (2020). doi: 10.1101/2020.11.22.20236398
115. Gaillard R. Maternal Obesity During Pregnancy and Cardiovascular Development and Disease in the Offspring. *Eur J Epidemiol* (2015) 30 (11):1141–52. doi: 10.1007/s10654-015-0085-7
116. Oken E, Gillman MW. Fetal Origins of Obesity. *Obes Res* (2003) 11(4):496–506. doi: 10.1038/oby.2003.69
117. Oken E, Rifas-Shiman SL, Field AE, Frazier AL, Gillman MW. Maternal Gestational Weight Gain and Offspring Weight in Adolescence. *Obstet Gynecol* (2008) 112(5):999–1006. doi: 10.1097/AOG.0b013e31818a5d50
118. Gaillard R, Durmus B, Hofman A, Mackenbach JP, Steegers EA, Jaddoe VW. Risk Factors and Outcomes of Maternal Obesity and Excessive Weight Gain During Pregnancy. *Obes (Silver Spring)* (2013) 21(5):1046–55. doi: 10.1002/oby.20088
119. Whitaker RC. Predicting Preschooler Obesity at Birth: The Role of Maternal Obesity in Early Pregnancy. *Pediatrics* (2004) 114(1):e29–36. doi: 10.1542/peds.114.1.e29
120. Tie HT, Xia YY, Zeng YS, Zhang Y, Dai CL, Guo JJ, et al. Risk of Childhood Overweight or Obesity Associated With Excessive Weight Gain During Pregnancy: A Meta-Analysis. *Arch Gynecol Obstet* (2014) 289(2):247–57. doi: 10.1007/s00404-013-3053-z
121. Catalano PM, Farrell K, Thomas A, Huston-Presley L, Mencin P, de Mouzon SH, et al. Perinatal Risk Factors for Childhood Obesity and Metabolic Dysregulation. *Am J Clin Nutr* (2009) 90(5):1303–13. doi: 10.3945/ajcn.2008.27416
122. Gaillard R, Steegers EA, Duijts L, Felix JF, Hofman A, Franco OH, et al. Childhood Cardiometabolic Outcomes of Maternal Obesity During Pregnancy: The Generation R Study. *Hypertension* (2014) 63(4):683–91. doi: 10.1161/HYPERTENSIONAHA.113.02671
123. Li S, Zhu Y, Yeung E, Chavarro JE, Yuan C, Field AE, et al. Offspring Risk of Obesity in Childhood, Adolescence and Adulthood in Relation to Gestational Diabetes Mellitus: A Sex-Specific Association. *Int J Epidemiol* (2017) 46(6):2104. doi: 10.1093/ije/dyx211
124. Joaquim AO, Coelho CP, Motta PD, Felicio LF, Bondan EF, Teodorov E, et al. Maternal Food Restriction in Rats of the F0 Generation Increases Retroperitoneal Fat, the Number and Size of Adipocytes and Induces Periventricular Astrogliosis in Female F1 and Male F2 Generations. *Reprod Fertil Dev* (2017) 29(7):1340–8. doi: 10.1071/RD15309
125. Lukaszewski MA, Mayeur S, Fajardy I, Delahaye F, Dutriez-Casteloot I, Montel V, et al. Maternal Prenatal Undernutrition Programs Adipose Tissue Gene Expression in Adult Male Rat Offspring Under High-Fat Diet. *Am J Physiol Endocrinol Metab* (2011) 301(3):E548–59. doi: 10.1152/ajpendo.00011.2011
126. Munoz-Valverde D, Rodriguez-Rodriguez P, Gutierrez-Arzapalo PY, Lopez de Pablo AL, Carmen Gonzalez M, Lopez-Gimenez R, et al. Effect of Fetal

Undernutrition and Postnatal Overfeeding on Rat Adipose Tissue and Organ Growth at Early Stages of Postnatal Development. *Physiol Res* (2015) 64 (4):547–59. doi: 10.33549/physiolres.932811
127. Zhu W, Gui W, Lin X, Yin X, Liang L, Li H. Maternal Undernutrition Modulates Hepatic Micrornas Expression in the Early Life of Offspring. *Exp Cell Res* (2021) 400(2):112450. doi: 10.1016/j.yexcr.2020.112450
128. de Oliveira JC, Gomes RM, Miranda RA, Barella LF, Malta A, Martins IP, et al. Protein Restriction During the Last Third of Pregnancy Malprograms the Neuroendocrine Axes to Induce Metabolic Syndrome in Adult Male Rat Offspring. *Endocrinology* (2016) 157(5):1799–812. doi: 10.1210/en.2015-1883
129. Xie L, Zhang K, Rasmussen D, Wang J, Wu D, Roemmich JN, et al. Effects of Prenatal Low Protein and Postnatal High Fat Diets on Visceral Adipose Tissue Macrophage Phenotypes and IL-6 Expression in Sprague Dawley Rat Offspring. *PloS One* (2017) 12(1):e0169581. doi: 10.1371/journal.pone.0169581
130. Thompson N, Huber K, Bedurftig M, Hansen K, Miles-Chan J, Breier BH. Metabolic Programming of Adipose Tissue Structure and Function in Male Rat Offspring by Prenatal Undernutrition. *Nutr Metab (Lond)* (2014) 11 (1):50. doi: 10.1186/1743-7075-11-50
131. Ware S, Voigt JP, Langley-Evans SC. Body Composition and Behaviour in Adult Rats Are Influenced by Maternal Diet, Maternal Age and High-Fat Feeding. *J Nutr Sci* (2015) 4:e3. doi: 10.1017/jns.2014.64
132. Hanafi MY, Saleh MM, Saad MI, Abdelkhalek TM, Kamel MA. Transgenerational Effects of Obesity and Malnourishment on Diabetes Risk in F2 Generation. *Mol Cell Biochem* (2016) 412(1-2):269–80. doi: 10.1007/s11010-015-2633-6
133. Matveyenko AV, Singh I, Shin BC, Georgia S, Devaskar SU. Differential Effects of Prenatal and Postnatal Nutritional Environment on Ss-Cell Mass Development and Turnover in Male and Female Rats. *Endocrinology* (2010) 151(12):5647–56. doi: 10.1210/en.2010-0978
134. Fall CH. Fetal Malnutrition and Long-Term Outcomes. *Nestle Nutr Inst Workshop Ser* (2013) 74:11–25. doi: 10.1159/000348384
135. Langley-Evans SC, Sherman RC, Welham SJ, Nwagwu MO, Gardner DS, Jackson AA. Intrauterine Programming of Hypertension: The Role of the Renin-Angiotensin System. *Biochem Soc Trans* (1999) 27(2):88–93. doi: 10.1042/bst0270088
136. de Gusmao Correia ML, Volpato AM, Aguila MB, Mandarim-de-Lacerda CA. Developmental Origins of Health and Disease: Experimental and Human Evidence of Fetal Programming for Metabolic Syndrome. *J Hum Hypertens* (2012) 26(7):405–19. doi: 10.1038/jhh.2011.61
137. Roseboom TJ, van der Meulen JH, Ravelli AC, Osmond C, Barker DJ, Bleker OP. Effects of Prenatal Exposure to the Dutch Famine on Adult Disease in Later Life: An Overview. *Twin Res* (2001) 4(5):293–8. doi: 10.1375/twin.4.5.293
138. Veenendaal MV, Painter RC, de Rooij SR, Bossuyt PM, van der Post JA, Gluckman PD, et al. Transgenerational Effects of Prenatal Exposure to the 1944-45 Dutch Famine. *BJOG* (2013) 120(5):548–53. doi: 10.1111/1471-0528.12136
139. Ravelli AC, van der Meulen JH, Osmond C, Barker DJ, Bleker OP. Obesity at the Age of 50 Y in Men and Women Exposed to Famine Prenatally. *Am J Clin Nutr* (1999) 70(5):811–6. doi: 10.1093/ajcn/70.5.811
140. Ravelli GP, Stein ZA, Susser MW. Obesity in Young Men After Famine Exposure *In Utero* and Early Infancy. *N Engl J Med* (1976) 295(7):349–53. doi: 10.1056/NEJM197608122950701
141. Hales CN, Barker DJ. Type 2 (Non-Insulin-Dependent) Diabetes Mellitus: The Thrifty Phenotype Hypothesis. *Diabetologia* (1992) 35(7):595–601. doi: 10.1007/BF00400248
142. Hales CN, Barker DJ, Clark PM, Cox LJ, Fall C, Osmond C, et al. Fetal and Infant Growth and Impaired Glucose Tolerance at Age 64. *BMJ* (1991) 303 (6809):1019–22. doi: 10.1136/bmj.303.6809.1019
143. Ong TP, Guest PC. Nutritional Programming Effects on Development of Metabolic Disorders in Later Life. *Methods Mol Biol* (2018) 1735:3–17. doi: 10.1007/978-1-4939-7614-0_1
144. Guo F, Jen KL. High-Fat Feeding During Pregnancy and Lactation Affects Offspring Metabolism in Rats. *Physiol Behav* (1995) 57(4):681–6. doi: 10.1016/0031-9384(94)00342-4
145. Rodriguez-Gonzalez GL, Reyes-Castro LA, Bautista CJ, Beltran AA, Ibanez CA, Vega CC, et al. Maternal Obesity Accelerates Rat Offspring Metabolic Ageing in a Sex-Dependent Manner. *J Physiol* (2019) 597(23):5549_63. doi: 10.1113/JP278232
146. Williams L, Seki Y, Vuguin PM, Charron MJ. Animal Models of *In Utero* Exposure to a High Fat Diet: A Review. *Biochim Biophys Acta* (2014) 1842 (3):507–19. doi: 10.1016/j.bbadis.2013.07.006
147. Zhang Q, Xiao X, Zheng J, Li M, Yu M, Ping F, et al. A Maternal High-Fat Diet Induces DNA Methylation Changes That Contribute to Glucose Intolerance in Offspring. *Front Endocrinol (Lausanne)* (2019) 10:871. doi: 10.3389/fendo.2019.00871
148. Cardenas-Perez RE, Fuentes-Mera L, de la Garza AL, Torre-Villalvazo I, Reyes-Castro LA, Rodriguez-Rocha H, et al. Maternal Overnutrition by Hypercaloric Diets Programs Hypothalamic Mitochondrial Fusion and Metabolic Dysfunction in Rat Male Offspring. *Nutr Metab (Lond)* (2018) 15:38. doi: 10.1186/s12986-018-0279-6
149. Chen H, Simar D, Lambert K, Mercier J, Morris MJ. Maternal and Postnatal Overnutrition Differentially Impact Appetite Regulators and Fuel Metabolism. *Endocrinology* (2008) 149(11):5348–56. doi: 10.1210/en.2008-0582
150. Bortolin RC, Vargas AR, Gasparotto J, Chaves PR, Schnorr CE, Martinello KB, et al. A New Animal Diet Based on Human Western Diet Is a Robust Diet-Induced Obesity Model: Comparison to High-Fat and Cafeteria Diets in Term of Metabolic and Gut Microbiota Disruption. *Int J Obes (Lond)* (2018) 42(3):525–34. doi: 10.1038/ijo.2017.225
151. Buyukdere Y, Gulec A, Akyol A. Cafeteria Diet Increased Adiposity in Comparison to High Fat Diet in Young Male Rats. *PeerJ* (2019) 7:e6656. doi: 10.7717/peerj.6656
152. Navarro ME, Santos KC, Nascimento AF, Francisqueti FV, Minatel IO, Pierine DT, et al. Renal Inflammatory and Oxidative and Metabolic Changes After 6 Weeks of Cafeteria Diet in Rats. *J Bras Nefrol* (2016) 38(1):9–14. doi: 10.5935/0101-2800.20160003
153. Reichelt AC, Stoeckel LE, Reagan LP, Winstanley CA, Page KA. Dietary Influences on Cognition. *Physiol Behav* (2018) 192:118–26. doi: 10.1016/j.physbeh.2018.02.052
154. Sampey BP, Vanhoose AM, Winfield HM, Freemerman AJ, Muehlbauer MJ, Fueger PT, et al. Cafeteria Diet Is a Robust Model of Human Metabolic Syndrome With Liver and Adipose Inflammation: Comparison to High-Fat Diet. *Obes (Silver Spring)* (2011) 19(6):1109–17. doi: 10.1038/oby.2011.18
155. Candler T, Kuhnen P, Prentice AM, Silver M. Epigenetic Regulation of POMC; Implications for Nutritional Programming, Obesity and Metabolic Disease. *Front Neuroendocrinol* (2019) 54:100773. doi: 10.1016/j.yfrne.2019.100773
156. Chowen JA, Argente-Arizon P, Freire-Regatillo A, Argente J. Sex Differences in the Neuroendocrine Control of Metabolism and the Implication of Astrocytes. *Front Neuroendocrinol* (2018) 48:3–12. doi: 10.1016/j.yfrne.2017.05.003
157. Sanchez-Garrido MA, Ruiz-Pino F, Velasco I, Barroso A, Fernandois D, Heras V, et al. Intergenerational Influence of Paternal Obesity on Metabolic and Reproductive Health Parameters of the Offspring: Male-Preferential Impact and Involvement of Kiss1-Mediated Pathways. *Endocrinology* (2018) 159(2):1005–18. doi: 10.1210/en.2017-00705
158. Gomes D, von Kries R, Delius M, Mansmann U, Nast M, Stubert M, et al. Late-Pregnancy Dysglycemia in Obese Pregnancies After Negative Testing for Gestational Diabetes and Risk of Future Childhood Overweight: An Interim Analysis From a Longitudinal Mother-Child Cohort Study. *PloS Med* (2018) 15(10):e1002681. doi: 10.1371/journal.pmed.1002681
159. Eriksson JG, Sandboge S, Salonen M, Kajantie E, Osmond C. Maternal Weight in Pregnancy and Offspring Body Composition in Late Adulthood: Findings From the Helsinki Birth Cohort Study (HBCS). *Ann Med* (2015) 47 (2):94–9. doi: 10.3109/07853890.2015.1004360
160. Bhandari R, Xiao J, Shankar A. Urinary Bisphenol a and Obesity in U.S. children. *Am J Epidemiol* (2013) 177(11):1263–70. doi: 10.1093/aje/kws391
161. Lee DH, Porta M, Jacobs DR Jr, Vandenberg LN. Chlorinated Persistent Organic Pollutants, Obesity, and Type 2 Diabetes. *Endocr Rev* (2014) 35 (4):557–601. doi: 10.1210/er.2013-1084
162. Lobstein T, Brownell KD. Endocrine-Disrupting Chemicals and Obesity Risk: A Review of Recommendations for Obesity Prevention Policies. *Obes Rev* (2021) 22(11):e13332. doi: 10.1111/obr.13332
163. Wu W, Li M, Liu A, Wu C, Li D, Deng Q, et al. Bisphenol a and the Risk of Obesity a Systematic Review With Meta-Analysis of the Epidemiological

Evidence. *Dose-Response* (2020) 18(2):155932582091949. doi: 10.1177/1559325820916949

164. Ashley-Martin J, Dodds L, Arbuckle TE, Ettinger AS, Shapiro GD, Fisher M, et al. A Birth Cohort Study to Investigate the Association Between Prenatal Phthalate and Bisphenol a Exposures and Fetal Markers of Metabolic Dysfunction. *Environ Health* (2014) 13:84. doi: 10.1186/1476-069X-13-84
165. Heindel JJ. The Developmental Basis of Disease: Update on Environmental Exposures and Animal Models. *Basic Clin Pharmacol Toxicol* (2019) 125 (Suppl 3):5–13. doi: 10.1111/bcpt.13118
166. Rodgers A, Sferruzzi-Perri AN. Developmental Programming of Offspring Adipose Tissue Biology and Obesity Risk. *Int J Obes (Lond)* (2021) 45 (6):1170–92. doi: 10.1038/s41366-021-00790-w
167. Rolfo A, Nuzzo AM, De Amicis R, Moretti L, Bertoli S, Leone A. Fetal-Maternal Exposure to Endocrine Disruptors: Correlation With Diet Intake and Pregnancy Outcomes. *Nutrients* (2020) 12(6):1744. doi: 10.3390/nu12061744
168. Anway MD, Cupp AS, Uzumcu M, Skinner MK. Epigenetic Transgenerational Actions of Endocrine Disruptors and Male Fertility. *Science* (2005) 308(5727):1466–9. doi: 10.1126/science.1108190
169. Jirtle RL, Skinner MK. Environmental Epigenomics and Disease Susceptibility. *Nat Rev Genet* (2007) 8(4):253–62. doi: 10.1038/nrg2045
170. Malik VS, Popkin BM, Bray GA, Despres JP, Willett WC, Hu FB. Sugar-Sweetened Beverages and Risk of Metabolic Syndrome and Type 2 Diabetes: A Meta-Analysis. *Diabetes Care* (2010) 33(11):2477–83. doi: 10.2337/dc10-1079
171. Talbot CPJ, Dolinsky VW. Sex Differences in the Developmental Origins of Cardiometabolic Disease Following Exposure to Maternal Obesity and Gestational Diabetes (1). *Appl Physiol Nutr Metab* (2019) 44(7):687–95. doi: 10.1139/apnm-2018-0667
172. Arnold AP, Lusis AJ. Understanding the Sexome: Measuring and Reporting Sex Differences in Gene Systems. *Endocrinology* (2012) 153(6):2551–5. doi: 10.1210/en.2011-2134
173. Arnold AP, van Nas A, Lusis AJ. Systems Biology Asks New Questions About Sex Differences. *Trends Endocrinol Metab* (2009) 20(10):471–6. doi: 10.1016/j.tem.2009.06.007
174. Krishnaveni GV, Hill JC, Leary SD, Veena SR, Saperia J, Saroja A, et al. Anthropometry, Glucose Tolerance, and Insulin Concentrations in Indian Children: Relationships to Maternal Glucose and Insulin Concentrations During Pregnancy. *Diabetes Care* (2005) 28(12):2919–25. doi: 10.2337/diacare.28.12.2919
175. Puttabyatappa M, Sargis RM, Padmanabhan V. Developmental Programming of Insulin Resistance: Are Androgens the Culprits? *J Endocrinol* (2020) 245(3):R23–48. doi: 10.1530/JOE-20-0044
176. Sir-Petermann T, Codner E, Perez V, Echiburu B, Maliqueo M, Ladron de Guevara A, et al. Metabolic and Reproductive Features Before and During Puberty in Daughters of Women With Polycystic Ovary Syndrome. *J Clin Endocrinol Metab* (2009) 94(6):1923–30. doi: 10.1210/jc.2008-2836
177. Tamhane S, Rodriguez-Gutierrez R, Iqbal AM, Prokop LJ, Bancos I, Speiser PW, et al. Cardiovascular and Metabolic Outcomes in Congenital Adrenal Hyperplasia: A Systematic Review and Meta-Analysis. *J Clin Endocrinol Metab* (2018) 103(11):4097–103. doi: 10.1210/jc.2018-01862
178. Sosa-Larios TC, AM-G A, Reyes-Castro LA, Morimoto S, Jaramillo-Flores ME. Alterations in Lipid Metabolism Due to a Protein-Restricted Diet in Rats During Gestation and/or Lactation. *Food Funct* (2017). doi: 10.1039/C7FO01513E
179. Lecoutre S, Breton C. Maternal Nutritional Manipulations Program Adipose Tissue Dysfunction in Offspring. *Front Physiol* (2015) 6:158. doi: 10.3389/fphys.2015.00158
180. Morris TJ, Vickers M, Gluckman P, Gilmour S, Affara N. Transcriptional Profiling of Rats Subjected to Gestational Undernourishment: Implications for the Developmental Variations in Metabolic Traits. *PloS One* (2009) 4(9): e7271. doi: 10.1371/journal.pone.0007271
181. Guan H, Arany E, van Beek JP, Chamson-Reig A, Thyssen S, Hill DJ, et al. Adipose Tissue Gene Expression Profiling Reveals Distinct Molecular Pathways That Define Visceral Adiposity in Offspring of Maternal Protein-Restricted Rats. *Am J Physiol Endocrinol Metab* (2005) 288(4): E663–73. doi: 10.1152/ajpendo.00461.2004
182. Palou M, Priego T, Romero M, Szostaczuk N, Konieczna J, Cabrer C, et al. Moderate Calorie Restriction During Gestation Programs Offspring for Lower BAT Thermogenic Capacity Driven by Thyroid and Sympathetic Signaling. *Int J Obes (Lond)* (2015) 39(2):339 45. doi: 10.1038/ijo.2014.56
183. Lussana F, Painter RC, Ocke MC, Buller HR, Bossuyt PM, Roseboom TJ. Prenatal Exposure to the Dutch Famine Is Associated With a Preference for Fatty Foods and a More Atherogenic Lipid Profile. *Am J Clin Nutr* (2008) 88 (6):1648–52. doi: 10.3945/ajcn.2008.26140
184. Hult M, Tornhammar P, Ueda P, Chima C, Bonamy AK, Ozumba B, et al. Hypertension, Diabetes and Overweight: Looming Legacies of the Biafran Famine. *PloS One* (2010) 5(10):e13582. doi: 10.1371/journal.pone.0013582
185. Li Y, He Y, Qi L, Jaddoe VW, Feskens EJ, Yang X, et al. Exposure to the Chinese Famine in Early Life and the Risk of Hyperglycemia and Type 2 Diabetes in Adulthood. *Diabetes* (2010) 59(10):2400–6. doi: 10.2337/db10-0385
186. Lakshmy R. Metabolic Syndrome: Role of Maternal Undernutrition and Fetal Programming. *Rev Endocr Metab Disord* (2013) 14(3):229–40. doi: 10.1007/s11154-013-9266-4
187. Roseboom T, de Rooij S, Painter R. The Dutch Famine and Its Long-Term Consequences for Adult Health. *Early Hum Dev* (2006) 82(8):485–91. doi: 10.1016/j.earlhumdev.2006.07.001
188. Painter RC, Roseboom TJ, van Montfrans GA, Bossuyt PM, Krediet RT, Osmond C, et al. Microalbuminuria in Adults After Prenatal Exposure to the Dutch Famine. *J Am Soc Nephrol* (2005) 16(1):189–94. doi: 10.1681/ASN.2004060474
189. Cianfarani S, Germani D, Branca F. Low Birthweight and Adult Insulin Resistance: The "Catch-Up Growth" Hypothesis. *Arch Dis Child Fetal Neonatal Ed* (1999) 81(1):F71–3. doi: 10.1136/fn.81.1.F71
190. Jaquet D, Gaboriau A, Czernichow P, Levy-Marchal C. Insulin Resistance Early in Adulthood in Subjects Born With Intrauterine Growth Retardation. *J Clin Endocrinol Metab* (2000) 85(4):1401–6. doi: 10.1210/jc.85.4.1401
191. Marciniak A, Patro-Malysza J, Kimber-Trojnar Z, Marciniak B, Oleszczuk J, Leszczynska-Gorzelak B. Fetal Programming of the Metabolic Syndrome. *Taiwan J Obstet Gynecol* (2017) 56(2):133–8. doi: 10.1016/j.tjog.2017.01.001
192. Ravelli AC, van der Meulen JH, Michels RP, Osmond C, Barker DJ, Hales CN, et al. Glucose Tolerance in Adults After Prenatal Exposure to Famine. *Lancet* (1998) 351(9097):173–7. doi: 10.1016/S0140-6736(97)07244-9
193. Roseboom TJ, van der Meulen JH, Ravelli AC, van Montfrans GA, Osmond C, Barker DJ, et al. Blood Pressure in Adults After Prenatal Exposure to Famine. *J Hypertens* (1999) 17(3):325–30. doi: 10.1097/00004872-199917030-00004
194. Finer S, Iqbal MS, Lowe R, Ogunkolade BW, Pervin S, Mathews C, et al. Is Famine Exposure During Developmental Life in Rural Bangladesh Associated With a Metabolic and Epigenetic Signature in Young Adulthood? A Historical Cohort Study. *BMJ Open* (2016) 6(11):e011768. doi: 10.1136/bmjopen-2016-011768
195. Armitage JA, Lakasing L, Taylor PD, Balachandran AA, Jensen RI, Dekou V, et al. Developmental Programming of Aortic and Renal Structure in Offspring of Rats Fed Fat-Rich Diets in Pregnancy. *J Physiol* (2005) 565(Pt 1):171–84. doi: 10.1113/jphysiol.2005.084947
196. Gopalakrishnan GS, Gardner DS, Dandrea J, Langley-Evans SC, Pearce S, Kurlak LO, et al. Influence of Maternal Pre-Pregnancy Body Composition and Diet During Early-Mid Pregnancy on Cardiovascular Function and Nephron Number in Juvenile Sheep. *Br J Nutr* (2005) 94(6):938–47. doi: 10.1079/BJN20051559
197. Morrison JL, Botting KJ, Dyer JL, Williams SJ, Thornburg KL, McMillen IC. Restriction of Placental Function Alters Heart Development in the Sheep Fetus. *Am J Physiol Regul Integr Comp Physiol* (2007) 293(1):R306–13. doi: 10.1152/ajpregu.00798.2006
198. Wang J, Ma H, Tong C, Zhang H, Lawlis GB, Li Y, et al. Overnutrition and Maternal Obesity in Sheep Pregnancy Alter the JNK-IRS-1 Signaling Cascades and Cardiac Function in the Fetal Heart. *FASEB J* (2010) 24 (6):2066–76. doi: 10.1096/fj.09-142315
199. Fan L, Lindsley SR, Comstock SM, Takahashi DL, Evans AE, He GW, et al. Maternal High-Fat Diet Impacts Endothelial Function in Nonhuman Primate Offspring. *Int J Obes (Lond)* (2013) 37(2):254–62. doi: 10.1038/ijo.2012.42
200. Cerf ME. High Fat Programming and Cardiovascular Disease. *Medicina (Kaunas)* (2018) 54(5):86. doi: 10.3390/medicina54050086
201. Moreira AS, Teixeira Teixeira M, da Silveira Osso F, Pereira RO, de Oliveira Silva-Junior G, Garcia de Souza EP, et al. Left Ventricular Hypertrophy

Induced by Overnutrition Early in Life. *Nutr Metab Cardiovasc Dis* (2009) 19 (11):805–10. doi: 10.1016/j.numecd.2009.01.008

202. Habbout A, Guenancia C, Lorin J, Rigal E, Fassot C, Rochette L, et al. Postnatal Overfeeding Causes Early Shifts in Gene Expression in the Heart and Long-Term Alterations in Cardiometabolic and Oxidative Parameters. *PloS One* (2013) 8(2):e56981. doi: 10.1371/journal.pone.0056981
203. Borengasser SJ, Zhong Y, Kang P, Lindsey F, Ronis MJ, Badger TM, et al. Maternal Obesity Enhances White Adipose Tissue Differentiation and Alters Genome-Scale DNA Methylation in Male Rat Offspring. *Endocrinology* (2013) 154(11):4113–25. doi: 10.1210/en.2012-2255
204. Liang X, Yang Q, Fu X, Rogers CJ, Wang B, Pan H, et al. Maternal Obesity Epigenetically Alters Visceral Fat Progenitor Cell Properties in Male Offspring Mice. *J Physiol* (2016) 594(15):4453–66. doi: 10.1113/JP272123
205. Van De Maele K, Devlieger R, Gies I. *In Utero* Programming and Early Detection of Cardiovascular Disease in the Offspring of Mothers With Obesity. *Atherosclerosis* (2018) 275:182–95. doi: 10.1016/j.atherosclerosis.2018.06.016
206. Agarwal P, Morriseau TS, Kereliuk SM, Doucette CA, Wicklow BA, Dolinsky VW. Maternal Obesity, Diabetes During Pregnancy and Epigenetic Mechanisms That Influence the Developmental Origins of Cardiometabolic Disease in the Offspring. *Crit Rev Clin Lab Sci* (2018) 55 (2):71–101. doi: 10.1080/10408363.2017.1422109
207. Neri C EA. Effects of Maternal Obesity on Fetal Programming: Molecular Approaches. *Cold Spring Harb Perspect Med* (2016) 6(2):a026591. doi: 10.1101/cshperspect.a026591
208. Elahi MM, Cagampang FR, Mukhtar D, Anthony FW, Ohri SK, Hanson MA. Long-Term Maternal High-Fat Feeding From Weaning Through Pregnancy and Lactation Predisposes Offspring to Hypertension, Raised Plasma Lipids and Fatty Liver in Mice. *Br J Nutr* (2009) 102(4):514–9. doi: 10.1017/S000711450820749X
209. Samuelsson AM, Morris A, Igosheva N, Kirk SL, Pombo JM, Coen CW, et al. Evidence for Sympathetic Origins of Hypertension in Juvenile Offspring of Obese Rats. *Hypertension* (2010) 55(1):76–82. doi: 10.1161/HYPERTENSIONAHA.109.139402
210. Khan IY, Dekou V, Douglas G, Jensen R, Hanson MA, Poston L, et al. A High-Fat Diet During Rat Pregnancy or Suckling Induces Cardiovascular Dysfunction in Adult Offspring. *Am J Physiol Regul Integr Comp Physiol* (2005) 288(1):R127–33. doi: 10.1152/ajpregu.00354.2004
211. Drake AJ, Reynolds RM. Impact of Maternal Obesity on Offspring Obesity and Cardiometabolic Disease Risk. *Reproduction* (2010) 140(3):387–98. doi: 10.1530/REP-10-0077
212. Godfrey KM, Reynolds RM, Prescott SL, Nyirenda M, Jaddoe VW, Eriksson JG, et al. Influence of Maternal Obesity on the Long-Term Health of Offspring. *Lancet Diabetes Endocrinol* (2017) 5(1):53–64. doi: 10.1016/S2213-8587(16)30107-3
213. Reynolds RM, Allan KM, Raja EA, Bhattacharya S, McNeill G, Hannaford PC, et al. Maternal Obesity During Pregnancy and Premature Mortality From Cardiovascular Event in Adult Offspring: Follow-Up of 1 323 275 Person Years. *BMJ* (2013) 347:f4539. doi: 10.1136/bmj.f4539
214. McMillen IC, Robinson JS. Developmental Origins of the Metabolic Syndrome: Prediction, Plasticity, and Programming. *Physiol Rev* (2005) 85 (2):571–633. doi: 10.1152/physrev.00053.2003
215. Mamun AA, O'Callaghan M, Callaway L, Williams G, Najman J, Lawlor DA. Associations of Gestational Weight Gain With Offspring Body Mass Index and Blood Pressure at 21 Years of Age: Evidence From a Birth Cohort Study. *Circulation* (2009) 119(13):1720–7. doi: 10.1161/CIRCULATIONAHA.108.813436
216. Oken E, Taveras EM, Kleinman KP, Rich-Edwards JW, Gillman MW. Gestational Weight Gain and Child Adiposity at Age 3 Years. *Am J Obstet Gynecol* (2007) 196(4):322 e1–8. doi: 10.1016/j.ajog.2006.11.027
217. Tam CHT, Ma RCW, Yuen LY, Ozaki R, Li AM, Hou Y, et al. The Impact of Maternal Gestational Weight Gain on Cardiometabolic Risk Factors in Children. *Diabetologia* (2018) 61(12):2539–48. doi: 10.1007/s00125-018-4724-x
218. West NA, Crume TL, Maligie MA, Dabelea D. Cardiovascular Risk Factors in Children Exposed to Maternal Diabetes In Utero. *Diabetologia* (2011) 54 (3):504–7. doi: 10.1007/s00125-010-2008-1
219. Salter A TE, Langley-Evans S. Influence of Maternal Nutrition on the Metabolic Syndrome and Cardiovascular Risk in the Offspring. *Clin Lipidol* (2009) 4(2):145–58. doi: 10.2217/clp.09.4
220. Chen P, Piaggi P, Traurig M, Bogardus C, Knowler WC, Baier LJ, et al. Differential Methylation of Genes in Individuals Exposed to Maternal Diabetes In Utero. *Diabetologia* (2017) 60(4):645–55. doi: 10.1007/s00125-016-4203-1
221. Ruchat SM, Houde AA, Voisin G, St-Pierre J, Perron P, Baillargeon JP, et al. Gestational Diabetes Mellitus Epigenetically Affects Genes Predominantly Involved in Metabolic Diseases. *Epigenetics* (2013) 8(9):935–43. doi: 10.4161/epi.25578
222. Kawamura M, Itoh H, Yura S, Mogami H, Fujii T, Makino H, et al. Isocaloric High-Protein Diet Ameliorates Systolic Blood Pressure Increase and Cardiac Remodeling Caused by Maternal Caloric Restriction in Adult Mouse Offspring. *Endocr J* (2009) 56(5):679–89. doi: 10.1507/endocrj.K08E-286
223. Mossa F, Carter F, Walsh SW, Kenny DA, Smith GW, Ireland JL, et al. Maternal Undernutrition in Cows Impairs Ovarian and Cardiovascular Systems in Their Offspring. *Biol Reprod* (2013) 88(4):92. doi: 10.1095/biolreprod.112.107235
224. Torrens C, Brawley L, Anthony FW, Dance CS, Dunn R, Jackson AA, et al. Folate Supplementation During Pregnancy Improves Offspring Cardiovascular Dysfunction Induced by Protein Restriction. *Hypertension* (2006) 47(5):982–7. doi: 10.1161/01.HYP.0000215580.43711.d1
225. Rexhaj E, Bloch J, Jayet PY, Rimoldi SF, Dessen P, Mathieu C, et al. Fetal Programming of Pulmonary Vascular Dysfunction in Mice: Role of Epigenetic Mechanisms. *Am J Physiol Heart Circ Physiol* (2011) 301(1): H247–52. doi: 10.1152/ajpheart.01309.2010
226. Vickers MH, Breier BH, McCarthy D, Gluckman PD. Sedentary Behavior During Postnatal Life Is Determined by the Prenatal Environment and Exacerbated by Postnatal Hypercaloric Nutrition. *Am J Physiol Regul Integr Comp Physiol* (2003) 285(1):R271–3. doi: 10.1152/ajpregu.00051.2003
227. Barros MA, De Brito Alves JL, Nogueira VO, Wanderley AG, Costa-Silva JH. Maternal Low-Protein Diet Induces Changes in the Cardiovascular Autonomic Modulation in Male Rat Offspring. *Nutr Metab Cardiovasc Dis* (2015) 25(1):123–30. doi: 10.1016/j.numecd.2014.07.011
228. Manning J, Vehaskari VM. Low Birth Weight-Associated Adult Hypertension in the Rat. *Pediatr Nephrol* (2001) 16(5):417–22. doi: 10.1007/s004670000560
229. Goyal R, Longo LD. Maternal Protein Deprivation: Sexually Dimorphic Programming of Hypertension in the Mouse. *Hypertens Res* (2013) 36(1):29–35. doi: 10.1038/hr.2012.129
230. Gilbert JS, Lang AL, Grant AR, Nijland MJ. Maternal Nutrient Restriction in Sheep: Hypertension and Decreased Nephron Number in Offspring at 9 Months of Age. *J Physiol* (2005) 565(Pt 1):137–47. doi: 10.1113/jphysiol.2005.084202
231. Tappia PS, Gabriel CA. Role of Nutrition in the Development of the Fetal Cardiovascular System. *Expert Rev Cardiovasc Ther* (2006) 4(2):211–25. doi: 10.1586/14779072.4.2.211
232. Gilbert JS, Lang AL, Nijland MJ. Maternal Nutrient Restriction and the Fetal Left Ventricle: Decreased Angiotensin Receptor Expression. *Reprod Biol Endocrinol* (2005) 3:27. doi: 10.1186/1477-7827-3-27
233. Cheema KK, Dent MR, Saini HK, Aroutiounova N, Tappia PS. Prenatal Exposure to Maternal Undernutrition Induces Adult Cardiac Dysfunction. *Br J Nutr* (2005) 93(4):471–7. doi: 10.1079/BJN20041392
234. Corstius HB, Zimanyi MA, Maka N, Herath T, Thomas W, van der Laarse A, et al. Effect of Intrauterine Growth Restriction on the Number of Cardiomyocytes in Rat Hearts. *Pediatr Res* (2005) 57(6):796–800. doi: 10.1203/01.PDR.0000157726.65492.CD
235. Jelinek DF, Andersson S, Slaughter CA, Russell DW. Cloning and Regulation of Cholesterol 7 Alpha-Hydroxylase, the Rate-Limiting Enzyme in Bile Acid Biosynthesis. *J Biol Chem* (1990) 265(14):8190–7. doi: 10.1016/S0021-9258(19)39056-8
236. Sun C, Denisenko O, Sheth B, Cox A, Lucas ES, Smyth NR, et al. Epigenetic Regulation of Histone Modifications and Gata6 Gene Expression Induced by Maternal Diet in Mouse Embryoid Bodies in a Model of Developmental Programming. *BMC Dev Biol* (2015) 15:3. doi: 10.1186/s12861-015-0053-1
237. Wang J, Wu Z, Li D, Li N, Dindot SV, Satterfield MC, et al. Nutrition, Epigenetics, and Metabolic Syndrome. *Antioxid Redox Signal* (2012) 17 (2):282–301. doi: 10.1089/ars.2011.4381
238. Khorram O, Chuang TD, Pearce WJ. Long-Term Effects of Maternal Undernutrition on Offspring Carotid Artery Remodeling: Role of Mir-29c. *J Dev Orig Health Dis* (2015) 6(4):342–9. doi: 10.1017/S2040174415001208

239. Bogdarina I, Welham S, King PJ, Burns SP, Clark AJ. Epigenetic Modification of the Renin-Angiotensin System in the Fetal Programming of Hypertension. *Circ Res* (2007) 100(4):520–6. doi: 10.1161/01.RES.0000258855.60637.58
240. Alexander BT, Dasinger JH, Intapad S. Fetal Programming and Cardiovascular Pathology. *Compr Physiol* (2015) 5(2):997–1025. doi: 10.1002/cphy.c140036
241. Alabduljabbar S, Zaidan SA, Lakshmanan AP, Terranegra A. Personalized Nutrition Approach in Pregnancy and Early Life to Tackle Childhood and Adult Non-Communicable Diseases. *Life (Basel)* (2021) 11(6):476. doi: 10.3390/life11060467
242. Li Y, Jaddoe VW, Qi L, He Y, Wang D, Lai J, et al. Exposure to the Chinese Famine in Early Life and the Risk of Metabolic Syndrome in Adulthood. *Diabetes Care* (2011) 34(4):1014–8. doi: 10.2337/dc10-2039
243. Roseboom TJ, van der Meulen JH, Osmond C, Barker DJ, Ravelli AC, Schroeder-Tanka JM, et al. Coronary Heart Disease After Prenatal Exposure to the Dutch Famine, 1944-45. *Heart* (2000) 84(6):595–8. doi: 10.1136/heart.84.6.595
244. Pearce WJ, Khorram O. Maturation and Differentiation of the Fetal Vasculature. *Clin Obstet Gynecol* (2013) 56(3):537–48. doi: 10.1097/GRF.0b013e31829e5bc9
245. Bilbo SD, Tsang V. Enduring Consequences of Maternal Obesity for Brain Inflammation and Behavior of Offspring. *FASEB J* (2010) 24(6):2104–15. doi: 10.1096/fj.09-144014
246. Contu L, Hawkes CA. A Review of the Impact of Maternal Obesity on the Cognitive Function and Mental Health of the Offspring. *Int J Mol Sci* (2017) 18(5):1093. doi: 10.3390/ijms18051093
247. Nizari S, Carare RO, Hawkes CA. Increased Abeta Pathology in Aged Tg2576 Mice Born to Mothers Fed a High Fat Diet. *Sci Rep* (2016) 6:21981. doi: 10.1038/srep21981
248. Mucellini AB, Laureano DP, Silveira PP, Sanvitto GL. Maternal and Post-Natal Obesity Alters Long-Term Memory and Hippocampal Molecular Signaling of Male Rat. *Brain Res* (2019) 1708:138–45. doi: 10.1016/j.brainres.2018.12.021
249. Page KC, Jones EK, Anday EK. Maternal and Postweaning High-Fat Diets Disturb Hippocampal Gene Expression, Learning, and Memory Function. *Am J Physiol Regul Integr Comp Physiol* (2014) 306(8):R527–37. doi: 10.1152/ajpregu.00319.2013
250. Edlow AG. Maternal Obesity and Neurodevelopmental and Psychiatric Disorders in Offspring. *Prenat Diagn* (2017) 37(1):95–110. doi: 10.1002/pd.4932
251. Tozuka Y, Wada E, Wada K. Diet-Induced Obesity in Female Mice Leads to Peroxidized Lipid Accumulations and Impairment of Hippocampal Neurogenesis During the Early Life of Their Offspring. *FASEB J* (2009) 23 (6):1920–34. doi: 10.1096/fj.08-124784
252. Moody L, Chen H, Pan YX. Early-Life Nutritional Programming of Cognition-the Fundamental Role of Epigenetic Mechanisms in Mediating the Relation Between Early-Life Environment and Learning and Memory Process. *Adv Nutr* (2017) 8(2):337–50. doi: 10.3945/an.116.014209
253. Ishikawa J, Ishikawa A, Nakamura S. Interferon-Alpha Reduces the Density of Monoaminergic Axons in the Rat Brain. *Neuroreport* (2007) 18(2):137–40. doi: 10.1097/WNR.0b013e328010231a
254. Naef L, Moquin L, Dal Bo G, Giros B, Gratton A, Walker CD. Maternal High-Fat Intake Alters Presynaptic Regulation of Dopamine in the Nucleus Accumbens and Increases Motivation for Fat Rewards in the Offspring. *Neuroscience* (2011) 176:225–36. doi: 10.1016/j.neuroscience.2010.12.037
255. Vucetic Z, Kimmel J, Totoki K, Hollenbeck E, Reyes TM. Maternal High-Fat Diet Alters Methylation and Gene Expression of Dopamine and Opioid-Related Genes. *Endocrinology* (2010) 151(10):4756–64. doi: 10.1210/en.2010-0505
256. Peleg-Raibstein D, Luca E, Wolfrum C. Maternal High-Fat Diet in Mice Programs Emotional Behavior in Adulthood. *Behav Brain Res* (2012) 233 (2):398–404. doi: 10.1016/j.bbr.2012.05.027
257. Sullivan EL, Grayson B, Takahashi D, Robertson N, Maier A, Bethea CL, et al. Chronic Consumption of a High-Fat Diet During Pregnancy Causes Perturbations in the Serotonergic System and Increased Anxiety-Like Behavior in Nonhuman Primate Offspring. *J Neurosci* (2010) 30(10):3826–30. doi: 10.1523/JNEUROSCI.5560-09.2010
258. Cordner ZA, Tamashiro KL. Effects of High-Fat Diet Exposure on Learning & Memory. *Physiol Behav* (2015) 152(Pt B):363 71. doi: 10.1016/j.physbeh.2015.06.008
259. Mehta SH KJ, Sokol RJ, Keating DP, Paneth N. The Association Between Maternal Obesity and Neurodevelopmental Outcomes of Offspring. *J Pediatr* (2014) 165(5):891–6. doi: 10.1016/j.jpeds.2014.07.003
260. Basatemur E, Gardiner J, Williams C, Melhuish E, Barnes J, Sutcliffe A. Maternal Prepregnancy BMI and Child Cognition: A Longitudinal Cohort Study. *Pediatrics* (2013) 131(1):56–63. doi: 10.1542/peds.2012-0788
261. Tanda R, Salsberry PJ, Reagan PB, Fang MZ. The Impact of Prepregnancy Obesity on Children's Cognitive Test Scores. *Matern Child Health J* (2013) 17(2):222–9. doi: 10.1007/s10995-012-0964-4
262. Mina TH, Lahti M, Drake AJ, Denison FC, Raikkonen K, Norman JE, et al. Prenatal Exposure to Maternal Very Severe Obesity Is Associated With Impaired Neurodevelopment and Executive Functioning in Children. *Pediatr Res* (2017) 82(1):47–54. doi: 10.1038/pr.2017.43
263. Mina TH, Lahti M, Drake AJ, Forbes S, Denison FC, Raikkonen K, et al. Maternal Lipids in Pregnancy Are Associated With Increased Offspring Cortisol Reactivity in Childhood. *Psychoneuroendocrinology* (2017) 83:79–83. doi: 10.1016/j.psyneuen.2017.04.018
264. Rodriguez A. Maternal Pre-Pregnancy Obesity and Risk for Inattention and Negative Emotionality in Children. *J Child Psychol Psychiatry* (2010) 51 (2):134–43. doi: 10.1111/j.1469-7610.2009.02133.x
265. Sullivan EL, Riper KM, Lockard R, Valleau JC. Maternal High-Fat Diet Programming of the Neuroendocrine System and Behavior. *Horm Behav* (2015) 76:153–61. doi: 10.1016/j.yhbeh.2015.04.008
266. Rodriguez A, Miettunen J, Henriksen TB, Olsen J, Obel C, Taanila A, et al. Maternal Adiposity Prior to Pregnancy Is Associated With ADHD Symptoms in Offspring: Evidence From Three Prospective Pregnancy Cohorts. *Int J Obes (Lond)* (2008) 32(3):550–7. doi: 10.1038/sj.ijo.0803741
267. Li M, Fallin MD, Riley A, Landa R, Walker SO, Silverstein M, et al. The Association of Maternal Obesity and Diabetes With Autism and Other Developmental Disabilities. *Pediatrics* (2016) 137(2):e20152206. doi: 10.1542/peds.2015-2206
268. Lamerz A, Kuepper-Nybelen J, Bruning N, Wehle C, Trost-Brinkhues G, Brenner H, et al. Prevalence of Obesity, Binge Eating, and Night Eating in a Cross-Sectional Field Survey of 6-Year-Old Children and Their Parents in a German Urban Population. *J Child Psychol Psychiatry* (2005) 46(4):385–93. doi: 10.1111/j.1469-7610.2004.00363.x
269. Stice E, Agras WS, Hammer LD. Risk Factors for the Emergence of Childhood Eating Disturbances: A Five-Year Prospective Study. *Int J Eat Disord* (1999) 25(4):375–87. doi: 10.1002/(SICI)1098-108X(199905)25:4<375::AID-EAT2>3.0.CO;2-K
270. Almeida SS, Tonkiss J, Galler JR. Prenatal Protein Malnutrition Affects Exploratory Behavior of Female Rats in the Elevated Plus-Maze Test. *Physiol Behav* (1996) 60(2):675–80. doi: 10.1016/S0031-9384(96)80047-3
271. Barra R, Morgan C, Saez-Briones P, Reyes-Parada M, Burgos H, Morales B, et al. Facts and Hypotheses About the Programming of Neuroplastic Deficits by Prenatal Malnutrition. *Nutr Rev* (2019) 77(2):65–80. doi: 10.1093/nutrit/nuy047
272. Belluscio LM, Berardino BG, Ferroni NM, Ceruti JM, Canepa ET. Early Protein Malnutrition Negatively Impacts Physical Growth and Neurological Reflexes and Evokes Anxiety and Depressive-Like Behaviors. *Physiol Behav* (2014) 129:237–54. doi: 10.1016/j.physbeh.2014.02.051
273. Francolin-Silva AL, da Silva Hernandes A, Fukuda MT, Valadares CT, Almeida SS. Anxiolytic-Like Effects of Short-Term Postnatal Protein Malnutrition in the Elevated Plus-Maze Test. *Behav Brain Res* (2006) 173 (2):310–4. doi: 10.1016/j.bbr.2006.06.042
274. Reyes-Castro LA, Rodriguez JS, Charco R, Bautista CJ, Larrea F, Nathanielsz PW, et al. Maternal Protein Restriction in the Rat During Pregnancy and/or Lactation Alters Cognitive and Anxiety Behaviors of Female Offspring. *Int J Dev Neurosci* (2012) 30(1):39–45. doi: 10.1016/j.ijdevneu.2011.10.002
275. Wang L, Xu RJ. The Effects of Perinatal Protein Malnutrition on Spatial Learning and Memory Behaviour and Brain Derived Neurotrophic Factor Concentration in the Brain Tissue in Young Rats. *Asia Pac J Clin Nutr* (2007) 16(Suppl 1):467–72.
276. Batista TH, Giusti-Paiva A, Vilela FC. Maternal Protein Malnutrition Induces Autism-Like Symptoms in Rat Offspring. *Nutr Neurosci* (2019) 22 (9):655–63. doi: 10.1080/1028415X.2018.1427660
277. Matos RJ, Orozco-Solis R, Lopes de Souza S, Manhaes-de-Castro R, Bolanos-Jimenez F. Nutrient Restriction During Early Life Reduces Cell Proliferation in the Hippocampus at Adulthood But Does Not Impair the Neuronal Differentiation Process of the New Generated Cells. *Neuroscience* (2011) 196:16 24. doi: 10.1016/j.neuroscience.2011.08.071

278. Zhang Y, Wei J, Yang Z. Perinatal Undernutrition Attenuates Field Excitatory Postsynaptic Potentials and Influences Dendritic Spine Density and Morphology in Hippocampus of Male Rat Offspring. *Neuroscience* (2013) 244:31–41. doi: 10.1016/j.neuroscience.2013.03.061
279. Chertoff M. Protein Malnutrition and Brain Development. *Brain Disord Ther* (2015) 4(3):171. doi: 10.4172/2168-975X.1000171
280. Feoli AM, Leite MC, Tramontina AC, Tramontina F, Posser T, Rodrigues L, et al. Developmental Changes in Content of Glial Marker Proteins in Rats Exposed to Protein Malnutrition. *Brain Res* (2008) 1187:33–41. doi: 10.1016/j.brainres.2007.10.035
281. Zhang Y, Li N, Yang Z. Perinatal Food Restriction Impaired Spatial Learning and Memory Behavior and Decreased the Density of Nitric Oxide Synthase Neurons in the Hippocampus of Adult Male Rat Offspring. *Toxicol Lett* (2010) 193(2):167–72. doi: 10.1016/j.toxlet.2010.01.002
282. Chang YM, Galler JR, Luebke JI. Prenatal Protein Malnutrition Results in Increased Frequency of Miniature Inhibitory Postsynaptic Currents in Rat CA3 Interneurons. *Nutr Neurosci* (2003) 6(4):263–7. doi: 10.1080/1028415031000151549
283. Soto-Moyano R, Fernandez V, Sanhueza M, Belmar J, Kusch C, Perez H, et al. Effects of Mild Protein Prenatal Malnutrition and Subsequent Postnatal Nutritional Rehabilitation on Noradrenaline Release and Neuronal Density in the Rat Occipital Cortex. *Brain Res Dev Brain Res* (1999) 116(1):51–8. doi: 10.1016/S0165-3806(99)00074-7
284. Chen J, Chen P, Bo T, Luo K. Cognitive and Behavioral Outcomes of Intrauterine Growth Restriction School-Age Children. *Pediatrics* (2016) 137 (4). doi: 10.1542/peds.2015-3868
285. Murray E, Fernandes M, Fazel M, Kennedy SH, Villar J, Stein A. Differential Effect of Intrauterine Growth Restriction on Childhood Neurodevelopment: A Systematic Review. *BJOG* (2015) 122(8):1062–72. doi: 10.1111/1471-0528.13435
286. Gibney ER, Nolan CM. Epigenetics and Gene Expression. *Heredity (Edinb)* (2010) 105(1):4–13. doi: 10.1038/hdy.2010.54
287. Duffy KA, Bale TL, Epperson CN. Germ Cell Drivers: Transmission of Preconception Stress Across Generations. *Front Hum Neurosci* (2021) 15:642762. doi: 10.3389/fnhum.2021.642762
288. Lane M, Robker RL, Robertson SA. Parenting From Before Conception. *Science* (2014) 345(6198):756–60. doi: 10.1126/science.1254400

17

Impact of Prepregnancy Overweight and Obesity on Treatment Modality and Pregnancy Outcome in Women with Gestational Diabetes Mellitus

*Tina Linder[1], Anna Eder[1], Cécile Monod[2], Ingo Rosicky[1], Daniel Eppel[1], Katharina Redling[2], Franziska Geissler[2], Evelyn A. Huhn[2], Irene Hösli[2] and Christian S. Göbl[1,2]**

[1] Department of Obstetrics and Gynaecology, Division of Obstetrics and feto-maternal Medicine, Medical University of Vienna, Vienna, Austria, [2] Department of Obstetrics and Gynaecology, University Hospital Basel, Basel, Switzerland

Correspondence:
Christian S. Göbl
christian.goebl@meduniwien.ac.at

Background: We aim to evaluate the impact of prepregnancy overweight on treatment modalities of Gestational Diabetes Mellitus (GDM). We assessed the association of increased pregravid Body Mass Index (BMI) with dosing of basal and rapid acting insulin as well as pregnancy outcome.

Methods: We included 509 gestational diabetic women (normal weight: 200, overweight: 157, obese: 152), attending the pregnancy outpatient clinic at the Department of Obstetrics and Gynecology, Medical University of Vienna, in this retrospective study. We used a prospectively compiled database to assess patient characteristics, treatment approaches – particularly maximum doses of basal and rapid acting insulin or metformin – and pregnancy outcome.

Results: Increased BMI was associated with the need of glucose lowering medication (odds ratio (OR): 1.08 for the increase of 1 kg/m² BMI, 95%CI 1.05–1.11, $p<0.001$). Mothers with pregestational obesity received the highest amount of insulin. Metformin was more often used in patients with obesity who also required higher daily doses. Maternal BMI was associated with increased risk of cesarean section (OR 1.04, 95%CI 1.01–1.07, $p<0.001$) and delivering large for gestational age offspring (OR 1.09, 95%CI 1.04–1.13, $p<0.001$). Birthweight percentiles were highest in patients with obesity who required glucose lowering therapy.

Conclusions: Treatment modalities and outcome in GDM pregnancies are closely related to the extent of maternal BMI. Patients with obesity required glucose lowering medication more often and were at higher risk of adverse pregnancy outcomes. It is crucial to further explore the underlying pathophysiologic mechanisms to optimize clinical management and individual treatment approaches.

Keywords: gestational diabetes (GDM), obesity, pharmacotherapy, pregnancy outcome, birth weight

INTRODUCTION

Growing evidence suggests that GDM comprises a broad spectrum of metabolic entities. It is crucial to identify factors which contribute to the observed heterogeneity in treatment modalities and outcomes of the disease (1), so that the clinical management can be tailored to individual patients.

Increased maternal BMI has a high prevalence in women developing GDM [approximately 65–75% are either overweight or obese (2, 3)] and was shown to be independently associated with pregnancy complications (such as fetal growth excess and adiposity) in the HAPO (Hyperglycaemia and Adverse Pregnancy Outcomes) study (4). Moreover, maternal obesity is associated with a higher level of insulin resistance, which is closely related to adverse pregnancy outcomes (like the development of large for gestational age offspring) (5, 6). In one of our previous studies we found that impaired insulin action at early pregnancy predicts the later requirement of glucose lowering medications, and therefore, an increased level of insulin resistance in mothers with overweight or obesity has possible impact on treatment modalities in those patients who develop GDM (7). While prepregnancy weight loss interventions are often not successful and are not recommended during pregnancy (8), a better understanding of the pathophysiological mechanisms linking pregestational BMI, the effectiveness of GDM treatment and adverse pregnancy outcomes could be used to further tailor the clinical pregnancy management of patients with obesity to their individual risk profile.

However, despite of major clinical importance, data on differences in treatment regimen and pregnancy outcomes in relation to the degree of maternal BMI in patients with GDM is sparsely available.

This study aims to evaluate differences in treatment modalities including use of insulin and metformin in relation to different degrees of obesity in pregnant women affected by GDM, taking into special consideration dosing regimens of basal insulin and rapid acting formulations. An analysis of pregnancy outcome and its association with maternal obesity is a further objective of this study.

METHODS

Study Design and Participants

In this study, we included a total of 509 digitally registered patients with GDM, attending the pregnancy outpatient clinic at the Department of Obstetrics and Gynecology, Medical University of Vienna, between May 2015 and December 2017. Of a total of 617 originally registered patients during this period, 68 women were excluded because of preexisting diabetes, 10 patients were excluded because of pregestational diabetes, which was unrecognized before pregnancy, 25 women were excluded because of unclear GDM diagnosis (e.g. reported as GDM but negative OGTT results) and 5 patients were excluded because of missing pregestational BMI. Study participants self-reported their pregestational BMI (BMIPG) at their first visit (9, 10) and were categorized into women with normal weight (BMIPG <25 kg/m^2), overweight (BMIPG ≥25 and <30 kg/m^2) or obesity (BMIPG ≥30 kg/m^2). GDM was diagnosed by use of a 75g 2h-OGTT according to the International Diabetes in Pregnancy Study Groups (IADPSG) recommendation (11). Glucose lowering medication (insulin and/or metformin) was started if glycemic targets were not achieved by lifestyle modification (i.e. if fasting or postprandial glucose levels exceeded 95 mg/dl or 140 mg/dl, according to international guidelines) (12). Data was assessed retrospectively; the following variables were extracted from a prospectively compiled database: age, height, weight before pregnancy, singleton or multiple pregnancy, OGTT glucose values (fasting, 60' and 120' after oral glucose load). Additionally, we assessed data on insulin treatment strategies: use and dose of metformin or insulin as well as details about insulin formulations (basal insulin such as intermediate or long-acting insulin analogues or rapid-acting insulin). All patients were treated with fixed insulin doses and the maximum doses per day were assessed. Moreover, neonatal outcome (birth weight, length and head circumference, gestational age at delivery (GAD), transfer to neonatal intensive care unit) and mode of delivery were assessed by referring to the medical history. Calculations of age and sex adjusted percentiles of the Austrian population were based on an analysis of the local growth standard curves. Small (SGA) and large for gestational age (LGA) were defined as bodyweight below the 10th and above the 90th percentile, respectively.

This study was approved by the local ethics committee and performed in accordance with the Declaration of Helsinki.

Statistical Analysis

Continuous variables were summarized by mean ± standard deviation or as median and interquartile ranges (IQR) in case of skewed distribution and compared by analysis of variance or rank based inference, respectively. Dichotomous variables were summarized by counts and percentages, and compared by binomial logistic regression. Odds ratios (OR) and 95% confidence intervals (95%CI) were additionally calculated for binary outcomes. Fisher protected Least Significant Difference (LSD) tests were used for multiple comparisons (k=3 groups) to achieve a 95% coverage probability. Statistical analysis was performed with R (version 4.0.2) and contributing packages (13). A two-sided p-value of ≤0.05 was considered statistically significant.

RESULTS

In **Table 1** main characteristics of the study sample are provided; categorized according to their pregestational BMI into GDM patients with normal weight (GDM-NW: n=200), overweight (GDM-OW: n=157) and obesity (GDM-OB: n=152). As compared to patients with normal weight, patients with overweight (mean difference, MD: 4.4 mg/dl, 95%CI 1.9 to 6.8, p<0.001) or obesity (MD: 6.7 mg/dl, 95%CI 4.3 to 9.2, p<0.001)

TABLE 1 | Characteristics of the study sample.

	GDM-NW (n=200)	GDM-OW (n=157)	GDM-OB (n=152)	p-value
Age (years)	31.6 ± 4.8	32.6 ± 4.9	32.0 ± 4.6	0.192
Height (cm)	164 ± 6.8	163 ± 6.8	164 ± 6.2	0.280
Weight, before pregnancy (kg)	59.0 ± 7.0	72.8 ± 6.7*	95.5 ± 15.3*†	<0.001
BMI, before pregnancy (kg/m^2)	21.9 ± 2.0	27.4 ± 1.3*	35.6 ± 4.8*†	<0.001
Multiple pregnancy (%)	23 (11.4)	15 (9.6)	10 (6.6)	0.295
OGTT Glucose 0' (mg/dl)	88.4 ± 12.2	92.8 ± 9.9*	95.2 ± 9.0*	<0.001
OGTT Glucose 60' (mg/dl)	174.6 ± 33.2	179.1 ± 34.4	180.3 ± 33.4	0.336
OGTT Glucose 120' (mg/dl)	135.2 ± 30.9	139.8 ± 31.4	138.8 ± 35.1	0.482
Gestational age at GDM diagnosis (weeks)	28.0 (26.0-29.5)	27.0 (25.0-30.0)	26.5 (23.0-28.0)*†	<0.001
Pharmacotherapy (Metformin and/or Insulin)	52 (26.0)	75 (47.8)*	84 (55.3)*	<0.001
Metformin only (%)	12 (6.0)	15 (9.6)	15 (9.9)	0.317
Metformin total (%)	16 (8.0)	19 (12.1)	27 (17.9)*	0.022
Metformin total (g/d)	1.50 (1.25-1.85)	1.50 (1.00-2.50)	2.50 (1.50-2.50)*	0.032
Insulin and Metformin (%)	4 (2.0)	4 (2.5)	12 (7.9)*†	0.016
Insulin BI or RAI total (%)	40 (20.0)	60 (38.2)*	69 (45.3)*	<0.001
Insulin BI or RAI total (IU/d)	24.0 (15.5-31.5)	30.0 (18.0-40.0)	40.0 (27.0-52.0)*†	0.019
Insulin BI total (%)	31 (15.5)	55 (35.0)*	63 (41.4)*	<0.001
Insulin BI total (IU/d)	12 (9-24)	12 (10-21)	16 (12-27)	0.122
Insulin RAI total (%)	24 (12.1)	31 (20.0)*	34 (22.4)*	0.026
Insulin RAI total (IU/d)	10 (4.5-15)	10 (5-19)	14 (10-26)*	0.029

Data are mean ± SD or median (IQR) and count (%) for patients with GDM and normal weight (GDM-NW) vs. overweight (GDM-OW) and obese patients (GDM-OB). BMI, body mass index; OGTT, oral glucose tolerance test; Insulin BI, basal insulin; insulin RAI, rapid acting insulin.
**p<0.05 vs. GDM-NW.*
†p<0.05 vs. GDM-OW.

had significantly higher fasting glucose concentrations, whereas OGTT glucose levels at 60' and 120' were comparable. Of note, obese women were diagnosed at an earlier gestational age. Higher pregestational BMI was significantly associated with the need of glucose lowering medications (OR: 1.08 for the increase of 1 kg/m^2 BMI, 95%CI 1.05 to 1.11, p<0.001), as visualized in **Figure 1A**. Insulin (basal or rapid acting) was more often prescribed for patients with overweight or obesity, whereby the latter showed the highest requirement of total insulin units per day (**Table 1**). There was no difference in the daily dose of basal insulin formulations between groups. However, GDM patients with obesity required a higher amount of rapid acting insulin as compared to normal weight patients. Metformin was more often used in patients with obesity who also required higher daily doses as compared to normal weight women. Moreover, a combination therapy with insulin and metformin was more often observed in gestational diabetic mothers with obesity. Glycemic control was evaluated in a subgroup of 220 patients at 38 (IQR: 37-39) weeks of gestation. Adequate glycemic control was protocolled in 74 (83%) normal weight, 49 (67%) overweight and 42 (72%) obese patients. Although there was a tendency that overweight and obese patients reached glycemic targets less often, the observed difference didn't reach significance (p=0.052). Moreover, weight gain was assessed in 340 women around delivery (median 1.0, IQR: 0.0-2.0 weeks before delivery). It was found that normal weight patients had a weight gain of 13.2 ± 6.7 kg vs. 12.2 ± 6.1 kg in overweight patients (p=0.504). Obese patients gained 10.7 ± 7.6 kg which was significantly lower as compared to overweight (p=0.04) or obese women (p=0.006).

Assessment of pregnancy outcome data showed that pregestational BMI was associated with an increased risk of delivering LGA offspring (OR 1.09 for the increase of 1 kg/m^2 BMI, 95%CI 1.04 to 1.13, p<0.001, **Figure 1B**) as well as with an increased cesarean section rate (OR 1.04 for the increase of 1 kg/m^2 BMI, 95%CI 1.01 to 1.07, p<0.001, **Figure 1C**). Consequently, offspring of mothers with obesity showed higher birth weight percentiles as compared to normal weight and overweight patients as provided in **Table 2**. However, analysis of interaction indicated that the association of obesity status and birth weight percentiles of newborns was modified if pharmacotherapy was necessary in these patients (p<0.001 for the interaction between overweight or obesity status and requirement of pharmacotherapy for GDM). As compared to not medicated mothers with obesity (which showed mean birth weight of 43.2 ± 28.2 Pct.), birthweight percentiles were increased in patients with obesity who received glucose lowering medication (63.0 ± 28.8 Pct.), leading to a significant interaction (**Figure 2**). However, weight gain during pregnancy showed no significant association with LGA development in our study (p=0.591).

DISCUSSION

We aimed to assess characteristics of treatment modalities, neonatal outcome and delivery mode in women with GDM, categorized according to their pregestational BMI into patients with normal-weight, overweight or obesity. We found that pregestational BMI was significantly associated with an earlier diagnosis of GDM and increased requirement of glucose lowering medication, with mothers with obesity needing the highest amount of insulin units per day. This observation is in

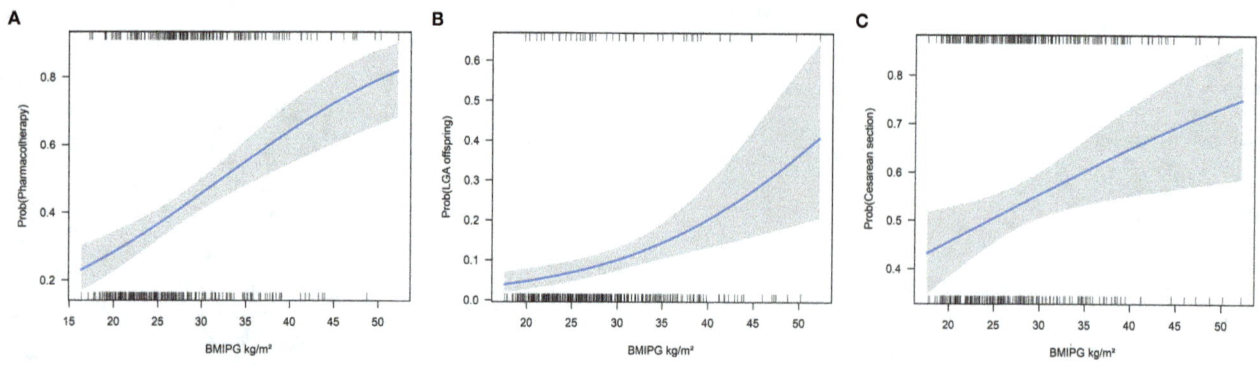

FIGURE 1 | Association of pregestational BMI (BMIPG) with the probability of receiving pharmacotherapy **(A)**, for delivering large for gestational age (LGA) offspring **(B)** and having delivery by cesarean section **(C)**.

line with previous publications: Langer and co-workers found that mothers with overweight and obesity required a significantly higher total daily insulin dose (88 and 121 IU/d) as compared to normal weight GDM patients (69 IU/d) (14). Of note, the number of patients who received pharmacotherapy (69% vs. 41%) as well as the amount of required insulin was markedly higher as compared to our study. This might be explained by the use of different diagnosis criteria. There is some data suggesting that the IADPSG approach (which was used in our study) identifies more, but also less severe, cases of GDM as compared to other approaches [such as the Carpenter-Coustan criteria, which were used by Langer et al. (14)] (15). More recently, Machado et al. evaluated the impact of pregestational obesity on pregnancy outcomes in GDM pregnancies and observed that the need of pharmacological intervention was higher in patients with obesity (54%) as compared to patients with overweight (42%) or normal weight (29%) (16). This is comparable to our findings; however, the amount of insulin or metformin doses per day were not reported. In line with the above mentioned findings, another retrospective cohort study concluded that maternal BMI was the only predictor for the need of treatment with glucose lowering agents in patients with GDM (17).

The higher need of pharmacotherapy in patients with obesity may be explained by impaired insulin action, which is often prevalent already before conception. With advancing pregnancy insulin sensitivity decreases, leading to manifest hyperglycemia in patients who do not adequately compensate impaired insulin action by increased insulin release from the pancreatic β-cells (18–20). In this context, we observed increased fasting plasma glucose levels in patients with overweight and obesity at the time of GDM diagnosis, whereas glucose levels after oral glucose load were comparable between groups. Higher fasting glucose concentrations are pointing towards a primary defect in hepatic insulin sensitivity [as fasting glucose is mostly regulated by the liver (21)] in GDM patients with overweight or obesity and may be an underlying reason why basal insulin [which suppresses hepatic gluconeogenesis (22)] was more often used in those patients in our study. The higher requirement of rapid acting insulin may be due to additional defects in β-cell function.

Interestingly, GDM patients with obesity were more often treated with metformin [which also suppresses hepatic gluconeogenesis (23)] and required a higher dosage of this medication. We also observed that obesity resulted in an increased complementary treatment with insulin. This may

TABLE 2 | Fetal biometry and pregnancy outcomes (multiple pregnancies and cases with missing pregnancy outcome data are excluded).

	GDM-NW (n=177)	GDM-OW (n=142)	GDM-OB (n=142)	p-value
Cesarean Section	79 (44.6)	76 (53.5)	90 (63.4)*	0.004
Neonatal Intensive Care	13 (7.3)	10 (7.2)	11 (7.9)	0.976
GAD (weeks)	40 (39-41)	39 (39-41)	39 (39-40)*	0.028
Preterm Delivery (<37 GW)	17 (9.6)	11 (7.7)	9 (6.3)	0.558
Birth Weight (Percentile)	42.5 ± 27.3	44.6 ± 28.6	54.4 ± 30.1*†	<0.001
Birth Length (Percentile)	46.9 ± 26.3	48.2 ± 26.9	49.2 ± 28.7	0.758
Birth Head Circumference (Percentile)	42.2 ± 27.1	44.1 ± 28.9	53.3 ± 29.4*†	0.002
SGA (<10. Pct)	20 (11.5)	18 (13.0)	15 (10.6)	0.819
LGA (>90. Pct)	10 (5.7)	10 (7.2)	23 (16.3)*†	0.005

Data are mean ± SD or median (IQR) and count (%) for patients with GDM and normal weight (GDM-NW) vs. overweight (GDM-OW) and obese patients (GDM-OB). GAD, gestational age at delivery; SGA, small for gestational age offspring; LGA, large for gestational age offspring.

**p<0.05 vs. GDM-NW.*

†p<0.05 vs. GDM-OW.

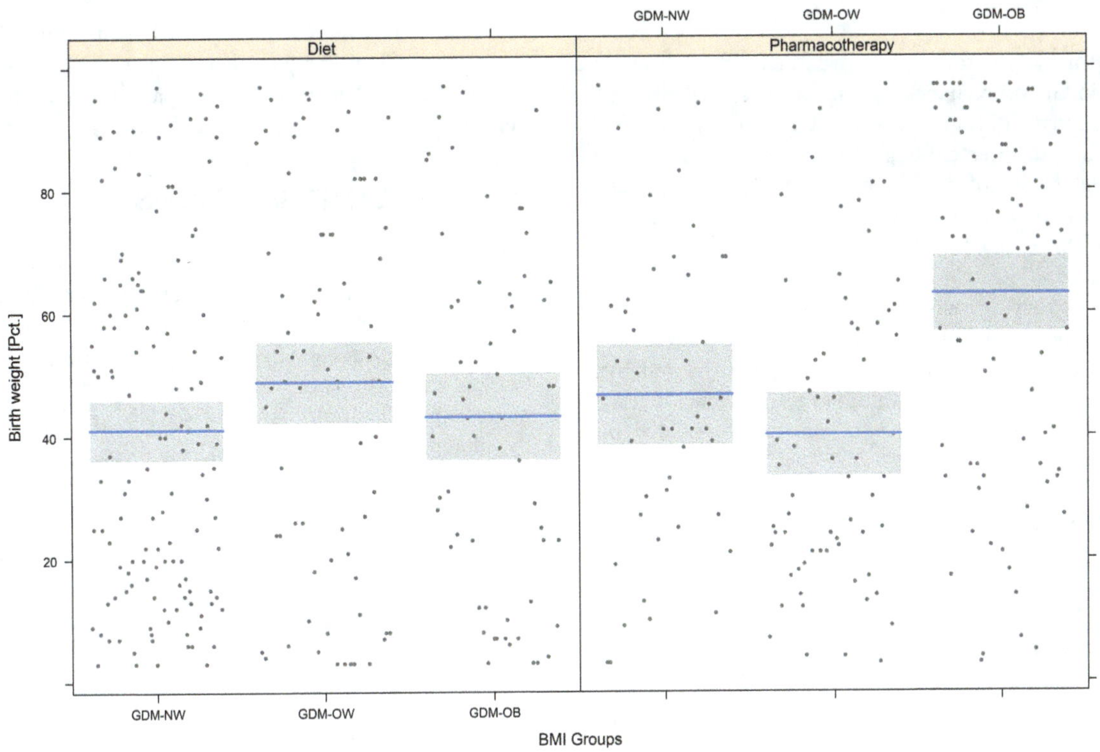

FIGURE 2 | Birth weight percentiles in normal weight (GDM-NW), overweight (GDM-OW) or obese patients with GDM (GDM-OB), categorized further into patients who received glucose lowering pharmacotherapy (PT) or diet only. The grey box represents the interquartile range. The median is indicated by a blue line.

possibly indicate an increased risk of secondary treatment failure of metformin in pregnant women with obesity. In this context, results from the MIG (Metformin in Gestational Diabetes) trial and other studies suggest that its use in pregnancy is save and has some advantages over insulin (especially being weight neutral and without risk of hypoglycemia) (24, 25). However, a significant treatment failure rate of metformin was already reported in the MIG trial, where 46% of the patients received supplemental insulin therapy (24). Other studies (26, 27) reported lower rates of metformin treatment failure. Previous research, aiming to assess the contributors to the observed failure rate of metformin monotherapy in pregnant women, concluded that the chance for responding to metformin was lower in patients with increased BMI (17, 28, 29) and higher fasting glucose levels (26, 28, 29). It is also noteworthy that large intervention studies failed to identify a protective effect of metformin on the risk of GDM, further suggesting that metformin is less effective in mothers with obesity (30, 31).

A number of studies indicated an increased risk of cesarean section delivery in mothers with obesity, potentially related to fetal adiposity (18). As shown in a secondary analysis of the HAPO study, the impact of increased maternal obesity on the risk of fetal growth excess is aggravated by hyperglycemia (32). This is in line with our results; however, our data further indicates that the well-known association between maternal and fetal adiposity is markedly increased in GDM patients with obesity who required glucose lowering therapy. There are two possible explanations for this observation: First; mothers with obesity have poor glycemic control despite receiving glucose lowering medication. Second; there is an underlying pathophysiologic factor (e.g. impaired insulin sensitivity) responsible for both, exceeded fetal growth as well as treatment failure of life-style modification, leading to the requirement of pharmacologic intervention in some patients. The latter theory is supported by observations suggesting that impaired insulin action in early pregnancy is per se contributing to fetal adiposity (due to hyperinsulinism and placental changes leading to increased nutrient supply to the offspring) but is also acting as a risk factor for the need of glucose lowering medication as described above (7, 18). We are not able to further elaborate those theories due to lack of detailed data about insulin sensitivity status in this retrospective study which is a limitation of this work. Impaired insulin sensitivity can possibly lead to increased maternal lipids, which can possibly explain the increased rates of LGA offspring in obese women (33, 34). We suggest further investigation of the possible interaction between the extent of insulin resistance (as well as other glucometabolic parameters in early pregnancy) and fetal development in patients with obesity. Also, the role of maternal body composition (especially the amount of visceral fat), lipid profiles and inflammatory markers should be further investigated to further disentangle the interaction between BMI, poor glycemic control and detrimental neonatal and maternal pregnancy outcomes in women with obesity.

In summary, we found that treatment modalities and outcomes in GDM pregnancies are strongly associated with the extent of maternal BMI and obesity status. Patients with obesity showed higher requirement of glucose lowering medication and were at higher risk of adverse pregnancy outcomes, such as cesarean section or LGA offspring. Our finding of markedly exceeded birth weight in infants of mothers with obesity who required glucose lowering medication is interesting and points towards an underlying role of early pregnancy insulin resistance, which interferes either with glycemic control or the development of fetal adiposity. It is crucial to further explore the underlying pathophysiologic mechanisms to optimize individual treatment approaches in these patients with particular risk for poor obstetric outcomes.

ETHICS STATEMENT

This study was reviewed and approved by the Ethics Committee of the Medical University of Vienna, Borschkegasse 8b/E06, 1090 Vienna, Austria. The patients/participants provided their written informed consent to participate in this study.

AUTHOR CONTRIBUTIONS

CG conceived the study. Data assessment was performed by CM, AE, IR, DE, TL and CG. Calculations and data interpretation were performed by CG. Statistical analysis was performed by CG. CSG prepared tables and figures. The manuscript was written by CG and TL. CM, IR, DE, FG, KR, IH, EH critically revised the manuscript. All authors contributed to the article and approved the submitted version.

REFERENCES

1. Wexler DJ, Powe CE, Barbour LA, Buchanan T, Coustan DR, Corcoy R, et al. Research Gaps in Gestational Diabetes Mellitus: Executive Summary of a National Institute of Diabetes and Digestive and Kidney Diseases Workshop. *Obstetrics Gynecol* (2018) 132:496–505. doi: 10.1097/AOG.0000000000002726
2. Black MH, Sacks DA, Xiang AH, Lawrence JM. Clinical Outcomes of Pregnancies Complicated by Mild Gestational Diabetes Mellitus Differ by Combinations of Abnormal Oral Glucose Tolerance Test Values. *Diabetes Care* (2010) 33:2524–30. doi: 10.2337/dc10-1445
3. Ouzounian JG, Hernandez GD, Korst LM, Montoro MM, Battista LR, Walden CL, et al. Pre-Pregnancy Weight and Excess Weight Gain Are Risk Factors for Macrosomia in Women With Gestational Diabetes. *J Perinatol* (2011) 31:717–21. doi: 10.1038/jp.2011.15
4. Study Cooperative Research Group. Hyperglycaemia HAPO. And Adverse Pregnancy Outcome (HAPO) Study: Associations With Maternal Body Mass Index. *BJOG* (2010) 117:575–84. doi: 10.1111/j.1471-0528.2009.02486.x
5. Powe CE, Allard C, Battista M-C, Doyon M, Bouchard L, Ecker JL, et al. Heterogeneous Contribution of Insulin Sensitivity and Secretion Defects to Gestational Diabetes Mellitus. *Dia Care* (2016) 39:1052–5. doi: 10.2337/dc15-2672
6. Benhalima K, Van Crombrugge P, Moyson C, Verhaeghe J, Vandeginste S, Verlaenen H, et al. Characteristics and Pregnancy Outcomes Across Gestational Diabetes Mellitus Subtypes Based on Insulin Resistance. *Diabetologia* (2019) 62:2118–28. doi: 10.1007/s00125-019-4961-7
7. Falcone V, Kotzaeridi G, Breil MH, Rosicky I, Stopp T, Yerlikaya-Schatten G, et al. Early Assessment of the Risk for Gestational Diabetes Mellitus: Can Fasting Parameters of Glucose Metabolism Contribute to Risk Prediction? *Diabetes Metab J* (2019) 43:785–93. doi: 10.4093/dmj.2018.0218
8. Institute of Medicine (US) and National Research Council (US) Committee to Reexamine IOM Pregnancy Weight Guidelines. *Weight Gain During Pregnancy: Reexamining the Guidelines* (2009). Washington (DC: National Academies Press (US. Available at: http://www.ncbi.nlm.nih.gov/books/NBK32813/ (Accessed August 31, 2021).
9. Natamba BK, Sanchez SE, Gelaye B, Williams MA. Concordance Between Self-Reported Pre-Pregnancy Body Mass Index (BMI) and BMI Measured at the First Prenatal Study Contact. *BMC Pregnancy Childbirth* (2016) 16:187. doi: 10.1186/s12884-016-0983-z
10. Holland E, Moore Simas TA, Doyle Curiale DK, Liao X, Waring ME. Self-Reported Pre-Pregnancy Weight Versus Weight Measured at First Prenatal Visit: Effects on Categorization of Pre-Pregnancy Body Mass Index. *Matern Child Health J* (2013) 17:1872–8. doi: 10.1007/s10995-012-1210-9
11. International Association of Diabetes and Pregnancy Study Groups Consensus Panel. International Association of Diabetes and Pregnancy Study Groups Recommendations on the Diagnosis and Classification of Hyperglycemia in Pregnancy. *Diabetes Care* (2010) 33:676–82. doi: 10.2337/dc09-1848
12. American Diabetes Association. Management of Diabetes in Pregnancy: *Standards of Medical Care in Diabetes—2020. Dia Care* (2020) 43:S183–92. doi: 10.2337/dc20-S014
13. *R: The R Project for Statistical Computing*. Available at: https://www.r-project.org/ (Accessed May 21, 2018).
14. Langer O, Yogev Y, Xenakis EMJ, Brustman L. Overweight and Obese in Gestational Diabetes: The Impact on Pregnancy Outcome. *Am J Obstetrics Gynecol* (2005) 192:1768–76. doi: 10.1016/j.ajog.2004.12.049
15. Huhn EA, Rossi SW, Hoesli I, Göbl CS. Controversies in Screening and Diagnostic Criteria for Gestational Diabetes in Early and Late Pregnancy. *Front Endocrinol (Lausanne)* (2018) 9:696. doi: 10.3389/fendo.2018.00696
16. Machado C, Monteiro S, Oliveira MJGrupo de Estudo de Diabetes e Gravidez da Sociedade Portuguesa de Diabetologia. Impact of Overweight and Obesity on Pregnancy Outcomes in Women With Gestational Diabetes - Results From a Retrospective Multicenter Study. *Arch Endocrinol Metab* (2020) 64:45–51. doi: 10.20945/2359-3997000000178
17. Ali A, Shastry S, Nithiyananthan R, Ali A, Ganapathy R. Gestational Diabetes–Predictors of Response to Treatment and Obstetric Outcome. *Eur J Obstetrics Gynecol Reprod Biol* (2018) 220:57–60. doi: 10.1016/j.ejogrb.2017.11.014
18. Catalano PM, Shankar K. Obesity and Pregnancy: Mechanisms of Short Term and Long Term Adverse Consequences for Mother and Child. *BMJ* (2017) 356:j1. doi: 10.1136/bmj.j1
19. Stopp T, Feichtinger M, Rosicky I, Yerlikaya-Schatten G, Ott J, Egarter HC, et al. Novel Indices of Glucose Homeostasis Derived From Principal Component Analysis: Application for Metabolic Assessment in Pregnancy. *J Diabetes Res* (2020) 2020:4950584. doi: 10.1155/2020/4950584
20. Catalano PM. Trying to Understand Gestational Diabetes. *Diabetes Med* (2014) 31:273–81. doi: 10.1111/dme.12381
21. Abdul-Ghani MA, Tripathy D, DeFronzo RA. Contributions of Beta-Cell Dysfunction and Insulin Resistance to the Pathogenesis of Impaired Glucose Tolerance and Impaired Fasting Glucose. *Diabetes Care* (2006) 29:1130–9. doi: 10.2337/diacare.2951130
22. Hedrington MS, Pulliam L, Davis SN. Basal Insulin Treatment in Type 2 Diabetes. *Diabetes Technol Ther* (2011) 13:S-33-S-42. doi: 10.1089/dia.2011.0062
23. Ferrannini E. The Target of Metformin in Type 2 Diabetes. *N Engl J Med* (2014) 371:1547–8. doi: 10.1056/NEJMcibr1409796
24. Rowan JA, Hague WM, Gao W, Battin MR, Moore MP. Metformin Versus Insulin for the Treatment of Gestational Diabetes. *N Engl J Med* (2008) 358:2003–15. doi: 10.1056/NEJMoa0707193
25. Butalia S, Gutierrez L, Lodha A, Aitken E, Zakariasen A, Donovan L. Short- and Long-Term Outcomes of Metformin Compared With Insulin Alone in Pregnancy: A Systematic Review and Meta-Analysis. *Diabetes Med* (2017) 34:27–36. doi: 10.1111/dme.13150

26. Ashoush S, El-Said M, Fathi H, Abdelnaby M. Identification of Metformin Poor Responders, Requiring Supplemental Insulin, During Randomization of Metformin Versus Insulin for the Control of Gestational Diabetes Mellitus: Metformin in GDM. *J Obstet Gynaecol Res* (2016) 42:640–7. doi: 10.1111/jog.12950
27. Silva JC, Fachin DRRN, Coral ML, Bertini AM. Perinatal Impact of the Use of Metformin and Glyburide for the Treatment of Gestational Diabetes Mellitus. *J Perinat Med* (2012) 40:225–8. doi: 10.1515/jpm-2011-0175
28. de Souza MLR, Silva R, Silva T, de Oliveira LC, Dienstmann G, do Nascimento IB, et al. Factors Associated With the Need for Insulin as a Complementary Treatment to Metformin in Gestational Diabetes Mellitus. *Rev Bras Ginecol Obstet* (2019) 41:697–702. doi: 10.1055/s-0039-1700796
29. Gante I, Melo L, Dores J, Ruas L, Almeida M do C. Metformin in Gestational Diabetes Mellitus: Predictors of Poor Response. *Eur J Endocrinol* (2018) 178:129–35. doi: 10.1530/EJE-17-0486
30. Syngelaki A, Nicolaides KH, Balani J, Hyer S, Akolekar R, Kotecha R, et al. Metformin Versus Placebo in Obese Pregnant Women Without Diabetes Mellitus. *N Engl J Med* (2016) 374:434 43. doi: 10.1056/NEJMoa1509819
31. Chiswick C, Reynolds RM, Denison F, Drake AJ, Forbes S, Newby DE, et al. Effect of Metformin on Maternal and Fetal Outcomes in Obese Pregnant Women (EMPOWaR): A Randomised, Double-Blind, Placebo-Controlled Trial. *Lancet Diabetes Endocrinol* (2015) 3:778–86. doi: 10.1016/S2213-8587(15)00219-3
32. Catalano PM, McIntyre HD, Cruickshank JK, McCance DR, Dyer AR, Metzger BE, et al. The Hyperglycemia and Adverse Pregnancy Outcome Study: Associations of GDM and Obesity With Pregnancy Outcomes. *Diabetes Care* (2012) 35:780–6. doi: 10.2337/dc11-1790
33. Bozkurt L, Göbl CS, Hörmayer AT, Lugert A, Pacini G, Kautzky-Willer A, et al. The impact of Preconceptional Obesity on Trajectories of Maternal Lipids During Gestation. *Sci Rep* (2016) 6:29971. doi: 10.1038/srep29971
34. Göbl CS, Handisurya A, Klein K, Bozkurt L, Luger A, Bancher-Todesca D, et al. Changes in Serum Lipid Levels During Pregnancy in Type 1 and Type 2 Diabetic Subjects. *Diabetes Care* (2010) 33:2071–3. doi: 10.2337/dc10-0484

18

Spatial Analysis of Incidence of Diagnosed Type 2 Diabetes Mellitus and its Association with Obesity and Physical Inactivity

Jinrong Wu[1,2†], *Yang Wang*[1†], *Xin Xiao*[1,3], *Xianwen Shang*[1], *Mingguang He*[1,4,5*‡] *and Lei Zhang*[1,6,7,8*‡]

[1] Centre for Eye Research Australia, Royal Victorian Eye and Ear Hospital, Melbourne, VIC, Australia, [2] Research Centre for Data Analytics and Cognition, La Trobe University, Melbourne, VIC, Australia, [3] Center for Optometry and Visual Science, Department of Optometry, People's Hospital of Guangxi Zhuang Autonomous Region, Guangxi, China, [4] Ophthalmology, Department of Surgery, University of Melbourne, Melbourne, VIC, Australia, [5] State Key Laboratory of Ophthalmology, Zhongshan Ophthalmic Center, Sun Yat-sen University, Guangzhou, China, [6] Melbourne Sexual Health Centre, Alfred Health, Melbourne, VIC, Australia, [7] Central Clinical School, Faculty of Medicine, Monash University, Melbourne, VIC, Australia, [8] Department of Epidemiology and Biostatistics, College of Public Health, Zhengzhou University, Zhengzhou, China

Correspondence:
Lei Zhang
Lei.zhang1@monash.edu
Mingguang He
mingguang.he@unimelb.edu.au

†These authors have contributed equally to this work and share first authorship

‡These authors have supervised equally

Objectives: To investigate the spatial distribution of 10-year incidence of diagnosed type 2 diabetes mellitus (T2DM) and its association with obesity and physical inactivity at a reginal level breakdown.

Methods: Demographic, behavioral, medical and pharmaceutical and diagnosed T2DM incidence data were collected from a cohort of 232,064 participants who were free of diabetes at enrolment in the 45 and Up Study, conducted in the state of New South Wales (NSW), Australia. We examined the geographical trend and correlation between obesity prevalence, physical inactivity rate and age-and-gender-adjusted cumulative incidence of T2DM, aggregated based on geographical regions.

Result: The T2DM incidence, prevalence of obesity and physical inactivity rate at baseline were 6.32%, 20.24%, and 18.7%, respectively. The spatial variation of T2DM incidence was significant (Moran's I=0.52; p<0.01), with the lowest incidence of 2.76% in Richmond Valley-Coastal and the highest of 12.27% in Mount Druitt. T2DM incidence was significantly correlated with the prevalence of obesity (Spearman r=0.62, p<0.001), percentage of participants having five sessions of physical activities or less per week (r=0.79, p<0.001) and percentage of participants walked to work (r=-0.44, p<0.001). The geographical variations in obesity prevalence and physical inactivity rate resembled the geographical variation in the incidence of T2DM.

Conclusion: The spatial distribution of T2DM incidence is significantly associated with the geographical prevalence of obesity and physical inactivity rate. Regional campaigns advocating the importance of physical activities in response to the alarming T2DM epidemic should be promoted.

Keywords: diabetes, incidence, GIS, Australian, risk factors, obesity, physical inactivity

INTRODUCTION

Diabetes is a key non-communicable disease (NCDs) targeted for global action (1, 2). The prevalence of diabetes has increased from 4.7% in 1980 to 8.5% in 2014 in the adult population globally (1). The World Health Organization (WHO) projected that the number of diabetes cases worldwide would reach 366 million by 2030 (3). Type 2 diabetes mellitus (T2DM), diagnosed when the pancreas could no longer produce sufficient insulin, accounts for 90-95% of all diabetic cases (4). The management of T2DM is complex and time-consuming, often involving regular health consultations, lifestyle modifications, frequent blood glucose and podiatry monitoring and complex medication regimes (5–8). The estimated annual spending on T2DM in Australia is around $6 billion. The average annual healthcare cost per person is as high as $4,025, even if there are no associated complications (9).

Previous studies (10–12) have revealed that the development of T2DM results from complex interactions between genetic, environmental, lifestyle and other risk factors. It is also revealed that obesity and physical inactivity are highly correlated with T2DM (13, 14). Most of these associated studies have been conducted on an individual level, providing essential information to identify key modifiable health behaviours for the general health of people living with T2DM. However, understanding the geographical trends of T2DM at a population level may provide important evidence to inform better health policies and population-based prevention programs.

Several existing studies have reported the geographical variance in T2DM disease burden (15–19). Angela et al. (16) evaluated the geographical variations of T2DM incidence among teenagers in the United States. Douglas et al. (17) identified regions with a high disease burden of T2DM in the city of London, UK. Similar studies were also conducted in Ukraine (19) and China (20). Geospatial correlation studies that focused on the association between the risk factors and population effects on T2DM were also conducted in Europe, the US and China as evidence to facilitate political commitment and implementation of community-based programs to curb the epidemic of T2DM (21–23). They reported the association of T2DM with obesity and physical activity, and some studies also highlighted that these geographical variances could result from social determinants, such as income and employment (24–26). In Australia, a typical developed country with the world's 12th largest economy, several government-issued reports unveiled the geographical variations of T2DM incidence nationwide but without in-depth spatial analysis of T2DM and its interaction with population risk factors (9, 27–29). In particular, more than 90% of T2DM in Australia were found in the middle-aged and elderly population of more than 45 years old. Therefore, understanding the geographical trends and the relevant population factors that contribute to T2DM in this group is key for the prevention of T2DM in the ageing Australian population.

We hypothesised that there are significant geographical variations in T2DM incidence across the Australian state of New South Wales, and these variations are potentially associated with the obesity prevalence and physical inactivity rate in the population. We used demographic, behavioural, medical, and pharmaceutical data from a ten-year follow-up study cohort with 266,896 participants to explore the geographical variation in the incidence of T2DM and associated population factors. Findings from this study will add new evidence to inform health policies to be modified based on geographical variations across Australia at a population level.

METHODS

Data Source

The data used in this study was mainly collected from the Sax Institute's 45 and Up Study, a population-based cohort study with participants aged 45 and over in NSW, Australia (30). A total of 266,896 participants, who were first randomly sampled from Services Australia's (formerly the Australian Government Department of Human Services) Medicare enrolment database, joined the Study between January 2006 and December 2009. Each participant completed a baseline questionnaire and provided signed consent for follow-up and linkage of one's information to a routine health database. The baseline questionnaire captured a broad range of information related to socioeconomic, health, and lifestyle factors. The 45 and Up Study data was also linked to the Medicare Benefits Schedule (MBS), and Pharmaceutical Benefits Scheme (PBS) claims from 2004 to 2016 with deterministic matching. Hence, detailed medical procedures (identified by MBS code) and medications prescribed by clinicians (identified by PBS code) could be tracked for each participant. Data of population walking to work was obtained from a census study by Zander et al. in 2011 (31), where they aggregated the raw data from the ABS.

Geographical Measures

Statistical Area Level 3 (SA3) is a regional breakdown of Australia based on the Australian Statistical Geography Standard (ASGS), using a standardised set of numeric codes issued by the ABS to uniformly identify geographical entities (32). The delimitation of a total of 91 SA3s in New South Wales was based on the relative homogeneity in the demographic, functional, geographical, and socioeconomic characteristics (32). SA3 code for each participant was derived from the self-reported baseline questionnaire in the 45 and Up Study, and the SA3 maps of Digital Boundaries for the year 2011 were downloaded from ABS website (32).

Ethics Considerations

Ethics approval for the 45 and Up Study was granted by the University of New South Wales Human Research Ethics Committee. Ethics approval for this specific study was granted by the Royal Victorian Eye and Ear Hospital Human Research Ethics Committee.

Inclusion and Exclusion Criteria

We excluded participants with established diabetes at baseline, defined as those who:

- self-reported to have established diabetes;
- applied diabetes medications before the baseline implied by the PBS database (33);
- defined as a diagnosis of diabetes earlier than the last childbirth, but without diabetes medication use subsequently;
- had missing or invalid BMI or Statistical Area 3 data;
- reported age of diabetes diagnosis older than the age at baseline survey. We also excluded participants who are from the SA3 regions with less than 100 participants (10702, 10803 and 12402).

After exclusions, a total of 232,064 residents were selected in this study (**Figure 1**).

Outcomes and Associated Factors

The SA3-level 10-year diabetes incidence rates were estimated in 232,064 residents for the period from 2006 to 2017. Age- and-gender adjusted diabetes incidence was calculated using the direct adjustment method, based on the age and gender distribution of 2011 census population data. We defined diabetes incidence as the first occurrence of any kind of medications prescribed for T2DM (including oral hypoglycaemic agents and insulin) with their corresponding PBS codes. As all participants were aged above 45 years, we assumed that all incident cases of new diabetes medication use were for T2DM rather than type 1 diabetes mellitus.

Each participants' body mass index (BMI) was derived from the self-reported baseline questionnaire in the 45 and Up Study. Definition of obesity is based on body mass index calculated from height and weight, which was previously validated in this study cohort (34, 35). According to the definition by WHO (34), a person with a BMI of more than 30kg/m^2 is considered obese in our study. Using this standard, we calculated the obesity prevalence for each SA3 region.

We applied two methods to evaluate physical inactivity in our study. Using the first method, we defined people who do physical activities of less than five sessions (metabolically adjusted) per week as participants "having insufficient physical activities", based on recommendations by the US Centers for Disease Control (CDC) (36, 37). Since information about the number of physical activity sessions for all participants were available in the self-reported baseline questionnaires in the 45 and Up Study, we aggregated the percentage of the population with insufficient physical activities for each SA3 region. To strengthen our physical inactivity measures, we applied a secondary indicator to measure physical inactivity. A previous study (31) conducted in Australia has shown that the percentage of the population walking to work, which is the ratio of the number of journeys to work by walking to the total number of journeys to work, is a good indicator of physical activity in Australia. A low percentage of the population walking to work presented the lack of physical activity in the population and a high rate of physical inactivity. Since the data from the previous study were aggregated based on a different region breakdown standard (38), we mapped each region in that study to the SA3 region in our study using the correspondence data from ABS and re-calculated the percentage of the population walking to work for each SA3 region.

ANALYSES FOR T2DM INCIDENCE

SAS version 9.4 (SAS Institute Incorporation) and R Studio was used for non-spatial data analyses. To understand the distributions in diabetes incidence across different regions in Australia,

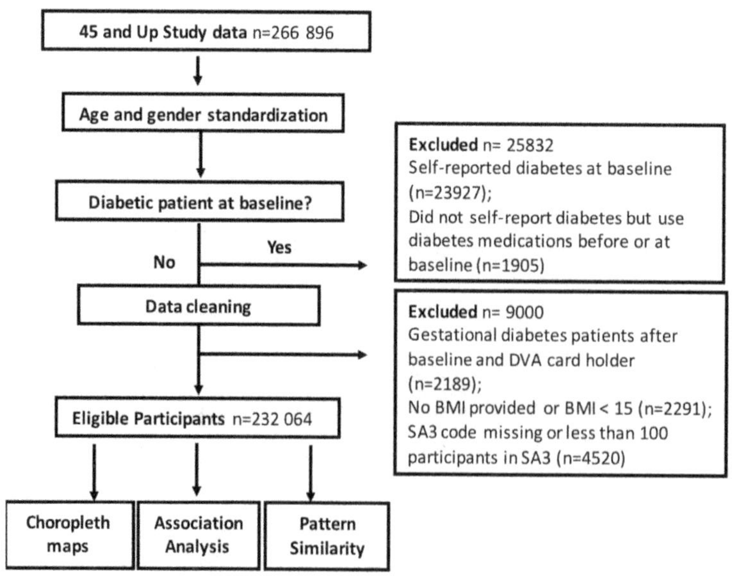

FIGURE 1 | Spatial Analysis of Diabetes Study Flow Diagram.

we calculated the range, mean and standard deviation for each potential association factor, including obesity prevalence, percentage of the population with insufficient physical activities and percentage of the population walking to walk. We further analysed the non-spatial correlation between diabetes incidence and each factor using Spearman correlation.

For spatial analysis, Choropleth maps of the outcome and associated factors were plotted using ArcGIS 10.4 (ESRI, Redlands, CA) and GeoDa 1.12. We applied univariate Moran' I to identify if there are significant geographical variations in diabetes incidence, obesity prevalence, percentage of the population with insufficient physical activities and percentage of the population walking to walk, respectively. If a univariate Moran' I value is close to 1, it indicates a significant geographical variation, whereas a value close to 0 indicates no clear geographical variations. To assess colocation between T2DM incidence and each of the association factors, we calculated the bivariate Moran's I and intraclass correlation coefficient for the associated factors and diabetes incidence. Bivariate Moran's I was a global measure of spatial correlation to measure the influence one variable has on the occurrence of another variable in close proximity (39). A value close to 1 represents a clear spatial correlation, whereas a value close to 0 means no clear spatial correlation.

RESULTS

Characteristics of Participants Based on SA3

Amongst the 232,064 individuals in the 88 SA3s aged 45 and over, the average 10-year incidence of diabetes in the period of 2006–2017 was 6.32% (95% CI, 2.76-12.27%). The average prevalence of obesity across all SA3s was 20.24% (10.36-31.40%). The average percentage of the population with insufficient physical activities was 18.70% (10.39-25.66%), and only 4.43% (1.45 -23.11%) of the population walk to work in metropolitan areas.

Correlation Between Diabetes and Associated Factors

As shown in **Figure 2**, the prevalence of obesity and the percentage of the population with insufficient physical activities showed a strong positive correlation with T2DM incidence (obesity prevalence: r=0.62, p<0.001, insufficient physical activities: r=0.79, p<0.001). The percentage of the population walking to work showed a negative correlation with T2DM incidence (r=-0.44, p<0.001) in metropolitan areas.

Geographical Variation of Diabetes Incidence and Associated Factors

Geographical variations in T2DM incidence and associated factors were shown in **Figure 3**. T2DM incidence presented a significant uneven geographical distribution (Univariate Moran's I=0.52; p=0.001). Similar findings were also identified in the geographical distribution of prevalence of obesity (Univariate Moran's I=0.67; p=0.001), percentage of the population with insufficient physical activities (Univariate Moran's I=0.59; p=0.001) and percentage of the population walking to work in metropolitan areas (Univariate Moran's I=0.44; p=0.001).

The choropleth maps (**Figure 3**) shows that the north-western regions of NSW and the western regions of Sydney had relatively high T2DM incidence, high obesity prevalence, a high percentage of the population with insufficient physical activities and a low percentage of the population walking to work. In comparison, areas along the coastal lines had relatively low T2DM incidence, low prevalence of obesity, low percentage of the population with insufficient physical activities and a high percentage of the population walking to work.

The highest T2DM incidence was found in Mount Druitt (**Figures 3A, E**), which also showed the highest obesity prevalence (**Figures 3B, F**) and the second-highest percentage of the population with insufficient physical activities (following its neighbour Blacktown-North, **Figures 3C, G**). Consistently, both Blacktown-North and Mount Druitt showed the lowest percentage of the population walking to walk (**Figures 3D, H**). In contrast, the lowest T2DM incidence was found in Richmond Valley-Coastal and Manly (**Figures 3A, E**), which also showed

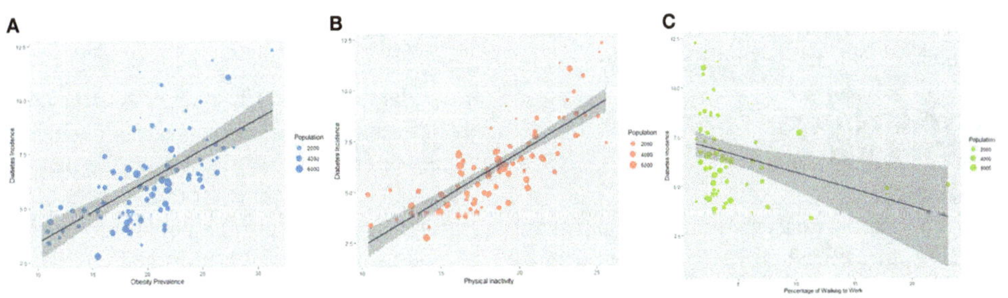

FIGURE 2 | Association in Prevalence of Obesity **(A)** and Physical Inactivity Rate **(B, C)** with Incidence of Diabetes **(A)** shows the correlation between T2DM incidence and obesity prevalence with a spearman correlation coefficient of 0.62 ($p < 0.001$); **(B)** shows the correlation between T2DM incidence and percentage of the population with insufficient physical activities with a spearman correlation coefficient of 0.79 ($p < 0.001$); **(C)** shows the correlation between T2DM incidence and percentage of the population walking to work with a spearman correlation coefficient of -0.44 ($p < 0.001$).

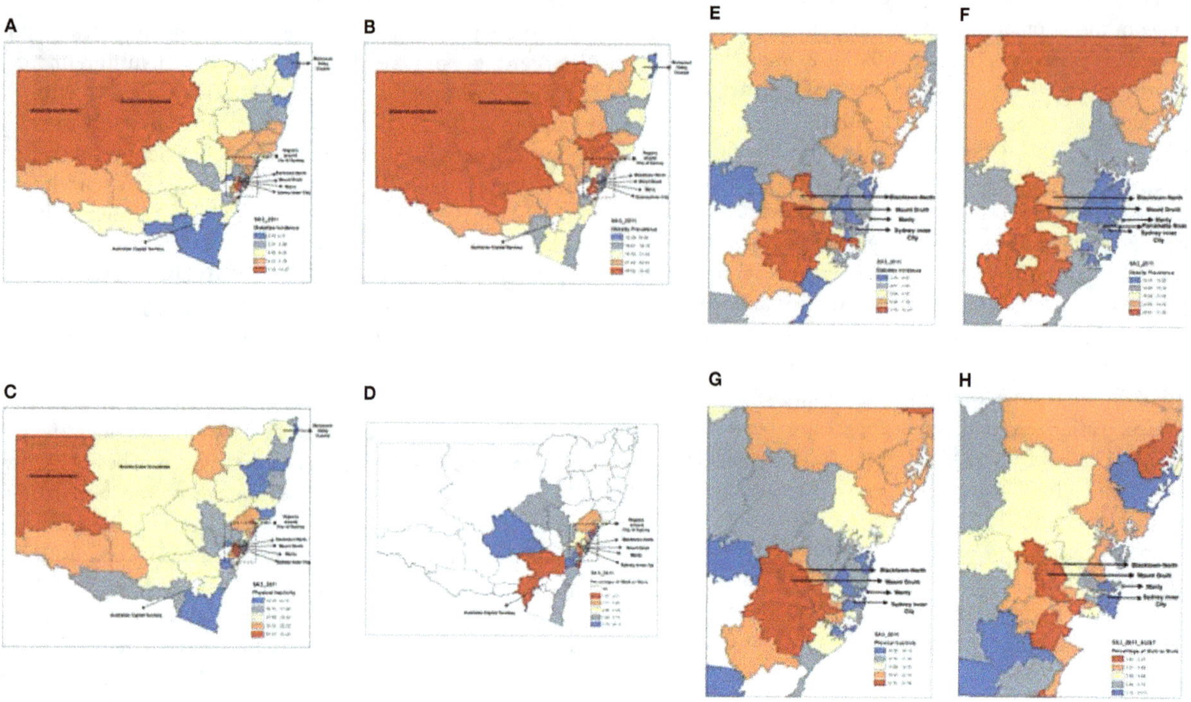

FIGURE 3 | Geographic Variations in the Incidence of Diabetes, Obesity Prevalence, Percentage of the Population with Insufficient Physical Activities and Percentage of the Population Walking to Work. **(A)** shows the variations in T2DM incidence at SA3 level with a Univariate Moran's I of 0.52 (p=0.001) while **(E)** shows T2DM incidence in the magnified Sydney region; **(B)** shows the variance of obesity prevalence at SA3 level with a Univariate Moran's I of 0.67 (p=0.001) while **(F)** shows obesity prevalence in the magnified Sydney region, and by comparing between **(A, B)**, it can be identified a very similar pattern between them with a Bivariate Moran's I of 0.37 (p=0.001) and an intraclass correlation coefficient of 0.6 (p<0.001); **(C)** shows the variance of the percentage of the population with insufficient physical activities at SA3 level with a Univariate Moran's I of 0.59 (p=0.001) while **(G)** shows the percentage of the population with insufficient physical activities in the magnified Sydney region, by comparing between **(A, C)**, it can be identified a very similar pattern between them with a Bivariate Moran's I of 0.54 (p=0.001) and an intraclass correlation coefficient of 0.8 (p < 0.001); **(D)** shows the variance of the percentage of the population walking to work at SA3 level with a Univariate Moran's I of 0.44 (p=0.001) while **(H)** shows the percentage of the population walking to work in the magnified Sydney region, and by comparing between **(E, H)**, it can be identified a similar pattern between them with a Bivariate Moran's I of -0.23 (p=0.001) and an intraclass correlation coefficient between T2DM incidence and percentage of the population walking to work of -0.47 (p < 0.001); by comparing between, it can be identified a very similar pattern between them with and an intraclass correlation coefficient of 0.61 (p < 0.001).

the lowest obesity prevalence. In addition, Sydney Inner City (**Figure 3G**) showed the lowest percentage of the population with insufficient physical activities. In Southeast Sydney, SA3s with high T2DM incidence also presented high obesity prevalence and physical inactivity rate (**Figures 3E–G**). Two SA3s, Bourke-Cobar-Coonamble, and Broken Hill, together with far west regions, showed very high T2DM incidence (**Figure 3A**).

Colocation Between the 10-Years Incidence of T2DM and Associated Factors

Results of the spatial correlation analyses indicate significant colocation between T2DM incidence and its associated factors, such as the prevalence of obesity (Bivariate Moran's I=0.37, p=0.001), the percentage of the population with insufficient physical activities (Bivariate Moran's I=0.54, p=0.001) and the percentage of the population walking to work in metropolitan areas (Bivariate Moran's I=-0.23, p=0.001, **Figure 3**). Similarly, intraclass correlation analysis based on the choropleth maps showed a significant spatial correlation between T2DM incidence and its associated factors (p<0.001 for all, **Figure 3**).

DISCUSSION

In this large-cohort GIS study of Australians aged 45 and above, we identified significant geographical variations in T2DM incidence across NSW, Australia. We demonstrate that T2DM incidence is significantly correlated with obesity prevalence and physical inactivity rate at a population level.

The geographical variation and spatial clustering of T2DM incidence identified in this study are consistent with the results from previous studies that compare the diabetes prevalence among major cities and remote areas in Australia (40). Besides, the very high T2DM incidence in the outback region of NSW could result from the arid local climate and the lack of health resources in these regions (41).

Our finding that the onset of T2DM was closely associated with obesity and physical inactivity is consistent with the findings from existing studies (13, 42, 43). Although multiple epidemiological studies identified obesity as the most significant associated factor for T2DM due to its pro-inflammatory contribution to the development of insulin resistance and disease progression (44, 45), our study revealed that physical inactivity rate is more important contributing factor to T2DM than obesity in an Australian population. This is supported by Ansari (42) who found that physical activities, including stair climbing and cycling, may reduce the risk of T2DM at a population level.

Previous studies have identified that the spatial variance of T2DM, obesity and physical inactivity can result from a few socioeconomic factors, such as income, education and occupational status (46, 47). It is found that one's education level is most likely to affect one's understanding and knowledge of the health benefits of preventative behaviors (48). Low income and education level have also shown to be associated with a high risk of metabolic system, leading to over-weight and obesity (49, 50). In addition, employment status categorized by occupation, has shown an inverse relation with glucose intolerance (47, 51). Therefore, more educational resources and occupational guidance can be provided to population in the high-risk regions for T2DM control.

The major contribution of this study is that we identified a significant colocation of T2DM incidence with obesity prevalence and physical inactivity rate at a population level. A population with a high prevalence of obesity (BMI>30kg/m^2) and a high percentage of insufficient activity (physical activities of <5 sessions/week) was strongly associated with a high incidence of T2DM. To our knowledge, our study was the first to investigate the spatial correlation of T2DM with its associated lifestyle factors, contributing to the sociocultural perspective of T2DM prevention. The advances in technology and transportation, long hours of sedentary office work, and increasing access to processed food increase the risk of obesity and physical inactivity (52), leading to an increased risk of T2DM onset in adults. For instance, in our study, the Mount Druitt region has the highest obesity prevalence, the second-highest percentage of population physical inactivity; therefore, substantial changes in public policies to create an environment that promotes the wellbeing of the whole community is a priority in the region. Further, the government may consider allocating resources for health promotion campaigns and increasing accessible exercise facilities at the workplace to reduce T2DM incidence (53). Another strength of this study is that the use of a sizable study cohort with 232,064 participants in Australia with a long follow-up period, and the comprehensiveness of the captured information for each participant, can lead to more reliable study findings. T2DM incidence was captured based on the Medicare record system, which effectively minimized the recall bias from the participants, especially the elderly.

However, the study has a number of limitations. First, our definition of T2DM might overlook cases of gestational diabetes. Second, our study was conducted based on the assumption that participants did not move to a new location, and their body weights were relatively stable during the study period. Third, the data of working to work used in this study only relates to the regions around the City of Sydney not the whole of NSW and is limited to the people who are employed. Fourth, data for obesity prevalence and physical inactivity rate were collected from individual-level questionnaires with the response rate of only 18%, raising issues regarding the overall representativeness of the recruited participants from each SA3 region. But we found that the characteristics of participants in our study are, in fact, very similar to the characteristics presented in the New South Wales Population Health Survey conducted by the NSW government (54).

In conclusion, this study is a large-scale GIS study that addressed the geographical disparities in T2DM incidence and its associations with the prevalence of obesity and physical inactivity across an Australian state. This study highlights that a high prevalence of obesity and physical inactivity in a population may contribute to a high incidence of T2DM in the population. Community-based intervention on healthy lifestyles and behaviors should be prioritized to help control T2DM incidence in a population.

AUTHOR CONTRIBUTIONS

JW was in charge of the project experiments and analysis, and writing the draft for the paper. YW was responsible for assuring the experiment the results are consistent and modifying the paper. XX was providing method advice and tool advice to make sure appropriate data analysis. XS is responsible for data preprocessing to extract proper data for our project. MH and LZ supervised the project, gave advice on the techniques and direction advice on the project, and helped in paper revision. All authors contributed to the article and approved the submitted version.

ACKNOWLEDGMENTS

This research was completed using data collected through the 45 and Up Study (www.saxinstitute.org.au) supplied by Services Australia and the Australian Bureau of Statistics (ABS). The 45 and Up Study is managed by the Sax Institute in collaboration with major partner Cancer Council NSW; and partners: the National Heart Foundation of Australia (NSW Division); NSW Ministry of Health; NSW Government Family & Community Services–Ageing, Carers and the Disability Council NSW; and the Australian Red Cross Blood Service. We thank the many thousands of people participating in the 45 and Up Study.

REFERENCES

1. World Health Organization. *Global Report on Diabetes*. Geneva: World Health Organization (2016).
2. Liu J, Ren ZH, Qiang H, Wu J, Shen M, Zhang L, et al. Trends in the Incidence of Diabetes Mellitus: Results From the Global Burden of Disease Study 2017 and Implications for Diabetes Mellitus Prevention. *BMC Public Health* (2020) 20(1):1415. doi: 10.1186/s12889-020-09502-x
3. Wild S, Roglic G, Green A, Sicree R, King H. Global Prevalence of Diabetes: Estimates for the Year 2000 and Projections for 2030. *Diabetes Care* (2004) 27 (5):1047–53. doi: 10.2337/diacare.27.5.1047
4. Tripathi BK, Srivastava AK. Diabetes Mellitus: Complications and Therapeutics. *Med Sci Monit* (2006) 12(7):RA130–47 www.medscimonit.com/.
5. Diabetes Prevention Program Research Group. Reduction in the Incidence of Type 2 Diabetes With Lifestyle Intervention or Metformin. *N Engl J Med* (2002) 346(6):393–403. doi: 10.1056/NEJMoa012512
6. Spann SJ, Nutting PA, Galliher JM, Peterson KA, Pavlik VN, Dickinson LM, et al. Management of Type 2 Diabetes in the Primary Care Setting: A Practice-Based Research Network Study. *Ann Fam Med* (2006) 4(1):23–31. doi: 10.1370/afm.420
7. Wu C, Han X, Yan X, Shang X, Zhang L, He M. Associations Between Physical Activity and Cataract Treated Surgically in Patients With Diabetes: Findings From the 45 and Up Study. *Br J Ophthalmol* (2019) 103(8):1099–105. doi: 10.1136/bjophthalmol-2018-312407
8. Shang X, Peng W, Hill E, Szoeke C, He M, Zhang L. Incidence of Medication-Treated Depression and Anxiety Associated With Long-Term Cancer, Cardiovascular Disease, Diabetes and Osteoarthritis in Community-Dwelling Women and Men. *EClinicalMedicine* (2019) 15:23–32. doi: 10.1016/j.eclinm.2019.08.010
9. Shaw J, Tanamas S. *Diabetes: The Silent Pandemic and its Impact on Australia*. Melbourne: Baker IDI Heart and Diabetes Institute (2012).
10. Tuomilehto J, Lindström J, Eriksson JG, Valle TT, Hämäläinen H, Ilanne-Parikka P, et al. Prevention of Type 2 Diabetes Mellitus by Changes in Lifestyle Among Subjects With Impaired Glucose Tolerance. *N Engl J Med* (2001) 344(18):1343–50. doi: 10.1056/NEJM200105033441801
11. Hu FB, Manson JE, Stampfer MJ, Colditz G, Liu S, Solomon CG, et al. Diet, Lifestyle, and the Risk of Type 2 Diabetes Mellitus in Women. *N Engl J Med* (2001) 345(11):790–7. doi: 10.1056/NEJMoa010492
12. Zhang L, Shang X, Sreedharan S, Yan X, Liu J, Keel S, et al. Predicting the Development of Type 2 Diabetes in a Large Australian Cohort Using Machine-Learning Techniques: Longitudinal Survey Study. *JMIR Med Inform* (2020) 8(7):e16850. doi: 10.2196/16850
13. Wu Y, Ding Y, Tanaka Y, Zhang W. Risk Factors Contributing to Type 2 Diabetes and Recent Advances in the Treatment and Prevention. *Int J Med Sci* (2014) 11(11):1185–200. doi: 10.7150/ijms.10001
14. Sato KK, Hayashi T, Kambe H, Nakamura Y, Harita N, Endo G, et al. Walking to Work is an Independent Predictor of Incidence of Type 2 Diabetes in Japanese Men: The Kansai Healthcare Study. *Diabetes Care* (2007) 30 (9):2296–8. doi: 10.2337/dc07-0090
15. Baker J, White N, Mengersen K. Spatial Modelling of Type II Diabetes Outcomes: A Systematic Review of Approaches Used. *R Soc Open Sci* (2015) 2(6):140460. doi: 10.1098/rsos.140460
16. Liese AD, Lawson A, Song HR, Hibbert JD, Porter DE, Nichols M, et al. Evaluating Geographic Variation in Type 1 and Type 2 Diabetes Mellitus Incidence in Youth in Four US Regions. *Health Place* (2010) 16(3):547–56. doi: 10.1016/j.healthplace.2009.12.015
17. Noble D, Smith D, Mathur R, Robson J, Greenhalgh T. Feasibility Study of Geospatial Mapping of Chronic Disease Risk to Inform Public Health Commissioning. *BMJ Open* (2012) 2(1):e000711. doi: 10.1136/bmjopen-2011-000711
18. Chaix B, Billaudeau N, Thomas F, Havard S, Evans D, Kestens Y, et al. Neighborhood Effects on Health: Correcting Bias From Neighborhood Effects on Participation. *Epidemiology* (2011) 22(1):18–26. doi: 10.1097/EDE. 0b013e3181fd2961
19. Kravchenko VI, Tronko ND, Pankiv VI, Venzilovich YM, Prudius FG. Prevalence of Diabetes Mellitus and its Complications in the Ukraine. *Diabetes Res Clin Pract* (1996) 34(Suppl):S73–8. doi: 10.1016/S0168-8227(96)90011-X
20. Zhou M, Astell-Burt T, Bi Y, Feng X, Jiang Y, Yi Y, et al. Geographical Variation in Diabetes Prevalence and Detection in China: Multilevel Spatial Analysis of 98,058 Adults. *Diabetes Care* (2015) 38(1):72–81. doi: 10.2337/dc14-1100
21. Uusitupa M, Tuomilehto J, Puska P. Are We Really Active in the Prevention of Obesity and Type 2 Diabetes at the Community Level? *Nutr Metab Cardiovasc Dis* (2011) 21(5):380–9. doi: 10.1016/j.numecd.2010.12.007
22. Saaristo T, Moilanen L, Korpi-Hyövälti E, Vanhala M, Saltevo J, Niskanen L, et al. Lifestyle Intervention for Prevention of Type 2 Diabetes in Primary Health Care: One-Year Follow-Up of the Finnish National Diabetes Prevention Program (FIN-D2D). *Diabetes Care* (2010) 33(10):2146–51. doi: 10.2337/dc10-0410
23. Zhuo X, Zhang P, Gregg EW, Barker L, Hoerger TJ, Pearson-Clarke T, et al. A Nationwide Community-Based Lifestyle Program Could Delay or Prevent Type 2 Diabetes Cases and Save $5.7 Billion in 25 Years. *Health Aff (Millwood)* (2012) 31(1):50–60. doi: 10.1377/hlthaff.2011.1115
24. Hill J, Nielsen M, Fox MH. Understanding the Social Factors That Contribute to Diabetes: A Means to Informing Health Care and Social Policies for the Chronically Ill. *Permanente J* (2013) 17(2):67. doi: 10.7812/TPP/12-099
25. Chang VW, Lauderdale DS. Income Disparities in Body Mass Index and Obesity in the United States, 1971-2002. *Arch Internal Med* (2005) 165 (18):2122–8. doi: 10.1001/archinte.165.18.2122
26. Allender S, Foster C, Boxer A. Occupational and Nonoccupational Physical Activity and the Social Determinants of Physical Activity: Results From the Health Survey for England. *J Phys Act Health* (2008) 5(1):104–16. doi: 10.1123/jpah.5.1.104
27. Australian Institute of Health and Welfare. *Diabetes Snapshot*. Canberra: AIHW (2018).
28. Australian Institute of Health and Welfare. *Incidence of Insulin-Treated Diabetes in Australia*. AIHW (2018).
29. Jiwa M, Gudes O, Varhol R, Mullan N. Impact of Geography on the Control of Type 2 Diabetes Mellitus: A Review of Geocoded Clinical Data From General Practice. *BMJ Open* (2015) 5(12):e009504. doi: 10.1136/bmjopen-2015-009504
30. 45 and Up Study Collaborators. Cohort Profile: The 45 and Up Study. *Int J Epidemiol* (2008) 37(5):941–7. doi: 10.1093/ije/dym184
31. Zander A, Rissel C, Rogers K, Bauman A. *Walking to Work in Sydney: Analysis of Journey-to-Work Census Data From 2001 and 2011*. Camperdown: Prevention Research CollaborationThe University of Sydney (2013).
32. ABo S. *Australian Statistical Geography Standard (ASGS): Volume 1—Main Structure and Greater Capital City Statistical Areas*. Canberra: Australian Bureau of Statistics (2011).
33. Comino EJ, Tran DT, Haas M, Flack J, Jalaludin B, Jorm L, et al. Validating Self-Report of Diabetes Use by Participants in the 45 and Up Study: A Record Linkage Study. *BMC Health Serv Res* (2013) 13:481. doi: 10.1186/1472-6963-13-481
34. World Health Organization. Obesity: Preventing and Managing the Global Epidemic. Report of a WHO Consultation. *Report of a WHO Consultation* Geneva:World Health Organization (2000). WHO Technical Report Series 894. p. 1–252.
35. Ng SP, Korda R, Clements M, Latz I, Bauman A, Bambrick H, et al. Validity of Self-Reported Height and Weight and Derived Body Mass Index in Middle-Aged and Elderly Individuals in Australia. *Aust N Z J Public Health* (2011) 35 (6):557–63. doi: 10.1111/j.1753-6405.2011.00742.x
36. Pate RR, Pratt M, Blair SN, Haskell WL, Macera CA, Bouchard C, et al. Physical Activity and Public Health. A Recommendation From the Centers for Disease Control and Prevention and the American College of Sports Medicine. *JAMA* (1995) 273(5):402–7. doi: 10.1001/jama.1995.03520290054029
37. Lai JK, Lucas RM, Armstrong M, Banks E. Prospective Observational Study of Physical Functioning, Physical Activity, and Time Outdoors and the Risk of Hip Fracture: A Population-Based Cohort Study of 158,057 Older Adults in the 45 and Up Study. *J Bone Miner Res* (2013) 28:2222–31. doi: 10.1002/jbmr.1963
38. Pink B. *Australian Statistical Geography Standard (ASGS): Volume 3-Non ABS Structures*. Australian: Australian Bureau of Statistics (2011).
39. Anselin L. Exploring Spatial Data With GeoDaTM: A Workbook. *Urbana* (2004) 51(61801):309.
40. Australian Health Ministers' Advisory Council. *Diabetes in Australia: Focus on the Future*. Canberra: Australian Government (2017).
41. National Rural Health Alliance. *Diabetes in Rural Australia - Fact Sheet 21*

Deakin West: National Rural Health Alliance (2011).

42. Ansari RM. Effect of Physical Activity and Obesity on Type 2 Diabetes in a Middle-Aged Population. *J Environ Public Health* (2009) 2009:195285. doi: 10.1155/2009/195285
43. Collins GS, Mallett S, Omar O, Yu LM. Developing Risk Prediction Models for Type 2 Diabetes: A Systematic Review of Methodology and Reporting. *BMC Med* (2011) 9:103. doi: 10.1186/1741-7015-9-103
44. Gillett M, Royle P, Snaith A, Scotland G, Poobalan A, Imamura M, et al. Non-Pharmacological Interventions to Reduce the Risk of Diabetes in People With Impaired Glucose Regulation: A Systematic Review and Economic Evaluation. *Health Technol Assess* (2012) 16(33):1–236, iii-iv. doi: 10.3310/hta16330
45. Holbrook TL, Barrett-Connor E, Wingard DL. The Association of Lifetime Weight and Weight Control Patterns With Diabetes Among Men and Women in an Adult Community. *Int J Obes* (1989) 13(5):723–9.
46. Robbins JM, Vaccarino V, Zhang H, Kasl SV. Socioeconomic Status and Diagnosed Diabetes Incidence. *Diabetes Res Clin pract* (2005) 68(3):230–6. doi: 10.1016/j.diabres.2004.09.007
47. Connolly V, Unwin N, Sherriff P, Bilous R, Kelly W. Diabetes Prevalence and Socioeconomic Status: A Population Based Study Showing Increased Prevalence of Type 2 Diabetes Mellitus in Deprived Areas. *J Epidemiol Community Health* (2000) 54(3):173–7. doi: 10.1136/jech.54.3.173
48. Chiolero A, Faeh D, Paccaud F, Cornuz J. Consequences of Smoking for Body Weight, Body Fat Distribution, and Insulin Resistance. *Am J Clin Nutr* (2008) 87:801–9. doi: 10.1093/ajcn/87.4.801
49. Brunner EJ, Marmot MG, Nanchahal K, Shipley MJ, Stansfeld SA, Juneja M, et al. Social Inequality in Coronary Risk: Central Obesity and the Metabolic Syndrome. Evidence From the Whitehall II Study. *Diabetologia* (1997) 40 (11):1341–9. doi: 10.1007/s001250050830
50. Welch R, Boorman S, Golding JF, Towell T, Roberts R. Variations in Self-Reported Health by Occupational Grade in the British Post Office: The Q-Health Project. *Occup Med* (1999) 49(8):491–7. doi: 10.1093/occmed/49.8.491
51. Rose G, Marmot MG. Social Class and Coronary Heart Dis- Ease. *Br Heart J* (1981) 45:13–9. doi: 10.1136/hrt.45.1.13
52. Zimmet P, Alberti KG, Shaw J. Global and Societal Implications of the Diabetes Epidemic. *Nature* (2001) 414(6865):782–7. doi: 10.1038/414782a
53. McKinlay J, Marceau L. US Public Health and the 21st Century: Diabetes Mellitus. *Lancet* (2000) 356(9231):757–61. doi: 10.1016/S0140-6736(00) 02641-6
54. Mealing NM, Banks E, Jorm LR, Steel DG, Clements MS, Rogers KD. Investigation of Relative Risk Estimates From Studies of the Same Population With Contrasting Response Rates and Designs. *BMC Med Res Methodol* (2010) 10:26. doi: 10.1186/1471-2288-10-26

Permissions

All chapters in this book were first published Frontiers; hereby published with permission under the Creative Commons Attribution License or equivalent. Every chapter published in this book has been scrutinized by our experts. Their significance has been extensively debated. The topics covered herein carry significant findings which will fuel the growth of the discipline. They may even be implemented as practical applications or may be referred to as a beginning point for another development.

The contributors of this book come from diverse backgrounds, making this book a truly international effort. This book will bring forth new frontiers with its revolutionizing research information and detailed analysis of the nascent developments around the world.

We would like to thank all the contributing authors for lending their expertise to make the book truly unique. They have played a crucial role in the development of this book. Without their invaluable contributions this book wouldn't have been possible. They have made vital efforts to compile up to date information on the varied aspects of this subject to make this book a valuable addition to the collection of many professionals and students.

This book was conceptualized with the vision of imparting up-to-date information and advanced data in this field. To ensure the same, a matchless editorial board was set up. Every individual on the board went through rigorous rounds of assessment to prove their worth. After which they invested a large part of their time researching and compiling the most relevant data for our readers.

The editorial board has been involved in producing this book since its inception. They have spent rigorous hours researching and exploring the diverse topics which have resulted in the successful publishing of this book. They have passed on their knowledge of decades through this book. To expedite this challenging task, the publisher supported the team at every step. A small team of assistant editors was also appointed to further simplify the editing procedure and attain best results for the readers.

Apart from the editorial board, the designing team has also invested a significant amount of their time in understanding the subject and creating the most relevant covers. They scrutinized every image to scout for the most suitable representation of the subject and create an appropriate cover for the book.

The publishing team has been an ardent support to the editorial, designing and production team. Their endless efforts to recruit the best for this project, has resulted in the accomplishment of this book. They are a veteran in the field of academics and their pool of knowledge is as vast as their experience in printing. Their expertise and guidance has proved useful at every step. Their uncompromising quality standards have made this book an exceptional effort. Their encouragement from time to time has been an inspiration for everyone.

The publisher and the editorial board hope that this book will prove to be a valuable piece of knowledge for researchers, students, practitioners and scholars across the globe.

List of Contributors

Peter Van Dyken
Neuroscience Program, Ottawa Hospital Research Institute, Ottawa, ON, Canada

Baptiste Lacoste
Neuroscience Program, Ottawa Hospital Research Institute, Ottawa, ON, Canada
Department of Cellular and Molecular Medicine, Faculty of Medicine, University of Ottawa, Ottawa, ON, Canada
Brain and Mind Research Institute, University of Ottawa, Ottawa, ON, Canada

Paige Rucker
School of Medicine, The University of Mississippi Medical Center, Jackson, MS, United States

Toshikazu Ikuta
Department of Communication Sciences and Disorders, The University of Mississippi, Oxford, MS, United States

Felipe Macedo, Lucas Souza dos Santos, Isaias Glezer and Fernanda Marques da Cunha
Departamento de Bioquímica, Escola Paulista de Medicina, Universidade Federal de São Paulo, São Paulo, Brazil

Leticia Forny-Germano and Marcelo Nunes do Nascimento Vieira
Institute of Medical Biochemistry Leopoldo de Meis, Federal University of Rio de Janeiro, Rio de Janeiro, Brazil

Fernanda G. De Felice
Institute of Medical Biochemistry Leopoldo de Meis, Federal University of Rio de Janeiro, Rio de Janeiro, Brazil
Centre for Neuroscience Studies, Department of Psychiatry, Queen's University, Kingston, ON, Canada

Arnaud Bessac, Gilles Dietrich and Claude Knauf
NeuroMicrobiota, European Associated Laboratory INSERM/UCLouvain, Brussels, Belgium
Institut National de la Santé et de la Recherche Médicale, U1220, Université Paul Sabatier, Institut de Recherche en Santé Digestive et Nutrition, Toulouse, France

Patrice D. Cani
NeuroMicrobiota, European Associated Laboratory INSERM/UCLouvain, Brussels, Belgium
Metabolism and Nutrition Research Group, Walloon Excellence in Life Sciences and Biotechnology, Louvain Drug Research Institute, UCLouvain, Université catholique de Louvain, Brussels, Belgium

Etienne Meunier
Institut de Pharmacologie et de Biologie Structurale, UMR 5089, Université Paul Sabatier, Toulouse, France

Eric H. Chang, Sangeeta S. Chavan and Valentin A. Pavlov
Center for Bioelectronic Medicine and Biomedical Sciences, Feinstein Institute for Medical Research, Northwell Health, Manhasset, NY, United States
Donald and Barbara Zucker School of Medicine at Hofstra/Northwell, Hempstead, NY, United States

Natália Prudente de Mello, Geovanni de Morais Lima and Elisa Mitiko Kawamoto
Laboratory of Molecular and Functional Neurobiology, Department of Pharmacology, Institute of Biomedical Sciences, University of São Paulo, São Paulo, Brazil

Ana Maria Orellana, Caio Henrique Mazucanti and Cristoforo Scavone
Laboratory of Molecular Neuropharmacology, Department of Pharmacology, Institute of Biomedical Sciences, University of São Paulo, São Paulo, Brazil

Eliana P. Araújo
School of Nursing, State University of Campinas, Campinas, Brazil
Laboratory of Cell Signaling, Obesity and Comorbidities Research Center, State University of Campinas, Campinas, Brazil

Natália F. Mendes
School of Nursing, State University of Campinas, Campinas, Brazil
Department of Medicine, Division of Endocrinology, Diabetes, and Metabolism - Beth Israel Deaconess Medical Center, Harvard Medical School, Boston, MA, United States
Laboratory of Cell Signaling, Obesity and Comorbidities Research Center, State University of Campinas, Campinas, Brazil

Young-Bum Kim
Department of Medicine, Division of Endocrinology, Diabetes, and Metabolism - Beth Israel Deaconess Medical Center, Harvard Medical School, Boston, MA, United States

Lício A. Velloso
Laboratory of Cell Signaling, Obesity and Comorbidities Research Center, State University of Campinas, Campinas, Brazil
National Institute of Science and Technology on Neuroimmunomodulation, Rio de Janeiro, Brazil

Felipe Azevedo Gomes and Rui Daniel Prediger
Postgraduate Program in Pharmacology, Federal University of Santa Catarina, Florianópolis, Brazil

Rafael Appel Flores and Maciel Alencar Bruxel
Multicenter Postgraduate Program in Physiological Sciences, Federal University of Santa Catarina, Florianópolis, Brazil

Eduardo Luiz Gasnhar Moreira
Multicenter Postgraduate Program in Physiological Sciences, Federal University of Santa Catarina, Florianópolis, Brazil
Department of Physiological Sciences, Center of Biological Sciences, Federal University of Santa Catarina, Florianópolis, Brazil

Flávia Natividade da Silva
Department of Physiological Sciences, Center of Biological Sciences, Federal University of Santa Catarina, Florianópolis, Brazil

Alex Rafacho
Postgraduate Program in Pharmacology, Federal University of Santa Catarina, Florianópolis, Brazil
Multicenter Postgraduate Program in Physiological Sciences, Federal University of Santa Catarina, Florianópolis, Brazil
Department of Physiological Sciences, Center of Biological Sciences, Federal University of Santa Catarina, Florianópolis, Brazil

Daniel Breseghello Zoccal
Department of Physiology and Pathology, School of Dentistry, São Paulo State University, Araraquara, Brazil

Douglas A. Formolo and Hiago M. Melo
Center for Applied Neuroscience, University Hospital, Federal University of Santa Catarina, Florianópolis, Brazil
Graduate Program in Neuroscience, Federal University of Santa Catarina, Florianópolis, Brazil

Joana M. Gaspar, Tuany Eichwald and Alexandra Latini
Laboratory of Bioenergetics and Oxidative Stress, Department of Biochemistry, Federal University of Santa Catarina, Florianópolis, Brazil
Graduate Program in Biochemistry, Department of Biochemistry, Federal University of Santa Catarina, Florianópolis, Brazil

Ramiro Javier Zepeda
Department of Neuroscience, Faculty of Medicine, Chile University and Health Science Institute, O'Higgins University, Santiago, Chile

Michael S. Okun
Fixel Institute for Neurological Diseases, Department of Neurology, University of Florida, Gainesville, FL, United States

Roger Walz
Center for Applied Neuroscience, University Hospital, Federal University of Santa Catarina, Florianópolis, Brazil
Graduate Program in Neuroscience, Federal University of Santa Catarina, Florianópolis, Brazil
Fixel Institute for Neurological Diseases, Department of Neurology, University of Florida, Gainesville, FL, United States
Graduate Program in Medical Sciences, Federal University of Santa Catarina, Florianópolis, Brazil
Department of Internal Medicine, University Hospital, Federal University of Santa Catarina, Florianópolis, Brazil

Ana Francisca Soares
Laboratory for Functional and Metabolic Imaging, École Polytechnique Fédérale de Lausanne, Lausanne, Switzerland

Blanca Lizarbe
Laboratory for Functional and Metabolic Imaging, École Polytechnique Fédérale de Lausanne, Lausanne, Switzerland
Instituto de Investigaciones Biomédicas "Alberto Sols", Consejo Superior de Investigaciones Científicas - Universidad Autónoma de Madrid, Madrid, Spain

Sara Larsson and João M. N. Duarte
Department of Experimental Medical Science, Faculty of Medicine, Lund University, Lund, Sweden
Wallenberg Centre for Molecular Medicine, Faculty of Medicine, Lund University, Lund, Sweden

Viviane José de Oliveira Bristot and Liziane Rosa Cardoso
Research Group on Biology of Exercise, Department of Health Sciences, Centro Araranguá, Federal University of Santa Catarina, Araranguá, Brazil

Ana Cristina de Bem Alves, Débora da Luz Scheffer and Aderbal Silva Aguiar Jr.
Research Group on Biology of Exercise, Department of Health Sciences, Centro Araranguá, Federal University of Santa Catarina, Araranguá, Brazil
Laboratório de Bioenergética e Estresse Oxidativo, Departamento de Bioquímica, Centro de Ciências Biológicas, Universidade Federal de Santa Catarina, Florianópolis, Brazil

Trevor Rajchgot, Sini Christine Thomas, Maryam Ahmadi, Mohammad Balood, Théo Crosson, Réjean Couture, Audrey Claing and Sébastien Talbot
Département de Pharmacologie et Physiologie, Faculté de Médecine, Université de Montréal, Montréal, QC, Canada

Jo-Chiao Wang
Graduate Institute of Microbiology, College of Medicine, National Taiwan University, Taipei, Taiwan

Jenny Pena Dias
Johns Hopkins University School of Medicine, Division of Endocrinology, Diabetes and Metabolism, Baltimore, MD, United States

Md Habibur Rahman and Kyoungho Suk
Department of Pharmacology, Brain Science and Engineering Institute, BK21 Plus KNU Biomedical Convergence Program, School of Medicine, Kyungpook National University, Daegu, South Korea

Min-Seon Kim
Division of Endocrinology and Metabolism, University of Ulsan College of Medicine, Seoul, South Korea

In-Kyu Lee
Department of Internal Medicine, Division of Endocrinology and Metabolism, School of Medicine, Kyungpook National University, Daegu, South Korea

Rina Yu
Department of Food Science and Nutrition, University of Ulsan, Ulsan, South Korea

Emilia Grzęda, Julia Matuszewska and Joanna H. Sliwowska
Laboratory of Neurobiology, Faculty of Veterinary Medicine and Animal Science, Poznań University of Life Sciences, Poznań, Poland

Kamil Ziarniak
Laboratory of Neurobiology, Faculty of Veterinary Medicine and Animal Science, Poznań University of Life Sciences, Poznań, Poland
Molecular and Cell Biology Unit, Poznań University of Medical Sciences, Poznań, Poland

Anna Gertig-Kolasa, Izabela Krzyśko-Pieczka and Bogda Skowrońska
Department of Paediatric Diabetes and Obesity, Poznań University of Medical Sciences, Poznań, Poland

Tina Linder, Anna Eder, Ingo Rosicky and Daniel Eppel
Department of Obstetrics and Gynaecology, Division of Obstetrics and feto-maternal Medicine, Medical University of Vienna, Vienna, Austria

Christian S. Göbl
Department of Obstetrics and Gynaecology, Division of Obstetrics and feto-maternal Medicine, Medical University of Vienna, Vienna, Austria
Department of Obstetrics and Gynaecology, University Hospital Basel, Basel, Switzerland

Cécile Monod, Katharina Redling, Franziska Geissler, Evelyn A. Huhn and Irene Hösli
Department of Obstetrics and Gynaecology, University Hospital Basel, Basel, Switzerland

Yang Wang and Xianwen Shang
Centre for Eye Research Australia, Royal Victorian Eye and Ear Hospital, Melbourne, VIC, Australia

Jinrong Wu
Centre for Eye Research Australia, Royal Victorian Eye and Ear Hospital, Melbourne, VIC, Australia
Research Centre for Data Analytics and Cognition, La Trobe University, Melbourne, VIC, Australia

Xin Xiao
Centre for Eye Research Australia, Royal Victorian Eye and Ear Hospital, Melbourne, VIC, Australia
Center for Optometry and Visual Science, Department of Optometry, People's Hospital of Guangxi Zhuang Autonomous Region, Guangxi, China

Mingguang He
Centre for Eye Research Australia, Royal Victorian Eye and Ear Hospital, Melbourne, VIC, Australia
Ophthalmology, Department of Surgery, University of Melbourne, Melbourne, VIC, Australia
State Key Laboratory of Ophthalmology, Zhongshan Ophthalmic Center, Sun Yat-sen University, Guangzhou, China

Lei Zhang
Centre for Eye Research Australia, Royal Victorian Eye and Ear Hospital, Melbourne, VIC, Australia
Melbourne Sexual Health Centre, Alfred Health, Melbourne, VIC, Australia
Central Clinical School, Faculty of Medicine, Monash University, Melbourne, VIC, Australia
Department of Epidemiology and Biostatistics, College of Public Health, Zhengzhou University, Zhengzhou, China

Index

www.ingramcontent.com/pod-product-compliance
Lightning Source LLC
LaVergne TN
LVHW081019210926
848485LV00004B/904